W9-ARJ-490

Computational Explorations in Cognitive Neuroscience

Computational Explorations in Cognitive Neuroscience

Understanding the Mind by Simulating the Brain

Randall C. O'Reilly and Yuko Munakata

A Bradford Book
The MIT Press
Cambridge, Massachusetts
London, England

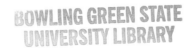
BOWLING GREEN STATE
UNIVERSITY LIBRARY

©2000 Massachusetts Institute of Technology

All rights reserved. No part of this book may be reproduced in any form by any electronic or mechanical means (including photocopying, recording, or information storage and retrieval) without permission in writing from the publisher.

This book was set in Times-Roman by the authors using LaTeX and was printed and bound in the United States of America.

Library of Congress Cataloging-in-Publication Data

O'Reilly, Randall C.
Computational explorations in cognitive neuroscience: Understanding the mind by simulating the brain / Randall
    C. O'Reilly and Yuko Munakata.
    p. cm.
    "A Bradford book."
    Includes bibliographical references and index.
                          ISBN 0-262-65054-1 (pb : alk. paper)
    1. Cognitive neuroscience – Computer simulation. 2. Neural networks (Neurobiology)
I. Munakata, Yuko. II. Title.

QP360.5 .O74 2000
612.8'01'13–dc21

                                                                                        99-086066

To our families

Brief Contents

1 Introduction and Overview   1

I   Basic Neural Computational Mechanisms   21
2   Individual Neurons   23
3   Networks of Neurons   71
4   Hebbian Model Learning   115
5   Error-Driven Task Learning   147
6   Combined Model and Task Learning, and Other Mechanisms   173

II Large-Scale Brain Area Organization and Cognitive Phenomena   203
7   Large-Scale Brain Area Functional Organization   205
8   Perception and Attention   227
9   Memory   275
10 Language   323
11 Higher-Level Cognition   379
12 Conclusions   411

III Simulator Details   425
A   Introduction to the PDP++ Simulation Environment   427
B   Tutorial for Constructing Simulations in PDP++   435
C   Leabra Implementation Reference   455
References   467
Author Index   485
Subject Index   491

Contents

Foreword xix
Preface xxv
Acknowledgments xxvii

1 Introduction and Overview   **1**
   1.1   Computational Cognitive Neuroscience 1
   1.2   Basic Motivations for Computational Cognitive Neuroscience 2
        1.2.1   Physical Reductionism 2
        1.2.2   Reconstructionism 3
        1.2.3   Levels of Analysis 4
        1.2.4   Scaling Issues 6
   1.3   Historical Context 8
   1.4   Overview of Our Approach 10
   1.5   General Issues in Computational Modeling 11
   1.6   Motivating Cognitive Phenomena and Their Biological Bases 14
        1.6.1   Parallelism 15
        1.6.2   Gradedness 15
        1.6.3   Interactivity 17
        1.6.4   Competition 17
        1.6.5   Learning 18
   1.7   Organization of the Book 19
   1.8   Further Reading 20

I Basic Neural Computational Mechanisms   **21**

2 Individual Neurons   **23**
   2.1   Overview 23
   2.2   Detectors: How to Think About a Neuron 24
        2.2.1   Understanding the Parts of the Neuron Using the Detector Model 26
   2.3   The Biology of the Neuron 27
        2.3.1   The Axon 29

	2.3.2	The Synapse	29
	2.3.3	The Dendrite	31
2.4	The Electrophysiology of the Neuron	32
	2.4.1	Basic Electricity	32
	2.4.2	Diffusion	33
	2.4.3	Electric Potential versus Diffusion: The Equilibrium Potential	34
	2.4.4	The Neural Environs and Ions	35
	2.4.5	Putting It All Together: Integration	37
	2.4.6	The Equilibrium Membrane Potential	38
	2.4.7	Summary	40
2.5	Computational Implementation of the Neural Activation Function	40
	2.5.1	Computing Input Conductances	42
	2.5.2	Point Neuron Parameter Values	45
	2.5.3	The Discrete Spiking Output Function	45
	2.5.4	The Rate Code Output Function	46
	2.5.5	Summary	48
2.6	Explorations of the Individual Neuron	48
	2.6.1	The Membrane Potential	49
	2.6.2	The Activation Output	53
	2.6.3	The Neuron as Detector	54
2.7	Hypothesis Testing Analysis of a Neural Detector	58
	2.7.1	Objective Probabilities and Example	59
	2.7.2	Subjective Probabilities	62
	2.7.3	Similarity of V_m and $P(h|d)$	65
2.8	The Importance of Keeping It Simple	65
2.9	Self-Regulation: Accommodation and Hysteresis	66
	2.9.1	Implementation of Accommodation and Hysteresis	67
2.10	Summary	69
2.11	Further Reading	70
3	**Networks of Neurons**		**71**
3.1	Overview	71
3.2	General Structure of Cortical Networks	72
3.3	Unidirectional Excitatory Interactions: Transformations	75
	3.3.1	Exploration of Transformations	79
	3.3.2	Localist versus Distributed Representations	82
	3.3.3	Exploration of Distributed Representations	84
3.4	Bidirectional Excitatory Interactions	85
	3.4.1	Bidirectional Transformations	86
	3.4.2	Bidirectional Pattern Completion	87
	3.4.3	Bidirectional Amplification	89
	3.4.4	Attractor Dynamics	92

3.5   Inhibitory Interactions 93
       3.5.1   General Functional Benefits of Inhibition 94
       3.5.2   Exploration of Feedforward and Feedback Inhibition 95
       3.5.3   The k-Winners-Take-All Inhibitory Functions 100
       3.5.4   Exploration of kWTA Inhibition 103
       3.5.5   Digits Revisited with kWTA Inhibition 104
       3.5.6   Other Simple Inhibition Functions 105
3.6   Constraint Satisfaction 106
       3.6.1   Attractors Again 108
       3.6.2   The Role of Noise 108
       3.6.3   The Role of Inhibition 109
       3.6.4   Explorations of Constraint Satisfaction: Cats and Dogs 109
       3.6.5   Explorations of Constraint Satisfaction: Necker Cube 111
3.7   Summary 112
3.8   Further Reading 114

4 Hebbian Model Learning   **115**
4.1   Overview 115
4.2   Biological Mechanisms of Learning 116
4.3   Computational Objectives of Learning 118
       4.3.1   Simple Exploration of Correlational Model Learning 121
4.4   Principal Components Analysis 122
       4.4.1   Simple Hebbian PCA in One Linear Unit 122
       4.4.2   Oja's Normalized Hebbian PCA 124
4.5   Conditional Principal Components Analysis 125
       4.5.1   The CPCA Learning Rule 127
       4.5.2   Derivation of CPCA Learning Rule 128
       4.5.3   Biological Implementation of CPCA Hebbian Learning 129
4.6   Exploration of Hebbian Model Learning 130
4.7   Renormalization and Contrast Enhancement 132
       4.7.1   Renormalization 133
       4.7.2   Contrast Enhancement 134
       4.7.3   Exploration of Renormalization and Contrast Enhancement in CPCA 135
4.8   Self-Organizing Model Learning 137
       4.8.1   Exploration of Self-Organizing Learning 138
       4.8.2   Summary and Discussion 142
4.9   Other Approaches to Model Learning 142
       4.9.1   Algorithms That Use CPCA-Style Hebbian Learning 143
       4.9.2   Clustering 143
       4.9.3   Topography 143
       4.9.4   Information Maximization and MDL 144
       4.9.5   Learning Based Primarily on Hidden Layer Constraints 144

           4.9.6   Generative Models   145
    4.10 Summary   145
    4.11 Further Reading   146

5   Error-Driven Task Learning   **147**
    5.1   Overview   147
    5.2   Exploration of Hebbian Task Learning   148
    5.3   Using Error to Learn: The Delta Rule   150
           5.3.1   Deriving the Delta Rule   152
           5.3.2   Learning Bias Weights   152
    5.4   Error Functions, Weight Bounding, and Activation Phases   154
           5.4.1   Cross Entropy Error   154
           5.4.2   Soft Weight Bounding   155
           5.4.3   Activation Phases in Learning   156
    5.5   Exploration of Delta Rule Task Learning   156
    5.6   The Generalized Delta Rule: Backpropagation   158
           5.6.1   Derivation of Backpropagation   160
           5.6.2   Generic Recursive Formulation   161
           5.6.3   The Biological Implausibility of Backpropagation   162
    5.7   The Generalized Recirculation Algorithm   162
           5.7.1   Derivation of GeneRec   163
           5.7.2   Symmetry, Midpoint, and CHL   165
    5.8   Biological Considerations for GeneRec   166
           5.8.1   Weight Symmetry in the Cortex   166
           5.8.2   Phase-Based Activations in the Cortex   167
           5.8.3   Synaptic Modification Mechanisms   168
    5.9   Exploration of GeneRec-Based Task Learning   170
    5.10 Summary   171
    5.11 Further Reading   172

6   Combined Model and Task Learning, and Other Mechanisms   **173**
    6.1   Overview   173
    6.2   Combined Hebbian and Error-driven Learning   173
           6.2.1   Pros and Cons of Hebbian and Error-Driven Learning   174
           6.2.2   Advantages to Combining Hebbian and Error-Driven Learning   175
           6.2.3   Inhibitory Competition as a Model-Learning Constraint   175
           6.2.4   Implementation of Combined Model and Task Learning   176
           6.2.5   Summary   177
    6.3   Generalization in Bidirectional Networks   178
           6.3.1   Exploration of Generalization   179
    6.4   Learning to Re-represent in Deep Networks   181
           6.4.1   Exploration of a Deep Network   183

6.5 Sequence and Temporally Delayed Learning 186

6.6 Context Representations and Sequential Learning 187

  6.6.1 Computational Considerations for Context Representations 188

  6.6.2 Possible Biological Bases for Context Representations 189

  6.6.3 Exploration: Learning the Reber Grammar 189

  6.6.4 Summary 193

6.7 Reinforcement Learning for Temporally Delayed Outcomes 193

  6.7.1 The Temporal Differences Algorithm 195

  6.7.2 Phase-Based Temporal Differences 198

  6.7.3 Exploration of TD: Classical Conditioning 199

6.8 Summary 202

6.9 Further Reading 202

II Large-Scale Brain Area Organization and Cognitive Phenomena 203

7 Large-Scale Brain Area Functional Organization 205

7.1 Overview 205

7.2 General Computational and Functional Principles 206

  7.2.1 Structural Principles 206

  7.2.2 Dynamic Principles 210

7.3 General Functions of the Cortical Lobes and Subcortical Areas 211

  7.3.1 Cortex 211

  7.3.2 Limbic System 212

  7.3.3 The Thalamus 212

  7.3.4 The Basal Ganglia, Cerebellum, and Motor Control 213

7.4 Tripartite Functional Organization 214

  7.4.1 Slow Integrative versus Fast Separating Learning 214

  7.4.2 Active Memory versus Overlapping Distributed Representations 215

7.5 Toward a Cognitive Architecture of the Brain 216

  7.5.1 Controlled versus Automatic Processing 217

  7.5.2 Declarative/Procedural and Explicit/Implicit Distinctions 218

7.6 General Problems 219

  7.6.1 The Binding Problem for Distributed Representations of Multiple Items 220

  7.6.2 Representing Multiple Instances of the Same Thing 222

  7.6.3 Comparing Representations 222

  7.6.4 Representing Hierarchical Relationships 222

  7.6.5 Recursion and Subroutine-like Processing 223

  7.6.6 Generalization, Generativity, and Abstraction 224

  7.6.7 Summary of General Problems 224

7.7 Summary 225

8 Perception and Attention   **227**
  8.1 Overview 227
  8.2 Biology of the Visual System 228
      8.2.1 The Retina 228
      8.2.2 The LGN of the Thalamus 230
      8.2.3 Primary Visual Cortex: V1 230
      8.2.4 Two Visual Processing Streams 232
      8.2.5 The Ventral Visual Form Pathway: V2, V4, and IT 233
      8.2.6 The Dorsal Where/Action Pathway 233
  8.3 Primary Visual Representations 234
      8.3.1 Basic Properties of the Model 235
      8.3.2 Exploring the Model 237
      8.3.3 Summary and Discussion 240
  8.4 Object Recognition and the Visual Form Pathway 241
      8.4.1 Basic Properties of the Model 243
      8.4.2 Exploring the Model 246
      8.4.3 Summary and Discussion 255
  8.5 Spatial Attention: A Simple Model 257
      8.5.1 Basic Properties of the Model 258
      8.5.2 Exploring the Simple Attentional Model 261
      8.5.3 Summary and Discussion 268
  8.6 Spatial Attention: A More Complex Model 269
      8.6.1 Exploring the Complex Attentional Model 269
      8.6.2 Summary and Discussion 272
  8.7 Summary 272
  8.8 Further Reading 273

9 Memory   **275**
  9.1 Overview 275
  9.2 Weight-Based Memory in a Generic Model of Cortex 277
      9.2.1 Long-Term Priming 278
      9.2.2 AB–AC List Learning 282
  9.3 The Hippocampal Memory System 287
      9.3.1 Anatomy and Physiology of the Hippocampus 287
      9.3.2 Basic Properties of the Hippocampal Model 289
      9.3.3 Explorations of the Hippocampus 293
      9.3.4 Summary and Discussion 296
  9.4 Activation-Based Memory in a Generic Model of Cortex 298
      9.4.1 Short-Term Priming 298
      9.4.2 Active Maintenance 299
      9.4.3 Robust yet Rapidly Updatable Active Maintenance 303
  9.5 The Prefrontal Cortex Active Memory System 305

        9.5.1   Dynamic Regulation of Active Maintenance 306
        9.5.2   Details of the Prefrontal Cortex Model 307
        9.5.3   Exploring the Model 310
        9.5.4   Summary and Discussion 312
    9.6 The Development and Interaction of Memory Systems 314
        9.6.1   Basic Properties of the Model 314
        9.6.2   Exploring the Model 315
        9.6.3   Summary and Discussion 317
    9.7 Memory Phenomena and System Interactions 318
        9.7.1   Recognition Memory 318
        9.7.2   Cued Recall 319
        9.7.3   Free Recall 319
        9.7.4   Item Effects 320
        9.7.5   Working Memory 320
    9.8 Summary 320
    9.9 Further Reading 321

10 **Language**   **323**
    10.1 Overview 323
    10.2 The Biology and Basic Representations of Language 325
        10.2.1 Biology 325
        10.2.2 Phonology 327
    10.3 The Distributed Representation of Words and Dyslexia 329
        10.3.1 Comparison with Traditional Dual-Route Models 330
        10.3.2 The Interactive Model and Division of Labor 331
        10.3.3 Dyslexia 331
        10.3.4 Basic Properties of the Model 333
        10.3.5 Exploring the Model 335
        10.3.6 Summary and Discussion 341
    10.4 The Orthography to Phonology Mapping 341
        10.4.1 Basic Properties of the Model 343
        10.4.2 Exploring the Model 344
        10.4.3 Summary and Discussion 349
    10.5 Overregularization in Past-Tense Inflectional Mappings 350
        10.5.1 Basic Properties of the Model 352
        10.5.2 Exploring the Model 353
        10.5.3 Summary and Discussion 357
    10.6 Semantic Representations from Word Co-occurrences and Hebbian Learning 358
        10.6.1 Basic Properties of the Model 360
        10.6.2 Exploring the Model 361
        10.6.3 Summary and Discussion 365
    10.7 Sentence-Level Processing 365

      10.7.1 Basic Properties of the Model 367

      10.7.2 Exploring the Model 370

      10.7.3 Summary and Discussion 375

  10.8 Summary 376

  10.9 Further Reading 377

11 Higher-Level Cognition   **379**

  11.1 Overview 379

  11.2 Biology of the Frontal Cortex 384

  11.3 Controlled Processing and the Stroop Task 385

      11.3.1 Basic Properties of the Model 387

      11.3.2 Exploring the Model 388

      11.3.3 Summary and Discussion 391

  11.4 Dynamic Categorization/Sorting Tasks 392

      11.4.1 Basic Properties of the Model 395

      11.4.2 Exploring the Model 397

      11.4.3 Summary and Discussion 402

  11.5 General Role of Frontal Cortex in Higher-Level Cognition 403

      11.5.1 Functions Commonly Attributed to Frontal Cortex 403

      11.5.2 Other Models and Theoretical Frameworks 407

  11.6 Interacting Specialized Systems and Cognitive Control 408

  11.7 Summary 409

  11.8 Further Reading 410

12 Conclusions   **411**

  12.1 Overview 411

  12.2 Fundamentals 411

  12.3 General Challenges for Computational Modeling 413

      12.3.1 Models Are Too Simple 414

      12.3.2 Models Are Too Complex 417

      12.3.3 Models Can Do Anything 418

      12.3.4 Models Are Reductionistic 418

      12.3.5 Modeling Lacks Cumulative Research 419

  12.4 Specific Challenges 419

      12.4.1 Analytical Treatments of Learning 419

      12.4.2 Error Signals 420

      12.4.3 Regularities and Generalization 420

      12.4.4 Capturing Higher-Level Cognition 421

  12.5 Contributions of Computation to Cognitive Neuroscience 421

      12.5.1 Models Help Us to Understand Phenomena 421

      12.5.2 Models Deal with Complexity 422

      12.5.3 Models Are Explicit 423

12.5.4 Models Allow Control 423
12.5.5 Models Provide a Unified Framework 423
12.6 Exploring on Your Own 424

III Simulator Details 425

A Introduction to the PDP++ Simulation Environment 427
A.1 Overview 427
A.2 Downloading and Installing the Software 427
A.3 Overall Structure of PDP++ 428
A.4 Buttons and Menu Commands 429
A.5 Edit Dialogs 430
A.6 Control Panels 430
A.7 Specs 431
A.8 Networks and NetViews 431
A.8.1 NetView 431
A.9 Environments and EnviroViews 431
A.10 Processes 432
A.10.1 Process Control Panels 432
A.10.2 Statistics 432
A.11 Logs 433
A.11.1 TextLog 433
A.11.2 GraphLog 433
A.11.3 GridLog 433
A.12 Scripts 434

B Tutorial for Constructing Simulations in PDP++ 435
B.1 Overview 435
B.2 Constructing a Basic Simulation 436
B.2.1 Creating a Project 436
B.2.2 Recording a Script 436
B.2.3 Creating a Network and Layers 437
B.2.4 Creating Projections and Connections 438
B.2.5 Specifying Layer Activity Levels 439
B.2.6 Creating an Environment 440
B.2.7 Creating Training Process 442
B.2.8 Creating a Training Log and Running the Model 443
B.3 Examining the Script 443
B.3.1 Object Paths 444
B.3.2 Object-Oriented Function Calls 444
B.3.3 Assigning Member Values 444

	B.3.4	Scoped Variables	445
	B.3.5	Running Processes from the Script	445
	B.3.6	Saving Files from the Script	446
	B.3.7	Compiling and Running the Script	446
B.4		Creating a Testing Process	447
	B.4.1	Monitoring Unit Activities	447
	B.4.2	Creating a New Statistic for Testing	448
	B.4.3	Automatically Testing during Training	449
B.5		Writing Script Code to Create an Environment	450
	B.5.1	Setting a Stopping Criterion for Training	451
B.6		Creating an Overall Control Panel	452
B.7		Creating SRN Context Layers	453

C   Leabra Implementation Reference   **455**

C.1	Overview	455
C.2	Pseudocode	456
C.3	Connection-Level Variables	456
C.4	Unit-Level Variables	459
C.5	Layer-Level Variables	463
C.6	Process-Level Variables	465

References   **467**

Author Index   **485**

Subject Index   **491**

Foreword

The Role of Computational Models in Cognitive Neuroscience

The publication of O'Reilly and Munakata's *Computational Explorations in Cognitive Neuroscience* comes at an opportune moment. The field is rapidly growing, with centers and institutes springing up everywhere. Researchers from backgrounds ranging from psychology to molecular biology are pouring into the field. Eric Kandel has suggested that "cognitive neuroscience—with its concern about perception, action, memory, language and selective attention—will increasingly come to represent the central focus of all neurosciences in the twentyfirst century."

Today, quite a bit of the excitement in the field surrounds the use of several important new experimental methodologies. For the study of the neural basis of cognition in humans, fMRI and other imaging modalities hold great promise to allow us to visualize the brain while cognition is occurring, and it is likely that there will be ongoing breakthroughs in spatial and temporal resolution. Working upward from the molecular level, new genetic methods for creating animals with alterations in the basic functional properties of specific groups of neurons and synapses is allowing detailed exploration of how these cellular and synaptic processes impact higher processes such as spatial learning in animals. Within neurophysiology, the use of multi-electrode arrays to record from as many as 100 separate neurons at a time has led to new insights into the representation of information during behavior, and the later reactivation of these representations from memory during sleep.

With all their marvelous tools, the question arises, do we really need computational models in cognitive neuroscience? Can we not learn everything we need to know about the neural basis of cognition through experimental investigation? Do we need a book like the present one to explore the principles of neural computation and apply them to the task of understanding how cognition arises from neuronal interactions?

The answer is: Yes, we do need computational models in cognitive neuroscience. To support this answer, I will begin by describing what I take to be one of the central goals of cognitive neuroscience. I will then describe what we mean by the phrase "a computational model" and consider the role such models can play in addressing the central goal. Along the way I hope to indicate some of the shortcomings of experimental research undertaken without the aid of computational models and how models can be used to go beyond these limitations. The goal is to make clear exactly what models are, and the role they are intended to play.

First, what is this central goal of cognitive neuroscience? To me, and I think to O'Reilly, Munakata, and many researchers in the field, the goal is to understand how neural processes give rise to cognition. Typically, cognition is broadly construed to include perception, attention, language, memory, problem solving, planning, reasoning, and the coordination and execution of action. And typically some task or tasks are used to make behavioral observations that tap these underlying processes; aspects of conscious experience are included, to the extent that they can be subjected to scientific scrutiny through observables (including verbal reports or other readout methods). The processes considered may be ones that take place in a brief interval of time, such as the processes that occur when a human observer reads a visually presented word. Or they may be ones that take place over longer periods of time, such as the processes that occur as a child progresses through various developmental stages in understanding the role of weight and distance, say, in balance. Processes occurring in individuals with disorders are often of interest, in part to understand the disorder and in part for the light the disorder may shed on the effort to understand the "normal" case. Cognition as it occurs in humans is often the main focus, but animal models are often used, in part because there are clear structure-function homologues between humans and nonhuman animals in many domains of cognition, and in part because we can manipulate the nervous systems of nonhuman animals and invade their nervous systems with probes we cannot use in humans.

Whatever the exact target phenomenon, the essential goal is to understand the mechanisms involved. Here, we must be extremely careful to distinguish different specific kinds of mechanistic goals. One might have the goal simply to provide a detailed characterization of the actual physical and chemical processes that underlie the cognitive processes in question. This is certainly a very worthwhile goal, and will be essential for medical applications of cognitive neuroscience. But most researchers who call themselves cognitive neuroscientists are probably looking for something more general; I think most researchers would like to say it is not the details themselves that matter but the principles that are embodied in these details. As one example, consider the phenomenon observed of depletion of neurotransmitter that occurs when a synapse is repeatedly activated by an incoming neural impulse. The exact details of the molecular mechanisms involved in this process are a focus of considerable interest in neuroscience. But for cognitive neuroscience, a key focus is on the fact that this depletion results in a temporary reduction in efficacy at the affected synapse. The principle that activity weakens synapses has been incorporated into several models, and then has been used to account for a variety of phenomena, including alternation between distinct interpretations of the same percept (also known as "bistable perception"). The point is that the basic principle can be built into a model that captures emergent perceptual phenomena without incorporating all of the underlying biophysical details.

It may be worth noting here that some researchers who call themselves cognitive neuroscientists disavow a concern for the neural processes themselves that form the underlying basis of cognition and focus instead on what they take to be more fundamental issues that transcend the details. For example, many researchers consider the task of cognitive neuroscience to be one of finding the correct partitioning of the brain into distinct modules with isolable functions. This is a highly seductive enterprise, one that is reinforced by the fact that damage to particular brain regions can produce a profound deficit in the ability to perform certain cognitive tasks or to carry out a task for a particular type of item, while largely sparing performance of other tasks or other types of items.

For example, damage to anterior language areas can have a large effect on the ability to produce the past tenses of words that exhibit the regular English past tense (such as "need" – "needed"), leaving performance on exception words (such as "take" – "took") largely intact. On the other hand, damage to more posterior areas can sometimes lead to a large deficit in producing the past tenses of the exception words, with relative sparing of the regular items and a tendency to "regularize" exceptions ("wear" – "weared"). Such findings have often enticed cognitive neuroscientists to attribute performance on the different tasks or classes of items to different cognitive modules, and fMRI and other brain imaging models showing differential activations of brain regions in different tasks or with different items are used in a similar way to assign functions to brain modules.

Thus, one interpretation of the findings on verb inflection is that the system of rules that is used in processing the regular items is subserved by some part or parts of the anterior language processing system, while a lexicon or list of word-specific information specifying the correct past tenses of exceptions is subserved by some part or parts of the affected posterior areas (Ullman, Corkin, & Pinker, 1997). As appealing intuitively as this sort of inference may seem, there are two problems. One problem is that, as stated, it isn't always clear whether the ideas are sufficient to provide a full account of the pattern of spared and impaired performance seen by both types of patients. An explicit model can help the scientific community work through in full detail the actual ability of a proposed set of modular mechanisms to account for the observed pattern of data. We will come back to this issue. Before doing so, it is important to consider the second problem with drawing inferences directly without an explicit model of the processes involved providing guidance.

The second problem is that in the absence of an explicit process model, investigators often have a tendency to reify aspects of task differences, stimulus types, or types of errors in their theorizing about the underlying modular organization. Here, models help to illustrate that other interpretations may be possible, ones that may require fewer modules or independent loci of damage in the resulting account for normal and disordered behavior. For example, the connectionist model of Joanisse and Seidenberg (1999) offers an alternative to the Ullman et al. account of the pattern of deficits in forming past tenses. According to this model, damage to the posterior system disrupts the semantic representations of all types of words, while damage to the anterior system disrupts phonological processing of all types of words. The reason why anterior lesions have a disproportionate impact on inflection of regular words is that the regular inflection is both subtler to perceive and harder to produce, making it more sensitive to a phonological disruption. The reason why posterior lesions have a disproportionate impact on exceptions is that the semantics of a word provides distinct, word specific input that is necessary for overriding the regular inflectional pattern that is typical of most words.

The key point here is that an explicit computational perspective often leads to new ways of understanding observed phenomena that are apparently not always accessible to those who seek to identify subsystems without giving detailed consideration to the mechanisms involved. To demonstrate how commonly this arises, I will mention three other cases in point, two of which are explored more fully by O'Reilly and Munakata. All three suggest how a computational perspective has led to new interpretations of neuropsychological phenomena:

- It has long been known that lesions in posterior parietal cortex lead to deficits in visual processing in the opposite visual field. Posner, Walker, Friedrich, and Rafal (1984) observed that patients with lateralized posterior parietal lesions had only a moderate deficit

in detecting targets in the opposite visual field, and that the deficit became much larger when the task required shifting away from the unaffected visual field into the affected field, and proposed that this reflected a deficit in a specific neural module for disengagement of attention from the opposite side of space. But as O'Reilly and Munakata explore in a model in chapter 8, Cohen, Romero, Farah, and Servan-Schreiber (1994) later demonstrated that in a simple neural network, in which there are pools of neurons on each side of the brain each responsible to attention to the opposite side of space, partial damage to the pool of neurons on one side led to a close fit to whole pattern of data; no separate module for disengagement, over and above the basic mechanism of attention itself, was required to account for the data.

- Several investigators have observed interesting patterns of disproportionate deficits in patients with problems with face recognition. For example, such patients can show profound deficits in the ability to name famous faces, yet show facilitation of reading a person's name aloud when the face is presented along with it. Such a finding was once interpreted as suggesting that the damage had affected only conscious face processing (or access to consciousness of the results of an intact unconscious process). But Farah, O'Reilly, and Vecera (1993) later demonstrated that in a simple neural network, partial damage can easily have a disproportionate impact of the ability to produce a complete, correct answer, while nevertheless leaving enough residual sensitivity to specific faces to bias processing in other parts of the system.

- The intriguing phenomenon of deep dyslexia was puzzling to neuropsychologists for many years (Coltheart, Patterson, & Marshall, 1980). An essential characteristic of this disorder is the fact that the patients sometimes make dramatic errors preserving meaning but completely failing to respect the visual or phonological aspects of the stimulus word. For example such a patient might read "ROSE" as "TULIP." This suggests a semantic deficit; yet at the same time all such patients also make visual errors, such as misreading "SYMPHONY" as "SYMPATHY," for example. Neuropsychologists working from a modular perspective were forced to propose at least two distinct lesion loci to account for these effects; and this was deeply troubling to the modelers, who considered being forced to postulate multiple lesions for every single case to be unparsimonious. As O'Reilly and Munakata explore in a model in chapter 10, a computational approach has led to a far more parsimonious account. Hinton and Shallice (1991) (and later Plaut & Shallice, 1993) were able to show that in a simple neural network model that maps representations of letters onto representations of word meanings, a lesion anywhere in the network led to both visual and semantic errors. Lesions "closer to orthography" led to a greater number of visual errors, and lesions "closer to semantics" led to a greater number of semantic errors, but crucially, both kinds of lesions led to some errors of both types. Thus, the model suggests that a single locus of lesion may be consistent with the data after all.

What these three examples and the earlier example about the past tense all illustrate is that the inference from data to the modular architecture of the mind is not at all straightforward, and that explicit computational models can provide alternatives to what in some cases appears to be a fairly simplistic reification of task or item differences into cognitive modules, and in other cases manifests as a reification of types of errors (semantic, visual) into lesion sights.

Given that thinking about the underlying mechanism leads to alternative accounts for patterns of data, then we must return to the the crucial question of deciding which of several alternative proposals provides the "right" account. The question is very hard to answer, without an implemented computational instantiation of all of the competing accounts, since it isn't clear in advance of a specification and implementation just what the detailed predictions of each of the accounts might really be. The point is that a computational approach can lead both to appealing alternatives to intuitive accounts as well as to explicit predictions that can be compared to all aspects of data to determine which account is actually able to offer an adequate account. For this reason, explicit computational models (whether based on neural networks or on other frameworks) are becoming more and more central to the effort to understand the nature of the underlying mechanisms of cognition.

Providing a detailed account of a body of empirical data has been the goal of a great deal of modeling work, but it is important to understand that models can be useful and informative, even when they are not fit in detail to a complex data set. Instead of viewing models only as data fitting tools, it seems preferable to view them as tools (implemented in a computer program) for exploring what a given set of postulates about some process or mechanism implies about its resulting behavior. In cognitive neuroscience, we are usually interested in understanding what mechanism or process might give rise to observables, either behavioral data obtained in a cognitive task or some observable neural phenomenon such as the receptive field properties and spatial distribution of neurons in visual cortex. We explore this by laying out a set of postulates that define an explicit computational process, its inputs and its initial conditions, and then we run the process on a computer to see how it behaves. Typically there will be outputs that are intended to correspond in some way to behavioral responses, and there may be internal variables that are intended to correspond to observable neural variables, such as neuronal firing rates.

A very important point is that in this particular kind of work, the postulates built into a model need not represent the beliefs of the modeler; rather, they may represent a particular set of choices the modeler has made to try to gain insight into the model and, by proxy, the associated behavioral or biological phenomenon. A key aspect of the process of making good choices is abstraction and simplification. Unless models are kept as minimal as possible, it can become extremely difficult to understand them, or even to run the simulations quickly enough for them to serve as useful part of the research process. On the other hand, it is essential that we maintain sufficient structure within the model to deal with the issues and phenomena that are of interest. The process of model development within cognitive neuroscience is an exploration—a search for the key principles that the models must embody, for the most direct and succinct way of capturing these principles, and for a clear understanding of how and why the model gives rise to the phenomena that we see exhibited in its behavior.

This book by O'Reilly and Munakata is an important step in the progress of these explorations. The book represents an evolution from the earlier explorations represented by the "PDP books" (*Parallel Distributed Processing: Explorations in the Microstructure of Cognition* by Rumelhart, McClelland, and the PDP Research Group, 1986, and the companion Handbook, *Explorations in Parallel Distributed Processing*, by McClelland and Rumelhart, 1988). O'Reilly and Munakata have built on a set of computational principles that arose from the effort to constrain the parallel distributed processing framework for modeling cognitive processes (McClelland, 1993), and have instantiated them within an integrated computational framework incorporating additional principles associated with O'Reilly's Leabra algorithm. They have taken the computational and psychological abstraction characteristic of the PDP work, while moving many of the properties of the framework closer to aspects of the underlying neural implementation. They have employed a powerful set of software tools, including a sophisticated graphical user interface and a full-featured scripting language to create an impressive, state-of-the art simulation tool. They have exploited the combined use of expository text and hands-on simulation exercises to illustrate the basic properties of processing, representation, and learning in networks, and they have used their integrated framework to implement close analogs of a number of the examples that were developed in the earlier PDP work to illustrate key aspects of the emergent behavior or neural networks. They have gone on to show how these models can be applied in a number of domains of cognitive neuroscience to offer alternatives to traditional approaches to a number of central issues. Overall this book represents an impressive effort to construct a framework for the further exploration of the principles and their implications for cognitive neuroscience.

It is important, however, to be aware that the computational exploration of issues in cognitive neuroscience is still very much in its infancy. There is a great deal that remains to be discovered about learning, processing, and representation in the brain, and about how cognition emerges from the underlying neural mechanisms. As with the earlier, PDP books, an important part of the legacy of this book is likely to be its influence on the next wave of researchers who will take the next steps in these explorations.

James L. McClelland
Center for the Neural Basis of Cognition
February, 2000

Preface

Computational approaches to cognitive neuroscience (computational cognitive neuroscience) focus on understanding how the brain embodies the mind, using biologically based computational models made up of networks of neuronlike units. Because this endeavor lies at the intersection of a number of different disciplines, including neuroscience, computation, and cognitive psychology, the boundaries of computational cognitive neuroscience are difficult to delineate, making it a subject that can be difficult to teach well. This book is intended to support the teaching of this subject by providing a coherent, principled introduction to the main ideas in the field. It is suitable for an advanced undergraduate or graduate course in one semester or quarter (the authors have each used this text for such courses at their respective universities), and also for researchers in related areas who want to learn more about this approach to understanding the relation between mind and brain.

Any introductory text on the subject of computational cognitive neuroscience faces a potentially overwhelming set of compromises — one could write volumes on each of the different component aspects of computation, cognition, and neuroscience. Many existing texts have avoided these compromises by focusing on specific issues such as the firing patterns of individual neurons (e.g., Reike, Warland, van Steveninck, & Bialek, 1996), mathematically oriented treatments of the computational properties of networks (e.g., Hertz, Krogh, & Palmer, 1991), or more abstract models of cognitive phenomena (e.g., Elman, Bates, Johnson, Karmiloff-Smith, Parisi, & Plunkett, 1996; Plunkett & Elman, 1997). However, we knew that our excitement in the field was based in large part on the wide scope of the issues involved in this endeavor — from biological and computational properties to cognitive function — which

requires a broader perspective (hand in hand with a greater compromise on some of the details) than is captured in these texts.

Thus, like many of our colleagues teaching similar courses, we continued to think that the original PDP (parallel distributed processing) volumes (Rumelhart, McClelland, & PDP Research Group, 1986c; McClelland, Rumelhart, & PDP Research Group, 1986; McClelland & Rumelhart, 1988) were the best texts for covering the broader scope of issues. Unlike many later works, these volumes present the computational and biological mechanisms from a distinctly cognitive perspective, and they make a serious attempt at modeling a range of cognitive phenomena. However, the PDP volumes are now somewhat dated and present an often confusing hodge-podge of different algorithms and ideas. Also, the simulation exercises were a separate volume, rather than being incorporated into the text to play an integral role in students' understanding of the complex behavior of the models. Finally, the neuroscience got short shrift in this treatment, because most of the models relied on very abstract and somewhat biologically implausible mechanisms.

Our objective in writing this text was therefore to replicate the scope (and excitement) of the original PDP volumes in a more modern, integrated, and unified manner that more tightly related biology and cognition and provided intuitive graphical simulations at every step along the way. We achieved this scope by focusing on a consistent set of principles that form bridges between computation, neuroscience, and cognition. Within this coherent framework, we cover a breadth and depth of simulations of cognitive phenomena unlike any other textbook that we know of. We provide a large number of modern, state-of-the-art, research-grade simulation models that readers explore in some detail as guided by the text, and that they can then explore further on their own.

We are well aware that there is a basic tradeoff between consistency and diversity (e.g., exploitation versus exploration as emphasized in the reinforcement-learning paradigm). The field of computational cognitive neuroscience has generally been characterized more by the diversity of theoretical approaches and models than by any kind of explicit consistency. This diversity has been cataloged in places like the encyclopedic Arbib (1995) volume, where readers can find overview treatments of widely varying perspectives. We view this book as a complementary resource to such encyclopedic treatments. We focus on consistency, striving to abstract and present as much as possible a consensus view, guided by a basic set of well-developed principles, with brief pointers to major alternative perspectives.

In summary, this book is an attempt to consolidate and integrate advances across a range of fields and phenomena into one coherent package, which can be digested relatively easily by the reader. At one level, the result can be viewed as just that — an integration and consolidation of existing knowledge. However, we have found that the process of putting all of these ideas together into one package has led to an emergent phenomenon in which the whole is greater than the sum of its parts. We come away with a sense of renewed excitement and interest in computational cognitive neuroscience after writing this book, and hope that you feel some of this, too.

Acknowledgments

This book has benefited greatly from the generous input of a number of individuals. First, we thank our students for working through early drafts of the text and simulations, and for providing useful feedback from the perspective of the primary target audience for this book. From the University of Denver: David Bauer, Nick Bitz, Rebecca Betjemann, Senia Bozova, Kristin Brelsford, Nomita Chhabildas, Tom Delaney, Elizabeth Griffith, Jeff Grubb, Leane Guzzetta, Erik Johnston, Gabe Lebovich, John McGoldrick, Jamie Ogline, Joan Ross, Robbie Rossman, Jeanne Shinskey, Tracy Stackhouse, Jennifer Stedron, Rachel Tunick, Tara Wass, and Julie Wilbarger. And from the University of Colorado, Boulder: Anita Bowles, Mike Emerson, Michael Frank, Naomi Friedman, Tom Helman, Josh Hemann, Darrell Laham, Noelle LaVoie, Bryan Loughry, Ben Pageler, Chris Ritacca, Alan Sanfey, Rodolfo Soto, Steve Romero, Mike Vanelzakker, Jim Vanoverschelde, Tor Wager, Rebecca Washlow, and Ting-Yu Wu.

We were very fortunate for the comments of the following colleagues who provided invaluable expertise and insight: Dan Barth, Lyle Bourne, Axel Cleeremans and colleagues, Martha Farah, Lew Harvey, Alex Holcombe, Jim Hoeffner, Jan Keenan, Akira Miyake, Mike Mozer, David Noelle, Ken Norman, Dick Olson, Bruce Pennington, Jerry Rudy, and Jack Werner. We reserve special thanks for M. Frank Norman for a very thorough reading of the entire manuscript and careful attention to the mathematical equations, and for Chad Marsolek who gave us extensive feedback after teaching from the book.

Michael Rutter at MIT Press was very supportive throughout the development, writing, and reviewing process of the book — he is good enough to make us almost feel like writing another book! We will have to see how this one does first. Katherine Almeida at MIT Press and the entire production staff made the production process remarkably smooth — thanks!

Peter Dayan deserves special gratitude for inspiring us to write this thing in the first place. Josh Dorman was very generous in agreeing to do the cover for the book, which is entitled "Yonder: Interior" — please buy his artwork (we did)! His work is represented by 55 Mercer Gallery in New York (212) 226-8513, and on the web at: www.sirius.com/ zknower/josh.

Finally, we owe the greatest debt to Jay McClelland, who was our mentor throughout graduate school and continues to inspire us. It will be obvious to all that many of the framing ideas in this book are based on Jay's pioneering work, and that he deserves extraordinary credit for shaping the field and maintaining a focus on cognitive issues.

RO and YM were supported by NSF KDI/LIS grant IBN-9873492. RO was supported by NIH Program Project MH47566, and YM was supported by NICHD 1R29 HD37163-01 and NIMH 1R03 MH59066-01.

Chapter 1

Introduction and Overview

Contents

1.1 Computational Cognitive Neuroscience 1
1.2 Basic Motivations for Computational Cognitive
Neuroscience 2
   1.2.1 Physical Reductionism 2
   1.2.2 Reconstructionism 3
   1.2.3 Levels of Analysis 4
   1.2.4 Scaling Issues 6
1.3 Historical Context 8
1.4 Overview of Our Approach 10
1.5 General Issues in Computational Modeling 11
1.6 Motivating Cognitive Phenomena and Their Biological Bases 14
   1.6.1 Parallelism 15
   1.6.2 Gradedness 15
   1.6.3 Interactivity 17
   1.6.4 Competition 17
   1.6.5 Learning 18
1.7 Organization of the Book 19
1.8 Further Reading 20

1.1 Computational Cognitive Neuroscience

How does the brain think? This is one of the most challenging unsolved questions in science. Armed with new methods, data, and ideas, researchers in a variety of fields bring us closer to fully answering this question each day. We can even watch the brain as it thinks, using modern neuroimaging machines that record the biological shadows of thought and transform them into vivid color images. These amazing images, together with the results from many other important techniques, have advanced our understanding of the neural bases of cognition considerably. We can consolidate these various different approaches under the umbrella discipline of **cognitive neuroscience**, which has as its goal answering this most important of scientific questions.

Cognitive neuroscience will remain a frontier for many years to come, because both thoughts and brains are incredibly complex and difficult to understand. Sequences of images of the brain thinking reveal a vast network of glowing regions that interact in complex ways with changing patterns of thought. Each picture is worth a thousand words — indeed, language often fails us in the attempt to capture the richness and subtlety of it all. **Computational** models based on biological properties of the brain can provide an important tool for understanding all of this complexity. Such models can capture the flow of information from your eyes recording these letters and words, up to the parts of your brain activated by the different word meanings, resulting in an integrated comprehension of this text. Although our understanding of such phenomena is still incomplete, these models enable us to explore their underlying mechanisms, which we can implement on a computer and manipulate, test, and ultimately understand.

This book provides an introduction to this emerging subdiscipline known as **computational cognitive neuroscience**: simulating human cognition using biologically based networks of neuronlike units (**neural networks**). We provide a textbook-style treatment of the central ideas in this field, integrated with computer simulations that allow readers to undertake their own **explorations** of the material presented in the text. An important and unique aspect of this book is that the explorations include a number of large-scale simulations used in recent original research projects, giving students and other researchers the opportunity to examine these models up close and in detail.

In this chapter, we present an overview of the basic motivations and history behind computational cognitive neuroscience, followed by an overview of the subsequent chapters covering basic neural computational mechanisms (part I) and cognitive phenomena (part II). Using the neural network models in this book, you will be able to explore a wide range of interesting cognitive phenomena, including:

Visual encoding: A neural network will view natural scenes (mountains, trees, etc.), and, using some basic principles of learning, will develop ways of encoding these visual scenes much like those your brain uses to make sense of the visual world.

Spatial attention: By taking advantage of the interactions between two different streams of visual processing, you can see how a model focuses its attention in different locations in space, for example to scan a visual scene. Then, you can use this model to simulate the attention performance of normal and brain-damaged people.

Episodic memory: By incorporating the structure of the brain area called the *hippocampus,* a neural network will become able to form new memories of everyday experiences and events, and will simulate human performance on memory tasks.

Working memory: You will see that specialized biological mechanisms can greatly improve a network's *working memory* (the kind of memory you need to multiply 42 by 17 in your head, for example). Further, you will see how the skilled control of working memory can be learned through experience.

Word reading: You can see how a network can learn to read and pronounce nearly 3,000 English words. Like human subjects, this network can pronounce novel nonwords that it has never seen before (e.g., "mave" or "nust"), demonstrating that it is not simply memorizing pronunciations — instead, it learns the complex web of regularities that govern English pronunciation. And, by damaging a model that captures the many different ways that words are represented in the brain, you can simulate various forms of dyslexia.

Semantic representation: You can explore a network that has "read" every paragraph in this textbook and in the process acquired a surprisingly good understanding of the words used therein, essentially by noting which words tend to be used together or in similar contexts.

Task directed behavior: You can explore a model of the "executive" part of the brain, the *prefrontal cortex,* and see how it can keep us focused on performing the task at hand while protecting us from getting distracted by other things going on.

Deliberate, explicit cognition: A surprising number of things occur relatively automatically in your brain (e.g., you are not aware of exactly how you translate these black and white strokes on the page into some sense of what these words are saying), but you can also think and act in a deliberate, explicit fashion. You'll explore a model that exhibits both of these types of cognition within the context of a simple categorization task, and in so doing, provides the beginnings of an account of the biological basis of conscious awareness.

1.2 Basic Motivations for Computational Cognitive Neuroscience

1.2.1 Physical Reductionism

The whole idea behind cognitive neuroscience is the once radical notion that the mysteries of human thought can be explained in much the same way as everything else in science — by reducing a complex phenomenon (cognition) into simpler components (the underlying biological mechanisms of the brain). This process is just **reductionism**, which has been and continues to be the standard method of scientific advancement across most fields. For example, all matter can be reduced to its atomic components, which helps to explain the various properties of different kinds of matter, and the ways in which they interact. Similarly, many biological phenomena can be explained in terms of the actions of underlying DNA and proteins.

Although it is natural to think of reductionism in terms of physical systems (e.g., explaining cognition in terms of the physical brain), it is also possible to achieve a form of reductionism in terms of more abstract components of a system. Indeed, one could argue that all forms of explanation entail a form of reductionism, in that they explain a previously inexplicable thing in terms of other, more familiar constructs, just as one can understand the definition of an unfamiliar word in the dictionary in terms of more familiar words.

There have been many attempts over the years to explain human cognition using various different languages and metaphors. For example, can cognition be explained by assuming it is based on simple logical operations? By assuming it works just like a standard serial computer? Although these approaches have borne some fruit, the idea that one should look to the brain itself for the language and principles upon which to explain human cognition seems more likely to succeed, given that the brain is ultimately responsible for it all. Thus, it is not just reductionism that defines the essence of cognitive neuroscience — it is also the stipulation that the components be based on the physical substrate of human cognition, the brain. This is **physical reductionism**.

As a domain of scientific inquiry matures, there is a tendency for constructs that play a role in that domain to become physically grounded. For example, in the biological sciences before the advent of modern molecular biology, ephemeral, vitalistic theories were common, where the components were posited based on a theory, not on any physical evidence for them. As the molecular basis of life was understood, it became possible to develop theories of biological function in terms of real underlying components (proteins, nucleic acids, etc.) that can be measured and localized. Some prephysical theoretical constructs accurately anticipated their physically grounded counterparts; for example, Mendel's theory of genetics anticipated many important functional aspects of DNA replication, while others did not fare so well. Similarly, many previous and current theories of hu-

man cognition are based on constructs such as "attention" and "working memory buffers" that are based on an analysis of behaviors or thoughts, and not on physical entities that can be independently measured. Cognitive neuroscience differs from other forms of cognitive theorizing in that it seeks to explain cognitive phenomena in terms of underlying **neurobiological** components, which can in principle be independently measured and localized. Just as in biology and other fields, some of the nonphysical constructs of cognition will probably fit well with the underlying biological mechanisms, and others may not (e.g., Churchland, 1986). Even in those that fit well, understanding their biological basis will probably lead to a more refined and sophisticated understanding (e.g., as knowing the biological structure of DNA has for understanding genetics).

1.2.2 Reconstructionism

However, reductionism in all aspects of science — particularly in the study of human cognition — can suffer from an inappropriate emphasis on the process of reducing phenomena into component pieces, without the essential and complementary process of using those pieces to reconstruct the larger phenomenon. We refer to this latter process as **reconstructionism**. It is simply not enough to say that the brain is made of neurons; one must explain how billions of neurons interacting with each other produce human cognition. Teitelbaum (1967) argued for a similar complementarity of scientific processes — analysis and synthesis — in the study of physiological psychology. Analysis entails dissecting and simplifying a system to understand its essential elements; synthesis entails combining elements and understanding their interactions.

The computational approach to cognitive neuroscience becomes critically important in reconstructionism: it is very difficult to use verbal arguments to reconstruct human cognition (or any other complex phenomenon) from the action of a large number of interacting components. Instead, we can implement the behavior of these components in a computer program and test whether they are indeed capable of reproducing the desired phenomena. Such simulations are crucial to developing our understanding of how neurons produce cog-

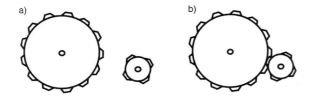

Figure 1.1: Illustration of the importance of reconstruction-ism — it is not enough to say that the system is composed of components (e.g., two gears as in **a**), one must also show how these components interact to produce overall behaviors. In **b**, the two gears interact to produce changes in rotational speed and torque — these effects emerge from the interaction, and are not a property of each component individually.

nition. This is especially true when there are **emergent phenomena** that arise from these interactions without obviously being present in the behavior of individual elements (neurons) — where the whole is greater than the sum of its parts. The importance of reconstruction-ism is often overlooked in all areas of science, not just cognitive neuroscience, and the process has really only recently become feasible with the advent of relatively affordable fast computers.

Figure 1.1 shows a simple illustration of the impor-tance of reconstructionism in understanding how sys-tems behave. Here, it is not sufficient to say that the system is composed of two components (the two gears shown in panel a). Instead, one must also specify that the gears interact as shown in panel b, because it is only through this interaction that the important "behavioral" properties of changes in rotational speed and torque can emerge. For example, if the smaller gear drives the larger gear, this achieves a decrease in rotational speed and an increase in torque. However, if this same driving gear were to interact with a gear that was even smaller than it, it would produce the opposite effect. This is essentially what it means for the behavior to emerge from the interaction between the two gears, because it is clearly not a property of the individual gears in isola-tion. Similarly, cognition is an emergent phenomenon of the interactions of billions of neurons. It is not suf-ficient to say that the cognitive system is composed of billions of neurons; we must instead specify how these neurons interact to produce cognition.

1.2.3 Levels of Analysis

Although the physical reductionism and reconstruction-ism motivations behind computational cognitive neuro-science may appear sound and straightforward, this ap-proach to understanding human cognition is challenged by the extreme complexity of and lack of knowledge about both the brain and the cognition it produces. As a result, many researchers have appealed to the notion of hierarchical **levels** of analysis to deal with this complex-ity. Clearly, some levels of underlying mechanism are more appropriate for explaining human cognition than others. For example, it appears foolhardy to try to ex-plain human cognition directly in terms of atoms and simple molecules, or even proteins and DNA. Thus, we must focus instead on higher level mechanisms. How-ever, exactly which level is the "right" level is an im-portant issue that will only be resolved through further scientific investigation. The level presented in this book represents our best guess at this time.

One approach toward thinking about the issue of lev-els of analysis was suggested by David Marr (1982), who introduced the seductive notion of **computational**, **algorithmic**, and **implementational** levels by forging an analogy with the computer. Take the example of a program that sorts a list of numbers. One can specify in very abstract terms that the computation performed by this program is to arrange the numbers such that the smallest one is first in the list, the next largest one is next, and so on. This abstract computational level of analysis is useful for specifying what different pro-grams do, without worrying about exactly how they go about doing it. Think of it as the "executive summary."

The algorithmic level then delves into more of the details as to how sorting actually occurs — there are many different strategies that one could adopt, and they have various tradeoffs in terms of factors such as speed or amount of memory used. Critically, the algorithm provides just enough information to implement the pro-gram, but does not specify any details about what lan-guage to program it in, what variable names to use, and so on. These details are left for the implementational level — how the program is actually written and exe-cuted on a particular computer using a particular lan-guage.

Marr's levels and corresponding emphasis on the computational and algorithmic levels were born out of the early movements of **artificial intelligence**, **cognitive psychology**, and **cognitive science**, which were based on the idea that one could ignore the underlying biological mechanisms of cognition, focusing instead on identifying important computational or cognitive level properties. Indeed, these traditional approaches were based on the assumption that the brain works like a standard computer, and thus that Marr's computational and algorithmic levels were much more important than the "mere details" of the underlying neurobiological implementation.

The **optimality** or **rational analysis** approach, which is widely employed across the "sciences of complexity" from biology to psychology and economics (e.g., Anderson, 1990), shares the Marr-like emphasis on the computational level. Here, one assumes that it is possible to identify the "optimal" computation or function performed by a person or animal in a given context, and that whatever the brain is doing, it must somehow be accomplishing this same optimal computation (and can therefore be safely ignored). For example, Anderson (1990) argues that memory retention curves are optimally tuned to the expected frequency and spacing of retrieval demands for items stored in memory. Under this view, it doesn't really matter how the memory retention mechanisms work, because they are ultimately driven by the optimality criterion of matching expected demands for items, which in turn is assumed to follow general laws.

Although the optimality approach may sound attractive, the definition of optimality all too often ends up being conditioned on a number of assumptions (including those about the nature of the underlying implementation) that have no real independent basis. In short, optimality can rarely be defined in purely "objective" terms, and so often what is optimal in a given situation depends on the detailed circumstances.

Thus, the dangerous thing about both Marr's levels and these optimality approaches is that they appear to suggest that the implementational level is largely irrelevant. In most standard computers and languages, this is true, because *they are all effectively equivalent at the implementational level*, so that the implementational is-

sues don't really affect the algorithmic and computational levels of analysis. Indeed, computer algorithms can be turned into implementations by the completely automatic process of compilation. In contrast, in the brain, the neural implementation is certainly not derived automatically from some higher-level description, and thus it is not obviously true that it can be easily described at these higher levels.

In effect, the higher-level computational analysis has already *assumed* a general implementational form, without giving proper credit to it for shaping the whole enterprise in the first place. However, with the advent of parallel computers, people are beginning to realize the limitations of computation and algorithms that assume the standard serial computer with address-based memory — entirely new classes of algorithms and ways of thinking about problems are being developed to take advantage of parallel computation. Given that the brain is clearly a parallel computer, having billions of computing elements (neurons), one must be very careful in importing seductively simple ideas based on standard computers.

On the other end of the spectrum, various researchers have emphasized the *implementational* level as primary over the computational and algorithmic. They have argued that cognitive models should be assembled by making extremely detailed replicas of neurons, thus guaranteeing that the resulting model contains all of the important biological mechanisms (e.g., Bower, 1992). The risk of this approach is complementary to those that emphasize a purely computational approach: without any clear understanding of which biological properties are functionally important and which are not, one ends up with massive, complicated models that are difficult to understand, and that provide little insight into the critical properties of cognition. Further, these models inevitably fail to represent *all* of the biological mechanisms in their fullest possible detail, so one can never be quite sure that something important is not missing.

Instead of arguing for the superiority of one level over the other, we adopt a fully **interactive, balanced** approach, which emphasizes forming connections between data across all of the relevant levels, and striking a reasonable balance between the desire for a simplified model and the desire to incorporate as much of the

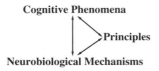

Figure 1.2: The two basic levels of analysis used in this text, with an intermediate level to help forge the links.

known biological mechanisms as possible. There is a place for both **bottom-up** (i.e., working from biological facts "up" to cognition), **top-down** (i.e., working from cognition "down" to biological facts), and, most important, interactive approaches, where one tries to simultaneously take into account constraints at the biological and cognitive levels.

For example, it can be useful to take a set of facts about how neurons behave, encode them in a set of equations in a computer program, and see how the kinds of behaviors that result depend on the properties of these neurons. It can also be useful to think about what cognition should be doing in a particular case (e.g., at the computational level, or on some other principled basis), and then derive an implementation that accomplishes this, and see how well that characterizes what we know about the brain, and how well it does the cognitive job it is supposed to do. This kind of interplay between neurobiological, cognitive and principled (computational and otherwise) considerations is emphasized throughout the text.

To summarize our approach, and to avoid the unintended associations with Marr's terminology, we adopt the following hierarchy of analytical levels (figure 1.2). At its core, we have essentially a simple bi-level physical reductionist/reconstructionist hierarchy, with a lower level consisting of *neurobiological mechanisms,* and an upper level consisting of *cognitive phenomena.* We will reduce cognitive phenomena to the operation of neurobiological mechanisms, and show, through simulations, how these mechanisms produce emergent cognitive phenomena. Of course, our simulations will have to rely on simplified, abstracted renditions of the neurobiological mechanisms.

To help forge links between these two levels of analysis, we have an auxiliary intermediate level consisting of *principles* presented throughout the text. We do not think that the brain nor cognition can be fully described by these principles, which is why they play an auxiliary role and are shown off to one side of the figure. However, they serve to highlight and make clear the connection between certain aspects of the biology and certain aspects of cognition. Often, these principles are based on computational-level descriptions of aspects of cognition. But, we want to avoid any implication that these principles provide some privileged level of description (i.e., like Marr's view of the computational level), that tempts us into thinking that data at the two basic empirical levels (cognition and neurobiology) are less relevant. Instead, these principles are fundamentally shaped by, and help to strike a good balance between, the two primary levels of analysis.

The levels of analysis issue is easily confused with different levels of *structure* within the nervous system, but these two types of levels are not equivalent. The relevant levels of structure range from molecules to individual neurons to small groups or columns of neurons to larger areas or regions of neurons up to the entire brain itself. Although one might be tempted to say that our cognitive phenomena level of analysis should be associated with the highest structural level (the entire brain), and our neurobiological mechanisms level of analysis associated with lower structural levels, this is not really accurate. Indeed, some cognitive phenomena can be traced directly to properties of individual neurons (e.g., that they exhibit a fatiguelike phenomenon if activated too long), whereas other cognitive phenomena only emerge as a result of interactions among a number of different brain areas. Furthermore, as we progress from lower to higher structural levels in successive chapters of this book, we emphasize that specific computational principles and cognitive phenomena can be associated with each of these structural levels. Thus, just as there is no privileged level of analysis, there is no privileged structural level — all of these levels must be considered in an interactive fashion.

1.2.4 Scaling Issues

Having adopted essentially two levels of analysis, we are in the position of using biological mechanisms operating at the level of individual neurons to explain even relatively complex, high-level cognitive phenomena. This raises the question as to why these basic neural mechanisms should have any relevance to understanding something that is undoubtedly the product of millions or even billions of neurons — certainly we do not include anywhere near that many neurons in our simulations! This **scaling issue** relates to the way in which we construct a scaled-down model of the real brain. It is important to emphasize that the need for scaling is at least partially a pragmatic issue having to do with the limitations of currently available computational resources. Thus, it should be possible to put the following arguments to the test in the future as larger, more complex models can be constructed. However, scaled-down models are also easier to understand, and are a good place to begin the computational cognitive neuroscience enterprise.

We approach the scaling problem in the following ways.

- The target cognitive behavior that we expect (and obtain) from the models is similarly scaled down compared to the complexities of actual human cognition.

- We show that one of our simulated neurons (units) in the model can approximate the behavior of many real neurons, so that we can build models of multiple brain areas where the neurons in those areas are simulated by many fewer units.

- We argue that information processing in the brain has a **fractal** quality, where the same basic properties apply across disparate physical scales. These basic properties are those of individual neurons, which "show through" even at higher levels, and are thus relevant to understanding even the large-scale behavior of the brain.

The first argument amounts to the idea that our neural network models are performing essentially the same type of processing as a human in a particular task, but on a reduced problem that either lacks the detailed information content of the human equivalent or represents a subset of these details. Of course, many phenomena can become qualitatively different as they get scaled up

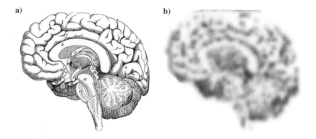

Figure 1.3: Illustration of scaling as performed on an image — the original image in (a) was scaled down by a factor of 8, retaining only 1/8th of the original information, and then scaled back up to the same size and averaged (blurred) to produce (b), which captures many of the general characteristics of the original, but not the fine details. Our models give us something like this scaled-down, averaged image of how the brain works.

or down along this content dimension, but it seems reasonable to allow that some important properties might be relatively scale invariant. For example, one could plausibly argue that each major area of the human cortex could be reduced to handle only a small portion of the content that it actually does (e.g., by the use of a $16x16$ pixel retina instead of 16 million x 16 million pixels), but that some important aspects of the essential computation on any piece of that information are preserved in the reduced model. If several such reduced cortical areas were connected, one could imagine having a useful but simplified model of some reasonably complex psychological phenomena.

The second argument can perhaps be stated most clearly by imagining that an individual unit in the model approximates the behavior of a population of essentially identical neurons. Thus, whereas actual neurons are discretely spiking, our model units typically (but not exclusively) use a continuous, graded activation signal. We will see in chapter 2 that this graded signal provides a very good approximation to the average number of spikes per unit time produced by a population of spiking neurons. Of course, we don't imagine that the brain is constructed from populations of identical neurons, but we do think that the brain employs overlapping distributed representations, so that an individual model unit can represent the centroid of a set of such representations. Thus, the population can encode much more information (e.g., many finer shades of meaning), and is probably different in other important ways (e.g., it might be more robust to the effects of noise). A visual analogy for this kind of scaling is shown in figure 1.3, where the sharp, high-resolution detail of the original (panel a) is lost in the scaled-down version (panel b), but the basic overall structure is preserved.

Finally, we believe that the brain has a fractal character for two reasons: First, it is likely that, at least in the cortex, the effective properties of long-range connectivity are similar to that of local, short-range connectivity. For example, both short and long-range connectivity produce a balance between excitation and inhibition by virtue of connecting to both excitatory and inhibitory neurons (more on this in chapter 3). Thus, a model based on the properties of short-range connectivity within a localized cortical area could also describe a larger-scale model containing many such cortical areas simulated at a coarser level. The second reason is basically the same as the one given earlier about averaging over populations of neurons: if on average the population behaves roughly the same as the individual neuron, then the two levels of description are self-similar, which is what it means to be fractal.

In short, these arguments provide a basis for optimism that models based on neurobiological data can provide useful accounts of cognitive phenomena, even those that involve large, widely distributed areas of the brain. The models described in this book substantiate some of this optimism, but certainly this issue remains an open and important question for the computational cognitive neuroscience enterprise. The following historical perspective on this enterprise provides an overview of some of the other important issues that have shaped the field.

1.3 Historical Context

Although the field of computational cognitive neuroscience is relatively young, its boundaries are easily blurred into a large number of related disciplines, some of which have been around for quite some time. Indeed, research in any aspect of cognition, neuroscience, or computation has the potential to make an important contribution to this field. Thus, the entire space of this book could be devoted to an adequate account of the relevant history of the field. This section is instead intended to merely provide a brief overview of some of the particularly relevant historical context and motivation behind our approach. Specifically, we focus on the advances in understanding how networks of simulated neurons can lead to interesting cognitive phenomena, which occurred initially in the 1960s and then again in the period from the late '70s to the present day. These advances form the main heritage of our approach because, as should be clear from what has been said earlier, the neural network modeling approach provides a crucial link between networks of neurons and human cognition.

The field of **cognitive psychology** began in the late 1950s and early '60s, following the domination of the behaviorists. Key advances associated with this new field included its emphasis on *internal mechanisms* for mediating cognition, and in particular the use of *explicit computational models* for simulating cognition on computers (e.g., problem solving and mathematical reasoning; Newell & Simon, 1972). The dominant approach was based on the **computer metaphor**, which held that human cognition is much like processing in a standard serial computer.

In such systems, which we will refer to as "traditional" or "symbolic," the basic operations involve **symbol manipulation** (e.g., manipulating logical statements expressed using dynamically-bound variables and operators), and processing consists of a sequence of **serial**, **rule-governed** steps. **Production systems** became the dominant framework for cognitive modeling within this approach. **Productions** are essentially elaborate if-then constructs that are activated when their if-conditions are met, and they then produce actions that enable the firing of subsequent productions. Thus, these productions control the sequential flow of processing. As we will see, these traditional, symbolic models serve as an important contrast to the neural-network framework, and the two have been in a state of competition from the earliest days of their existence.

Even though the computer metaphor was dominant, there was also considerable interest in neuronlike processing during this time, with advances like: (a) the

McCulloch and Pitts (1943) model of neural processing in terms of basic logical operations; (b) Hebb's (1949) theory of **Hebbian learning** and the **cell assembly**, which holds that connections between coactive neurons should be strengthened, joining them together; and (c) Rosenblatt's (1958) work on the **perceptron** learning algorithm, which could learn from **error signals**. These computational approaches built on fundamental advances in neurobiology, where the idea that the neuron is the primary information processing unit of the brain became established (the "neuron doctrine"; Shepherd, 1992), and the basic principles of neural communication and processing (action potentials, synapses, neurotransmitters, ion channels, etc.) were being developed. The dominance of the computer metaphor approach in cognitive psychology was nevertheless sealed with the publication of the book *Perceptrons* (Minsky & Papert, 1969), which proved that some of these simple neuronlike models had significant computational limitations — they were unable to learn to solve a large class of basic problems.

While a few hardy researchers continued studying these neural-network models through the '70s (e.g., Grossberg, Kohonen, Anderson, Amari, Arbib, Willshaw), it was not until the '80s that a few critical advances brought the field back into real popularity. In the early '80s, psychological (e.g., McClelland & Rumelhart, 1981) and computational (Hopfield, 1982, 1984) advances were made based on the activation dynamics of networks. Then, the backpropagation learning algorithm was rediscovered by Rumelhart, Hinton, and Williams (1986b) (having been independently discovered several times before: Bryson & Ho, 1969; Werbos, 1974; Parker, 1985) and the *Parallel Distributed Processing (PDP)* books (Rumelhart et al., 1986c; McClelland et al., 1986) were published, which firmly established the credibility of neural network models. Critically, the backpropagation algorithm eliminated the limitations of the earlier models, enabling essentially any function to be learned by a neural network. Another important advance represented in the PDP books was a strong appreciation for the importance of **distributed representations** (Hinton, McClelland, & Rumelhart, 1986), which have a number of computational advantages over symbolic or localist representations.

Backpropagation led to a new wave of cognitive modeling (which often goes by the name **connectionism**). Although it represented a step forward computationally, backpropagation was viewed by many as a step backward from a biological perspective, because it was not at all clear how it could be implemented by biological mechanisms (Crick, 1989; Zipser & Andersen, 1988). Thus, backpropagation-based cognitive modeling carried on without a clear biological basis, causing many such researchers to use the same kinds of arguments used by supporters of the computer metaphor to justify their approach (i.e., the "computational level" arguments discussed previously). Some would argue that this deemphasizing of the biological issues made the field essentially a reinvented computational cognitive psychology based on "neuronlike" processing principles, rather than a true computational cognitive neuroscience.

In parallel with the expanded influence of neural network models in understanding cognition, there was a rapid growth of more biologically oriented modeling. We can usefully identify several categories of this type of research. First, we can divide the biological models into those that emphasize learning and those that do not. The models that do not emphasize learning include detailed biophysical models of individual neurons (Traub & Miles, 1991; Bower, 1992), information-theoretic approaches to processing in neurons and networks of neurons (e.g., Abbott & LeMasson, 1993; Atick & Redlich, 1990; Amit, Gutfreund, & Sompolinsky, 1987; Amari & Maginu, 1988), and refinements and extensions of the original Hopfield (1982, 1984) models, which hold considerable appeal due to their underlying mathematical formulation in terms of concepts from statistical physics. Although this research has led to many important insights, it tends to make less direct contact with cognitively relevant issues (though the Hopfield network itself provides some centrally important principles, as we will see in chapter 3, and has been used as a framework for some kinds of learning).

The biologically based learning models have tended to focus on learning in the early visual system, with an emphasis on Hebbian learning (Linsker, 1986; Miller, Keller, & Stryker, 1989; Miller, 1994; Kohonen, 1984; Hebb, 1949). Importantly, a large body of basic neuroscience research supports the idea that Hebbian-like mechanisms are operating in neurons in most cognitively important areas of the brain (Bear, 1996; Brown, Kairiss, & Keenan, 1990; Collingridge & Bliss, 1987). However, Hebbian learning is generally fairly computationally weak (as we will see in chapter 5), and suffers from limitations similar to those of the 1960s generation of learning mechanisms. Thus, it has not been as widely used as backpropagation for cognitive modeling because it often cannot learn the relevant tasks.

In addition to the cognitive (connectionist) and biological branches of neural network research, considerable work has been done on the computational end. It has been apparent that the mathematical basis of neural networks has much in common with statistics, and the computational advances have tended to push this connection further. Recently, the use of the Bayesian framework for statistical inference has been applied to develop new learning algorithms (e.g., Dayan, Hinton, Neal, & Zemel, 1995; Saul, Jaakkola, & Jordan, 1996), and more generally to understand existing ones. However, none of these models has yet been developed to the point where they provide a framework for learning that works reliably on a wide range of cognitive tasks, while simultaneously being implementable by a reasonable biological mechanism. Indeed, most (but not all) of the principal researchers in the computational end of the field are more concerned with theoretical, statistical, and machine-learning kinds of issues than with cognitive or biological ones.

In short, from the perspective of the computational cognitive neuroscience endeavor, the field is in a somewhat fragmented state, with modelers in computational cognitive psychology primarily focused on understanding human cognition without close contact with the underlying neurobiology, biological modelers focused on information-theoretic constructs or computationally weak learning mechanisms without close contact with cognition, and learning theorists focused at a more computational level of analysis involving statistical constructs without close contact with biology or cognition. Nevertheless, we think that a strong set of cognitively relevant computational and biological principles has emerged over the years, and that the time is ripe for an attempt to consolidate and integrate these principles.

1.4   Overview of Our Approach

This brief historical overview provides a useful context for describing the basic characteristics of the approach we have taken in this book. Our core mechanistic principles include both backpropagation-based error-driven learning and Hebbian learning, the central principles behind the Hopfield network for interactive, constraint-satisfaction style processing, distributed representations, and inhibitory competition. The neural units in our simulations use equations based directly on the ion channels that govern the behavior of real neurons (as described in chapter 2), and our neural networks incorporate a number of well-established anatomical and physiological properties of the neocortex (as described in chapter 3). Thus, we strive to establish detailed connections between biology and cognition, in a way that is consistent with many well-established computational principles.

Our approach can be seen as an integration of a number of different themes, trends, and developments (O'Reilly, 1998). Perhaps the most relevant such development was the integration of a coherent set of neural network principles into the *GRAIN* framework of McClelland (1993). GRAIN stands for graded, random, adaptive, interactive, (nonlinear) network. This framework was primarily motivated by (and applied to) issues surrounding the dynamics of activation flow through a neural network. The framework we adopt in this book incorporates and extends these GRAIN principles by emphasizing learning mechanisms and the architectural properties that support them.

For example, there has been a long-standing desire to understand how more biologically realistic mechanisms could give rise to error-driven learning (e.g., Hinton & McClelland, 1988; Mazzoni, Andersen, & Jordan, 1991). Recently, a number of different frameworks for achieving this goal have been shown to be variants of a common underlying error propagation mechanism (O'Reilly, 1996a). The resulting algorithm, called *GeneRec*, is consistent with known biological mechanisms of learning, makes use of other biological properties of the brain (including interactivity), and allows for realistic neural activation functions to be used. Thus, this algorithm plays an important role in our integrated framework by allowing us to use the principle of back-propagation learning without conflicting with the desire to take the biology seriously.

Another long-standing theme in neural network models is the development of inhibitory competition mechanisms (e.g., Kohonen, 1984; McClelland & Rumelhart, 1981; Rumelhart & Zipser, 1986; Grossberg, 1976). Competition has a number of important functional benefits emphasized in the GRAIN framework (which we will explore in chapter 3) and is generally required for the use of Hebbian learning mechanisms. It is technically challenging, however, to combine competition with distributed representations in an effective manner, because the two tend to work at cross purposes. Nevertheless, there are good reasons to believe that the kinds of sparse distributed representations that should in principle result from competition provide a particularly efficient means for representing the structure of the natural environment (e.g., Barlow, 1989; Field, 1994; Olshausen & Field, 1996). Thus, an important part of our framework is a mechanism of neural competition that is compatible with powerful distributed representations and can be combined with interactivity and learning in a way that was not generally possible before (O'Reilly, 1998, 1996b).

The emphasis throughout the book is on the facts of the biology, the core computational principles just described, which underlie most of the cognitive neural network models that have been developed to date, and their interrelationship in the context of a range of well-studied cognitive phenomena. To facilitate and simplify the hands-on exploration of these ideas by the student, we take advantage of a particular implementational framework that incorporates all of the core mechanistic principles called *Leabra* (**l**ocal, **e**rror-driven and **a**ssociative, **b**iologically **r**ealistic **a**lgorithm). Leabra is pronounced like the astrological sign Libra, which emphasizes the *balance* between many different objectives that is achieved by the algorithm.

To the extent that we are able to understand a wide range of cognitive phenomena using a consistent set of biological and computational principles, one could consider the framework presented in this book to be a "first draft" of a coherent framework for computational cog-

nitive neuroscience. This framework provides a useful consolidation of existing ideas, and should help to identify the limitations and problems that will need to be solved in the future.

Newell (1990) provided a number of arguments in favor of developing unified theories of cognition, many of which apply to our approach of developing a coherent framework for computational cognitive neuroscience. Newell argued that it is relatively easy (and thus relatively uninformative) to construct specialized theories of specific phenomena. In contrast, one encounters many more constraints by taking on a wider range of data, and a theory that can account for this data is thus much more likely to be true. Given that our framework bears little resemblance to Newell's SOAR architecture, it is clear that just the process of making a unified architecture does not guarantee convergence on some common set of principles. However, it is clear that casting a wider net imposes many more constraints on the modeling process, and the fact that the single set of principles can be used to model the wide range of phenomena covered in this book lends some measure of validity to the undertaking.

Chomsky (1965) and Seidenberg (1993) also discussed the value of developing *explanatory* theories that explain phenomena in terms of a small set of independently motivated principles, in contrast with *descriptive* theories that essentially restate phenomena.

1.5 General Issues in Computational Modeling

The preceding discussion of the benefits of a unified model raises a number of more general issues regarding the benefits of computational modeling[1] as a methodology for cognitive neuroscience. Although we think the benefits generally outweigh the disadvantages, it is also important to be cognizant of the potential traps and problems associated with this methodology. We will just provide a brief summary of these advantages and problems here.

---

[1] We consider both models that are explicitly simulated on a computer and more abstract mathematical models to be computational models, in that both are focused on the computational processing of information in the brain.

Advantages:

Models help us to understand phenomena. A computational model can provide novel sources of insight into behavior, for example by providing a counter-intuitive explanation of a phenomenon, or by reconciling seemingly contradictory phenomena (e.g., by complex interactions among components). Seemingly different phenomena can also be related to each other in nonobvious ways via a common set of computational mechanisms.

Computational models can also be lesioned and then tested, providing insight into behavior following specific types of brain damage, and in turn, into normal functioning. Often, lesions can have nonobvious effects that computational models can explain.

By virtue of being able to translate between functional desiderata and the biological mechanisms that implement them, computational models enable us to understand not just how the brain is structured, but *why* it is structured in the way it is.

Models deal with complexity. A computational model can deal with complexity in ways that verbal arguments cannot, producing satisfying explanations of what would otherwise just be vague hand-wavy arguments. Further, computational models can handle complexity across multiple levels of analysis, allowing data across these levels to be integrated and related to each other. For example, the computational models in this book show how biological properties give rise to cognitive behaviors in ways that would be impossible with simple verbal arguments.

Models are explicit. Making a computational model forces you to be explicit about your assumptions and about exactly how the relevant processes actually work. Such explicitness carries with it many potential advantages.

First, explicitness can help in deconstructing psychological concepts that may rely on *homunculi* to do their work. A homunculus is a "little man," and many theories of cognition make unintended use of them by embodying particular components (often "boxes") of the theory with magical powers that end up doing all the work in the theory. A canonical example is

the "executive" theory of prefrontal cortex function: if you posit an executive without explaining how it makes all those good decisions and coordinates all the other brain areas, you haven't explained too much (you might as well just put pinstripes and a tie on the box).

Second, an explicitly specified computational model can be run to generate novel predictions. A computational model thus forces you to accept the consequences of your assumptions. If the model must be modified to account for new data, it becomes very clear exactly what these changes are, and the scientific community can more easily evaluate the resulting deviance from the previous theory. Predictions from verbal theories can be tenuous due to lack of specificity and the flexibility of vague verbal constructs.

Third, explicitness can contribute to a greater appreciation for the complexities of otherwise seemingly simple processes. For example, before people tried to make explicit computational models of object recognition, it didn't seem that difficult or interesting a problem — there is an anecdotal story about a scientist in the '60s who was going to implement a model of object recognition over the summer. Needless to say, he didn't succeed.

Fourth, making a computational model forces you to confront aspects of the problem that you might have otherwise ignored or considered to be irrelevant. Although one sometimes ends up using simplifications or stand-ins for these other aspects (see the list of problems that follows), it can be useful to at least confront these problems.

Models allow control. In a computational model you can control many more variables much more precisely than you can with a real system, and you can replicate results precisely. This enables you to explore the causal role of different components in ways that would otherwise be impossible.

Models provide a unified framework. As we discussed earlier, there are many advantages to using a single computational framework to explain a range of phenomena. In addition to providing a more stringent test of a theory, it encourages parsimony and also enables one to relate two seemingly disparate phenomena by understanding them in light of a common set of basic principles.

Also, it is often difficult for people to detect inconsistency in a purely verbal theory — we have a hard time keeping track of everything. However, a computational model reveals inconsistencies quite readily, because everything has to hang together and actually *work*.

Problems:

Models are too simple. Models, by necessity, involve a number of simplifications in their implementation. These simplifications may not capture all of the relevant details of the biology, the environment, the task, and so on, calling into question the validity of the model.

Inevitably, this issue ends up being an empirical one that depends on how wrong the simplifying assumptions are and how much they influence the results. It is often possible for a model to make a perfectly valid point while using a simplified implementation because the missing details are simply not relevant — the real system will exhibit the same behavior for any reasonable range of detailed parameters. Furthermore, simplification can actually be an important benefit of a model — a simple explanation is easier to understand and can reveal important truths that might otherwise be obscured by details.

Models are too complex. On the flip side, other critics complain that models are too complex to understand why they behave the way they do, and so they contribute nothing to our understanding of human behavior. This criticism is particularly relevant if a modeler treats a computational model as a theory, and it points to the mere fact that the model reproduces a set of data as an explanation of this data.

However, this criticism is less relevant if the modeler instead identifies and articulates the critical principles that underly the model's behavior, and demonstrates the relative irrelevance of other factors. Thus, a model should be viewed as a concrete instantiation

of broader principles, not as an end unto itself, and the way in which the model "uses" these principles to account for the data must be made clear. Unfortunately, this essential step of making the principles clear and demonstrating their generality is often not taken. This can be a difficult step for complex models (which is, after all, one of the advantages of modeling in the first place!), but one made increasingly manageable with advances in techniques for analyzing models.

Models can do anything. This criticism is inevitably leveled at successful models. Neural network models do have a very large number of parameters in the form of the adaptable weights between units. Also, there are many degrees of freedom in the architecture of the model, and in other parameters that determine the behavior of the units. Thus, it might seem that there are so many parameters available that fitting any given set of behavioral phenomena is uninteresting. Relatedly, because of the large number of parameters, sometimes multiple different models can provide a reasonable account of a given phenomenon. How can one address this *indeterminacy* problem to determine which is the "correct" model?

The general issues of adopting a principled, explanatory approach are relevant here — to the extent that the model's behavior can be understood in terms of more general principles, the success of the model can be attributed to these principles, and not just to random parameter fitting. Also, unlike many other kinds of models, many of the parameters in the network (i.e., the weights) are determined by principled learning mechanisms, and are thus not "free" for the modeler to set. In this book, most of the models use the same basic parameters for the network equations, and the cases where different parameters were used are strongly motivated.

The general answer to the *indeterminacy* problem is that as you apply a model to a wider range of data (e.g., different tasks, newly discovered biological constraints), and in greater detail on each task (e.g., detailed properties of the learning process), the models will be much more strenuously tested. It thus becomes much less likely that two different models can fit all the data (unless they are actually isomorphic in some way).

Models are reductionistic. One common concern is that the mechanistic, reductionistic models can never tell us about the real essence of human cognition. Although this will probably remain a philosophical issue until very large-scale models can be constructed that actually demonstrate realistic, humanlike cognition (e.g., by passing the *Turing test*), we note that *reconstructionism* is a cornerstone of our approach. Reconstructionism complements reductionism by trying to reconstruct complex phenomena in terms of the reduced components.

Modeling lacks cumulative research. There seems to be a general perception that modeling is somehow less cumulative than other types of research. This perception may be due in part to the relative youth and expansive growth of modeling — there has been a lot of territory to cover, and a breadth-first search strategy has some obvious pragmatic benefits for researchers (e.g., "claiming territory"). As the field begins to mature, cumulative work is starting to appear (e.g., Plaut, McClelland, Seidenberg, & Patterson, 1996 built on earlier work by Seidenberg & McClelland, 1989, which in turn built on other models) and this book certainly represents a very cumulative and integrative approach.

The final chapter in the book will revisit some of these issues again with the benefit of what comes in between.

1.6 Motivating Cognitive Phenomena and Their Biological Bases

Several aspects of human cognition are particularly suggestive of the kinds of neural mechanisms described in this text. We briefly describe some of the most important of these aspects here to further motivate and highlight the connections between cognition and neurobiology. However, as you will discover, these aspects of cognition are perhaps not the most obvious to the average person. Our introspections into the nature of our own cognition tend to emphasize the "conscious" aspects (because this is by definition what we are aware

of), which appear to be *serial* (one thought at a time) and *focused* on a subset of things occurring inside and outside the brain. This fact undoubtedly contributed to the popularity of the standard serial computer model for understanding human cognition, which we will use as a point of comparison for the discussion that follows.

We argue that these conscious aspects of human cognition are the proverbial "tip of the iceberg" floating above the waterline, while the great mass of cognition that makes all of this possible floats below, relatively inaccessible to our conscious introspection. In the terminology of Rumelhart et al. (1986c), neural networks focus on the *microstructure* of cognition. Attempts to understand cognition by only focusing on what's "above water" may be difficult, because all the underwater stuff is necessary to keep the tip above water in the first place — otherwise, the whole thing will just sink! To push this metaphor to its limits, the following are a few illuminating shafts of light down into this important underwater realm, and some ideas about how they keep the "tip" afloat. The aspects of cognition we will discuss are:

- Parallelism
- Gradedness
- Interactivity
- Competition
- Learning

Lest you get the impression that computational cognitive neuroscience is unable to say anything useful about conscious experience, or that we do not address this phenomenon in this book, we note that chapter 11 deals specifically with "higher-level cognition," which is closely associated with conscious experience. There we present a set of ideas and models that provide the bridge between the basic mechanisms and principles developed in the rest of the book, and the more sequential, discrete, and focused nature of conscious experience. We view these properties as arising partly due to specializations of particular brain areas (the prefrontal cortex and the hippocampus), and partly as a result of the *emergent phenomena* that arise from the basic properties of neural processing as employed in a coordinated processing system. This chapter emphasizes that there is really a continuum between what we have been referring to as conscious and subconscious processing.

1.6.1 Parallelism

Everyone knows the old joke about not being able to walk and chew gum at the same time. This is a simple case of processing multiple things in parallel (doing more than one thing at the same time). In our everyday experience, there are lots of examples of a situation where this kind of parallel processing is evident: having a conversation while driving or doing anything else (cooking, eating, watching TV, etc.); hearing your name at a cocktail party while talking to someone else (the aptly named "cocktail party effect"); and speaking what you are reading (reading aloud), to name just a few.

What may come as a surprise to you is that each of the individual processes from the above examples is itself the product of a large number of processes working in parallel. At the lowest level of analysis, we know that the human brain contains something like 10 *billion* neurons, and that each one contributes its little bit to overall human cognition. Thus, biologically, cognition must emerge from the parallel operation of all these neurons. We refer to this as parallel *distributed* processing (PDP) — the processing for any given cognitive function is distributed in parallel across a large number of individual processing elements. This parallelism occurs at many different levels, from brain areas to small groups of neurons to neurons themselves.

For example, when you look at a visual scene, one part of your brain processes the visual information to identify *what* you are seeing, while another part identifies *where* things are. Although you are not aware that this information is being processed separately, people who have lesions in one of these brain areas but not the other can only do one of these things! Thus, the apparently seamless and effortless way in which we view the world is really a product of a bunch of specialized brain areas, operating "under the hood" in a tightly coordinated fashion. As this hood is being opened using modern neuroimaging techniques, the parallelism of the brain is becoming even more obvious, as multiple brain areas are inevitably activated in most cognitive tasks.

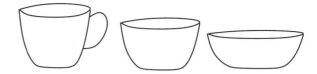

Figure 1.4: Example of graded nature of categorical representations: Is the middle item a cup or a bowl? It could be either, and lies in between these two categories.

Parallel processing can make it challenging to understand cognition, to figure out how all these subprocesses coordinate with each other to end up doing something sensible as a whole. In contrast, if cognition were just a bunch of discrete sequential steps, the task would be much easier: just identify the steps and their sequence! Instead, parallelism is more like the many-body problem in physics: understanding any pairwise interaction between two things can be simple, but once you have a number of these things all operating at the same time and mutually influencing each other, it becomes very difficult to figure out what is going on.

One virtue of the approach to cognition presented in this book is that it is based from the start on parallel distributed processing, providing powerful mathematical and intuitive tools for understanding how collective interactions between a large number of processing units (i.e., neurons) can lead to something useful (i.e., cognition).

1.6.2 Gradedness

In contrast with the discrete boolean logic and binary memory representations of standard computers, the brain is more **graded** and analog in nature. We will see in the next chapter that neurons integrate information from a large number of different input sources, producing essentially a *continuous, real valued* number that represents something like the relative *strength* of these inputs (compared to other inputs it could have received). The neuron then communicates another graded signal (its rate of firing, or *activation*) to other neurons as a function of this relative strength value. These graded signals can convey something like the *extent* or *degree* to which something is true. In the example in

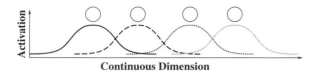

Figure 1.5: Graded activation values are important for representing continuous dimensions (e.g., position, angle, force, color) by coarse coding or basis-function representations as shown here. Each of the four units shown gives a graded activation signal roughly proportional to how close a point is along the continuous dimension to the unit's preferred point, which is defined as the point where it gives its maximal response.

figure 1.4, a neuron could convey that the first object pictured is almost definitely a cup, whereas the second one is maybe or sort-of a cup and the last one is not very likely to be a cup. Similarly, people tend to classify things (e.g., *cup* and *bowl*) in a graded manner according to how close the item is to a *prototypical* example from a category (Rosch, 1975).

Gradedness is critical for all kinds of perceptual and motor phenomena, which deal with continuous underlying values like position, angle, force, and color (wavelength). The brain tends to deal with these continua in much the same way as the continuum between a cup and a bowl. Different neurons represent different "prototypical" values along the continuum (in many cases, these are essentially arbitrarily placed points), and respond with graded signals reflecting how close the current exemplar is to their preferred value (see figure 1.5). This type of representation, also known as *coarse coding* or a *basis function* representation, can actually give a precise indication of a particular location along a continuum, by forming a *weighted estimate* based on the graded signal associated with each of the "prototypical" or basis values.

Another important aspect of gradedness has to do with the fact that each neuron in the brain receives inputs from many thousands of other neurons. Thus, each individual neuron is not critical to the functioning of any other — instead, neurons contribute as part of a graded overall signal that reflects the number of other neurons contributing (as well as the strength of their individual contributions). This fact gives rise to the phenomenon of *graceful degradation*, where function degrades "gracefully" with increasing amounts of damage to neural tissue. Simplistically, we can explain this by saying that removing more neurons reduces the strength of the signals, but does not eliminate performance entirely. In contrast, the CPU in a standard computer will tend to fail catastrophically when even one logic gate malfunctions.

A less obvious but equally important aspect of gradedness has to do with the way that processing happens in the brain. Phenomenologically, all of us are probably familiar with the process of trying to remember something that does not come to mind immediately — there is this fuzzy sloshing around and trying out of different ideas until you either hit upon the right thing or give up in frustration. Psychologists speak of this in terms of the "tip-of-the-tongue" phenomenon, as in, "its just at the tip of my tongue, but I can't quite spit it out!" Gradedness is critical here because it allows your brain to float a bunch of relatively weak ideas around and see which ones get stronger (i.e., *resonate* with each other and other things), and which ones get weaker and fade away. Intuition has a similar flavor — a bunch of relatively weak factors add up to support one idea over another, but there is no single clear, discrete reason behind it.

Computationally, these phenomena are all examples of **bootstrapping** and **multiple constraint satisfaction**. Bootstrapping is the ability of a system to "pull itself up by its bootstraps" by taking some weak, incomplete information and eventually producing a solid result. Multiple constraint satisfaction refers to the ability of parallel, graded systems to find good solutions to problems that involve a number of constraints. The basic idea is that each factor or constraint pushes on the solution in rough proportion to its (graded) strength or importance. The resulting solution thus represents some kind of compromise that capitalizes on the convergence of constraints that all push in roughly the same direction, while minimizing the number of constraints that remain unsatisfied. If this sounds too vague and fuzzy to you, don't worry — we will write equations that express how it all works, and run simulations showing it in action.

1.6.3 Interactivity

Another way in which the brain differs from a standard serial computer is that processing doesn't just go in only one direction at a time. Thus, not only are lots of things happening at the same time (parallelism), but they are also going both forward and backward too. This is known as *interactivity*, or *recurrence*, or *bidirectional connectivity*. Think of the brain as having hierarchically organized processing areas, so that visual stimuli, for example, are first processed in a very simple, low-level way (e.g., in terms of the little oriented lines present in the image), and then in subsequent stages more sophisticated features are represented (combinations of lines, parts, objects, configurations of objects, etc.). This is at least approximately correct. In such a system, interactivity amounts to simultaneous *bottom-up* and *top-down* processing, where information flows from the simple to the more complex, and also from the more complex down to the simple. When combined with parallelism and gradedness, interactivity leads to a satisfying solution to a number of otherwise perplexing phenomena.

For example, it was well documented by the 1970s that people are faster and more accurate at identifying letters in the context of words than in the context of random letters (the *word superiority effect*). This finding was perplexing from the unidirectional serial computer perspective: Letters must be identified before words can be read, so how could the context of a word help in the identification of a letter? However, the finding seems natural within an interactive processing perspective: Information from the higher word level can come back down and affect processing at the lower letter level. Gradedness is critical here too, because it allows weak, first-guess estimates at the letter level to go up and activate a first-guess at the word level, which then comes back down and resonates with the first-guess letter estimates to home in on the overall representation of the word and its letters. This explanation of the word superiority effect was proposed by McClelland and Rumelhart (1981). Thus, interactivity is important for the bootstrapping and multiple constraint satisfaction processes described earlier, because it allows constraints from all levels of processing to be used to bootstrap and converge on a good overall solution.

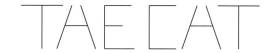

Figure 1.6: Ambiguous letters can be disambiguated in the context of words (Selfridge, 1955), demonstrating interactivity between word-level processing and letter-level processing.

There are numerous other examples of interactivity in the psychological literature, many of which involve stimuli that are ambiguous in isolation, but not in context. A classic example is shown in figure 1.6, where the words constrain an ambiguous stimulus to look more like an H in one case and an A in the other.

1.6.4 Competition

The saying, "A little healthy competition can be a good thing," is as true for the brain as it is for other domains like economics and evolution. In the brain, competition between neurons leads to the *selection* of certain representations to become more strongly active, while others are weakened or suppressed (e.g., in the context of bootstrapping as described above). In analogy with the evolutionary process, the "survival of the fittest" idea is an important force in shaping both learning and processing to encourage neurons to be better adapted to particular situations, tasks, environments, and so on. Although some have argued that this kind of competition provides a sufficient basis for learning in the brain (Edelman, 1987), we find that it is just one of a number of important mechanisms. Biologically, there are extensive circuits of *inhibitory interneurons* that provide the mechanism for competition in the areas of the brain most central to cognition.

Cognitively, competition is evident in the phenomenon of *attention*, which has been most closely associated with perceptual processing, but is clearly evident in all aspects of cognition. The phenomenon of *covert* spatial attention, as demonstrated by the Posner task (Posner, 1980) is a good example. Here, one's attention is drawn to a particular region of visual space by a *cue* (e.g., a little blinking bar on a computer screen), and then another stimulus (the *target*) is presented shortly thereafter. The target appears either near the cue or in the opposite region of space, and the subject must respond (e.g., by pressing a key on the computer) whenever they detect the onset of the target stimulus. The target is detected significantly faster in the cued location, and significantly slower in the noncued location, relative to a baseline of target detection without any cues at all. Thus, the processing of the cue competes with target detection when they are in different locations, and facilitates it when they are in the same location. All of this happens faster than one can move one's eyes, so there must be some kind of internal ("covert") attention being deployed as a result of processing the cue stimulus. We will see in section 8.5 that these results, and several other related ones, can be accounted for by a simple model that has competition between neurons (as mediated by the inhibitory interneurons).

1.6.5 Learning

The well-worn nature versus nurture debate on the development of human intelligence is inevitably decided in terms of both. Thus, both the genetic configuration of the brain and the results of learning make important contributions. However, this fact does nothing to advance our understanding of exactly *how* genetic configuration and learning interact to produce adult human cognition. Attaining this understanding is a major goal of computational cognitive neuroscience, which is in the unique position of being able to simulate the kinds of complex and subtle interdependencies that can exist between certain properties of the brain and the learning process.

In addition to the developmental learning process, learning occurs constantly in adult cognition. Thus, if it were possible to identify a relatively simple learning mechanism that could, with an appropriately instantiated initial architecture, organize the billions of neurons in the human brain to produce the whole range of cognitive functions we exhibit, this would obviously be the "holy grail" of cognitive neuroscience. For this reason, this text is dominated by a concern for the properties of such a learning mechanism, the biological and cognitive environment in which it operates, and the results it might produce. Of course, this focus does not diminish

the importance of the genetic basis of cognition. Indeed, we feel that it is perhaps only in the context of such a learning mechanism that genetic parameters can be fully understood, much as the role of DNA itself in shaping the phenotype must be understood in the context of the emergent developmental process.

A consideration of what it takes to learn reveals an important dependence on gradedness and other aspects of the biological mechanisms discussed above. The problem of learning can be considered as the problem of *change*. When you learn, you change the way that information is processed by the system. Thus, it is much easier to learn if the system responds to these changes in a graded, proportional manner, instead of radically altering the way it behaves. These graded changes allow the system to try out various new ideas (ways of processing things), and get some kind of graded, proportional indication of how these changes affect processing. By exploring lots of little changes, the system can evaluate and strengthen those that improve performance, while abandoning those that do not. Thus, learning is very much like the *bootstrapping* phenomenon described with respect to processing earlier: both depend on using a number of weak, graded signals as "feelers" for exploring possibly useful directions to proceed further, and then building on those that look promising.

None of this kind of bootstrapping is possible in a discrete system like a standard serial computer, which often responds catastrophically to even small changes. Another way of putting this is that a computer program typically only works if everything is right — a program that is missing just one step typically provides little indication of how well it would perform if it were complete. The same thing is true of a system of logical relationships, which typically unravels into nonsense if even just one logical assertion is incorrect. Thus, discrete systems are typically too *brittle* to provide an effective substrate for learning.

However, although we present a view of learning that is dominated by this bootstrapping of small changes idea, other kinds of learning are more discrete in nature. One of these is a "trial and error" kind of learning that is more familiar to our conscious experience. Here, there is a discrete "hypothesis" that governs behavior during a "trial," the outcome of which ("error") is used to update the hypothesis next time around. Although this has a more discrete flavor, we find that it can best be implemented using the same kinds of graded neural mechanisms as the other kinds of learning (more on this in chapter 11). Another more discrete kind of learning is associated with the "memorization" of particular discrete facts or events. It appears that the brain has a specialized area that is particularly good at this kind of learning (called the *hippocampus*), which has properties that give its learning a more discrete character. We will discuss this type of learning further in chapter 9.

1.7 Organization of the Book

This book is based on a relatively small and coherent set of mechanistic principles, which are introduced in part I of the text, and then applied in part II to understanding a range of different cognitive phenomena. These principles are implemented in the Leabra algorithm for the exploration simulations. These explorations are woven throughout the chapters where the issues they address are discussed, and form an integral part of the text. To allow readers to get as much as possible out of the book without doing the simulations, we have included many figures and have carefully separated the procedural aspects from the content using special typesetting.

Because this book emphasizes the linkages and interactions between biology, computational principles, and a wide variety of human cognitive phenomena, we cannot provide exhaustive detail on all potentially relevant aspects of neuroscience, computation, or cognition. We do attempt to provide references for deeper exploration, however. Relatedly, all of the existing supporting arguments and details are not presented for each idea in this book, because in many cases the student would likely find this tedious and relatively uninformative. Thus, we expect that expert neuroscientists, computational/mathematical researchers, and cognitive psychologists may find this book insufficiently detailed in their area of expertise. Nevertheless, we provide a framework that spans these areas and is consistent with well-established facts in each domain.

Thus, the book should provide a useful means for experts in these various domains to bridge their knowledge into the other domains. Areas of current debate in which we are forced to make a choice are presented as such, and relevant arguments and data are presented. We strive above all to paint a coherent and clear picture at a pace that moves along rapidly enough to maintain the interest (and fit within the working memory span) of the reader. As the frames of a movie must follow in rapid enough succession to enable the viewer to perceive motion, the ideas in this book must proceed cleanly and rapidly from neurobiology to cognition for the coherence of the overall picture to emerge, instead of leaving the reader swimming in a sea of unrelated facts.

Among the many tradeoffs we must make in accomplishing our goals, one is that we cannot cover much of the large space of existing neural network algorithms. Fortunately, numerous other texts cover a range of computational algorithms, and we provide references for the interested reader to pursue. Many such algorithms are variants on ideas covered here, but others represent distinct frameworks that may potentially provide important principles for cognition and/or neurobiology. As we said before, it would be a mistake to conclude that the principles we focus on are in any way considered final and immutable — they are inevitably just a rough draft that covers the domain to some level of satisfaction at the present time.

As the historical context (section 1.3) and overview of our approach (section 1.4) sections made clear, the Leabra algorithm used in this book incorporates many of the important ideas that have shaped the history of neural network algorithm development. Throughout the book, these principles are introduced in as simple and clear a manner as possible, making explicit the historical development of the ideas. When we implement and explore these ideas through simulations, the Leabra implementation is used for coherence and consistency. Thus, readers acquire a knowledge of many of the standard algorithms from a unified and integrated perspective, which helps to understand their relationship to one another. Meanwhile, readers avoid the difficulties of learning to work with the various implementations of all these different algorithms, in favor of investing effort into fully understanding one integrated algorithm at a practical hands-on level. Only algebra and simple calculus concepts, which are reviewed where necessary, are required to understand the algorithm, so it should be accessible to a wide audience.

As appropriate for our focus on cognition (we consider perception to be a form of cognition), we emphasize processing that takes place in the human or mammalian **neocortex**, which is typically referred to simply as the **cortex**. This large, thin, wrinkled sheet of neurons comprising the outermost part of the brain plays a disproportionally important role in cognition. It also has the interesting property of being relatively homogeneous from area to area, with the same basic types of neurons present in the same basic types of connectivity patterns. This is principally what allows us to use a single type of algorithm to explain such a wide range of cognitive phenomena.

Interactive, graphical computer simulations are used throughout to illustrate the relevant principles and how they interact to produce important features of human cognition. Detailed, step-by-step instructions for exploring these simulations are provided, together with a set of exercises for the student that can be used for evaluation purposes (an answer key is available from the publisher). Even if you are not required to provide a written answer to these questions, it is a good idea to look them over and consider what your answer might be, because they do raise important issues. Also, the reader is strongly encouraged to go beyond the step-by-step instructions to explore further aspects of the model's behavior.

In terms of the detailed organization, part I covers *Basic Neural Computational Mechanisms* across five chapters (*Individual Neurons*, *Networks of Neurons*, and three chapters on *Learning Mechanisms*), and part II covers *Large-Scale Brain Area Organization and Cognitive Phenomena* across five chapters (*Perception and Attention, Memory, Language,* and *Higher-Level Cognition*, with an introductory chapter on *Large-Scale Brain Area Functional Organization*). Each chapter begins with a detailed table of contents and an introductory overview of its contents, to let the reader know the scope of the material covered. When key words are defined or first used extensively, they are highlighted in **bold** font for easy searching, and can always be found in the index. `Simulation terms` are in the font as shown.

↪ Procedural steps to be taken in the explorations are formatted like this, so it is easy to see exactly what you have to do, and allows readers who are not running the model to skip over them.

Summaries of the chapters appear at the end of each one (this chapter excluded), which encapsulate and interrelate the contents of what was just read. After that, a list of references for further reading is provided. We hope you enjoy your explorations!

1.8 Further Reading

The original PDP (parallel-distributed processing) volumes, though somewhat dated, remain remarkably relevant: Rumelhart, McClelland, and PDP Research Group (1986c), McClelland, Rumelhart, and PDP Research Group (1986).

An excellent collection of the important early papers in neural networks can be found in Anderson and Rosenfeld (1988).

For other views on the basic premises of cognitive neuroscience and levels of analysis, we suggest: Marr (1982), chapter 1; Sejnowski and Churchland (1989); Shallice (1988), chapter 2; Posner, Inhoff, Friedrich, and Cohen (1987); Farah (1994); Kosslyn (1994).

For a developmentally-focused treatment of computational neural network modeling, see: Elman et al. (1996) and Plunkett and Elman (1997).

For other treatments of computational modeling using artificial neural networks, see: Hertz, Krogh, and Palmer (1991), Ballard (1997), Anderson (1995), McCleod, Plunkett, and Rolls (1998), and Bishop (1995).

For an encyclopedic collection of computational neural network models and more general brain-level theories, see Arbib (1995).

Part I

Basic Neural Computational Mechanisms

Chapter 2

Individual Neurons

Contents

2.1 Overview **23**

2.2 Detectors: How to Think About a Neuron **24**

   2.2.1 Understanding the Parts of the Neuron Using the Detector Model *26*

2.3 The Biology of the Neuron **27**

   2.3.1 The Axon *29*

   2.3.2 The Synapse *29*

   2.3.3 The Dendrite *31*

2.4 The Electrophysiology of the Neuron **32**

   2.4.1 Basic Electricity *32*

   2.4.2 Diffusion *33*

   2.4.3 Electric Potential versus Diffusion: The Equilibrium Potential *34*

   2.4.4 The Neural Environs and Ions *35*

   2.4.5 Putting It All Together: Integration *37*

   2.4.6 The Equilibrium Membrane Potential *38*

   2.4.7 Summary *40*

2.5 Computational Implementation of the Neural Activation Function **40**

   2.5.1 Computing Input Conductances *42*

   2.5.2 Point Neuron Parameter Values *45*

   2.5.3 The Discrete Spiking Output Function . . . *45*

   2.5.4 The Rate Code Output Function *46*

   2.5.5 Summary *48*

2.6 Explorations of the Individual Neuron **48**

   2.6.1 The Membrane Potential *49*

   2.6.2 The Activation Output *53*

   2.6.3 The Neuron as Detector *54*

2.7 Hypothesis Testing Analysis of a Neural Detector **58**

   2.7.1 Objective Probabilities and Example *59*

   2.7.2 Subjective Probabilities *62*

   2.7.3 Similarity of V_m and $P(h|d)$ *65*

2.8 The Importance of Keeping It Simple **65**

2.9 Self-Regulation: Accommodation and Hysteresis **66**

   2.9.1 Implementation of Accommodation and Hysteresis *67*

2.10 Summary **69**

2.11 Further Reading **70**

2.1 Overview

The **neuron** (or a **unit** in more abstract computational models) provides the basic information-processing mechanisms that are the foundation for all of human cognition. Biological neurons are tiny but very complex electrochemical systems. To use simulated neurons in models of cognitive phenomena, we need to simplify the neuron greatly while extracting its basic functional characteristics. Thus, perhaps even more so than in other chapters, this chapter places great demands on the delicate balancing act between the different levels of analysis that we talked about in the introduction. We can think about the essential function of a neuron from a computational perspective in terms of a **detector** (e.g., like a smoke detector): A neuron integrates information from many different sources (**inputs**) into a single real-valued number that reflects how well this information matches what the neuron has become specialized to detect, and then sends an **output** that reflects the results of this evaluation. This is the well-known **integrate-and-fire** model of neural function. The output then provides the input to other neurons, continuing the information-processing cascade through a network of interconnected neurons.

This chapter provides an overview of the computational-level description of a neuron (as a detector), and the biological mechanisms that underlie this neural information processing. We focus on the canonical **pyramidal** neuron in the **cortex**, which is consistent with the general focus throughout this book on the cortex. The sum of these biological mechanisms is known as the **activation function**, as the resulting output of a neuron is called its **activation** value. There is actually quite a bit known about the neural activation function, and the Leabra algorithm strikes a balance between using biologically based mechanisms on the one hand, and keeping the computational implementation relatively simple and tractable on the other. Thus, we use a **point neuron** activation function, which uses the same basic dynamics of information processing as real biological neurons, while shrinking the spatial extent (geometry) of the neuron to a single point, which vastly simplifies the computational implementation. Simulations in this chapter illustrate the basic properties of the activation function, and how it arises from the underlying biological properties of neurons. Further, we show how this activation function can be understood in terms of a mathematical analysis based on Bayesian hypothesis testing.

2.2 Detectors: How to Think About a Neuron

In a standard serial computer, the basic information processing operations are simple arithmetic and memory manipulations (e.g., storage and retrieval). Although it is conceivable that the brain could have been based on the same kinds of operations, this does not appear to be the case. Thus, to understand what functions the biological mechanisms of the neuron are serving, we need to come up with a *computational level* description of what the neuron is doing. That is the purpose of this section, which uses the standard computer as a point of contrast.

In a standard computer, memory and processing are separated into distinct modules, and processing is centralized in the **central processing unit** or **CPU**. Thus,

information must be retrieved from the memory module, sent to the CPU, processed, and then stored back into memory. In contrast, the brain appears to employ **parallel distributed processing** (**PDP**), where processing occurs simultaneously (in parallel) across billions of neurons distributed throughout the brain. Memory, like processing, is similarly distributed throughout the brain. Thus, our computational level description of neural processing must explain how each neuron provides memory and processing functions in a distributed way, while still producing something useful when all the neurons work together.

The central idea we use to explain what the neuron is doing is that of a **detector**. As a simplification, we can think of a neuron as detecting the existence of some set of conditions, and responding with a signal that communicates the extent to which those conditions have been met. Think of a smoke detector, which is constantly sampling the air looking for conditions that indicate the presence of a fire. In the brain, there are neurons in the early stages of the visual system that are constantly sampling the visual input looking for conditions that indicate the presence of very simple visual features such as bars of light at a given position and orientation in the visual scene. Higher up in the visual system, there are neurons that detect different sets of objects.

We must emphasize that although it is useful to view the *function* of a neuron as a detector, the *content* of exactly what it is detecting is not well captured by the relatively simplistic notions evoked by things like smoke detectors. In contrast with most synthetic detectors, a neuron is considerably more complex, having many thousands of different inputs, and living in a huge and dynamic network of other neurons. Thus, although it is sometimes possible to describe roughly what a neuron is detecting, this need not necessarily be the case — as we will see later, neurons can contribute usefully to the overall computation if a number of them are detecting different hard-to-label subsets or combinations.

A neuron's response is also often **context sensitive**, in that it depends on other things that you might not have otherwise anticipated. For example, one of the oriented bar detectors in the early visual system may not respond in some visual scenes that have a bar of light appropriately oriented and positioned for that detector, as a result of the other aspects of the scene (i.e., the "context" that surrounds this one bar of light). Further, this detector may respond one time a scene is viewed and not the next, as a result of dynamic changes in the network that determine one's focus of attention.

One way to think about this context sensitivity is that it can make a neuron act more like a *dynamic* detector that plays multiple roles in different situations, instead of the more *static* model conveyed by the smoke detector analogy. Further, although detection is more obviously appropriate for sensory processing, it can also be used to describe processing in the motor or output pathways of the brain, or purely internal processing. Thus, a neuron can detect when a given motor response should be executed, and its output then leads to the execution of that response. More abstract, internal actions (e.g., engaging an attentional system, or thinking of an appropriate word to describe something) can also be thought of in terms of detecting the appropriate conditions for doing these things. A virtue of the detector model is that it can easily accommodate all of this complexity and subtlety within a basic framework that can nevertheless be understood initially in very simple and intuitive terms by analogy with simple devices like smoke detectors.

The detector model of a neuron emphasizes several important properties. First, it emphasizes that neurons are **dedicated**, **specialized** processors (like smoke detectors), not the general purpose memory cells of a standard computer, which can be filled with any arbitrary piece of information. By virtue of the way each neuron is connected up with other neurons within the network, it becomes dedicated to detecting some specific set of things (no matter how dynamic or difficult it may be to describe exactly what this set of things is).

It is this dedication that enables a neuron to simultaneously perform memory and processing functions: its memory amounts to remembering the conditions that it applies to its inputs to detect whatever it detects, and its processing is the way that it goes about evaluating those conditions and communicating its results to other neurons. Thus, neurons are much more like the workers on a traditional assembly line who specialize in doing one little step of the manufacturing process, whereas conventional computers are much more like craftspeople who skillfully build and assemble all the different

parts themselves. This analogy helps to explain how something useful can emerge from the actions of a large number of individual neurons. It also captures the efficiency gains that can be achieved by parallel processing as compared to serial processing.

The specialized nature of neural detectors is also important in enabling us to refer to the **representation** of a given neuron. This term has a somewhat controversial history, but it is widely used in a way that is roughly consistent with the idea that the a neuron's representation is simply that which it detects. Thus, the neuron that detects an oriented bar at a given position is said to *represent* an oriented bar at a given position. Because neurons tend to be dedicated and specialized, one can think of the representation as a somewhat permanent property of each neuron. Nevertheless, a neuron must become active to affect directly the activation of other neurons, so it is useful to distinguish between the sense of representation denoting the relatively permanent specializations of the neurons (i.e., the *latent* or *weight-based* representations), and the active representation produced by those neurons that are presently active. We will talk more about these issues later in this chapter, in the next chapter, and in chapter 9.

Finally, it is important to note that although the view of the brain as a standard serial computer is inconsistent with the biological facts that give rise to the detector model, the **production system** model of cognition is potentially quite consistent, at least in general spirit. Here, cognition is simulated by the chaining together of *productions,* each of which can be seen as detectors (albeit often very sophisticated ones). These productions *fire* (are activated) when they *detect* an appropriate configuration of information active in the system, and the result of their firing is then to alter the activation state in some appropriate way. For example, the production for adding two numbers will detect the presence of two digits' being active (and the intention to add them), and when it fires it will replace these digits with their sum. Then, this altered state provides the appropriate configuration for activating another production, and so on. We will revisit this issue in chapter 11, where we will see how neurons can implement productionlike operations (though they do so within the constraints of dedicated, specialized representations).

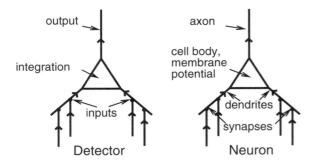

Figure 2.1: The detector model can be used to understand the function of corresponding neural components.

2.2.1   Understanding the Parts of the Neuron Using the Detector Model

The neuron, though tiny, is a highly complex biochemical and electrical structure. Any attempt to incorporate all of its complexity into a cognitive-level simulation would be impossible using current computational technology. Thus, simplifications are necessary on purely practical grounds. Furthermore, these simplifications can help us figure out which aspects of the neuron's complex biology are most cognitively relevant — these simplifications constitute an important part of the scientific endeavor (witness the popularity of the fictional frictionless plane in physics). One of the most commonly used simplifications of the neuron is the **integrate-and-fire** model (Abbott, 1999). As shown in figure 2.1 and elaborated below, the detector model maps quite nicely onto the integrate-and-fire model of the neuron.

First, a detector needs **inputs** that provide the information on which it bases its detection. A neuron receives its inputs via **synapses** that typically occur on its **dendrites**, which are branching fingers that can extend for somewhat large distances from the cell body of the neuron. In the human brain, only a relatively few neurons are directly connected with sensory inputs, with the rest getting their inputs from earlier stages of processing. The chaining of multiple levels of detectors can lead to more powerful and efficient detection capabilities than if everything had to work directly off of the raw sensory inputs. However, this also makes the neurosci-

entist's job that much more difficult, because it quickly becomes hard to figure out what kinds of input information a given neuron is basing its detection decision on when it is so indirectly related to the sensory inputs.

Regardless of where it gets them, the detector then performs processing on its inputs. In a smoke detector, this might involve combining and weighing the inputs from different types of smoke receptors to provide the best overall assessment of the likelihood of a fire. In the detector model of the neuron, the relative contribution of the different inputs to the overall detection decision is controlled by **weights**, which correspond in the neuron to the relative efficiency with which a synapse communicates inputs to the neuron (also known as **synaptic efficacies** or **synaptic strengths**). Thus, some inputs "weigh" more heavily into the detection decision than do others. These weights provide the critical parameters for specifying what the neuron detects — essentially, neurons can detect **patterns of activity** over their inputs, with those input patterns that best fit the pattern of weights producing the largest detection response.

It does not appear that much neural effort is spent analyzing individual inputs as such, treating them instead as just a part of the overall input pattern. This is done by combining or **integrating** over all the weighted inputs to form some sort of aggregate measure of the degree to which the input pattern fits the expected one. This happens through the electronic properties of the dendrites, resulting eventually in a **membrane potential** (electrical voltage) at the **cell body** (the central part of the neuron), which reflects the results of this combination. Thus, as we will see below, the neuron can be thought of as a little electronic system.

After integrating its inputs, a detector needs to communicate the results of its processing in the form of an **output** that informs anyone or anything that is listening if it has detected what it is looking for. In a smoke detector, this is the alarm siren or buzzer. Instead of directly communicating the value of the integrated inputs, many detectors have a **threshold** or **criterion** that is applied first. In a smoke detector, the threshold is there so that you are not constantly bombarded with the information that there is not sufficient smoke to be concerned about. You only want to hear from a smoke detector when there really is a likely cause for alarm —

in other words, when it has detected enough smoke to send it over the threshold for genuine concern.

The neuron also has a thresholding mechanism that keeps it quiet until it has detected something with sufficient strength or confidence to be worth communicating to other neurons. At a biological level, it takes metabolic resources for a neuron to communicate with other neurons, so it makes sense that this is reserved for important events. When the integrated input (as reflected in the membrane potential) goes over threshold, the neuron is said to *fire,* completing the integrate-and-fire model. The neural threshold is applied right at the start of a long and branching finger or process extending from the cell body called the **axon**. This axon then forms synapses on other neuron's dendrites, providing them with the inputs described earlier and repeating the great chain of neural processing.

Because of the good fit between the detector model and the integrate-and-fire view of neural function, we can use this detector model as a computational-level description of what a neuron is doing. However, for the detector model of the neuron to be of real use, it must be consistent with some larger understanding of how networks of such detectors can perform useful computations and exhibit humanlike cognition. The details of this larger picture will be spelled out in subsequent chapters.

To foreshadow one of the main ideas, we will see that *learning* can provide a means of getting a network of neural detectors to do something useful. Learning in neurons involves modifying the weights (synaptic efficacies) that provide the main parameters specifying what a neuron detects. Thus, by shaping the weights, learning shapes what neurons detect. There are powerful ways of making sure that each neuron learns to detect something that will end up being useful for the larger task performed by the entire network. The overall result is that the network after learning contains a number of detectors that are chained together in such a way as to produce appropriate outputs given a set of inputs (and to do so, it is hoped, using internal detectors that are related in some way to those used by humans in the way they perform a task).

2.3 The Biology of the Neuron

Having described the overall function of a neuron and the functions of its basic parts in terms of the detector model, we will now see how these functions are implemented in the underlying biological machinery of the neuron. In this section, we will provide a general overview of the biology of the neuron. In the next section, we will go into more detail on the **electrophysiology** of the neuron — how the electrical and physiological properties of the neuron serve to integrate inputs, and trigger the thresholded communication of outputs to other neurons.

Figure 2.2 shows a picture of a biological neuron, with the parts labeled as described in the previous section. Perhaps the most important biological fact about a neuron is that it is a single **cell**. Thus, it has a **cell body** with a **nucleus**, and is filled with fluid and cellular organelles and surrounded by a **cell membrane**, just like any other cell in the body. However, the neuron is unique in having very extended fingerlike processes of dendrites and axons. As noted previously, most of the input coming into a neuron enters in the dendrites, and the axon, which originates at the cell body, sends the output signal to other neurons.

To enable different neurons to communicate with each other despite being encased in membranes, there are little openings in the membrane called **channels** (imagine a cat door). The basic mechanisms of information processing (i.e., for integrating inputs, thresholding, and communicating outputs) in a neuron are based on the movement of charged atoms (**ions**) in and out of these channels, and within the neuron itself. As we will see in greater detail in the next section, we can understand how and why these ions move according to basic principles of electricity and **diffusion** (diffusion is the natural tendency of particles to spread out in a liquid or a gas, as is evident when you pour cream into coffee, for example). By applying these principles and their associated equations, we can develop a mathematical picture of how a neuron responds to inputs from other neurons.

A key element in the electrical model of the neuron is the difference in electrical charge (voltage) of the neuron relative to its external environment. This electrical

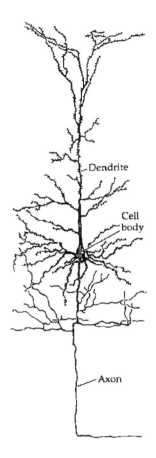

Figure 2.2: Image of a cortical pyramidal neuron, showing the major structures. Reproduced from Sejnowski and Churchland (1989).

difference is known as the *membrane potential* (as we mentioned previously), because it is the cell membrane that separates the inside and outside of the neuron, and thus it is across this membrane that the difference in electrical charge exists. As ions flow into and out of the neuron through channels, this changes the membrane potential. These changes in potential in one part of the neuron will propagate to other parts of the neuron, and integrate with the potentials there. This propagation and integration can be understood by treating the dendrites like *cables*, and analyzing their **cable properties**.

Thus, when ions flow through channels in the dendrites, these signals are integrated as they propagate up to the cell body. At the point where the cell body transitions into the axon, the membrane potential determines whether the neuron will fire. The thresholded property of this firing process is due to the sensitivity of a set of special channels to the membrane potential — these channels open up only when the membrane potential is sufficiently elevated. Such channels are called **voltage-gated** channels, of which there are many different types.

Although neural information processing is based fundamentally on electricity and diffusion, many chemical processes are necessary to make everything work. Indeed, many types of neurons rely on chemicals to send their outputs to other neurons, instead of directly passing an electrical signal (but other types of neurons do send electrical signals directly). The cortical neurons that we are primarily interested in use this chemical signaling. These chemicals, called **neurotransmitters**, are released at the parts of the axon that are connected to the dendrites of other neurons (i.e., at the synapses). Their release is triggered by an electrical pulse coming down the axon (called the **action potential**), and after being released, they diffuse over to the dendrites, and chemically bind to **receptors** on the dendritic part of the synapse, resulting in the opening of channels.

Thus, inputs are transmitted in the cortex when the neurotransmitters open particular types of channels on the receiving neurons, which then allow specific types of ions to flow, which then triggers the electrical propagation and integration in the receiving neuron as described previously. The great chain of neural communication thus contains alternating links of electrical and chemical processes. At a longer time scale, the construction, maintenance, and adaptation of the neuron is based on a complex interaction between genetics, cellular chemistry, and electrical signals, which is beyond the scope of this book.

In the next sections, we cover the biology of the axon, dendrite, and the synaptic connection between them in somewhat more detail, and then we explore the electrical mechanisms after that. It is difficult to describe the chain of neural communication one link at a time, inasmuch as each piece is so intimately interconnected

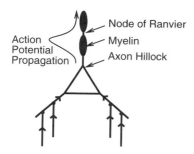

Figure 2.3: Illustration of the principal aspects of the axonal output system, including the axon hillock where the action potential (spike) is initiated, and the myelin separated by nodes of Ranvier that propagates the spike using a combination of passive and active properties.

with the others. That said, we will just jump in at the point where a *sending* neuron has gone over its threshold, and is *firing* an output signal to a *receiving* neuron. Thus, we will trace in more detail the chain of events as the signal moves down the axon of the sending neuron, through the synapse, and to the dendrite of the receiving neuron. We will also refer to the sending neuron as the **presynaptic** neuron (before the synapse), and the receiving neuron as the **postsynaptic** neuron (after the synapse).

2.3.1 The Axon

The action of neural firing is variously called **spiking**, or *firing a spike,* or triggering an *action potential.* As we have said, the spike is initiated at the very start of the axon, in a place called the **axon hillock** (figure 2.3). Here, there is a large concentration of two kinds of voltage-gated channels that only become activated when the membrane potential reaches a specific threshold value. Thus, it is the value of the membrane potential at this point where the threshold is applied, determining the spiking of the neuron.

When one type of voltage-gated channels at the hillock opens, they cause the neuron to become even more excited. This further excitation causes the other type of channels to open, and these channels act to inhibit the neuron. This results in a spike of excitation followed by inhibition. When the membrane potential is

brought back down by the inhibitory channels, it tends to *overshoot* the basic resting potential slightly. This causes a **refractory period** following a spike, where it is unable to fire another spike until the membrane potential climbs back up to the threshold level again. The refractory period can also be caused by the lingering inactivation of the voltage-gated channels that initiate the spike. This refractory period effectively results in a fixed maximum rate at which a neuron can fire spikes (more on this later).

This spike impulse is communicated down the length of the axon by the combination of two different mechanisms, *active* and *passive.* The active mechanism amounts to a chain-reaction involving the same kinds of voltage-gated channels distributed along the length of the axon. A spike triggered at the start of the axon will increase the membrane potential a little bit further down the axon, resulting in the same spiking process taking place there, and so on (think of the domino effect). However, this active mechanism requires a relatively large amount of energy, and is also relatively slow because it requires the opening and closing of channels. Thus, most neurons also have sections of the axon that propagate the spike using the passive mechanism. This mechanism is essentially the same as the one that takes place in the dendrites, based on the *cable properties* of electrical propagation. This passive propagation is much faster, because it is a purely electrical process.

Because the passive mechanism suffers from attenuation (weakening signal strength) over distances, the neuron has some *relay stations* along the way where the active spiking mechanism reamplifies the signal. These relay stations are called the **nodes of Ranvier**. To make the passive conduction in between these relay-station nodes more efficient, the axon is covered by an insulating sheath called **myelin**. With this combination of propagation mechanisms, the neuron can efficiently send signals over very long distances in the cortex (e.g., several centimeters) in a relatively short amount of time (on the order of a millisecond).

2.3.2 The Synapse

Now we move from the electrical pulse coursing down the axon as a result of spiking to the release of neuro-

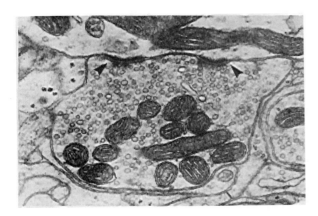

Figure 2.4: Electron-microscope image of a synapse. The arrows show the location of two synaptic release sites, with the terminal button extending below (the orientation is the same as in figure 2.5). The small circles are the synaptic vesicles containing neurotransmitter. The large dark structures in the terminal button are cellular organelles. Reproduced from Kandel et al. (1991).

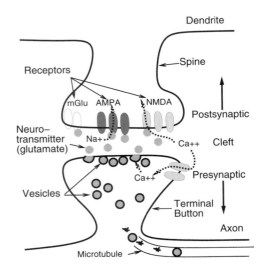

Figure 2.5: Diagram of the synapse. The action potential causes Ca^{++} ions to be mobilized in the button, causing vesicles to bind with the presynaptic membrane and release neurotransmitter (NT) into the cleft. NT (e.g., glutamate) then binds with the postsynaptic receptors, which are either associated with channels and thus allow ions to flow (e.g., Na^+ ions for AMPA channels or Ca^{++} ions for NMDA channels), or cause postsynaptic chemical processes to take place (e.g., the metabotropic glutamate receptor, mGlu). NT is produced in the soma and transported to the terminal via microtubules.

transmitter at the synapse. As we have said, the synapse is the junction between the sending neuron's axon and the receiving neuron's dendrite (figures 2.5 and 2.4). The end of the axon that enters into the synapse is called the **axon terminal** or **button** (pronounced "boo-tohn"). In some types of synapses, there is a special process called a **spine** on the dendrite where the synapse is formed. In other cases, the synapse is formed directly with the dendritic membrane.

When the electrical pulse reaches the terminal button, it mobilizes calcium ions (Ca^{++}) by opening voltage-sensitive channels that allow Ca^{++} ions to flow into the terminal, and also possibly by releasing internal stores of these ions. These calcium ions then promote the binding of little sacks or **vesicles** of neurotransmitter (*NT*) to the membrane of the terminal (this process is not yet fully understood at a detailed level). Upon binding with the membrane, the vesicles then release the NT into the **synaptic cleft** (the *very narrow* gap between the axon and dendrite).

After diffusing across the cleft, the released NT then binds to the postsynaptic receptors on the receiving neuron. This binding either causes a channel associated

with the receptor to open, allowing ions to flow (for **ionotropic** receptors), or results in the initiation of various chemical processes in the postsynaptic neuron (for **metabotropic** receptors that are not associated with channels). There are different types of NT chemicals that are released by different types of sending neurons, and these different chemicals bind to different receptors, causing different kinds of effects in the receiving neuron. We will discuss later some of the different types of NTs in the context of the different dendritic receptors.

To maintain the continued release of NT over many spikes, the vesicle material that gets bound to the membrane is later recycled to make new vesicles, and new NT and other important molecules are sent in from the cell body via **microtubules**. Once the NT is released into the cleft, it must also be broken down or taken back into the axon terminal for reuse (**reuptake**). Indeed, if NT is allowed to linger in the cleft (e.g., by inhibiting these reuptake mechanisms), then it will keep activating receptors, which can cause problems. There are many drugs that can affect various stages of this process, including blocking receptor activation, reuptake, and the postsynaptic chemical processes activated by receptors. These are important for studying the components of this complex biochemical system.

The synapse has a number of dynamic properties that affect the way it behaves as a function of prior activity. One commonly noted effect is *paired-pulse facilitation*, where the second of two spikes coming in reasonably rapid succession will be stronger, which can be caused by residual calcium ions in the terminal or residual binding of vesicles to the membrane as a result of the prior release episode. It is also likely that extended high rates of firing will deplete synaptic resources (e.g., NT, Ca^{++}), resulting in increased numbers of *release failures*, where NT fails to be released during a spike. This may contribute to the saturating nonlinearity of the neural output function, as discussed in a later section.

There are a couple of important features of the biology of the synapse that should be emphasized. First, there are a number of ways in which the different components of the synapse can affect the overall efficacy or strength of transmission of information from the sender to the receiver. As we have mentioned, the net effect of these biological components is summarized in the computational model by the *weight* between the two neurons. Furthermore, the modification of one or more of these weight factors can produce learning.

The main presynaptic components of the weight are the number of vesicles released with each action potential, the amount of NT within each vesicle (which is believed not to vary that much), and the efficacy of the reuptake mechanism. The main postsynaptic factors include the total number of channel receptors exposed to the neurotransmitter, the alignment and proximity of these receptors with the presynaptic release sites, and the efficacy of the individual channels in allowing ions to flow. Various researchers have also argued that the shape of the dendritic spine may have an important impact on the conductance of electrical signals from the synapse to the dendrite as a whole (Shep-

herd, 1990). Exactly which of these factors are modified during learning is a matter of considerable debate, but it appears that there may be multiple contributors, on both the pre- and postsynaptic side of things (Malenka & Nicoll, 1993).

2.3.3   *The Dendrite*

To continue the chain of communication, the dendritic end of the synapse houses the receptors and associated channels that allow ions to flow through the postsynaptic membrane. As the electrical effects of these ions propagate through the dendrites and up to the cell body, the process of communication can begin again in the axon of this receiving neuron. We discuss the electrical integration of inputs in detail in the next section, so the main things to point out here are the different types of dendritic receptors, and the NTs that activate them.

In the cortex, there are two primary types of NT/receptor combinations (along with many others that we will not discuss). One such type uses the NT **glutamate**, which in turn binds to the **AMPA**, **NMDA**, and **mGlu** receptors on the dendrite (as illustrated in figure 2.5). As we see in the next section, the AMPA receptor activated channel provides the primary **excitatory** input because it allows sodium (Na^+) ions to flow into the dendrite. These ions elevate (excite) the postsynaptic membrane potential and make the receiving neuron more likely to fire a spike. When excitatory channels are opened, the resulting change in the postsynaptic membrane potential is called an excitatory postsynaptic potential or **EPSP**.

The NMDA receptor activated channel is also excitatory, but it is probably more important for its effects on learning, because it allows calcium (Ca^{++}) ions to enter, which can then trigger chemical processes that lead to learning. The mGlu (metabotropic glutamate) receptor may also be important for learning by activating various chemical processes in the postsynaptic neuron when NT binds to it. We will discuss these learning effects in greater detail in chapters 4–6.

The other main type of NT/receptor combination uses the NT **GABA**, which in turn binds to and activates GABA receptors on the dendrite. These GABA receptors open channels that allow chlorine (Cl^-) ions to enter, which produces an **inhibitory** effect on the postsynaptic neuron, meaning that the receiving neuron becomes less likely to fire a spike. Individual inhibitory inputs from GABA receptors are called **IPSP**s: inhibitory postsynaptic potentials. There are two different subtypes of GABA receptors, GABA-A and GABA-B, which have different temporal dynamics (the B type stays open for a longer time period, thus having a more protracted inhibitory effect).

An important fact of biology is that, at least in the cortex, a given type of neuron releases only one type of neurotransmitter substance, which in turn activates only particular types of postsynaptic receptors. This means that cortical neurons either send excitatory inputs or inhibitory inputs to other neurons, but not both. We will see later that this has important implications for computational models. Note that this constraint of excitatory-only or inhibitory-only applies only to the type of output produced by a neuron — cortical neurons can (and do) receive both excitatory and inhibitory inputs. Indeed, we will emphasize the idea that one of the most important functions of neurons and networks of neurons is establishing an appropriate balance between excitatory and inhibitory inputs. In the next section, we will begin to see how this is accomplished by the electrical properties of neurons.

2.4 The Electrophysiology of the Neuron

The neuron can be understood using some basic principles of electricity. These mechanisms are all based on the movement of *ions* (charged atoms) into and out of the neuron, generating electric currents and electric potentials (voltages). In addition to these electrical concepts, we need to understand the behavior of concentrations (i.e., areas of relatively high or low density) of ions in a liquid, which is governed by the process of *diffusion* (e.g., the mixing of cream into coffee as mentioned previously). The basic ideas are introduced first, and then applied toward understanding how the neuron works. We will see that the neuron has different concentrations of ions inside and outside the cell, and this enables these electric and diffusion forces, working together and in opposition, to do something useful.

2.4.1 Basic Electricity

Electricity is all about the behavior and movement of **charge** carried by the basic constituents of matter, which (for our purposes) are electrons and protons. Electrons have **negative charge** and protons have **positive charge**, both of which are the same magnitude but opposite sign. Atoms are made of both electrons and protons, and most of them have equal numbers of electrons and protons, so that they have no *net* charge. However *ions* are atoms that have more electrons than protons, or vice versa, so that they carry a negative or positive net charge. Typically, there is only a difference of one or two, and this is indicated by writing the name of the ion with the corresponding number of plus or minus signs. The ions that are most relevant to neural functioning are sodium (Na^+), chloride (Cl^-), potassium (K^+), and calcium (Ca^{++}).

Charge obeys an *opposites attract* rule, so that negative charges like to be as close as possible to positive charges and vice versa. This means that if there is a larger concentration of positively charged ions somewhere, then any negative ions nearby will be drawn toward this positively charged area. When this happens you get electrical *current*, simply the movement of charge from one place to another. Conversely, same-sign charges repel each other, so positively charged ions concentrated in one area will move away from each other. Assuming that both positive and negative ions are mobile (e.g., like ions in a liquid, as is the case with neurons), the same type of current could be caused by positive ions leaving or negative ions arriving. This would be a *negative* current, while the opposite case of positive ions arriving or negative charges leaving a given area would be a *positive* current.

The extent of the disparity in amount of positive or negative charge in one place is called its electrical *potential* — it reflects the potential amount of opposite charge that can be attracted to that area. An excess of negative charges gives rise to a negative potential, while an excess of positive charges gives a positive potential. Note that as a given area starts attracting opposite charges, it starts losing its potential to attract more because these new opposite charges cancel out its net charge disparity! Thus, the potential of a given area

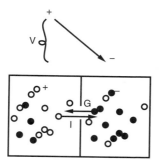

Figure 2.6: Sketch of Ohm's law in action, where an imbalance of charges leads to a potential V (with the difference in charge in the two chambers represented by the height of the line) that drives a current I through a channel with conductance G.

changes as a function of the current coming into that area. This will play an important role in how the neuron behaves when excited by incoming charges.

Usually, ions (like everything else) encounter **resistance** when they move, caused by being stuck in a viscous liquid, or by their path being blocked by a wall (membrane) with only small *channels* or *pores* they can pass through. The greater the resistance encountered by the ions when they move, the greater amount of potential required to get them there. Imagine an inclined plane with a ball on the top and a bunch of junk lying in its path. The more junk (resistance), the higher you have to tilt the plane (potential) to get the ball (ion) to go down the plane. This relationship is known as **Ohm's law** (figure 2.6):

$$I = \frac{V}{R} \qquad (2.1)$$

where I is the current (amount of motion), V is the electrical potential, and R is the resistance. This equation can be expressed in a slightly more convenient form in terms of the inverse of resistance, called **conductance** ($G = \frac{1}{R}$). Conductance G represents how easily ions can be *conducted* from one place to the other. Ohm's law written in these terms is just:

$$I = VG \qquad (2.2)$$

We will see that Ohm's law forms the basis for the equation describing how the neuron integrates informa-

tion! In brief, the opening and closing of membrane channels determines the conductances (G) for each type of ion as a function of the input it receives. The potential V is just the membrane potential that we discussed previously. We will see below that this potential can be updated by computing the current I using Ohm's law (equation 2.2) — this will tell us how many charges are moving into or out of the neuron, and thus how the membrane potential will change. By *iteratively* (repeatedly) applying Ohm's law, we can compute the changes in potential over time, resulting in a model of how the neuron computes. Owing to the combined forces of diffusion (explained below) and the electrical potential, each ion will respond to a given membrane potential in a different way. Thus, each ion makes a unique contribution to the overall current.

2.4.2 Diffusion

In addition to electrical potentials, the main other factor that causes ions to move into or out of the neuron is a somewhat mysterious "force" called **diffusion**. Recall that electrical potentials are caused by imbalanced concentrations of positive and negative ions in a given location. Diffusion also comes into play when there are imbalanced concentrations. Put simply, diffusion causes particles of a given type to be evenly distributed throughout space. Thus, any time there is a large concentration of some particle in one location, diffusion acts to spread out (*diffuse*) this concentration as evenly as possible.

Though diffusion may sound simple enough, the underlying causes of it are somewhat more complicated. Diffusion results from the fact that atoms in a liquid or gas are constantly moving around, and this results in a *mixing* process that tends (on average) to cause everything to be evenly mixed. Thus, diffusion is not a direct force like the electrical potential, but rather an indirect effect of stuff bouncing around and thus tending to get well mixed.

The key thing about diffusion is that *each* type of particle that can move independently gets evenly mixed, so having a large concentration of one type of ion in one place (e.g., Na^+) cannot be compensated for by having an equally large concentration of another ion with the

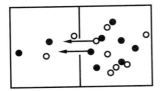

Figure 2.7: Sketch of diffusion in action, where both types of particles (ions) move in the same direction, each independent of the other, due to the accumulated effects of random motion.

same charge (e.g., K^+) somewhere else (figure 2.7). In contrast, electricity doesn't care about different types of ions (any positive charge is the same as any other) — it would be perfectly happy to attract all Na^+ ions and leave a large concentration of K^+ somewhere else.

Because it is just as reliable an effect as the electrical force, and it is convenient to write similar force-like equations for diffusion, we will treat diffusion as though it were a direct force even though technically it is not. Thus, we can use essentially the same terminology as we did with electricity to describe what happens to ions as a result of *concentration* differences (instead of charge differences).

Imagine that we have a box with two compartments of liquid separated by a removable barrier. With the door closed, we insert a large number of a particular type of ion (imagine blue food coloring in water) in one compartment. Thus, there is a concentration difference or *gradient* between the two compartments, which results in something like a *concentration potential* that will cause these ions to move into the other compartment. Thus, when the barrier is removed, a *diffusion current* is generated as these ions move to the other side, which, as is the case with electricity, reduces the concentration potential and eventually everything is well mixed. The *diffusion coefficient* acts much like the electrical conductance (inverse of resistance), and a relationship analogous to Ohm's law holds:

$$I = -DC \qquad (2.3)$$

This diffusion version of Ohm's law is called **Fick's first law**, where I is the movement of ions (diffusion current), D is the diffusion coefficient, and C is the concentration potential.

2.4.3 Electric Potential versus Diffusion: The Equilibrium Potential

To compute the current that a given ion will produce, we need some way of summarizing the results of both the electric and diffusion forces acting on the ion. This summarization can be accomplished by figuring out the special *equilibrium point* where the electric and diffusion forces balance each other out and the concentration of ions will stay exactly as it is (even though individual ions will be moving about randomly). At this point, there will be zero current with respect to this type of ion, because current is a function of the net motion of these ions. Of course, in a simple system with only electrical forces, the equilibrium point is where the electrical potential is actually zero. However, with different concentrations of ions inside and outside the neuron and the resulting diffusion forces, the equilibrium point is not typically at zero electrical potential.

Because the absolute levels of current involved are generally relatively small, we can safely assume that the relative concentrations of a given ion inside and outside the cell, which are typically quite different from each other, remain relatively constant over time. In addition, we will see that the neuron has a special mechanism for maintaining a relatively fixed set of relative concentrations. Thus, the equilibrium point can be expressed as the amount of electrical potential necessary to counteract an effectively constant diffusion force. This potential is called the **equilibrium potential**, or the **reversal potential** (because the current changes sign [*reverses*] on either side of this zero point), or the **driving potential** (because the flow of ions will *drive* the membrane potential toward this value).

The equilibrium potential (E) is particularly convenient because it can be used as a correction factor in Ohm's law, by simply subtracting it away from the actual potential V, resulting in the **net potential** ($V - E$):

$$I = G(V - E) \qquad (2.4)$$

We will call this the *diffusion corrected* version of Ohm's law, which can be applied on an ion-by-ion basis to get the current contributed by each type of ion, as we will see.

2.4.4 The Neural Environs and Ions

We can now put the basic principles of electricity and diffusion to work in understanding how the neuron integrates information. To do this, we must understand the nature of the internal and external environment of the neuron, specifically in terms of the types and concentrations of ions present. Neurons live in a liquid environment in the brain called the **extracellular space** that is very similar to seawater (which is interesting because life is thought to have originated in seawater). Thus, as in seawater, there is a certain amount of dissolved *salt* (NaCl), which results in a reasonable concentration of the ions Na^+ and Cl^-. The other major ions of relevance to the neuron are potassium (K^+) and calcium (Ca^{++}).

If these ions were simply allowed to flow at will across open membrane channels, the ion concentration on the inside of a neuron would end up being very similar to that of the extracellular space. However, there are two critical factors that create and preserve an imbalance in ion concentrations across the cell membrane. The first such factor is a mechanism called the **sodium-potassium pump** that actively works to create an imbalance in the concentrations of the sodium and potassium ions. It does this by pumping Na^+ ions out of the neuron and a smaller amount of K^+ ions into it. The second factor is the **selective permeability** of channels, where a given channel will only allow one or a few types of ions to pass. Furthermore, many of these channels are usually closed unless specifically activated (e.g., by neurotransmitter released by a sending neuron). Thus, the sodium-potassium pump creates an imbalance of ion concentrations, and the selective channels serve to both maintain this imbalance and dynamically alter it (and thus the membrane potential) by opening and closing as a function of inputs coming into the neuron.

The sodium-potassium pump uses energy, and can be thought of as charging up the battery that runs the neuron. As we will see in a moment, just by creating an imbalance in two types of ions, other imbalances are also created. Thus, in some sense, everything follows from this initial imbalance. Perhaps the most direct consequence of the relatively low internal concentration of Na^+ that is produced by the pump is the negative **rest-**

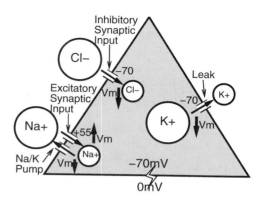

Figure 2.8: Summary of the three major activation ions and their channels.

ing potential of the neuron. The resting potential is the membrane potential that holds when no inputs are coming into the neuron, and because there are more positive Na^+ ions outside the cell than inside, the inside of the neuron will have a net negative charge. This negative charge is typically around -70 millivolts or $-70mV$, where $1mV$ is one thousandth of a volt — not much!

In the following listing, we will enumerate the internal and external concentrations of each of the four main ions, assess the electrical and diffusion forces acting on it, and discuss the channels that allow it to flow into or out of the neuron (also see figure 2.8).

Na^+ Because of the sodium-potassium pump, sodium exists in greater concentration outside the neuron than inside. Thus, the diffusion force pushes it into the neuron. To counteract this diffusion force with an electrical force, the neuron would have to have a positive charge inside relative to outside (thus repelling any other positive charges that might otherwise want to come in). Thus, the equilibrium potential of Na^+ is positive, with a typical value of around $+55mV$.

There are two primary types of channels that pass Na^+. The most important for our purposes is the excitatory synaptic input channel that is usually closed (preserving the imbalance), but is opened by the binding of the neurotransmitter **glutamate**, as discussed previously. There is also a voltage-gated Na^+ channel (i.e., its opening and closing is dependent on the level of the membrane potential) that plays a central role in triggering the action potential, as described previously. In general, Na^+ plays the central role in the *excitation* or *activation* of the neuron, because diffusion forces tend to push it into the neuron, resulting in the elevation of the membrane potential. Excitation is also referred to as **depolarization**, because it makes the membrane potential less polarized (i.e., closer to having a $0mV$ potential).

Cl^- Because of the negative resting potential created by the sodium-potassium pump, the negatively charged chloride ions are repelled out of the neuron, resulting in a concentration imbalance with more ions outside than inside. Thus, as with Na^+, the diffusion force pushes Cl^- into the neuron. However, this diffusion force is exactly counteracted by the negative resting potential, which creates the imbalance in the first place, so that the equilibrium potential for Cl^- is just the resting potential of the neuron, typically $-70mV$.

The main Cl^- channel is the inhibitory synaptic input channel that is opened by the neurotransmitter **GABA** as described previously. Note that because the equilibrium potential for Cl^- is the same as the resting potential, the inhibition delivered by these neurons does not have much of an effect (i.e., not much current is generated) until the neuron starts to get excited and its membrane potential rises. This phenomenon is often described as **shunting** inhibition.

K^+ The concentration of potassium is a function of both the direct and indirect effects of the sodium-potassium pump. The direct effect is that some amount of K^+ is actively pumped into the cell. In addition, the fact that the pump results in a negative resting potential will cause this positively charged ion to be drawn into the neuron as well. Thus, there is a much greater concentration of potassium inside than outside the cell. As a result, its diffusion force pushes it out of the neuron (unlike the previous two ions). This diffusion force is mostly countered by the negative resting potential, but because it is also actively pumped into the neuron, its internal concentration is even higher than would be expected from just

the negative resting potential, so that its equilibrium potential is typically around $-90mV$.

There are many different types of K^+ channels, but the most relevant for our purposes is the **leak** channel, which is constantly open and lets out small amounts of potassium. However, this channel also lets in small amounts of Na^+, so that the equilibrium potential for the conductance of this channel is not quite the same as that for the K^+ ion — it is instead the same as the resting potential, or roughly $-70mV$. There is also a voltage-gated K^+ channel that counteracts the effects of the excitation produced during the action potential by letting out larger amounts of K^+ when the neuron becomes very excited. A third type of K^+ channel opens as a function of the amount of calcium ion present in a neuron, which is indicative of extended periods of activity. Thus, this channel produces an *accommodation* or fatiguelike effect by inhibiting overactive neurons, as discussed further in the last section of this chapter. In general, K^+ plays a largely *regulatory* role in the neuron.

Ca^{++} The calcium ion is present in only minute concentrations inside the neuron due to another type of active pump that pumps Ca^{++} out, and other intracellular mechanisms that absorb or *buffer* calcium. Thus, the diffusion force on Ca^{++} is inward, requiring a positive internal potential to push it back out. This potential is somewhere on the order of $+100mV$, due to the relatively large concentration differences involved. Note also that by having two extra positive charges instead of one, a given electrical potential acts twice as strongly on this ion as on ions with only one net charge difference.

Perhaps the most important channel that conducts Ca^{++} is the NMDA channel, triggered by glutamate released by excitatory neurons as mentioned previously. This channel is critical for the learning mechanisms described in chapters 4–6. Also, the accommodation effect (and its opposite, the sensitization effect) depends on the presence of Ca^{++} ions in the neuron as a measure of neural activity. These ions enter the neuron through voltage-gated channels, so that their presence indicates recent neural activity, and they exist in such small amounts in the neuron that their concentration provides a reasonable indication of the average level of neural activity over the recent time period. This makes them useful for causing other things to happen in the neuron.

2.4.5 Putting It All Together: Integration

Having covered all the major ions and channels affecting neural processing, we are now in a position to put them all together into one equation that reflects the neural integration of information. The result of this will be an equation for updating the membrane potential, which is denoted by the variable V_m (V for voltage, and m for membrane). All we have to do is use Ohm's law to compute the current for each ion channel, and then add all these currents together. For each type of ion channel (generically denoted by the subscript c for now), we need to know three things: (1) its equilibrium potential as given above, E_c, (2) the fraction of the total number of channels for that ion that are open at the present time, $g_c(t)$), and (3) the maximum conductance that would result if all the channels were open (i.e., how many ions the channels let through), $\bar{g}_c$. The product of $g_c(t)$ and $\bar{g}_c$ then gives us the total conductance.

The current for the channel is then given by the diffusion corrected Ohm's law described above, which is just the total conductance (fraction open times maximum conductance) times the net potential (difference between the membrane potential at the present time ($V_m(t)$) and the equilibrium potential):

$$I_c = g_c(t)\bar{g}_c(V_m(t) - E_c) \qquad (2.5)$$

The three basic channels that do most of the activation work in the neuron are: (a) the excitatory synaptic input channel activated by glutamate and passing the Na$^+$ ion (subscript e), (b) the inhibitory synaptic input channel activated by GABA and passing the Cl$^-$ ion (subscript i), and (c) the leak channel that is always open and passing the K$^+$ ion (subscript l). The total or **net current** for these three channels is:

$$
\begin{aligned}
I_{net} = \ & g_e(t)\bar{g}_e(V_m(t) - E_e) + \\
& g_i(t)\bar{g}_i(V_m(t) - E_i) + \\
& g_l(t)\bar{g}_l(V_m(t) - E_l)
\end{aligned}
$$
$$(2.6)$$

As we said, this net current affects the membrane potential because the movement of charges decreases the net charge difference, which causes the potential in the first place. The following equation updates the membrane potential V_m (v_m in the simulator) in our model based on the previous membrane potential and net current:

$$
\begin{aligned}
V_m(t+1) & = V_m(t) - dt_{vm} I_{net} \\
& = V_m(t) - dt_{vm}[\\
& \quad g_e(t)\bar{g}_e(V_m(t) - E_e) + \\
& \quad g_i(t)\bar{g}_i(V_m(t) - E_i) + \\
& \quad g_l(t)\bar{g}_l(V_m(t) - E_l)] \qquad (2.7)
\end{aligned}
$$

The **time constant** $0 < dt_{vm} < 1$ (dt_vm in the simulator) slows the potential change, capturing the corresponding slowing of this change in a neuron (primarily as a result of the *capacitance* of the cell membrane, but the details of this are not particularly relevant here beyond the fact that they slow down changes).

In understanding the behavior of neurons, it is useful to think of increasing membrane potential as resulting from positive current (i.e., "excitation"). However, equation 2.7 shows that according to the laws of electricity, increasing membrane potential results from negative current. To match the more intuitively appealing relationship between potential and current, we simply change the sign of the current in our model ($I_{net-} = -I_{net}$) and add it to the previous membrane potential instead of subtracting it:

$$
\begin{aligned}
V_m(t+1) & = V_m(t) + dt_{vm} I_{net-} \\
& = V_m(t) + dt_{vm}[\\
& \quad g_e(t)\bar{g}_e(E_e - V_m(t)) + \\
& \quad g_i(t)\bar{g}_i(E_i - V_m(t)) + \\
& \quad g_l(t)\bar{g}_l(E_l - V_m(t))] \qquad (2.8)
\end{aligned}
$$

Equation 2.8 is of course mathematically equivalent to equation 2.7, but it captures the more intuitive relationship between potential and current. From now on, we will just use I_{net} (I_net in the simulator) to refer to I_{net-} to simplify our notation.

Equation 2.8 provides the means for integrating all the inputs into a neuron, which show up here as the different values of the conductances for the different ion

channels. For example, the amount of excitatory input
determines what fraction of the excitatory synaptic input channels are open ($g_e(t)$), and thus how much the
neuron's membrane potential is driven toward the excitatory reversal potential ($+55mV$). However, to accurately represent what happens in a real neuron, one
would need to apply equation 2.8 at every point along
the dendrites and cell body of the neuron, along with
additional equations that specify how the membrane potential spreads along neighboring points of the neuron.
The details of how to do this are beyond the scope of
this text — see Johnston and Wu (1995) for a detailed
treatment, and Bower and Beeman (1994) or Hines and
Carnevale (1997) for software that implements such detailed models.

To avoid the need to implement hundreds or thousands of equations to simulate a single neuron, we will
take advantage of a useful simplifying approximation
that enables us to directly use equation 2.8 to compute
the membrane potential of a simulated neuron. This approximation is based on the fact that a large part of what
happens to the electrical signals as they propagate from
the dendrites to the cell body is that they get *averaged*
together (though see section 2.5.1 for notable exceptions to this generalization). Thus, we can just use the
average fraction of open channels of the various types
across the entire dendrite as a very crude but efficient
approximation of the total conductance of a particular
type of channel, and plug these numbers directly into a
single equation (equation 2.8) that summarizes the behavior of the entire neuron.

This approximation is the essence of the *point neuron*
approximation mentioned previously, where we have
effectively shrunk the entire spatial extent of the neuron down to a single point, which can then be modeled
by a single equation. We see later that our computational model actually captures some important aspects
of the spatial structure of the dendrites in the way the
excitatory input conductance ($g_e(t)$) is computed.

To illustrate how a point neuron would behave in the
face of different amounts of excitatory input, we can
plot the results of repeatedly using equation 2.8 to update the membrane potential in response to fixed levels
of input as determined by specified values of the various
conductances. Figure 2.9 shows a graph of the net cur-

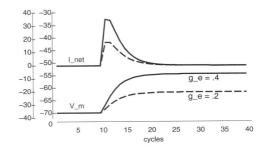

Figure 2.9: Two traces of the computed net current (I_{net})
and membrane potential (V_m) updated by excitatory inputs at
time 10, one of total conductance ($g_e(t)\bar{g}_e$, labeled as g_e) of
.4 and the other of .2.

rent and membrane potential (starting at 0 current with
the rest potential of $-70mV$) responding to two different inputs that come in the form of a $g_e(t)$ value of .4 or
.2 starting at time step 10 (with a $\bar{g}_e$ of 1). The $\bar{g}_l$ value
is a constant 2.8 (and $g_l(t)$ is always 1 because the leak
is always on), there is no inhibitory conductance, and
$dt_{vm} = .1$ (you will run this example yourself in section 2.6).

The important thing to note about this figure is that
the membrane potential becomes elevated in response
to an excitatory input, and that the level of elevation is
dependent on the strength (conductance) of the excitation compared to the leak conductance (and other conductances, if present). This membrane potential elevation then provides the basis for the neuron's subsequent
output (i.e., if it gets over the threshold, the neuron will
fire). Although the firing mechanism is not reflected in
the graph, the stronger of these inputs put our simulated
neuron just over its threshold for responding, which was
$-55mV$, while the weaker was clearly *sub-threshold*.

This figure also shows that the value of I_{net} represents the amount of change in the value of V_m. Thus,
I_{net} represents the **derivative** of V_m (i.e., I_{net} is large
when V_m is rising rapidly, and settles back toward 0 as
V_m settles into a steady or *equilibrium* value).

2.4.6 The Equilibrium Membrane Potential

The notion of an equilibrium membrane potential is an
important concept that we will explore in more detail

in this section. We will see later that this concept will be used in determining how long to present patterns to a network, and in the analysis presented in section 2.7 showing the relationship between the biology of a neuron and the mathematics of hypothesis testing.

Within a reasonably short period of time after excitatory and/or inhibitory channels are opened (and barring the effects of any voltage-gated channels that subsequently become activated), the membrane potential will always settle into a new stable value that reflects the new balance of forces acting on the neuron. At this new equilibrium membrane potential, the *net* current (I_{net}) will return to zero, even though the individual currents for particular channels will have non-zero values (they will all just add up to zero, thereby canceling each other out). Thus, a net current is present only when changes are taking place, not when the membrane potential is steady (as would be expected given that current is the mathematical derivative of the membrane potential).

It is useful to be able to compute a value of this equilibrium membrane potential for a given configuration of steady conductances. Clearly the equation for computing the value of V_m (equation 2.8) is relevant for figuring out what the equilibrium membrane potential should be. However the V_m equation is a *recursive* equation for computing the membrane potential — the membrane potential is a function that depends on itself! Thus, it provides a recipe for updating the membrane potential, but it doesn't tell you directly what value the membrane potential will settle on if you provided a constant input to the neuron.

Nevertheless, we can easily solve for the equilibrium membrane potential equation by noting that when I_{net} is equal to zero, then the value of V_m doesn't change (as should be obvious from equation 2.8). Thus, setting the equation for I_{net} (equation 2.6) equal to zero and solving for the value of V_m (which appears in several places in this equation) should give us the equilibrium value of the membrane potential. When we do this, and solve for the value of V_m (which is no longer a function of time, because everything is steady-state), we get:

$$V_m = \frac{g_e \bar{g}_e E_e + g_i \bar{g}_i E_i + g_l \bar{g}_l E_l}{g_e \bar{g}_e + g_i \bar{g}_i + g_l \bar{g}_l} \qquad (2.9)$$

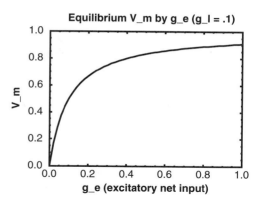

Figure 2.10: Plot of the equilibrium membrane potential as a function of level of excitatory input g_e, assuming no inhibitory current and a leak current of .1. For simplicity, $E_e = 1$ and $E_l = 0$, so V_m goes from 0 to approaching 1 as the strength of the excitatory input increases.

We can now use equation 2.9 to directly solve for the equilibrium membrane potential for any fixed set of inputs, just by plugging in the appropriate conductance values (and the reversal potential constants). Also, we will see in section 2.7 that the form of this equation can be understood in terms of a hypothesis testing analysis of a detector. Even without the benefit of that analysis, this equation shows that the membrane potential is basically just a *weighted average* based on the magnitude of the conductances for each type of channel. This can be made somewhat more obvious by rewriting equation 2.9 as follows:

$$
\begin{aligned}
V_m \;=\; & \frac{g_e \bar{g}_e}{g_e \bar{g}_e + g_i \bar{g}_i + g_l \bar{g}_l} E_e + \\[6pt]
& \frac{g_i \bar{g}_i}{g_e \bar{g}_e + g_i \bar{g}_i + g_l \bar{g}_l} E_i + \\[6pt]
& \frac{g_l \bar{g}_l}{g_e \bar{g}_e + g_i \bar{g}_i + g_l \bar{g}_l} E_l \qquad (2.10)
\end{aligned}
$$

Thus, the membrane potential moves toward the driving potential for a given channel c (E_c) in direct proportion to the fraction that the current for that channel is of the total current (figure 2.10). For example, let's examine a simple case where excitation drives the neuron toward a membrane potential (in arbitrary units) of 1 (i.e., $E_e = 1$) and leak and inhibition drive it toward 0 (i.e.,

$E_i = E_l = 0$). Then, let's assume that all three channels have the same conductance level (i.e., $g_e \bar{g}_e = 1$, $g_i \bar{g}_i = 1$, and $g_l \bar{g}_l = 1$). So, the total current is 3, and excitation makes up only $1/3$ of this total. Thus, the neuron will move $1/3$ of the way toward maximal excitation (i.e., $V_m = .333..$).

Perhaps the most important point to take away from equation 2.10 is that the neuron's membrane potential reflects a balance between excitation on the one hand, and leak plus inhibition on the other. Thus, both leak and inhibition provide *counterweights* to excitation. We will see in the next chapter how important these counterweights are for enabling a network of neurons to perform effectively.

2.4.7 Summary

By elaborating and exploring the electrical principles that underlie neural information processing, we have been able to develop a relatively simple equation (equation 2.8) that approximates the response of a neuron to excitatory and inhibitory inputs from other neurons. In the next section, we will see that we can use this equation (together with some additional equations for the thresholded firing process) to describe the behavior of the basic unit in our computational models of cognition. The fact that cognitive function can be so directly related in this way to the actions of charged atoms and basic physical principles of electricity and diffusion is a very exciting and important aspect of our overall physical reductionist approach to cognition.

Of course, we will find that we cannot actually describe cognitive phenomena directly in terms of ions and channels — we will see that there are a number of important emergent phenomena that arise from the interactions of individual neurons, and it is these higher levels of analysis that then provide a more useful language for describing cognition. Nevertheless, these higher levels of emergent phenomena can ultimately be traced back to the underlying ions, and our computer simulations of reading, word meaning, memory, and the like will all spend most of their time computing equation 2.8 and other associated equations!

2.5 Computational Implementation of the Neural Activation Function

In this section, we describe how the Leabra framework implements a simplified approximation to the biological mechanisms discussed in the previous sections. As mentioned previously, the major challenge we confront in developing this computational framework is striking an appropriate balance between the facts of biology on one hand, and simplicity and efficiency on the other. We first highlight some of the main features of the framework first, and then cover the details in subsequent subsections.

To contextualize properly our neural activation function, we first describe the most commonly used activation function for more abstract artificial neural networks (ANNs). This function is very simple, yet shares some basic properties with our more biologically based function. Thus, we view our activation function as providing a bridge between the more abstract, computationally motivated artificial activation function and the way that neurons actually do things.

There are only two equations in the abstract ANN activation function. The first defines the **net input** to the unit, which is just a sum of the individual weighted inputs from other units:

$$\eta_j = \sum_i x_i w_{ij} \qquad (2.11)$$

where η_j is the net input for receiving unit j, x_i is the activation value for sending unit i, and w_{ij} is the weight value for that input into the receiving unit. The other equation transforms this net input value into an activation value, which is then sent on to other units:

$$y_j = \frac{1}{1 + e^{-\eta_j}} \qquad (2.12)$$

where y_j is the activation value of the receiving unit j, and the form of this equation is known as a **sigmoid** (more specifically the **logistic**), because it is an S-shaped function as shown in box 2.1.

Among the most important computational properties of the sigmoid function is the fact that it has a **saturating nonlinearity**, such that ever stronger excitatory net

Box 2.1: Sigmoidal Activation Function

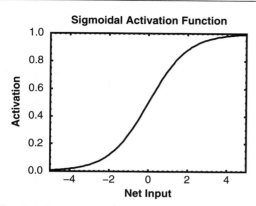

Sigmoidal Activation Function

The sigmoidal activation function, pictured in the above figure, is the standard function for abstract neural network models. The net input is computed using a linear sum of weighted activation terms:

$$\eta_j = \sum_i x_i w_{ij}$$

where η_j is the net input for receiving unit j, x_i is the activation value for sending unit i, and w_{ij} is the weight value for that input into the receiving unit.

The sigmoidal function transforms this net input value into an activation value (y_j), which is then sent on to other units:

$$y_j = \frac{1}{1 + e^{-\eta_j}}$$

input values approach a fixed upper limit of activation, and likewise for the lower limit on strongly inhibitory net inputs. Nonlinearity is important because this allows sequences of neurons chained together to achieve more complex computations than single stages of neural processing can — with a linear activation function, anything that can be done with multiple stages could actually be done in a single stage. Thus, as long as our more biologically based activation function also exhibits a similar kind of saturating nonlinearity, it should be computationally effective.

To implement the neural activation function, we use the point neuron approximation discussed previously,

which provides a crude but very efficient approximation to the neural dynamics of integrating over inputs. Thus, we use equation 2.8 to compute a single membrane potential value V_m for each simulated neuron, where this value reflects a balance of excitatory and inhibitory inputs. This membrane potential value then provides the basis for computing an activation output value as discussed in a moment. First, we highlight some of the important differences between this point neuron model and the more abstract ANN approach.

Perhaps one of the most important differences from a biological perspective is that the point neuron activation function requires an explicit separation between excitatory and inhibitory inputs, as these enter into different conductance terms in equation 2.8. In contrast, the abstract ANN net input term just directly adds together inputs with positive and negative weights. These weights also do not obey the biological constraint that all the inputs produced by a given sending neuron have the same sign (i.e., either all excitatory or all inhibitory). Furthermore, the weights often change sign during learning.

In our model, we obey the biological constraints on the separation of excitatory and inhibitory inputs by typically only directly simulating excitatory neurons (i.e., the pyramidal neurons of the cortex), while using an efficient approximation developed in the next chapter to compute the inhibitory inputs that would be produced by the cortical inhibitory interneurons (more on these neuron types in the next chapter). The excitatory input conductances ($g_e(t)$) is essentially an average over all the weighted inputs coming into the neuron (although the actual computation is somewhat more complicated, as described below), which is much like the ANN net input computation, only it is automatically normalized by the total number of such inputs:

$$g_e(t) = \langle x_i w_{ij} \rangle = \frac{1}{n} \sum_i x_i w_{ij} \qquad (2.13)$$

Another important difference between the ANN activation function and the point neuron model is that whereas the ANN goes straight from the net input to the activation output in one step (via the sigmoidal function), the point neuron model computes an intermediate integrated input term in the form of the membrane potential V_m, which reflects a balance between the aggregated excitatory and inhibitory inputs. There is then a second step that produces an activation output as a function of V_m. From a computational perspective, we will see in the next chapter that by computing an excitatory/inhibitory balance in this way, the point neuron function makes it easier to implement inhibitory competition dynamics among neurons efficiently.

In an actual neuron, we know that the output consists of a spike produced when V_m exceeds the firing threshold. We provide a simple implementation of this kind of discrete spiking output function in Leabra, which summarizes all of the biological machinery for producing a spike with a single binary activation value (1 if V_m is over threshold, and 0 otherwise).

However, most of our models use a **rate code** approximation to discrete spiking. Here, the output of the neuron is a continuous, real-valued number that reflects the instantaneous rate at which an otherwise equivalent spiking neuron would produce spikes. In the context of the scaling issues discussed in the introduction (section 1.2.4), we can think of this rate code output as representing the average output of a population of similarly configured spiking neurons (i.e., something like the proportion of neurons that are spiking over some relatively small time interval). Section 2.8 provides further justification for using this approximation.

The principal computational advantage of the rate code output is that it smoothes over the noise that is otherwise present with discrete spiking — we will see that the thresholded nature of the spike output makes the detailed timing of spike outputs very sensitive to even small fluctuations in membrane potential, and this sensitivity is manifest as noise. This kind of noise would tend to get averaged out with thousands of neurons, but not in the smaller-scale models that we often use.

We will see below that a thresholded, sigmoidal function provides a good continuous-valued approximation to the spiking rate produced by the discrete spiking version of our model. Thus, we can see here the link between the continuous-valued sigmoidal activation function used in the ANN models and the discrete spiking characteristic of biological neurons. Indeed, we will occasionally use the simpler ANN equations for the purposes of analysis, because they have been extensively

studied and have some important mathematical properties. Because one can switch between using either a discrete spiking or continuous rate code output in Leabra, the impact of the rate code approximation can be empirically evaluated more easily.

In the following subsections, we describe in greater detail the computation of the excitatory input ($g_e(t)$), the parameters used for the point neuron membrane potential update equation, the discrete spiking output function, and the continuous rate code output function. Then we will go on to explore the neural activation function in action!

2.5.1 Computing Input Conductances

We showed in equation 2.13 that the excitatory input conductance is essentially an average over the weighted inputs. However, there are some practical and biological details that require us to compute this average in a somewhat more elaborated fashion.

In a typical cortical neuron, excitatory synaptic inputs come from synaptic channels located all over the dendrites. There can be up to ten thousand or more synaptic inputs onto a single neuron, with each synaptic input having many individual Na^+ channels! Typically, a neuron receives inputs from a number of different brain areas. These different groups of inputs are called **projections**. Inputs from different projections are often grouped together on different parts of the dendritic tree. The way we compute the excitatory input is sensitive to this projection-level structure, allowing for different projections to have different levels of overall impact on the neuron, and allowing for differences in expected activity level in different projections (which is often the case in our models) to be automatically compensated for.

Another important component of the excitatory input in the model comes from the **bias input**, which summarizes the baseline differences in excitability between different neurons. It is likely that neurons have individual differences in their leak current levels or other differences (of which there are many candidates in the biology) that could give rise to such differences or *biases* in overall level of excitability (e.g., Desai, Rutherford, & Turrigiano, 1999). Thus, some neurons may require very strong inputs to fire (e.g., many inputs active and closely matching the weight pattern), while others may only require very weak inputs (e.g., only a few inputs active and/or not too closely matching the weights). Both types (and everything in between) can be useful and/or necessary in solving particular tasks, so it is important to include these differences in excitability in the model. It is also important to enable these biases to adapt with learning so that they can become tuned to the problem at hand (see section 3.3.1 in the next chapter for further discussion).

To keep the implementation simple, and because of the uncertainty regarding which biological mechanism is responsible, we implement the bias input in the way that most artificial neural network models do, as an additional *bias input* term in the input equation. Specifically, we introduce a **bias weight** (β), which determines the amount of bias input, and is modified with learning much like the other weights in the network.

We also include **time averaging** in the net input computation, which reflects the sluggishness involved in propagating and aggregating synaptic inputs over the entire dendritic membrane. Time averaging is also important when discrete spiking is used for having a window of **temporal summation**, where spiking inputs that arrive around the same time period will produce a larger excitatory effect than if those same inputs were distributed across time. In more pragmatic terms, time averaging smoothes out rapid transitions or fluctuations that might otherwise cause the network to oscillate or generally fail to propagate activation effectively.

The next subsection presents the details of the excitatory input computation. These details are mostly implementational, not conceptual, so you may wish to skip this section on your first pass through the book, returning to it later if necessary. The main features of the implementation are that inputs are averaged together by projections, and then combined using various *scaling* parameters that allow the different projections to be differentially weighted relative to each other. This scaling is much more important in the Leabra model than in more abstract ANN models because the weight values are naturally bounded between 0 and 1, and thus cannot grow arbitrarily large through learning to achieve a useful balance of influences from different inputs.

Details of Input Conductance Computation

At each synaptic input, the fraction of excitatory input channels open is computed as just the sending activation times the weight: $x_i w_{ij}$ (weights are `wt` in the simulator). All of the individual synaptic conductances that come from the same input projection k are then averaged together:

$$\langle x_i w_{ij} \rangle_k = \frac{1}{n} \sum_i x_i w_{ij} \qquad (2.14)$$

(note that we assume that all of the variables discussed in this section are a function of time (except the constants as noted), and so we generally omit the explicit time dependency (t) for simplicity, unless different time states of the variable are used within an equation).

The $\frac{1}{n}$ factor in the above equation is usually, but not always, equal to the number of connections a unit has within a given projection. When a given projection has *partial* connectivity from a sending layer, it is typically useful to treat the missing connections as though they simply have weights permanently set to 0. Thus, the $\frac{1}{n}$ factor is set to be the number of units in the sending layer of the projection by default, and not the number of actual connections in the projection. By so doing, one can easily use mechanisms for automatically configuring the network connectivity as a shortcut for setting a pattern of weights, without affecting the normalization properties of the net input compared to an otherwise identical network with full connectivity. Where this is not appropriate, the `div_gp_n` flag in the simulator divides by the actual number of connections in a projection (group).

The excitatory conductance value for a given projection k, which we write as g_{e_k}, is just the average of the individual inputs times a normalizing factor based on the expected activity level of the sending projection, which is represented by the variable α_k:

$$g_{e_k} = \frac{1}{\alpha_k} \langle x_i w_{ij} \rangle_k \qquad (2.15)$$

This normalization is useful because the different projections into a neuron may have very different baseline levels of activity due to relatively arbitrary aspects of the model, but as noted previously the weights cannot grow arbitrarily to establish a good balance across these different inputs. Thus, by automatically normalizing this baseline difference away, the default is that all projections have roughly the same level of influence.

In most cases, we can then compute the overall excitatory conductance $g_e(t)$, which we also refer to as the *net input* (net in the simulator) by analogy with the simpler ANN formalisms, as an average of the projection-level conductances together with the bias weight β (bias.wt in the simulator), with a time-averaging time constant dt_{net} ($0 < dt_{net} < 1$, dt_net in the simulator) for integrating $g_e(t)$ over time:

$$\begin{aligned}
g_e(t) &= (1 - dt_{net})g_e(t-1) + \\
&\quad dt_{net}\left(\frac{1}{n_p}\sum_k g_{e_k} + \frac{\beta}{N}\right) \\
&= (1 - dt_{net})g_e(t-1) + \\
&\quad dt_{net}\left(\frac{1}{n_p}\sum_k \frac{1}{\alpha_k}\langle x_i w_{ij}\rangle_k + \frac{\beta}{N}\right)
\end{aligned}$$

$$(2.16)$$

where n_p is the number of projections. The default dt_{net} value is .7, making for relatively fast temporal integration. Note that because the bias input is treated essentially as just another projection, it would have a disproportionately large impact relative to the other synaptic inputs if it were not scaled appropriately. We achieve this scaling by dividing by the total number of input connections N, which gives the bias weight roughly the same impact as one normal synaptic input.

Differential Projection-Level Scaling

In some cases, we need to introduce scaling constants that alter the balance of influence among the different projections. In cortical neurons for example, some projections may connect with the more *distal* (distant from the cell body) parts of the dendrites, and thus have a weaker overall impact on the neuron than more *proximal* (near to the cell body) inputs. We implement scaling constants by altering equation 2.15 as follows:

$$g_{e_k} = s_k \frac{r_k}{\sum_p r_p}\frac{1}{\alpha_k}\langle x_i w_{ij}\rangle_k \qquad (2.17)$$

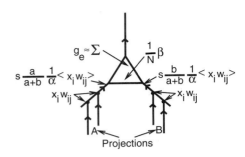

Figure 2.11: Computing the excitatory synaptic input. Individual weighted inputs at each synapse ($x_i w_{ij}$) coming from the same projection (A or B, as represented by the branches of the dendritic tree), are averaged together ($\langle x_i w_{ij}\rangle$). This average is normalized by the expected sending activity level for the projection (α), and scaled by arbitrary constants (absolute scale s and relative scales a and b). The bias input β (shown as a property of the soma) is treated like another projection, and is scaled by one over the total number of inputs N, making it equivalent to one input value. All the projection values (including bias) are then added up to get the overall excitatory conductance g_e (with the time-averaging also factored in).

where s_k (wt_scale.abs in the simulator) provides an *absolute* scaling parameter for projection k, and r_k (wt_scale.rel in the simulator) provides a *relative* scaling parameter that is normalized relative to the scaling parameters for all the other projections. When these parameters are all set to 1, as is typically the case, the equation reduces to equation 2.15. When they are used, relative scaling is almost always used because it maintains the same overall level of input to the neuron. However, absolute scaling can be useful for temporarily "lesioning" a projection (by setting $s_k = 0$) without affecting the contributions from other projections. Figure 2.11 shows a schematic for computing the excitatory input with these scaling constants.

How Much of Dendritic Integration in Real Neurons Does Our Model Capture?

The way we compute the excitatory input to our simulated neurons incorporates some of the important properties of dendritic integration in real neurons in a way that is not usually done with simplified point neuron level models. For example, our computations are sensitive to the projection-level organization of inputs, and they allow for the differential scaling of distal versus proximal inputs. Furthermore, we use time averaging to simulate the sluggishness of real neurons. Nevertheless, we are still ignoring a number of known properties of dendritic integration in real neurons.

For example, we now know that dendrites have a number of *active* voltage-gated channels that can potentially dramatically affect the way that information is integrated (e.g., Cauller & Connors, 1994). One result of these channels might be that weak, distal signals might be amplified and thus equalized to stronger, proximal inputs, which could be easily handled in our computation of the inputs. However, these channels may also impose thresholds and other nonlinearities that are not included in our simple model. These active channels may also communicate the output spikes produced at the axon hillock all the way back into the dendrites, which could be useful for learning based on the overall activity of the postsynaptic neuron (Amitai, Friedman, Connors, & Gutnick, 1993; Stuart & Sakmann, 1994).

Some researchers have emphasized the complex, logiclike interactions that can occur between inputs on the dendritic *spines* (where most excitatory inputs occur) and other branching aspects of the dendrites (e.g., Shepherd & Brayton, 1987). If these played a dominant role in the integration of inputs, our averaging model could be substantially inaccurate. However, these effects have not been well demonstrated in actual neurons, and may actually be mitigated by the presence of active channels. Furthermore, some detailed analyses of dendritic integration support the point neuron approximation, at least for some dendritic configurations (Jaffe & Carnevale, 1999). See section 2.8 for more discussion of the relative advantages and disadvantages of this kind of logiclike processing.

2.5.2 Point Neuron Parameter Values

The next step in the activation function after the input conductances are computed is to apply the membrane potential update equation (equation 2.8). We literally use this equation, but we typically use parameter values that range between 0 and 1, based on nor-

Parameter	mV	$(0-1)$	$\bar{g}$
E_a (K$^+$)	-90	0.00	0.50
E_l (K$^+$, Na$^+$)	-70	0.15	0.10
V_{rest}	-70	0.15	—
E_i (Cl$^-$)	-70	0.15	1.00
Θ	-55	0.25	—
E_e (Na$^+$)	+55	1.00	1.00
E_h (Ca^{++})†	+100	1.00	0.10

Table 2.1: Reversal potentials (in mV and $0-1$ normalized values) and maximum conductance values for the channels simulated in Leabra, together with other biologically based constants including the resting potential V_{rest} and the nominal firing threshold Θ (thr in the simulator). E_a and E_h are the accommodation and hysteresis currents discussed in greater detail in section 2.9. † Note that this value is clipped to 1.0 range based on -90 to +55.

malized biologically based values. The normalized values are easier to visualize on a common axis, are more intuitively meaningful, and can be related more easily to probability-like values (see section 2.7). Table 2.1 shows a table of all the basic parameters used in our simulations (including some that will be introduced in subsequent sections), with both the biological and normalized values. Normalization was performed by subtracting the minimum (-90) and dividing by the range (55 to -90), and rounding to the nearest .05. Also, we note that the dt_{vm} parameter in equation 2.8 is called dt_vm in the simulator, with a typical value of .2.

2.5.3 The Discrete Spiking Output Function

After updating the membrane potential, we need to compute an output value as a function of this potential. In this section we describe one of the two options for computing this output — the more biologically realistic discrete spiking output. The next section then discusses the other option, which is the continuous, real-valued rate code approximation to discrete spiking.

Recall that in a real neuron, spiking is caused by the action of two opposing types of voltage-gated channels, one that excites the membrane potential (by letting in Na$^+$ ions), and another that counters this excitement and restores the negative resting potential (by letting out

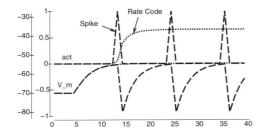

Figure 2.12:   Simple discrete spiking output, showing that as the membrane potential (V_m) exceeds the threshold ($-55mV$), the activation output (act) goes to 1. On the next time step, the membrane potential is reset to a hyperpolarized value, and the activation returns to 0. Also shown for comparison is the equivalent rate-code output activation (dotted line) that would be produced by this level of input excitation.

K^+ ions). A set of detailed mathematical equations derived by Hodgkin and Huxley (1952) describe the way that the two voltage-gated channels open and close as a function of the membrane potential. However, these equations provide more detail than our model requires.

Instead, we use a simple threshold mechanism that results in an activation value (act in the simulator) of 1 if the membrane potential exceeds the threshold (Θ, thr in the simulator), and a zero otherwise (figure 2.12). On the time step following the spike, the membrane potential is reset to a sub-resting level (determined by parameter v_m_r in the simulator), which captures the refractory effect seen in real neurons. Also, to simulate the temporally extended effects that a single spike can have on a postsynaptic neuron (e.g., due to extended activation of the receptors by neurotransmitter and/or delay in receptor closing after being opened) the spike activation can be extended for multiple cycles as determined by the dur parameter.

For ease of comparison with the rate-code function described next, and to enable learning to operate on continuous valued numbers, we also need to compute a time-averaged version of the firing rate, which we call the *rate-code equivalent* activation (y_j^{eq}, act_eq in the simulator). This is computed over a specified period of updates (*cycles*), as follows:

$$y_j^{eq} = \gamma_{eq} \frac{N_{spikes}}{N_{cycles}} \qquad (2.18)$$

where N_{spikes} is the number of spikes fired during that time period, N_{cycles} is the total number of cycles, and γ_{eq} (eq_gain in the simulator) is a gain factor that rescales the value to better fill the 0 to 1 range used by the rate code activations (the result is also clipped to ensure it stays within the $0 - 1$ range). The neuron might actually have something like this rate-code equivalent value in the form of the concentration of internal calcium ions, which may be what learning is based on (more on this in chapters 4–6).

2.5.4   The Rate Code Output Function

As we have stated, a rate code output function can provide smoother activation dynamics than the discrete spiking function, and constitutes a reasonable approximation to a population of neurons. To compute a rate code output, we need a function that takes the membrane potential at the present time and gives the expected instantaneous firing rate associated with that membrane potential (assuming it were to remain constant). Because there is no spiking, this membrane potential is not reset, so it continuously reflects the balance of inputs to the neuron as computed by the membrane potential update equation.

In the simple discrete spiking mechanism described in the previous section, the main factor that determines the spiking rate is the time it takes for the membrane potential to return to the threshold level after being reset by the previous spike (figure 2.12). Although we were unable to write a closed-form expression for this time interval as a function of a non-resetting membrane potential, simulations reveal that it can be summarized reasonably accurately with a function of the **X-over-X-plus-1** (XX1) form (suggested by Marius Usher in personal communication):

$$y_j = \frac{\gamma[V_m - \Theta]_+}{\gamma[V_m - \Theta]_+ + 1} \qquad (2.19)$$

where y_j is the activation (act in the simulator), Θ is again the threshold value, γ is a *gain* parameter (act_gain in the simulator), and the expression $[x]_+$ means the positive component of x and zero if negative.

Interestingly, equation 2.19 is of the same general form as that used to compute V_m itself (and can be given a similar Bayesian interpretation in terms of comparing the thresholded V_m value to the constant *null hypothesis* represented arbitrarily by the number 1, as described in section 2.7). This equation can also be written somewhat more simply as:

$$y_j = \frac{1}{1 + (\gamma[V_m - \Theta]_+)^{-1}} \qquad (2.20)$$

which makes clear the relationship between this function and the standard sigmoidal activation function (equation 2.12) commonly used in artificial neural network models, as discussed previously.

Equation 2.20 by itself does not provide a particularly good fit to actual discrete spiking rates, because it fails to take into account the presence of noise in the spiking model. Although our simulated spiking neuron will fire spikes at completely regular intervals with a constant input (figure 2.12), the detailed spike timing is very sensitive to small fluctuations in membrane potential, as we will see in explorations described later. Thus, once any noise enters into a network of spiking neurons, the resulting fluctuations in membrane potential will tend to propagate the noise throughout the network. This is consistent with the finding that neural spike timing indeed appears to be quite random (e.g., Shadlen & Newsome, 1994). Note however that just because the detailed timing appears to be random, the firing rate averaged over a suitable time window can nevertheless be relatively steady, as we will see.

One effect that this kind of noise would have is that the neuron would sometimes fire even when its average membrane potential is below threshold, due to random noise fluctuations. Thus, we might expect that the very sharp threshold in the XX1 function would be softened by the presence of noise. We will see that this is indeed what happens.

Perhaps the most direct way to capture the effects of noise in our rate code model would be to literally add noise to the membrane potential, resulting in a model that exhibits **stochastic** (noisy) behavior. However, this slows processing and results in the need for averaging over large samples to obtain reliable effects, which are some of the things we had hoped to avoid by using a rate code output in the first place. Thus, we instead use a modified rate-code activation function that

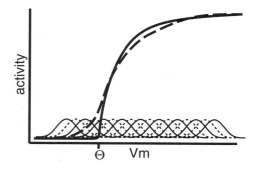

Figure 2.13: Illustration of convolution, where each point in the the new function (dashed line) is produced by adding up the values of a normalized Gaussian centered on that point multiplied times the original function (solid line).

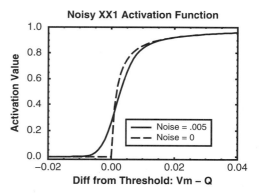

Figure 2.14: Noisy XX1 (X/X+1) activation function (threshold written as Q instead of Θ), showing effects of convolving with Gaussian noise of $\sigma = .005$ to the case with no noise. The gain (γ) is the standard 600 for membrane potentials in the $0 - -1$ range.

directly incorporates the average effect of noise. The result is that we still have **deterministic** (nonstochastic, perfectly predictable) units, which nevertheless reflect the expected or average effects of noise.

The averaging of the noise into the activation function is done by *convolving* a Gaussian-distributed noise function with the XX1 activation function given by equation 2.20. Convolving, illustrated in figure 2.13, simply amounts to multiplying a bell-shaped Gaussian noise function times a neighborhood of points surround-

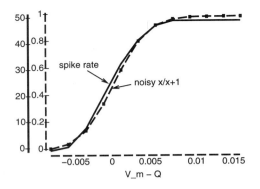

Figure 2.15: Average spiking rate as a function of equilibrium membrane potential above threshold (threshold written
as Q instead of Θ) with constant excitatory and inhibitory
conductances, compared with the noisy x/x+1 function for the
same conditions (equation 2.20). Note that due to aliasing effects resulting from the discretization of time, parameters had
to be altered from their standard values (e.g., as shown in figure 2.14). Nevertheless, the general form of the function is
obviously well captured by the noisy x/x+1 function.

ing (and including) each point in the activation function, and adding these multiplied neighbors together to
give the new value at that point. Thus, these new values
reflect the probabilities with which neighboring points
could jump (up or down) to a given point when noise
is added. This is the same process used in the "blur-
ring" or "smoothing" operations in computerized image manipulation programs. The result of this operation
is shown in figure 2.14. We call this new function the
noisy-X-over-X-plus-1 or **noisy XX1** function.

As we expected, the noisy XX1 function has a *softer*
threshold, which gradually curves up from zero instead
of starting sharply at the threshold point as in the original function. This is important for giving the neurons
a graded overall activation function, imparting all the
advantages of gradedness as discussed in section 1.6.2.
Note that this also means that there is some activity associated with subthreshold membrane potentials (i.e.,
due to noise occasionally sending it above threshold).
Another effect is that noise somewhat reduces the gain
(sharpness) of the activation function.

Figure 2.15 shows that the noisy XX1 function provides a good overall fit to the rate of discrete spiking in a

unit with noise added to the membrane potential. Thus,
we can use the noisy XX1 activation function to simulate the average or expected effects of a spiking neuron,
or to represent the collective effects of a population of
spiking neurons.

Figure 2.15 also shows that the noisy XX1 function
has the key property of a sigmoidal activation function
(e.g., box 2.1), namely the saturating nonlinearity discussed previously. The saturation is due in the spiking
case to the increasingly limiting effects of the refractory
period, where the potential must recover to threshold after being reset following a spike. Similar kinds of saturating nonlinearities have been suggested by other analyses of the neural spiking mechanism and other synaptic effects (Ermentrout, 1994; Abbott, Varela, Sen, &
Nelson, 1997). Another aspect of the noisy XX1 function is that it emphasizes small differences in the membrane potential in the vicinity of the threshold, at the
expense of representing differences well above or below the threshold. The gain parameter γ can shrink or
expand this sensitive region around the threshold. We
will see the importance of these aspects of the activation
function when we put neurons together in networks in
the next chapter.

2.5.5   Summary

We have now covered all the major components of computation at the level of the individual neuron, including the computation of excitatory inputs as a weighted
function of sending unit activity, the integration of excitatory, inhibitory, and leak forces (conductances), and
the thresholded, saturating activation output. We refer
to the collection of these equations as the *point neuron
activation function* or just the Leabra activation function. The major steps in this function are summarized
in box 2.2.

2.6   Explorations of the Individual Neuron

Now we will use the simulator to explore the properties of individual neurons as implemented by the point
neuron activation function just described. Before you
begin, there are two important prerequisites: First, the
software must be properly installed, and second, it will

Box 2.2: Point Neuron Activation Function

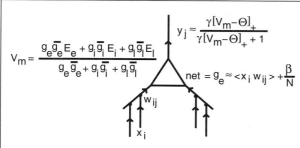

Activation flows from the sending units (x_i) through the weights (w_{ij}) resulting in the excitatory net input g_e over all inputs, and including the bias weight β:

$$g_e(t) = (1 - dt_{net})g_e(t-1) +$$
$$dt_{net}\left(\frac{1}{n_p}\sum_k \frac{1}{\alpha_k}\langle x_i w_{ij}\rangle_k + \frac{\beta}{N}\right)$$

Projection-level averages are normalized by expected sending-layer activity levels α_k and then averaged (optionally subject to differential scaling, not shown here) and subject to time-averaging with time constant dt_{net}. In the simulator, the variable `net` actually represents $g_e\bar{g}_e$, not just g_e.

Excitatory input is combined with inhibition and leak, each with their own driving or reversal potentials E, to compute the membrane potential V_m:

$$V_m(t+1) = V_m(t) + dt_{vm}[$$
$$g_e(t)\bar{g}_e(E_e - V_m(t)) +$$
$$g_i(t)\bar{g}_i(E_i - V_m(t)) +$$
$$g_l(t)\bar{g}_l(E_l - V_m(t))]$$

which has a weighted-average equilibrium form:

$$V_m = \frac{g_e\bar{g}_e E_e + g_i\bar{g}_i E_i + g_l\bar{g}_l E_l}{g_e\bar{g}_e + g_i\bar{g}_i + g_l\bar{g}_l}$$

Activation y_j is a thresholded ($[]_+$) sigmoidal function of the membrane potential:

$$y_j = \frac{\gamma[V_m - \Theta]_+}{\gamma[V_m - \Theta]_+ + 1}$$

which is convolved by a Gaussian noise kernel in the noisy XX1 function to soften the threshold and produce a smooth, continuous sigmoidal curve that closely approximates the firing rate of a discrete spiking neuron.

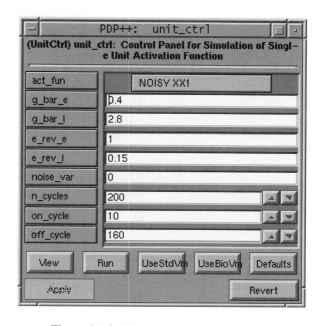

Figure 2.16: The `unit_ctrl` control panel.

be very useful for you to orient yourself to the organization and use of the simulator. Consult appendix A for an introduction to the simulator.

Once these prerequisites have been taken care of, you can proceed to the individual neuron simulations. You'll find these in `chapter_2`, so move into it now.

2.6.1 The Membrane Potential

↪ Open the project `unit.proj.gz` in `chapter_2`.

All projects start out with three windows: the **PDP++ Root** window (where you can quit the program or load a different project), the **NetView** (`Network_0`) window (which shows the network), and the **control panel** (`unit_ctrl`, which holds key parameters and controls all the basic tasks of the simulation; figure 2.16). In addition, some other windows will open up in an *iconified* (minimized) state — the control panel will allow us to activate these windows as needed.

The NetView shows how this simulation is configured — it consists of just a single input unit projecting to a single receiving unit. We will see this single input being turned on and then off again, and observe the response of the receiving unit. To see this, we can run the simulation.

↪ Press the Run button on the control panel.

You should see that very shortly after the input unit comes on (indicated by the yellow color), the receiving unit is activated by this input. To get a better idea of the precise trajectory of this activation, it is much more convenient to use the **GraphLog**, which displays the information graphically over time, allows multiple variables to be viewed at the same time, and even allows multiple runs (e.g., with different parameters) to be compared with each other.

↪ *Iconify* (minimize) the NetView window.

Software Tip: Iconify using your window manager's buttons (typically on the upper right-hand corner of the window), or using the Iconify menu option in the Object menu at the very left-hand side of the window. **Never use the** Object/Close **menu option to iconify** — it will destroy the object and cause a crash!

↪ Press View on the control panel, and select GRAPH_LOG to open up the GraphLog display.

The plots produced by this simulation are much like that shown in figure 2.9. Only the excitatory and leak currents are operating here, with their conductances (g_bar_e, g_bar_l) and reversal potentials (e_rev_e, e_rev_l) as shown in the control panel.

↪ Press the Run button on the control panel.

This produces a plot using the current parameters (figure 2.17). You should see various lines plotted over 200 time steps (*cycles*) on the X axis. Note that the standard $0 - 1$ normalized parameters are used by default (we can switch to the biological values later).

First, let's focus on the net line (it's the red one, displayed as a solid line in figure 2.17). This shows the *net input* to the unit, which starts out at 0, and then rapidly jumps to .4, remaining there until around 160 time steps, where it goes back to 0 again. Recall that this net input is just another name for the total excitatory input to the neuron (i.e., $net = g_e \bar{g}_e$). In this simulation, the sending unit always sends a g_e value of 1 when it's on, and a 0 when off. Later, we will manipulate the value of $\bar{g}_e$ (g_bar_e in the control panel) to control the magnitude of the net input (it is .4 because the default value of g_bar_e is .4). The timing of the input is controlled by the parameters on_cycle and off_cycle (the total number of cycles is controlled by n_cycles).

The second line, I_net (in orange/dashed), shows the *net current* in the unit. As expected, this shows an excitatory (upward) current when the input comes on, and an inhibitory (downward) one when the input goes off. This line is plotted using its own special vertical (Y) axis going from -1 to 1 (shown in orange), while all the other lines share the $0-1$ Y axis with the net-input (red). Note that the axis used by each line is color-coded to the right of the variable buttons.

The third line, v_m (in yellow/dotted), shows the *membrane potential*, which starts at the resting potential of .15, then increases with the excitation, and decreases back to rest when the input goes off.

The fourth line, act (in green/dash-dot), shows the *activation* value (using the NOISY_XX1 rate-coded activation function) that results from the membrane potential. It goes from 0 up to roughly .72 and back down again. Note that the activation rise trails the net input by several cycles — this is due to the time it takes for the membrane potential to reach threshold.

Software Tip: You can click with the left mouse button on any line in the graph to get the precise numerical value at a given point.

↪ Use the mouse to verify that the activation rise does indeed occur right around the threshold value for the membrane potential (.25).

The fifth line, act_eq (in blue), is the rate-code equivalent activation value for discrete spiking units. When an actual rate-code activation function (noisy XX1) is used, act_eq is just equivalent to act. This line is not turned on by default in the graph — we will use it later when we switch to spiking units.

Now we will use some of the parameters in the control panel to explore the properties of the point neuron activation function.

↪ Take a moment to familiarize yourself with the parameters (you can click on the label for each parameter to view a brief description of what it is).

Software Tip: All *edit dialogs* like the control panel have at least two buttons across the bottom: Apply (which applies any changes you have made to actually set the parameters) and Revert (which reverts to the previously applied values, which is useful if you have

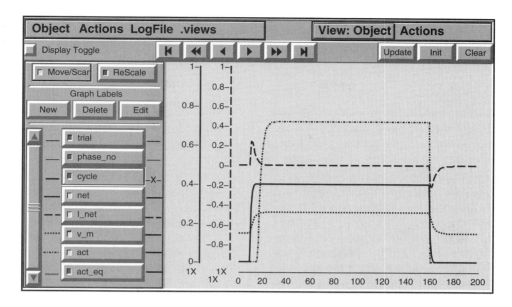

Figure 2.17: The GraphLog display of a run with standard parameters. The solid line (net) is red in the actual display, dashed (I_net) = orange, dotted (v_m) = yellow, and dash-dot (act) = green.

accidentally typed in a value that you didn't want). In addition, there are various special-purpose buttons that are specific to a given simulation. For more information on using these edit dialogs, see appendix A.5.

First, we will focus on g_bar_e, which controls the amount of excitatory conductance as described earlier. In general, we are interested in seeing how the unit membrane potential reflects a balance of the different inputs coming into it (here just excitation and leak), and how the output activation responds to the resulting membrane potential.

↪ Increase g_bar_e from .4 to .5 (and press the Apply and Run buttons to see the effects). Then observe the effects of decreasing g_bar_e to .3.

Question 2.1 (a) *Describe the effects on the neural response of increasing* g_bar_e *to .5, and of decreasing it to .3.* (b) *Is there a qualitative difference in the unit activation (act) between these two changes of magnitude .1 away from the initial .4 value?* (c) *What important aspect of the point neuron activation function does this reveal?*

Software tip: It is often useful to overlay different Runs on top of each other in the graph log, which will happen naturally. When you want to clear the log, press the Clear button. Also, if for any reason the graph goes blank or is somehow garbled, pressing the Init button should fix things.

By systematically searching the parameter range for g_bar_e between .3 and .4, you should be able to locate the point at which the membrane potential just reaches threshold (recall that this is at $V_m = .25$ in the normalized units). To make it easier to locate the threshold, we will switch from the noisy XX1 activation function (which has a *soft* threshold due to the effects of the convolved noise) to the XX1 activation function (which has a hard threshold due to the absence of noise).

↪ Switch the act_fun setting on the control panel from NOISY_XX1 to XX1 and press Apply.

Question 2.2 (a) *To 3 decimal places, what value of* g_bar_e *puts the unit just over threshold? Can you think of a better way of finding this value (Hint: Do you remember an equation for the equilibrium membrane potential given a particular set of inputs?)* (b) *Compute* *the exact value of excitatory input required to just reach threshold, showing your math (note that: g_l is always 1 because the leak channels are always open; g_e is 1 when the input is on; inhibition is not present here and can be ignored). Does this agree with your empirically determined value? (Hint: It should!)*

You can also play around with the value of the leak conductance, g_bar_l, which controls the size of the leak current.

↪ Press the Defaults button on the control panel to restore the default parameters, and then see what happens when you increase or decrease the leak.

Question 2.3 (a) *How does the response of the unit change when you change* g_bar_l? *Why?* **(b)** *How does this differ from changes to* g_bar_e? **(c)** *Use the same technique you used in the previous question to compute the exact amount of leak current necessary to put the membrane potential exactly at threshold when the* g_bar_e *value is at the default of .4 (show your math).*

↪ Press Defaults to restore the default parameters.

Now that we have a sense of how the unit responds to different currents, and computes a resulting membrane potential that reflects the balance of these currents, we can explore the role of the reversal potentials (e_rev_e and e_rev_l).

Question 2.4 (a) *What happens to the unit's activity if you change the leak reversal potential* e_rev_l *from .15 to 0?* **(b)** *What about when you increase it to .2? For both questions, explain the results, taking note of what happens before the input goes on as well as what happens while it is on.* **(c)** *What can you conclude about the relationship between the resting potential and the leak reversal potential?*

↪ Press Defaults to restore the default parameters.

Question 2.5 (a) *What happens to the unit's activity if you change the excitatory reversal potential* e_rev_e *from 1 to .5? Why does this happen?* **(b)** *Can you compensate for this by changing the value of* g_bar_e? *To two decimal places, use the simulator to find the value*

of g_bar_e *that gives essentially the same activation value as the default parameters.* **(c)** *Then use the same approach as in question 2.2 to solve for the exact value of* g_bar_e *that will compensate for this change in* e_rev_e *(use .256 for the membrane potential under the default parameters, and show your math).*

At this point, you should have a good idea about how the conductance and reversal potential parameters influence the resulting membrane potential. Just to demonstrate that it does not make a real difference in the behavior of the unit (and to satisfy the neuroscientists out there), we can switch from using the normalized $0 - 1$ reversal potential values to the biologically based ones.

↪ Click the UseBioVm button to switch to using the biological values, and then click Run.

The new GraphLog display should appear similar to the previous one, except that now the membrane potential is plotted on a scale from -90 to $+55$, instead of $0 - 1$, and the I_net is also on a larger scale. We changed the scaling (gain) of the activation function so that it is identical to that used before.

↪ Click the UseStdVm button to switch to back to using the normalized values.

If you are adventurous, you can look into the "guts" of the simulation to see exactly what we did to switch from normalized to biological parameters. The way a unit behaves in the simulator is controlled by something called the **UnitSpec** (*unit specifications*).

↪ Select View on the control panel, and then pick UNIT_SPECS. Two complex edit dialog will appear, one named UnitSpec_0 and the other named BioUnitSpec_0. Arrange the two edit dialogs side-by-side.

Going down the parameters from top to bottom, you can see which have different values, and hopefully make sense of the differences. You can also click on the parameter label for a helpful comment or explanation of the parameter. The values you manipulated in the control panel in the previous exercises are just a small subset of those in the full UnitSpec — see if you can locate them there.

↪ Press Cancel on the unit specs before continuing, which will close the edit dialog and not apply any changes you might have accidentally made.

2.6.2 The Activation Output

In this section, we explore the way in which the unit computes its activation output. The main objective is to understand the relationship between the spiking and rate-code activation functions. We will use the same project as the previous section.

↪ Press `Defaults` to start out with default parameters.

From the previous section, we know that changing the level of excitatory input will affect the membrane potential, and the resulting rate coded activation value. Now let's explore this relationship in the spiking activation function.

↪ Set `act_fun` to `SPIKE`, and press `Apply` and then `Run`.

Instead of the steady values during the input presentation period, you now see the oscillations caused by the spiking mechanism (as we saw previously in figure 2.12). Thus, as soon as the membrane potential crosses the threshold, the activation spikes, and the membrane potential is reset (to a sub-resting potential of 0, reflecting the overshoot of the spiking mechanism). Then, the potential climbs back up, and the process repeats itself.

The spacing between the spikes is inversely proportional to the firing rate, but it can be hard to eyeball this from the graph. Let's look at `act_eq`, the rate-code equivalent spike-rate value as a function of the spike train (see equation 2.18).

↪ Click on the `act_eq` graph line (plotted in blue).

↪ Next, observe the effects of changing `g_bar_e` from .4, first to .38 and then to .42.

Question 2.6 *Describe and explain the effects on the spike rate of decreasing* `g_bar_e` *to .38, and of increasing it to .42.*

The empirically-measured rate-code equivalent for the spiking activation function (`act_eq`) compares fairly closely with the rate-code value computed directly as a function of the membrane potential (act for `NOISY_XX1`), as we saw in figure 2.15.

↪ To explore this relationship in the simulation, you can switch between `SPIKE` and `NOISY_XX1` for different values of `g_bar_e`.

You should observe a reasonably close fit between the final values of `act_eq` for `SPIKE` with that of `NOISY_XX1`. However, with smaller `g_bar_e` values (e.g., .38), the `NOISY_XX1` is somewhat below the spiking `act_eq`. Achieving a much closer fit between spiking and rate coded activations such as that displayed in figure 2.15 requires different parameter values that are not otherwise appropriate for this exploration. This is due to the *aliasing* effects of discrete-time updating (i.e., coarse-grained digitization effects, like when trying to display a photograph on a low-resolution display), which the spiking model is very sensitive to.

↪ Change `g_bar_e` back to its default value of .4., and make sure `act_fun` is set to `SPIKE`.

An important aspect of spiking in real neurons is that the timing and intervals between spikes can be quite random, although the overall rate of firing remains predictable. This is obviously not evident with the single constant input used so far, which results in regular firing. However, if we introduce noise by adding small randomly generated values to the membrane potential, then we can see some of this kind of effect, although it is still not as dramatic as it would be with multiple spiking inputs coming into the cell. Note that this additional noise plays a similar role as the convolution of noise with the XX1 function in the noisy XX1 function, but in the case of the noisy XX1 we have a deterministic function that incorporates the averaged effects of noise, while here we are actually adding in the random values themselves, making the behavior stochastic.

↪ Change the variance of the noise generator (`noise_var` in the control panel) from 0 to .005, and press `Apply` and then `Run`.

It can be difficult to tell from a single run whether the spike timing is random — the unit still fires with some regularity.

↪ Do many `Run`s on top of each other in the graph log.

Now you should see that the spike timing was actually so random that there is essentially a uniform distribution of spike times across these different runs (i.e., a spike could occur at any time step), but the rate code equivalent activation (`act_eq`) nevertheless remained relatively constant (i.e., it had only a few different values at the end of a run). This happens because the precise time at which a spike fires depends greatly on whether the noise happens to move the membrane potential up or down when it approaches the threshold, which can delay or advance the spike timing in a random fashion. Thus, the threshold greatly magnifies small differences in membrane potential by making a large distinction between subthreshold and superthreshold potentials. On average, however, the spikes are equally likely to be early or late, so these random timing differences end up canceling out in the rate code average. This *robustness* of the rate code in the face of random noise (relative to the detailed spike timing) is one important argument for why it is reasonable to think that neurons rely primarily on rate code information (see section 2.8 for more discussion).

Now, let's explore some of the properties of the noisy XX1 rate-code activation function, compared to other possible such functions. We will compare XX1 (equation 2.20), which is the non-noisy version of noisy XX1, and LINEAR, which is just a threshold-linear function of the difference between the membrane potential and the threshold:

$$y_j = \gamma[V_m - \Theta]_+ \qquad (2.21)$$

where $[x]_+$ is again the positive component of x or 0 if x is negative (i.e., if the membrane potential is below threshold).

↪ Press Defaults. Then, change the excitatory input g_bar_e from .4 to .375, and press Apply and then Run. Then, run XX1 with the same parameters (under act_fun, select XX1, press Apply and then Run). Next run LINEAR in the same way.

Notice that NOISY_XX1 starts earlier than XX1 or LINEAR, because it has a soft threshold. This results from convolving the XX1 function with noise, such that even at sub-threshold values, there is a certain chance of getting above threshold, as reflected in a small positive activation value in the rate code.

↪ Change the excitatory input g_bar_e from .375 to .42, and press Apply and then Run. Then, as in the previous procedure, run the other two activation functions with the same parameters.

Notice that LINEAR goes up to ceiling (where it is clipped at a maximum of 1), while XX1 and NOISY_XX1 increase but stay below their maximum

values. Thus, the two XX1 based functions have a saturating nonlinearity that allows them to gradually approach a maximal value, instead of just being clipped off at this maximum. However, these XX1 functions approximate the threshold-linear function for lower levels of excitation.

You should also notice that XX1 and NOISY_XX1 get closer to each other as g_e gets larger. The noise convolution has much less of an effect when the function gets flatter, as it does in the saturating nonlinearity region. Convolving noise with a linear function gives you back the linear function itself, so wherever the function is approximately linear, noise has much less of an effect.

When you are done with this simulation, you can either close this project in preparation for loading the next project, or you can quit completely from the simulator.
↪ Locate the PDP++Root window. To continue on to the next simulation, close this project first by selecting .projects/Remove/Project_0. Or, if you wish to stop now, quit by selecting Object/Quit.

2.6.3 *The Neuron as Detector*

Having explored the basic equations that govern the point neuron activation function, we can now explore the basic function of the neuron: detecting input patterns. We will see how a particular pattern of weights makes a simulated neuron respond more to some input patterns than others. By adjusting the level of excitability of the neuron, we can make the neuron respond only to the pattern that best fits its weights, or in a more graded manner to other patterns that are close to its weight pattern. This provides some insight into why the point neuron activation function works the way it does.

↪ Open the project detector.proj.gz in chapter_2 to begin. (If you closed the previous project and did not quit completely from the simulator, do PDP++Root/.projects/OpenIn/root and select detector.proj.gz.)

As before, the three main windows (NetView, PDP++ Root, control panel) will open up. We begin by examining the NetView window. The network has an *input* which will have patterns of activation in the shape of

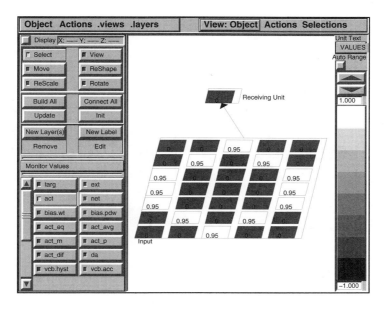

Figure 2.18: The NetView display of the detector network.

different digits, and these input units are connected to the receiving unit via a set of weighted synaptic connections (figure 2.18). Be sure you are familiar with the operation of the NetView, which is explained in appendix A.8. We can view the pattern of weights (synaptic strengths) that this receiving unit has from the input, which should give us an idea about what this unit will detect.

↪ Press the r.wt button on the lower left-hand side of the NetView window (you will probably have to use the scroll bar to find it — it's near the bottom of the list), and then click on the receiving unit.

You should now see the input grid lit up in the pattern of an 8. This is the weight pattern for the receiving unit for connections from the input units, with the weight value displayed in the corresponding sending (input) unit. Thus, when the input units have an activation pattern that matches this weight pattern, the receiving unit will be maximally activated. Input patterns that are close to the target '8' input will produce graded activations as a function of how close they are. Thus, this pattern of weights determines what the unit detects, as we will see. First, we will examine the patterns of

inputs that will be presented to the network.

↪ Press View on the main control panel (detect_ctrl) and select EVENTS.

The window that comes to the foreground (an **EnviroView** window, titled Environment_0) shows all of the different **Events** in the **Environment** that will be presented to a unit to measure its detection responses (figure 2.19). The patterns that are presented to units (and later to networks of units) are contained in an *environment* because it is the environment in the real world that provides the external inputs to brains. Each individual pattern is contained in an *event,* which represents one distinct possible state in the environment. As you can see, the environment in this case contains the digits from 0 to 9, represented in a simple font on a $5x7$ grid of pixels (picture elements). Each pixel in a given event (digit) will drive the corresponding input unit in the network.

To see the unit respond to these input patterns, we will present them one-by-one, and determine why the unit responds as it does given its weights. Thus, we need to view the activations again in the network window.

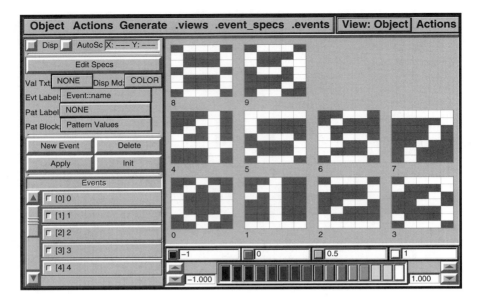

Figure 2.19: The EnviroView display of the input events for the detector network.

↪ Select the `act` button in the lower left hand part of the window (you will probably have to scroll back up, because act is near the top).

↪ Press the `Step` button in the control panel to process the first event in the environment (the digit 0). You will not actually see anything happen. Press `Step` one more time, and you will see the next digit (1) presented.

Each `Step` causes the input units to have their activation values fixed or **clamped** to the values given in the input pattern of the event, followed by a **settling** process where the activation of the receiving unit is iteratively updated over a series of **cycles** according to the point neuron activation function (just as the unit in the previous simulation was updated over time). This settling process continues until the activations in the network approach an *equilibrium* (i.e., the change in activation from one cycle to the next, shown as variable `da` in the simulator, is below some tolerance level). The network view is then updated at the end of settling so that we may view this equilibrium activation state that resulted from processing the input.

You should have seen the input pattern of the digits 0 and 1 in the input layer. However, the receiving unit showed an activity value of 0 for both inputs, meaning that it was not activated above threshold by these input patterns. Before getting into the nitty-gritty of why the unit responded this way, let's proceed through the remaining digits and observe how it responds to other inputs.

↪ Continue to press `Step` until the digit 9 has been presented.

You should have seen the receiving unit activated when the digit 8 was presented, with an activation of zero for all the other digits. Thus, as expected, the receiving unit acts like an "8" detector.

We can use a GraphLog to view the pattern of receiving unit activation across the different input patterns.

↪ Press `View` on the control panel and select `GraphLog`.

The graph shows the activation for the unit as a function of event (and digit) number along the X axis. You should see a flat line with a single peak at 8.

Now, let's try to understand exactly why the unit responds as it does. The key to doing so is to understand the relationship between the pattern of weights and the input pattern. Thus, we will configure the NetView to display both the weights and the current input pattern.

↪ First click on the `act` button (this will probably already be selected, but just make sure). Then, select the `r.wt` as before, except this time use the *middle* mouse button (or hold down the shift key and use the left button). Then, select the receiving unit (it may already have been selected, in which case you can either do nothing, or click twice because your first click will deselect it).

You should now see each unit in the display divided into two, with the left half displaying the activation, and the right half displaying the weight value. Note that activations provided by the environment are clipped to a maximum of .95, so you can use this to tell the difference between the weights (which are at 1) and the activations.

↪ Now `Step` to present the digit 0 again.

Question 2.7 (a) *For each digit, report the number of input units where there is a weight of 1 and the input unit is also active. This should be easily visually perceptible in the display. You should find some variability in these numbers across the digits.* **(b)** *Why does the activation value of the receiving unit not reflect any of this variability?* **(c)** *What would be a better variable to examine in order to view this underlying variability, and why?*

↪ Now, click on the `net` variable in the GraphLog window, to display the net input of the receiving unit in response to each of the digit inputs.

Question 2.8 (a) *What is the general relationship between the plot of the net input and the numbers you computed in the previous question?* **(b)** *Use equation 2.15 in section 2.5.1 to explain exactly how the net input is computed such that it results in the values plotted in the graph for each digit — verify this for a couple of digits. Remember that you can click on the line in the graph to obtain exact numerical values to check your work. The α_k for the input layer projection has been set to $\frac{17}{35}$. (You can use the simplified equation 2.15 rather than equation 2.16, because we are looking at the asymptotic values after settling rather than time-averaging,* `net` *is the same as $g_e(t)\bar{g}_e$, but $\bar{g}_e$ is set to the default of 1 in this case, and the bias weights are 0 and can be ignored (i.e, $\beta = 0$).)*

As a result of working through the above questions, you should now have a detailed understanding of how the net excitatory input to the neuron reflects the degree of match between the input pattern and the weights. You have also observed how the activation value can ignore much of the graded information present in this input signal. Now, we will explore how we can change how much information is conveyed by the activation signal. We will manipulate the leak current (`g_bar_l`), which has a default value of 7, which is sufficient to oppose the strength of the excitatory inputs for all but the strongest (best fitting) input pattern (the 8).

↪ Locate the `detect_ctrl` control panel. Notice the `g_bar_l` variable there, with its default value of 7. Reduce `g_bar_l` to 6. (Note that you can just hit the `Run` button in the control panel to both apply the new value of `g_bar_l` and run the epoch process for one sweep through the digits).

Question 2.9 (a) *What happens to the pattern of receiving unit activity when you reduce* `g_bar_l` *to 6?* **(b)** *What happens with* `g_bar_l` *values of 4, 1, and 8?* **(c)** *Explain the effect of changing* `g_bar_l` *in terms of the point neuron activation function.* **(d)** *What might the consequences of these different response patterns have for other units that might be listening to the output of this receiving unit? Try to give some possible advantages and disadvantages for both higher and lower values of* `g_bar_l`.

It is clearly important how responsive the neuron is to its inputs. However, there are tradeoffs associated with different levels of responsivity. The brain solves this kind of problem by using many neurons to code each input, so that some neurons can be more "high threshold" and others can be more "low threshold" types, providing their corresponding advantages and disadvantages in specificity and generality of response. The bias weights can be an important parameter in determining this behavior. As we will see in the next chapter, our tinkering with the value of the leak current `g_bar_l` is also partially replaced by the inhibitory input, which plays an important role in providing a dynamically adjusted level of inhibition for counteracting the excitatory net input. This ensures that neurons are generally in the right responsivity range for conveying useful information, and it makes each neuron's responsivity dependent on other neurons, which has many important consequences as one can imagine from the above explorations.

Finally, we can peek under the hood of the simulator to see how events are presented to the network. This is done using something called a **process**, which is like a conductor that orchestrates the presentation of the events in the environment to the network. We interact with processes through process *control panels* (not to be confused with the overall simulation control panels; see section A.10.1 in appendix A for more details).

↪ To see the process control panel for this simulation, press `View` on the `detect_ctrl` overall control panel and select `PROCESS_CTRL`.

The `Epoch_0` **EpochProcess** control panel will appear. The `Run` and `Step` buttons on our overall control panel work by essentially pressing the corresponding buttons on this process control panel. Try it. The `ReInit` and `NewInit` buttons initialize the process (to start back at digit 0 in this case) — the former reuses the same random values as the previous run (i.e., starting off with the same random seed), while the latter generates new random values. You can also `Stop` the process, and `GoTo` a specific event. Although the simulation exercises will not typically require you to access these process control panels directly, they are always an option if you want to obtain greater control, and you will have to rely on them when you make your own simulations.

↪ Go to the `PDP++Root` window. To continue on to the next simulation, close this project first by selecting `.projects/Remove/Project_0`. Or, if you wish to stop now, quit by selecting `Object/Quit`.

2.7 Hypothesis Testing Analysis of a Neural Detector

[Note: This section contains more abstract, mathematical ideas that are not absolutely essential for understanding subsequent material. Thus, it could be skipped, but at a loss of some depth and perspective.]

One of the primary ways of expressing and using a computational level description is via mathematical expressions and manipulations. The mathematical language of probability and statistics is particularly appropriate for describing the behavior of individual neurons as detectors. The relevant parts of this language are introduced here. We will see that they provide an interesting explanation for the basic form of the point neuron activation function described previously, which is the main objective of the formalization provided here. Note that there are other more complicated ways of analyzing things that provide a more precise definition of things like the weight values and the net input, which we are less concerned about here (e.g., Hinton & Sejnowski, 1983; McClelland, 1998).

The most relevant branch of statistics here is **hypothesis testing**. The general idea is that you have a **hypothesis** (or two) and some relevant **data** or **evidence**, and you want to determine how well the hypothesis is supported by these data. This provides an alternate language for the same basic operation that a detector performs: the data is the input, and the processing performed by the detector evaluates the hypothesis that the thing (or things) that the detector detects are present given the data (or not). We can identify two important hypotheses for a detector: 1) the hypothesis that the detected thing is really "out there," which we will label h; and 2) the **null hypothesis** that this thing is *not* out there, labeled $\overline{h}$. What we really want to do is compare the relative probabilities of these hypotheses being true, and produce some output that reflects the extent to which our detection hypothesis (h) wins out over the null hypothesis ($\overline{h}$) given the current input.

The result after the detailed derivation that follows is that the probability of h given the current input data d (which is written as $P(h|d)$) is a simple ratio function of two other functions of the relationship between the hypotheses and the data (written here as $f(h, d)$ and $f(\overline{h}, d)$):

$$P(h|d) = \frac{f(h, d)}{f(h, d) + f(\overline{h}, d)} \qquad (2.22)$$

Thus, the resulting probability is just a function of how strong the support for the detection hypothesis h is over the support for the null hypothesis $\overline{h}$. This ratio function may be familiar to some psychologists as the **Luce choice ratio** used in mathematical psychology models for a number of years. We will explore how this functional form maps onto the equilibrium membrane potential equation (equation 2.9), but you can already see that it has the same weighted average quality to it.

Another way of putting the objective of this analysis is that we want to evaluate to what extent a rational agent should believe in one of these hypotheses over the other. This rephrasing can be important because, although it is sometimes possible to actually go around and measure the **objective probabilities** that some hypothesis was true given a particular set of data, this is typically impossible for a number of reasons. Thus, we usually have to settle for a more **subjective** definition of probability that refers to **belief** instead of objective fact. In our analysis, we will start with the case where we know the objective probabilities, so that everything is perfectly clear. However, we will see that using such probabilities quickly becomes intractable due to combinatorial explosion, so we have to rely on subjective probabilities instead.

In either case, probabilities are simply numbers between 0 and 1, where 0 means something never happens (is never true, should never be believed in), and 1 means something always happens (is always true, should always be believed in). Intermediate values mean something in between, with .5 meaning that something happens half the time on average (like flipping a coin and getting "heads"). These intermediate probabilities correspond to intermediate truth or belief values, so that a value of .5 means that something is half-true, or that it should only be half-believed.[1] Another way of putting this is that you should believe in something to a graded extent p, where p is the probability value.

2.7.1 Objective Probabilities and Example

For the purposes of concretely instantiating the probabilistic hypothesis testing framework, we will use the simple detector example shown in figure 2.20. This detector receives inputs from three sources, which we assume are driven by the world, so that when a vertical

---

[1] The distinction between half-believing something and fully believing it half the time is an important one, but we are ultimately concerned here with real-valued, time-averaged numbers that are more consistent with something more like half-belief.

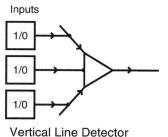

Figure 2.20: Simple vertical line detector that detects presence of vertical line (which amounts to all 3 inputs active). Each input can either be on or off (1 or 0). It is assumed that the inputs are driven in some way by visual signals, and that when there is a vertical line in the visual inputs, all 3 inputs will tend to light up. However, the system is noisy and inputs can be spuriously active or inactive.

			data		
freq	h	h̄	1	2	3
3	0	1	0	0	0
2	0	1	1	0	0
2	0	1	0	1	0
2	0	1	0	0	1
1	0	1	1	1	0
1	0	1	0	1	1
1	0	1	1	0	1
0	0	1	1	1	1
0	1	0	0	0	0
1	1	0	1	0	0
1	1	0	0	1	0
1	1	0	0	0	1
2	1	0	1	1	0
2	1	0	0	1	1
2	1	0	1	0	1
3	1	0	1	1	1
24					

Figure 2.21: All possible states of the world for the vertical line detector. *freq* gives the frequency (number of times) the state occurs in the world. h is the hypothesis that a line exists in the world, n is the null hypothesis that it doesn't exist, and the numbers are for the 3 inputs (data). The given frequencies show that states where more inputs are active are more likely to have the hypothesis true, and vice versa. The bottom line contains the total number of states, which is used in computing probabilities.

line is present, all three sources are likely to be activated. The hypothesis represented by this detector is that a vertical line is actually present in the world. We will represent this hypothesis with the variable h, which is 1 if the hypothesis is true, and 0 if not. The null hypothesis $\overline{h}$ is that a vertical line is not present in the world, and is just the complement (opposite) of h, so that if $h = 1$, then $\overline{h} = 0$ and vice-versa. Another way of putting this is that h and $\overline{h}$ are **mutually exclusive** alternatives: their summed probability is always 1.

To compute objective, **frequency-based probabilities** (as opposed to subjective probabilities) for our example, we need a table of states of the world and their frequencies of occurring. Figure 2.21 shows the table of states that will define our little world for the purposes of this example. Each state consists of values for all of the variables in our world: the two hypotheses and the three data inputs, together with a *frequency* associated with each state that determines how many times this state actually occurs in the world. These frequencies can be seen as a simple shorthand for the objective probabilities of the corresponding events. For example, the events that have a frequency of 3 have an objective probability of 3/24 or .125, where we simply divide by the total frequency over all events (24) to convert from frequency to probability.

There are three basic probabilities that we are interested in that can be computed directly from the world state table. The first is the overall probability that the hypothesis h is true, which is written $P(h = 1)$ or just $P(h)$ for short. This can be computed in the same way as we compute the probability for a single event in the table — just add up all the frequencies associated with states that have $h = 1$ in them, and divide the result by the total frequency (24). This computation is illustrated in figure 2.22a, and gives a result of 12/24 or .5. The next is the probability of the current input data (what we are receiving from our inputs at the present time). To compute this, we need to first pick a particular data state to analyze. Let's choose $d = 110$, which is the case with the first two inputs are active. Figure 2.22b shows that the probability of this data state ($P(d = 110)$ or $P(d)$ for short) is 3/24 (.125) because this condition occurs 1 time when the hypothesis is false, and 2 times when it is true in our little world.

The third probability that we need to know is just the *intersection* of the first two. This is also called the **joint probability** of the hypothesis *and* the data, and is written $P(h = 1, d = 110)$ or $P(h, d)$. Figure 2.22c shows that this is 2/24 (.083).

Our detector is primarily interested in how predictive the data is of the hypothesis being true: it gets some inputs and it wants to know if something is really "out there" or not. The joint probability of the hypothesis and the data clearly seems like an important quantity in this regard, as it indicates how often the hypothesis and data occur together. However, it doesn't quite give us the right information — if we actually got input data of *1 1 0*, we would tend to think that the hypothesis is quite likely to be true, but $P(h = 1, d = 110)$ is only 2/24 or .083, not a particularly large probability. The problem is that we haven't properly *scoped* (limited, restricted — think of a magnifying scope zooming in on a subset of the visual field) the space over which we are computing probabilities — the joint probability tells us how often these two co-occur compared to all other possible states, but we really just want to know how often the hypothesis is true *when we receive the particular input data* we just got. This is given by the **conditional probability** of the hypothesis given the data, which is written as $P(h|d)$, and is defined as follows:

$$P(h|d) = \frac{P(h, d)}{P(d)} \qquad (2.23)$$

So, in our example where we got d=*1 1 0*, we want to know

$$P(h = 1|d = 110) = \frac{P(h = 1, d = 110)}{P(d = 110)} \qquad (2.24)$$

which is (2/24) / (3/24), or .67 according to our table. Thus, matching our intuitions, this tells us that having 2 out of 3 inputs active indicates that it is more likely than not that the hypothesis of a vertical line being present is true. The basic information about how well correlated this input data and the hypothesis are comes from the joint probability in the numerator, but the denominator is critical for scoping this information to the appropriate context (cases where the particular input data actually occurred).

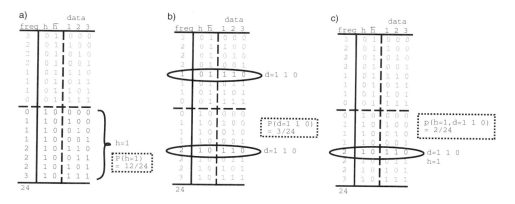

Figure 2.22: The three relevant probabilities computed from the table: **a)** $P(h = 1) = 12/24 = .5$. **b)** $P(d = 110) = 3/24 = .125$. **c)** $P(h = 1, d = 110) = 2/24 = .0833$.

Equation 2.23 is the basic equation that we want the detector to solve, and if we had a table like the one in figure 2.21, then we have just seen that this equation is easy to solve. However, we will see in the next section that having such a table is nearly impossible in the real world. Thus, in the remainder of this section, we will do some algebraic manipulations of equation 2.23 that result in an equation that will be much easier to solve without a table. We will work through these manipulations now, with the benefit of our table, so that we can plug in objective probabilities and verify that everything works. We will then be in a position to jump off into the world of subjective probabilities.

The key player in our reformulation of equation 2.23 is another kind of conditional probability called the **likelihood**. The likelihood is just the opposite conditional probability from the one in equation 2.23: the conditional probability of the data given the hypothesis,

$$P(d|h) = \frac{P(h, d)}{P(h)} \qquad (2.25)$$

It is a little bit strange to think about computing the probability of the *data*, which is, after all, just what was given to you by your inputs (or your experiment), based on your hypothesis, which is the thing you aren't so sure about! However, it all makes perfect sense if instead you think about how likely you would have *predicted* the data based on the assumptions of your hypothesis.

In other words, the likelihood simply computes how well the data fit with the hypothesis. As before, the basic data for the likelihood come from the same joint probability of the hypothesis and the data, but they are scoped in a different way. This time, we scope by all the cases where the hypothesis was true, and determine what fraction of this total had the particular input data state:

$$P(d = 110|h = 1) = \frac{P(h = 1, d = 110)}{P(h = 1)} \qquad (2.26)$$

which is (2/24) / (12/24) or .167. Thus, one would expect to receive this data .167 of the time when the hypothesis is true, which tells you how likely it is you would predict getting this data knowing only that the hypothesis is true.

The main advantage of a likelihood function is that we can often compute it directly as a function of the way our hypothesis is specified, without requiring that we actually know the joint probability $P(h, d)$ (i.e., without requiring a table of all possible events and their frequencies). This makes sense if you again think in terms of predicting data — once you have a well-specified hypothesis, you should in principle be able to predict how likely any given set of data would be under that hypothesis (i.e., assuming the hypothesis is true). We will see more how this works in the case of the neuron-as-detector in the next section.

Assuming that we have a likelihood function that can be computed directly, we would like to be able to write equation 2.23 in terms of these likelihood functions. The following algebraic steps take us there. First, we note that the definition of the likelihood (equation 2.25) gives us a new way of expressing the joint probability term that appears in equation 2.23:

$$P(h, d) = P(d|h)P(h) \qquad (2.27)$$

which can be substituted back into equation 2.23, giving:

$$P(h|d) = \frac{P(d|h)P(h)}{P(d)} \qquad (2.28)$$

This last equation is known as **Bayes formula**, and it provides the starting point for a whole field known as Bayesian statistics. It allows you to write $P(h|d)$, which is called the **posterior** in Bayesian terminology, in terms of the likelihood times the **prior**, which is what $P(h)$ is called. The prior basically indicates how likely the hypothesis is to be true without having seen any data at all — some hypotheses are just more plausible (true more often) than others, and this can be reflected in this term. Priors are often used to favor *simpler* hypotheses as more likely, but this is not necessary. In our application here, the prior terms will end up being constants, which can actually be measured (at least approximately) from the underlying biology.

As in equation 2.23, the likelihood times the prior is normalized by the probability of the data $P(d)$ in Bayes formula. We can replace $P(d)$ with an expression involving only likelihood and prior terms if we make use of our null hypothesis $\overline{h}$. Again, we want to use likelihood terms because they can often be computed directly. Because our hypothesis and null hypothesis are mutually exclusive and sum to 1, we can write the probability of the data in terms of the part of it that overlaps with the hypothesis plus the part that overlaps with the null hypothesis:

$$P(d) = P(h, d) + P(\overline{h}, d) \qquad (2.29)$$

In figure 2.21, this amounts to computing $P(d)$ in the top and bottom halves separately, and then adding these results to get the overall result.

As we did before to get Bayes formula, these joint probabilities can be turned into conditional probabilities with some simple algebra on the conditional probability definition (equation 2.23), giving us the following:

$$P(d) = P(d|h)P(h) + P(d|\overline{h})P(\overline{h}) \qquad (2.30)$$

which can then be substituted into Bayes formula, resulting in:

$$P(h|d) = \frac{P(d|h)P(h)}{P(d|h)P(h) + P(d|\overline{h})P(\overline{h})} \qquad (2.31)$$

This is now an expression that is strictly in terms of just the likelihoods and priors for the two hypotheses! Indeed, this is the equation that we showed at the outset (equation 2.22), with $f(h, d) = P(d|h)P(h)$ and $f(\overline{h}, d) = P(d|\overline{h})P(\overline{h})$. It has a very simple $\frac{h}{h+\overline{h}}$ form, which reflects a *balancing* of the likelihood in favor of the hypothesis with that against it. It is this form that the biological properties of the neuron implement, as we will see more explicitly in a subsequent section.

Before continuing, let's verify that equation 2.31 produces the same result as equation 2.23 for the case we have been considering all along ($P(h = 1|d = 110)$). First, we know that the likelihood $P(d = 110|h = 1)$ according to the table is (2/24) / (12/24) or .167. Also, $P(h) = .5$, and $P(\overline{h}) = .5$ as well. The only other thing we need is $P(d|\overline{h})$, which we can see from the table is (1/24)/(12/24) or .083. The result is thus:

$$\begin{aligned} P(h|d) &= \frac{P(d|h)P(h)}{P(d|h)P(h) + P(d|\overline{h})P(\overline{h})} \\ &= \frac{.167 * .5}{.167 * .5 + .083 * .5} = .67 \end{aligned} \qquad (2.32)$$

So, we can see that this result agrees with the previously computed value. Obviously, if you have the table, this seems like a rather indirect way of computing things, but we will see in the next section how the likelihood terms can be computed without a table.

2.7.2 Subjective Probabilities

Everything we just did was quite straightforward because we had a world state table, and could therefore compute objective probabilities. However, when more than just a few inputs are present, a table like that in figure 2.21 becomes intractably large due to the huge number of different unique combinations of input states. For example, if the inputs are binary (which is not actually true for neurons, so it's even worse), the table requires 2^{n+1} entries for n inputs, with the extra factor of two (accounting for the +1 in the exponent) reflecting the fact that all possibilities must be considered twice, once under each hypothesis. This is roughly $1.1x10^{301}$ for just 1,000 inputs (and our calculator gives Inf as a result if we plug in a conservative guess of 5,000 inputs for a cortical neuron). This is the main reason why we need to develop subjective ways of computing probabilities.

As we have stated, the main way we avoid using a table of objective probabilities is to use likelihood terms that can be computed *directly as a function of the input data and the specification of the hypothesis*, without reference to objective probabilities and the requisite table. When we directly compute a likelihood function, we effectively make a set of *assumptions* about the nature of the hypothesis and its relationship with the data, and then compute the likelihood under these assumptions. In general, we have no way of validating these assumptions (which would require the intractable table), so we must instead evaluate the *plausibility* of the assumptions and their relationship to the hypotheses.

One plausible assumption about the likelihood function for a detector is that it is directly (linearly) proportional to the number of inputs that match what the detector is trying to detect. Thus, we use a set of parameters to specify to what extent each input source is representative of the hypothesis that something interesting is "out there." These parameters are just our standard weight parameters w. Together with the linear proportionality assumption, this gives a likelihood function that is a normalized linear function of the weighted inputs:

$$P(d|h) = \frac{1}{z} \sum_i d_i w_i \qquad (2.33)$$

where d_i is the value of one input source i (e.g., $d_i = 1$ if that source detected something, and 0 otherwise), and the normalizing term $\frac{1}{z}$ ensures that the result is a valid probability between 0 and 1. We will see in a moment

that we need not be too concerned with the value of z. First, we want to emphasize what has been done here.

Equation 2.33 means that input patterns d become more probable when there is activity on input sources d_i that are thought to reflect the presence of something of interest in the world, as parameterized by the weight value w_i. Thus, if $w_i = 1$, we care about that input, but if it is 0, we don't care (because it is not relevant to our hypothesis). Furthermore, the overall likelihood is just the (normalized) sum of all these individual source-level contributions — our detector does not represent *interactions* among the inputs. The beauty of the Bayesian framework is that it enables us to use these definitions (or any others that we might also find plausible), to then compute in a rational manner the extent to which we should believe a given hypothesis to be true in the context of a particular data input. Of course, garbage-in gives garbage-out, so the whole thing rests on how good (plausible) the likelihood definition is.

In effect, what we have done with equation 2.33 is provided a *definition* of exactly what the hypothesis h is, by explicitly stating how likely any given input pattern would be assuming this hypothesis were true. The fact that we are defining probabilities, not measuring them, makes these probabilities subjective. They no longer correspond to frequencies of objectively measurable events in the world. Nevertheless, by working out our equations in the previous section *as if* we had objective probabilities, and establishing a self-consistent mathematical framework via Bayes formula, we are assured of using our subjective probabilities in the most "rational" way possible.

The objective world defined by the state table in figure 2.21 corresponds to the definition of the likelihood given by equation 2.33, because the frequency (objective probability) of each input state when the hypothesis h is true is proportional to the number of active inputs in that state — this is exactly what our assumption was in constructing equation 2.33. As you can verify yourself, the equation for the likelihood in the objective world is

$$P(d|h) = \frac{1}{12} \sum_i x_i w_i \qquad (2.34)$$

where we assume that the weights for the 3 input sources are all 1 (figure 2.23). To illustrate the impor-

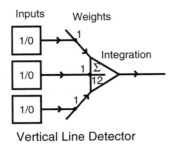

Figure 2.23: Computing of likelihood by integrating weighted input values. Inputs (x_i) are connected to the detector with a weight (w_i) of 1, and integrated using $\frac{1}{12} \sum_i x_i w_i$, resulting in the likelihood value $P(d|h)$.

tance of weights, we could add additional inputs with w_i parameters of 0 (e.g., from nonvertical input sources), and add corresponding entries in the table. We would just have to ensure that the probabilities (frequencies) of these new entries retained the property of proportionality with the number of active inputs *that matter* (i.e., that have $w_i = 1$, meaning that they correspond to a vertical line, and not some other angle of line).

To use our Bayesian equation (equation 2.31), it is equally important to establish a definition of the likelihood of the *null* hypothesis $\overline{h}$. As we can see from this equation, the **null likelihood** $P(d|\overline{h})$ serves as a **counterweight** that balances against the strength of the likelihood term to give a reasonable overall probability. One possible definition of this null likelihood is that it is linearly proportional to the extent that inputs that should be on are not in fact on. This is the form of the null likelihood that corresponds with our world state table:

$$P(d|\overline{h}) = \frac{1}{12} \sum_i (1 - x_i) w_i \qquad (2.35)$$

Now, let's plug our likelihood equations into equation 2.31, together with the simple assumption that the prior probabilities are equal, $P(h) = P(\overline{h}) = .5$:

$$
\begin{aligned}
P(h|d) &= \frac{P(d|h)P(h)}{P(d|h)P(h) + P(d|\overline{h})P(\overline{h})} \\
&= \frac{\frac{.5}{12} \sum_i x_i w_i}{\frac{.5}{12} \sum_i x_i w_i + \frac{.5}{12} \sum_i (1 - x_i) w_i}
\end{aligned}
$$

$$
= \frac{\sum_i x_i w_i}{\sum_i x_i w_i + \sum_i (1 - x_i) w_i} \qquad (2.36)
$$

Note that the normalizing factors of $\frac{1}{z}$ canceled out, which is why we said that we don't really need to be too concerned with them.

Equation 2.36 can be directly evaluated by plugging in x_i values (and weight parameters), without any need to consult a world state table. For our previous example of $d = 110$, we get $2/(2 + 1) = 2/3 = .67$, just as we found previously. As we will see in a moment, our point neuron model is actually using something very much like this computation. Thus, we can say that, conditional upon accepting the plausibility of the relevant assumptions, the neuron can be a rational detector!

Before continuing, we should also note that there are a variety of alternative assumptions that one could make about how the likelihood is computed, which also have relevance for neural network models. For example, Hinton and Sejnowski (1983) showed that the more abstract artificial neural network activation function of a sigmoidal function of the net input (summed weighted inputs) results from a particular kind of *independence* assumption in computing the likelihood term (see McClelland, 1998 for an updated treatment of these ideas). Their analysis also assumes that the weights have the property that $w_{ij} = \log \frac{p(d_i|h)}{p(d_i|\overline{h})} \frac{p(\overline{d}_i|h)}{p(\overline{d}_i|\overline{h})}$, which in addition to being a somewhat complex assumption about the weights, also requires the weights to take on arbitrary positive and negative values. This unfortunately violates the biologically based notion that weights are positive-valued or negative-valued, but not both.

The essential difference between the approach we have taken here and that of Hinton and Sejnowski (1983) is that we have separated out the contributions of the likelihood and the null likelihood, whereas they have combined them together into a ratio. This difference is consistent with the essential difference between the point neuron function and the sigmoid — the point neuron separates out the excitatory (likelihood) and inhibitory/leak (null likelihood) terms, whereas the sigmoid just combines them both together. In the broad scheme of hypothesis testing, either framework is equally valid (although the Hinton & Sejnowski, 1983 approach has the advantage of making more rigorous probabilistic assumptions about the weight values), but the particular assumptions of our approach end up being more applicable to what the biological neuron seems to be doing.

2.7.3 Similarity of V_m and $P(h|d)$

Finally, we can compare the equation for the equilibrium membrane potential (equation 2.9 from section 2.4.6) with the hypothesis testing function we just developed (equation 2.31). For ease of reference the equilibrium membrane potential equation is:

$$V_m = \frac{g_e \bar{g}_e E_e + g_i \bar{g}_i E_i + g_l \bar{g}_l E_l}{g_e \bar{g}_e + g_i \bar{g}_i + g_l \bar{g}_l} \qquad (2.37)$$

The general idea is that excitatory input plays the role of something like the likelihood or support for the hypothesis, and the inhibitory input and leak current both play the role of something like support for null hypotheses. Because we have considered only one null hypothesis in the preceding analysis (though it is easy to extend it to two), we will just ignore the leak current for the time being, so that the inhibitory input will play the role of the null hypothesis.

To compare the biological equation with our hypothesis testing equation, we need to use appropriate values of the reversal potentials, so that the resulting membrane potential lives on the same $0 - 1$ range that probabilities do. Thus, we will assume that excitatory input drives the potential toward 1 (i.e., $E_e = 1$), and that the inhibitory (and leak) currents drive the potential toward 0 (i.e., $E_i = E_l = 0$). This makes sense considering that complete support (i.e., only excitation) for the hypothesis should result in a probability of 1, and complete absence of support (i.e., no excitation, all inhibition/leak) should result in a probability of 0. If we substitute these values into the biological equation, we get the following relationship:

$$V_m \approx P(h|d)$$
$$\frac{g_e \bar{g}_e}{g_e \bar{g}_e + g_i \bar{g}_i} \approx \frac{P(d|h)P(h)}{P(d|h)P(h) + P(d|\bar{h})P(\bar{h})}$$
$$(2.38)$$

The equations are identical under the following assumptions: 1) excitation can be equated with the hy-

pothesis that the neuron is detecting and inhibition with the null hypothesis (as we assumed above); 2) the fraction of channels open gives the corresponding likelihood value ($g_e \approx P(d|h)$ for excitation and $g_i \approx P(d|\bar{h})$ for inhibition), which is essentially what we assumed already by computing the likelihood as a function of the sending activations times the weights; 3) the baseline conductance levels, $\bar{g}_e$ and $\bar{g}_i$, represent the prior probability values, $P(h)$ and $P(\bar{h})$, respectively. Note that the ratio form of the equation ensures that any uniform linear scaling of the parameters cancels out. Thus, even though the actual values of the relevant biological parameters are not on a $0 - 1$ scale and have no other apparent relationship to probabilities, we can still interpret them as computing a rationally motivated detection computation.

The full equation for V_m with the leak current (equation 2.9) can be interpreted as reflecting the case where there are two different (and independent) null hypotheses, represented by inhibition and leak. As we will see in more detail in chapter 3, inhibition dynamically changes as a function of the activation of other units in the network, whereas leak is a constant that sets a basic minimum standard against which the detection hypothesis is compared. Thus, each of these can be seen as supporting a different kind of null hypothesis. Although neither of these values is computed in the same way as the null likelihood in our example (equation 2.35), this just means that a different set of assumptions, which can be explicitly enumerated, are being used.

Taken together, this analysis provides a satisfying computational-level interpretation of the biological activation mechanism, and assures us that the neuron is integrating its information in a way that makes good statistical sense.

2.8   The Importance of Keeping It Simple

So far, we have articulated a very simple view of the neuron as a detector, and shown how this is consistent with its biological properties, and with a mathematical description of neural function based on hypothesis testing. Thus, this detector model, together with the importance of graded processing and learning, provide a basis for thinking that the neuron performs a relatively simple task. However, conspiring against this idea is the huge amount of biological complexity present in the neuron, and the vast amount of information processing power that a neuron could potentially exhibit. For example, Shepherd and Brayton (1987) and others have argued that the dendrites of a neuron could potentially perform complex processing on neural inputs, including various logical operations (AND, OR, NOT, etc.). Further, a sequence of output spikes from a neuron could potentially convey a huge amount of information by varying the timing between spikes in systematic ways (c.f., Reike et al., 1996). Thus, each individual neuron could be more like a complex CPU instead of a simpler detector.

Although there is clearly room for different perspectives on the relative complexity of neural processing, our view is motivated by the following considerations:

- Learning requires a graded, proportional response to bootstrap changes, as described in the introduction and later in chapters 4–6. The more a neuron is viewed as performing lots of discrete logical operations, or communicating via precise spike timing, the more *brittle* it becomes to the changes induced by learning, and the less likely there will be a robust, powerful learning algorithm for such neurons. Without such a learning mechanism, it becomes overwhelmingly difficult to organize networks of such neurons to perform effectively together.

- The brain is evidently quite robust to noise and damage. For example, the constant pumping of blood through the brain results in significant movement of neural tissue, which undoubtedly introduces some kinds of noise into processing, and there are many other known sources of noise due to the unreliability of various biological mechanisms (e.g., neurotransmitter release). In addition, many drugs have substantial effects on the detailed firing properties of individual neurons, but their effect on cognition is graded, not catastrophic. Further, surprisingly high levels of diffuse damage (e.g., loss of neurons) can be sustained before it has any measurable effects on cognition. As we saw earlier, the rate code is very robust to noise, while the detailed spike timing is not.

- Each neuron receives as many as 10,000 or even 100,000 inputs from other neurons, and yet it only sends one output signal. If it is computing detailed logical operations on these inputs or paying attention to the detailed spike timing of individual inputs, the complexity and difficulty of organizing such a large number of such operations would be tremendous. Further, all this complexity and detail must somehow be reduced down to a single output signal in the end, which will provide just one tiny fraction of the total input to other neurons, so it is not clear what the point of all this complex processing would be in the end.

Finally, the bottom line is that we are able to model a wide range of cognitive phenomena with the simple detector-style neurons, so any additional complexity does not appear to be necessary, at least at this point.

2.9   Self-Regulation: Accommodation and Hysteresis

[Note: This section is optional, because the mechanisms described herein are applicable to a more limited range of phenomena, and are not active by default in most simulations. Readers may wish to come back to this material later when they find a need for these mechanisms.]

In addition to the integration of inputs and thresholded communication of outputs, neurons have more complex activation dynamics that can result in the modification of responses to subsequent inputs as a function of prior activation history. These can be thought of as a form of **self-regulation** of the neuron's response. Although we think that these dynamics make an important contribution to behavior, and we incorporate them into some of our simulations (e.g., sections 3.6.5, 8.5.2, and 8.6.1), most of the time we just ignore them for the sake of simplicity. We can partially justify this simplification on the grounds that most simulations are concerned only with the activation state produced in roughly the first several hundred milliseconds of processing on a given input pattern, and these self-regulatory dynamics do not enter into the picture until after that.

Perhaps the most important source of what we have termed self-regulatory dynamics in the neuron are voltage and calcium gated channels, of which a large number have been described (see Johnston & Wu, 1995 for a textbook treatment). These channels open and close as a function of the instantaneous activity (voltage-gated) and averaged prior activity (calcium-gated, where internal calcium concentrations reflect prior activation history). Consistent with the need for simplification in cognitive-level models, we summarize more complicated biological mechanisms into two broad categories of self-regulatory effects: **accommodation** and **hysteresis**.

We use the term *accommodation* to refer to any inhibitory current (typically a K^+ channel) that is typically opened by increasing calcium concentrations, resulting in the subsequent inhibition of the neuron. The longer acting GABA-B inhibitory synaptic channel may also play a role in accommodation. Thus, a neuron that has been active for a while will *accommodate* or *fatigue* and become less and less active for the same amount of excitatory input. In contrast, hysteresis refers to excitatory currents (mediated by Na^+ or Ca^{++} ions) that are typically opened by elevated membrane potentials, and cause the neuron to remain active for some period of time even if the excitatory input fades or disappears.

The opposition between the two forces of accommodation and hysteresis, which would otherwise seem to cancel each other out, is resolved by the fact that hysteresis appears to operate over a shorter time period based on membrane potential values, whereas accommodation appears to operate over longer time periods based on calcium concentrations. Thus, neurons that have been active have a short-term tendency to remain active (hysteresis), but then get fatigued if they stay active longer (accommodation). Indeed, some of the hysteresis-type channels are actually turned off by increasing calcium concentrations. We will see in later chapters that the longer-term accommodation results in a tendency for the network to switch to a different interpretation, or locus of attention, for a given input pattern.

The detailed implementation of these processes in the simulator is spelled out in the following section.

2.9.1 Implementation of Accommodation and Hysteresis

As we stated, our implementation of self-regulatory dynamics represents a simplification of the underlying biological mechanisms. We use the same basic equations for accommodation and hysteresis, with the different effects dictated by the parameters. The basic approach is to capture the delayed effects of accommodation and hysteresis by using a *basis* variable b that represents the gradual accumulation of activation pressure for the relevant channels (e.g., calcium concentration, or persistently elevated membrane potential). The actual activation of the channel is then a function of this basis variable. Once the basis variable gets above an *activation threshold* value Θ_a, the conductance of the channel begins to increase with a specified time constant (dt_g). Then, once the basis falls below a second (lower) *deactivation threshold* value Θ_d, the conductance decreases again with the same time constant.

First, we will go through the example of the computation of the accommodation conductance $g_a(t)$ with basis variable $b_a(t)$, and then show how the same equations can be used for hysteresis. The gated nature of the channel is captured by the following function:

$$g_a(t) = \begin{cases} g_a(t-1) + dt_{g_a}(1 - g_a(t-1)); & \text{if}(b_a(t) > \Theta_a) \\ g_a(t-1) + dt_{g_a}(0 - g_a(t-1)); & \text{if}(b_a(t) < \Theta_d) \end{cases}$$

$$(2.39)$$

This accommodation conductance $g_a(t)$ is then used in a diffusion-corrected current equation:

$$I_a(t) = g_a(t)\bar{g}_a(V_m(t) - E_a) \qquad (2.40)$$

which is then added together with the other standard conductances (excitation, inhibition, and leak) to get the net current (see equation 2.6). Note that accommodation has an inhibitory effect because E_a is set to be at the resting potential (as is appropriate for a K^+ channel). Finally, the basis variable for accommodation, $b_a(t)$, is updated as a function of the activation value of the neuron:

$$b_a(t) = b_a(t-1) + dt_{b_a}(y_j(t) - b_a(t-1)) \quad (2.41)$$

where $y_j(t)$ is the activation value of the neuron. Thus, the basis value is just a time average of the activation state, with a time constant of dt_{b_a}.

The computation of hysteresis is the same as that of accommodation, except that the basis variable time constant is faster (dt_{b_h} is typically .05 compared to a typical value of .01 for dt_{b_a}), and the reversal potential E_h is excitatory (see table 2.1 for typical values).

Exploration of Accommodation and Hysteresis

↪   Open the project `self_reg.proj.gz` in `chapter_2` to begin.

It looks pretty much like the `unit.proj.gz` simulation you explored earlier, except that it plots more variables (the basis and conductance values for accommodation and hysteresis), and contains more parameters to control these self-regulatory channels in the control panel. On the `self_reg_ctrl` overall control panel, you should notice at the bottom that there are `on_cycle` and `off_cycle` parameters for two "stimuli."

↪   Iconify the NetView window, and `View` the `GRAPH_LOG`.

Note that the graph log has the same variables as before, plus four new ones. We will examine them in a moment, but first let's run the simulation.

↪ Press the `Run` button.

You should see that the activation result (without either accommodation or hysteresis turned on yet) is just as one would expect — a bump at 10 cycles lasting until 100, and another from 300 to 400. Note in particular that there is no apparent effect of the prior activation on the response to the latter one.

Now, let's turn on accommodation.

↪ Click the `on` button in the `acc` field (which contains the accommodation channel parameters) of the control panel and press `Apply`. Then, in the graph log window, click on the `vcb.acc` and `gc.a` buttons, which will cause the basis variable for accommodation (`vcb.acc`) and the net conductance for accommodation (`gc.a`) to be displayed in the graph. Press `Run` again.

You should observe that the `vcb.acc` line increases when the unit becomes active, but that it does not quite reach the activation threshold, which is set to .7 (see `a_thr` in the `acc` field of the control panel).

The unit needs to remain active for a little bit longer for the basis variable to accumulate to the point of ac-

tivation. One way we could achieve this is to set the `off_cycle` time for the first stimulus (`stim1`) to be somewhat later.

↪   Set the `off_cycle` time for the first stimulus (`stim1`) to 150 instead of 100, and then press `Run` again.

Now you should observe that the `gc.a` accommodation conductance starts to increase just before the stimulus goes off. Even though the unit becomes inactive, it takes a while for the basis variable to decrease to the deactivation threshold (.1, in `d_thr` of the `acc` field). Indeed, it takes so long that by the time the next input stimulus comes in at 300 cycles, there is still a strong accommodation current (`gc.a`), and the unit is not immediately activated by the input. Only at around 350 cycles, when the basis variable finally goes below the deactivation threshold, and thus `gc.a` starts to decrease, does the unit then become active.

Had this unit been in a network with other units that received input from the second stimulus, but some of these were not activated by the first stimulus, then these other units would get active immediately because they were not "fatigued," and they would produce a different representation of the input. Thus, accommodation provides one means for a network to respond differently to subsequent inputs based on prior activity.

At this point, you can explore the various parameters in the `acc` field, to make sure you understand what they do.

↪   For example, play with `g_bar_acc`, which determines the strength of the overall accommodation current. Change `g_bar_acc` from .5 to .3, and you should see that this is too weak to completely prevent the unit from immediately becoming active when the second stimulus comes in at 300 cycles.

Now, let's add hysteresis into the mix.

↪   First press the `Defaults` button to return to the default parameters. Then click on the `vcb.hyst` and `gc.h` buttons in the graph log, click the `on` button in the `hyst` field and press `Apply`, and then `Run`.

You should see that the unit remains active for some time after the input stimulus goes off at 100 cycles — this is caused by the hysteresis. Further, this additional period of activation causes the accommodation current to get activated, which eventually turns the unit off. As a result of this accommodation, as we saw before, the unit does not then get activated immediately by the second input.

↪ Now, you can play with the `hyst` parameters and see what they do to the unit's response properties.

In summary, you can see that there is considerable potential for complex dynamics to emerge from the interactions of these different channels. The fact that actual neurons have many such channels with even more complex dynamics suggests that our basic point neuron model is probably a lot simpler than the real thing. Due to pragmatic constraints, we typically ignore much of this complexity. As the simulations later in the text demonstrate, such simplifications do not make that much of a difference in the core aspects of behavior that we are modeling.

↪ To stop now, quit by selecting `Object/Quit` in the `PDP++Root` window.

2.10 Summary

Neuron as Detector

The biological and functional properties of a neuron are consistent with it being a **detector**, which constantly evaluates the information available to it looking for conditions that match those that it has become specialized to detect. Whereas standard serial computers are relatively *general purpose* computational devices, a neuron is relatively **specialized** or **dedicated** to detecting some particular set of things. We emphasize that it is typically difficult to describe exactly what a neuron detects with simple verbal terms (e.g., unlike "smoke" for the smoke detector), and that there is an important dynamic component to its behavior. Neurons exist in huge numbers and operate in **parallel** with one another, whereas a standard computer operates in serial performing one operation at a time. There are good reasons to think that neurons perform a relatively simple computation. A mathematical description of a neuron as a detector can be given using the framework of Bayesian statistical hypothesis testing, which produces the same form of mathematical activation function as the point neuron activation function. In sum, the detector model of the neuron provides a good intuitive model of how they

function, and can help to make sense of their underlying biological properties.

Biology of the Neuron

The neuron is an **electrophysiological** entity that can be understood using the principles of electricity and diffusion. **Inputs** come into the neuron primarily through **channels** located in **synapses**, allowing charged atoms or **ions** into and out of the neuron. Different ions have different **concentrations** on the inside and outside of a neuron, and this leads to the generation of **electrical current** when channels open and allow ions to flow along their concentration gradients (because of **diffusion**) into or out of the cell. Thus, neurons become **excited** when positively charged sodium ions (Na^+) enter the cell through synaptic channels in their receiving areas called **dendrites**. These synaptic channels are opened by the **neurotransmitter** known as **glutamate**, which is released by the sending or **presynaptic** neuron. Different inputs can provide different amounts of activation depending on both how much neurotransmitter is released by the sender and how many channels on the **postsynaptic** (receiving) neuron open as a result. These different **synaptic efficacies** for different inputs, which we refer to as **weights**, are critical for determining what it is that a neuron detects. Neurons become **inhibited** when negatively charged chloride ions (Cl^-) enter the neuron through channels that are opened by the neurotransmitter **GABA**, which is released by **inhibitory interneurons**. They also have a basic negative current caused by positive ions (potassium, K^+) *leaving* the neuron via **leak** channels that are always open. A simple equation describes the way in which the overall electrical voltage of the cell, known as its **membrane potential**, integrates all these currents into one real-valued number.

The membrane potential that results from integrating neural inputs in turn determines whether a given neuron will produce an **action potential** or **spike**, which causes neurotransmitter to be released at the ends of a neuron's sending projection or **axon**, which then forms **synapses** onto other neuron's dendrites (see above). The action potential is **thresholded**, meaning that it only occurs when the membrane potential (at the start of the axon, called the **axon hillock**) gets above a certain critical value, called the *threshold*. Thresholding means that neurons only communicate when they have detected something with some level of confidence, which is biologically and computationally efficient.

Computational Implementation of the Neural Activation Function

Leabra uses a simple **point neuron** activation function based on shrinking the geometry of the neuron to a point, but retaining some of the properties of the dendritic structure in the way the **net input** is computed. The resulting membrane potential update equation is taken straight from the biology, and produces the same **equilibrium potential** values as an equation derived from first principles based on the computational level detector model of a neuron. To compute an **output activation** value as a function of the membrane potential, we can either use a very simple spiking mechanism, or a **rate code** function, which provides a real-valued number representing the instantaneous frequency (rate) with which the cell would produce spikes based on a given membrane potential. The rate code also represents a *scaling assumption* where individual units in the model represent a number of roughly similar neurons, such that the average impact of many such spiking neurons is approximated by the rate code value. The spike rate function has a **saturating nonlinearity**, which is biologically determined by a number of factors including the **refractory period** just after a spike (where it is essentially impossible to fire another), and the rate at which the synapses can release neurotransmitter. The nonlinearity of the activation function is important for the computational power of neural networks, and for producing stable activation states in interactive networks.

Self-Regulation

Neurons have a number of **voltage gated** and **calcium gated** channels that affect the way the neuron responds based on its prior history of activity. Two such mechanisms are included in Leabra, though they are not essential aspects of the algorithm and are not used in most

simulations. One is **accommodation**, which causes a neuron which has been active for a while to "get tired" and become less and less active for the same amount of excitatory input. The other is **hysteresis**, which causes a neuron that has been active to remain active for some period of time even when its excitatory input disappears. These two mechanisms are obviously in conflict with each other, but this is not a problem because hysteresis operates over a shorter time period, and accommodation over a longer one.

2.11   Further Reading

Johnston and Wu (1995) provides a very detailed and mathematically sophisticated treatment of neurophysiology, starting from basic physical principles and covering issues of dendritic morphology, cable properties, active channels, synaptic release, and the like.

Koch and Segev (1998) provides a recent update to a watershed collection of papers on biophysical models of the neuron.

Shepherd (1990) has a strong synaptic focus, and represents the "complex neuron" hypothesis, in contrast to the "simple neuron" hypothesis developed here.

The *Neuron* (Hines & Carnevale, 1997) and *Genesis* (Bower & Beeman, 1994) simulators are two of the most popular computational tools used to construct complex, biophysically realistic neuron-level models.

Chapter 3

Networks of Neurons

Contents

3.1	Overview	**71**
3.2	**General Structure of Cortical Networks**	**72**
3.3	**Unidirectional Excitatory Interactions: Transformations**	**75**
	3.3.1 Exploration of Transformations	*79*
	3.3.2 Localist versus Distributed Representations	*82*
	3.3.3 Exploration of Distributed Representations .	*84*
3.4	**Bidirectional Excitatory Interactions**	**85**
	3.4.1 Bidirectional Transformations	*86*
	3.4.2 Bidirectional Pattern Completion	*87*
	3.4.3 Bidirectional Amplification	*89*
	3.4.4 Attractor Dynamics	*92*
3.5	**Inhibitory Interactions**	**93**
	3.5.1 General Functional Benefits of Inhibition . .	*94*
	3.5.2 Exploration of Feedforward and Feedback Inhibition	*95*
	3.5.3 The k-Winners-Take-All Inhibitory Functions	*100*
	3.5.4 Exploration of kWTA Inhibition	*103*
	3.5.5 Digits Revisited with kWTA Inhibition . . .	*104*
	3.5.6 Other Simple Inhibition Functions	*105*
3.6	**Constraint Satisfaction**	**106**
	3.6.1 Attractors Again	*108*
	3.6.2 The Role of Noise	*108*
	3.6.3 The Role of Inhibition	*109*
	3.6.4 Explorations of Constraint Satisfaction: Cats and Dogs	*109*
	3.6.5 Explorations of Constraint Satisfaction: Necker Cube	*111*
3.7	**Summary**	**112**
3.8	**Further Reading**	**114**

3.1 Overview

Although the neuron provides the basic unit of processing, a **network** of such neurons is required to accomplish everything but the most simple tasks. In the previous chapter we were able to describe the essential computation performed by the neuron in terms of the detector model. No such simple, overarching computational metaphor applies to the computation performed by the entire network. Instead, we adopt a two-pronged approach to understanding how networks work: first, in this chapter, we identify and explore several important principles that govern the general behavior of networks; second, in the next chapter, we show how learning, which is responsible for setting the detailed weight values that specify what each unit detects, can shape the behavior of networks according to various principles that build upon those developed in this chapter.

We begin with a summary of the general structure and patterns of connectivity within the mammalian *cortex* (neocortex), which establishes a biological basis for the general types of networks we use. There are many commonalities across all cortical areas in terms of neuron types and general patterns of connectivity, which give rise to a canonical or generic cortical network structure that can be used for modeling all kinds of different psychological phenomena. As explained in the previous chapter (section 2.3.3), excitation and inhibition are separated in the cortex, because they are implemented by different types of neurons with different patterns of connectivity. This separation is useful for understanding the basic principles governing network function.

We explore the properties of two major types of excitatory connectivity, *unidirectional* and *bidirectional*. The unidirectional or *feedforward* processing of information via excitatory interactions performs information processing *transformations* essential for cognition. Bidirectional connectivity has many advantages over unidirectional connectivity, and is predominant in the cortex. However, it requires inhibition to control positive excitatory feedback.

The effects of cortical inhibition can be summarized by a simplifying inhibitory function, which we then use to explore bidirectional excitation in the context of inhibition. In the end, it will become clear how both excitation and inhibition, although separable, are intricately intertwined in overall network behavior. It is possible to summarize the overall effects of these interactions in terms of *constraint satisfaction*, where networks achieve a state of activation that simultaneously maximizes the satisfaction of external constraints from the environment and internal constraints from patterns of weights connecting the neurons.

3.2   General Structure of Cortical Networks

The cerebral cortex or **neocortex** forms the outer part of the brain and is most enlarged in humans relative to other mammals. An abundance of data supports the idea that this is where much of the neural activity underlying cognition takes place (nevertheless, it is important to remember that the cortex depends critically on many other **subcortical** brain areas for its proper functioning). The cortex can be divided into a number of different **cortical areas** that are specialized for different kinds of processing — as we will see in the second half of this book, some areas are critical for recognizing objects, others process spatial information, and still others perform language processing, higher level planning, and the like.

Despite the apparent functional specialization of the cortex, we are able to use a common set of principles in modeling the cognitive functions associated with a wide range of cortical areas. This can be attributed to the fact that the cortex has a fairly consistent general structure that applies across all of the different cortical areas. Thus, the functional specializations of the cortex seem to take place within a common network structure, which can be simulated within a common computational framework. The properties of this structure are the topic of this section.

The detailed description of the biological properties of cortex is the topic of entire books (e.g., White, 1989a) — we will condense these details considerably here. First, there are two general classes of neurons that have been identified in the cortex: **excitatory neurons** that release the excitatory neurotransmitter **glutamate**, and **inhibitory neurons** that release the inhibitory neurotransmitter **GABA** (see section 2.4.4 for details on these transmitters).

There are two primary subtypes of excitatory neurons, the **pyramidal** and **spiny stellate** neurons, and a larger number of different subtypes of inhibitory neurons, with the **chandelier** and **basket** being some of the most prevalent (figure 3.1). The excitatory neurons constitute roughly 85 percent of the total number of neurons in the cortex (White, 1989a), and are apparently responsible for carrying much of the information flow, because they form long-range projections to different areas of the cortex and to subcortical areas. Thus, most of the following discussion of connectivity is focused on these excitatory neurons. Although the inhibitory neurons receive both long-range and localized inputs, they project within small localized areas of cortex, which is consistent with their hypothesized role of providing inhibitory regulation of the level of excitation in the cortex (section 3.5).

Cortical neurons are organized into six distinct layers (figure 3.2). The six cortical layers have been identified on anatomical grounds and are important for understanding the detailed biology of the cortex. However, for our purposes, we can simplify the picture by considering three **functional layers**: the **input**, **hidden**, and **output** layers (figure 3.3). We will use the term *layer* to refer to these functional layers, and the term *cortical layer* for the biologically based layers. As with the kinds of simplifications of the biology that we made in the previous chapter, one should regard this simplification into functional layers as only a rough (but useful) approximation to the underlying biology.

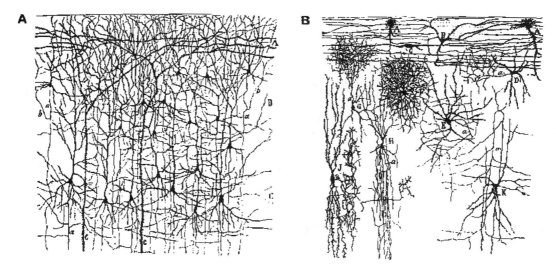

Figure 3.1: Images of the neural structure of the cortex. A) shows the dense web of connectivity among pyramidal neurons. B) shows a number of the other different neuron types, including chandelier and basket interneurons. Reproduced from Crick and Asanuma (1986).

The input layer corresponds to cortical layer 4, which usually receives the sensory input by way of a subcortical brain area called the **thalamus**, which receives information from the retina and other sense organs. The output layer corresponds to the *deep* cortical layers 5 and 6, which send motor commands and other outputs to a wide range of subcortical areas, including the **basal ganglia**. The hidden layer corresponds to the *superficial* (upper) cortical layers 2 and 3 (cortical layer 1 is largely just axons). These layers receive inputs locally from the other cortical layers and also from other more distant superficial cortical layers. The superficial layers usually project outputs back to these same more distant cortical areas, and to the deep (output) layers locally.

We view the role of the hidden layer (so named because it is not directly "visible" (connected) to either the noncortical input or output areas) as mediating the transformation from input to output. As we will see in the next section (and throughout the remainder of the text), much of what goes on in cognition can be thought of in terms of transforming input patterns in ways that emphasize some distinctions and deemphasize others. Having one or more hidden layers intervening between

the input and the output allows much richer and more complex transformations to be computed, which in turn enables much "smarter" behavior.

Essentially the same functional classification of the cortical layers was suggested as long ago as Bolton (1910) and is supported by several different types of data. First, the anatomical connectivity between the different areas (e.g., White, 1989a; Zilles, 1990) suggests that information coming into the input layer is next transmitted primarily to the hidden layer, and then on to the output layer (figure 3.3). In addition, recordings of the firing properties of neurons in the different cortical layers shows that the hidden and output layer neurons have more complex responses than those in the input layers (reviewed in White, 1989a).

Nevertheless, it is difficult to be certain of exactly what is connected to what in the cortex. One complication is that the dendrites of neurons extend over multiple cortical layers (figure 3.1), so one would need to identify not only what layer an input projection terminates in, but also which specific sets of neurons actually receive that input. Although this has been done in some cases, it is exceedingly difficult and tedious work, and

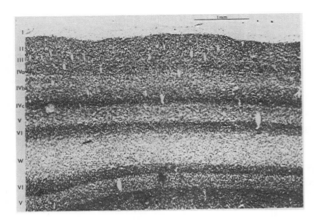

Figure 3.2: Image of a slice through the visual cortex of a cat, with the neuron cell bodies stained, showing the six primary layers, plus the different sublayers of the input layer 4. Reproduced from Sejnowski and Churchland (1989).

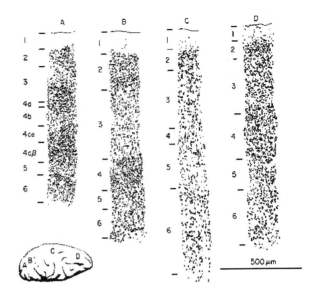

Figure 3.4: Different laminar structure of cortex from different areas. A) shows specialization for the input layer 4 in the primary visual input area. B) shows emphasis on hidden layers 2/3 in a hidden area (extrastriate cortex) higher up in the visual processing stream. C) shows emphasis on output layers 5/6 in a motor output area. D) shows a relatively even blend of layers in a prefrontal area. Reproduced from Shepherd (1990).

much remains to be done.

The view of the cortex presented in figure 3.3 has been simplified to emphasize the distinctive laminar (layered) structure of the cortex. In reality, the cortical areas that process sensory input are not the same ones that produce motor output, and there are a large number of areas which have neither direct sensory input nor direct motor output. Thus, figure 3.5 presents a more accurate (though still abstracted) picture of the structure of the three main different kinds of cortical areas, which correspond to the three functional layer types (*input, hidden,* and *output*). Each of these different types of areas emphasizes the corresponding functional layers (figure 3.4) — input areas have a well developed cortical layer 4 (including different sublayers of layer 4 in the primary visual input area of the monkey), and output areas have well developed output layers. The hidden

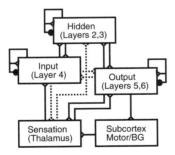

Figure 3.3: A simple, three-layer interpretation of cortical structure that is consistent with general connectivity patterns and provides a useful starting point for modeling. Direct excitatory connectivity is shown by the open triangular connections. Inhibitory interneurons are indicated by the filled circular connections; these operate within each cortical layer and receive the same types of excitatory connections as the excitatory neurons do. Dotted lines indicate connections that may exist but are not consistent with the flow of information from input to hidden to output. Limited data make it difficult to determine how prevalent and important these connections are.

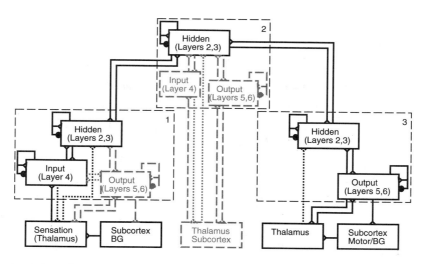

Figure 3.5: Larger scale version of cortical circuitry, showing the three different types of cortical areas: **1)** is an *input area*, which has a well-developed layer 4 receiving sensory input from the thalamus, but not producing motor output directly. **2)** is a *hidden area* (often called a higher-level association area), which receives input from input areas (or other hidden areas) and sends outputs to output areas (or other hidden areas). It has reduced input and output layers, and communicates primarily via layer 2–3 connectivity. **3)** is an *output area* (motor control area), projecting to subcortical brain areas that drive the motor system, which has no real layer 4 (and a larger layer 5). Dashed lines indicate layers and connections that are reduced in importance for a given area, and dotted lines again represent connections which may exist but are not consistent with the input-hidden-output model of information flow.

areas have reduced but still extant input and output layers. We will explore some ideas about what function these might be serving in later chapters.

The picture that emerges from the above view of cortical structure is a very sensible one — information comes into the network in specialized areas and layers, is processed by a potentially long sequence of internal processing areas (the hidden layers), and the results are then output to drive the motor system. However, we must add two important wrinkles of complexity to this otherwise simple picture — the excitatory connections are almost universally bidirectional within the cortex, and within each cortical layer there are a number of inhibitory neurons whose function has not yet been discussed. The importance of these features will be made clear later. Finally, the possible role of the connectivity with the thalamus and other subcortical structures in the hidden areas, which is somewhat puzzling under this simple view, is discussed in later chapters.

3.3 Unidirectional Excitatory Interactions: Transformations

In this and subsequent sections we explore the basic types of computations that networks of neurons with excitatory interactions can perform. We start with the simpler case of *unidirectional* or *feedforward* connections. Though these are rare in the cortex (see chapter 9 for a relevant exception in the *hippocampus*), we will see that the basic computations generalize to the bidirectionally connected case.

Unidirectional or **feedforward** excitatory connectivity causes information to flow "forward" in one direction (**bottom-up**) through the network. We covered one essential aspect of the computation performed by this type of connectivity in chapter 2, when we discussed the role of a neuron as a detector, and explored the process of detection in section 2.6.3. In this section we explore the collective effects of a number of detectors operating in parallel, in terms of how they **transform** patterns of activity over the input. We think of this transformation process as altering the **similarity structure** of the input activity patterns — making patterns more or less similar to each other. Specifically, a given transformation will tend to **emphasize** some distinctions among patterns, while **deemphasizing** or **collapsing** across others.

Thus, to understand the transformation process, we need to take into account the activities of *multiple detectors*, and how these activities vary over *multiple different input patterns*. We will extend our use of the term **representation** from the individual detector case to this multiple detector case by using it to refer to the properties of the pattern of activity over a set of multiple detector units, and across a set of different input patterns. Thus, this notion of representation is much more complex than the simple idea that a representation is what a detector detects. We will see however that there is some relationship between these two uses of the term.

To build up to the case of multiple detectors, we can start with the simpler example of the single '8' detector explored in section 2.6.3. Here, the patterns of activity over the input images (representing the different digits in a $5x7$ grid) were transformed into a pattern of activity of the detector unit over the different input patterns. This activity pattern reflected the extent to which each input pattern resembled an 8. Thus, the specific weight values of this detector imposed a transformation that emphasized similarity to the 8 pattern, while at the same time deemphasizing many of the other different ways in which the input patterns could be considered similar (e.g., according to whether they have a particular feature element like a vertical or horizontal line in a particular location).

The example that we explore here extends this single 8-detector network to the case where there are multiple units in the second layer (i.e., a *hidden* layer) containing detectors for all of the different digits (figure 3.6). Thus, when an image of any digit is presented, the unit in this *digit network* that represents that digit would be activated.

To see how this network transforms the input, we have to consider in general all possible input patterns that could be presented to the network. Specifically, there will be inputs that look like noisy versions of each of the digits (figure 3.7). If a noisy version is sufficiently

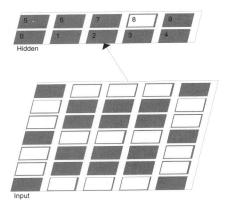

Figure 3.6: The digit network, with an input layer for digit images, and a hidden layer with units that represent the different digits.

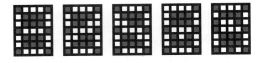

Figure 3.7: Noisy versions of an "8" input image (the original and weight template is the first image).

similar to the weight pattern of a digit detector, then that detector will fire. Importantly, just by looking at the activity of the hidden layer units, we will not in general be able to tell the difference between any of many different input patterns that fire a given detector. If we instead looked directly at the input pattern, we could tell the differences between the different noisy versions.

Thus, the hidden layer detectors have deemphasized the distinctions among all the noisy versions of the digits, while at the same time emphasizing the distinctions between the different digits (which are represented by different units). Although many other possible kinds of transformations could be implemented by configuring the detector weights in different ways, this particular type of transformation is beneficial if you happen to be concerned with the identity of the digit in question (e.g., for the purposes of doing mathematical calculations), and not the image details of the particular rendition of that digit (e.g., the "noisy" versions could amount to differences in font, color, size, etc.). We can think of this as being a *categorical representation* of the digits, where the activation of each digit detector corresponds to an entire category of possible input patterns.

Ideally, it would be useful to be able to visualize the transformation process somehow. In the detector exploration from the previous chapter (section 2.6.3), we could get a sense of the transformation being performed by plotting the response profile of the unit across each of the input patterns. Unfortunately, it is considerably more difficult to do this for an entire hidden layer with many units. One useful tool we have at our disposal is a **cluster plot** of the similarities of different activity patterns over the input and hidden layers.

A cluster plot recursively groups together the patterns or groups of patterns that are most similar to each other. Specifically, the two most similar patterns are grouped together first, and then the similarity of this group with respect to the other patterns is computed as the average of the similarities of the two patterns in the group. The grouping process continues by combining the next two most similar patterns (or groups) with each other, and so on until everything has been put into groups (clusters).

The similarity between patterns is typically computed using Euclidean distance:

$$d = \sqrt{\sum_i (x_i - y_i)^2} \qquad (3.1)$$

where x_i is the value of element i in one pattern, and y_i is the value of this same element in another pattern. The data necessary to produce a cluster plot is contained in a **distance matrix**, which represents all pairwise distances between patterns as the elements of the matrix. The advantage of a cluster plot over the raw distance matrix is that the visual form of the cluster plot often makes the similarity information more easy to see. Nevertheless, because the cluster plot reduces the high-dimensionality of the hidden unit representation into a two-dimensional figure, information is necessarily lost, so sometimes it is useful to also use the distance matrix itself.

Figure 3.8 shows two cluster plots that illustrate how the digit network transformation emphasizes some distinctions and deemphasizes others. The different groups are shown as horizontal *leaves* off of a vertical *branch* that denotes the grouping. These groups are the critical things to focus on for understanding how the network represents the digits. Note that the Y axis here is just an index across the different patterns and does not convey any meaningful information (e.g., one could randomly permute the orders of items within a group without changing the meaning of the plot). The X axis shows distance, with the distance among items within a cluster represented by the length of the horizontal line along the X axis coming out from their common vertical grouping line. Note also that the X axis is *auto-scaled*, so be sure to look at the actual values there (don't assume that all X axes across different plots are the same length).

Figure 3.8a shows a cluster plot of input patterns where there are three noisy versions of each digit (for example, the first three patterns in figure 3.7 were the inputs for the digit 8). There are two important features of this plot. First, you can see that the noisy versions of each digit are all clustered in groups, indicating that they are more similar to each other than to any other digit. Second, the fact that the different digits form an elaborate hierarchy of cluster groups indicates that there is a relatively complex set of similarity relationships among the different digits as represented in their input images.

Figure 3.8b shows a cluster plot of the hidden unit activation patterns for the same set of input images. Two things have happened here. First, the distinctions among the different noisy versions of the same digit have been *collapsed* (deemphasized) — the fact that the digit labels are flush against the vertical bar depicting the cluster group means that there is zero distance between the elements of the group (i.e., they all have an identical representation in the hidden layer). Second, the complex hierarchical structure of similarities among the different digits has been eliminated in favor of a very uniform similarity structure where each digit is equally distinct from every other. One can think of this as emphasizing the fact that each digit is equally distinct from the others, and that all of the digits form a single group of equals.

A conceptual sketch of the transformation performed by the digit network is shown in figure 3.9, which is intended to roughly capture the similarity structure shown

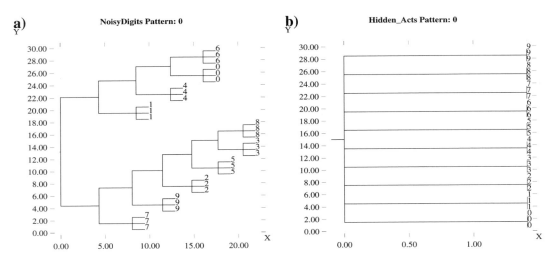

Figure 3.8: Cluster plots of digits with three different images of each digit. **a)** Shows cluster plot of the noisy digit images. **b)** Shows cluster plot of hidden layer digit detectors when shown these images. Note that the zero-length lines for the digit subclusters here indicates that these all have exactly the same pattern, with zero distance between them. While the input represents each image as a distinct pattern (though clustered nicely by digit), the hidden layer collapses across the differences within a given digit category, but preserves distinctions between categories.

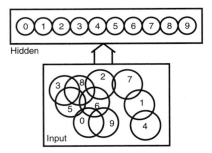

Figure 3.9: Sketch summarizing results of previous figure showing the transformation from the overlapping patterns of digit representations in the input layer to the categorical digit representations in the hidden layer. Each circle in the input loosely represents the collection of pixels that make up the different versions of a digit image, with overlap indicating similarity resulting from shared pixels. The hidden layer representations have no overlap, so that the digits are more clearly and categorically represented.

in the cluster plots of figure 3.8 as a function of overlap between the circles (though doing so accurately is impossible in two dimensions). Thus, the overlapping circles in the input indicate the similarity relationships (shared pixels) among the images of different digits, with each such circle corresponding to the set of different images of a digit that will activate the corresponding detector. The hidden layer circles do not overlap, indicating distinctions emphasized between digits.

One way to see how the transformations implemented by our digit network detectors emphasize distinctions between digits at the expense of deemphasizing other distinctions is to present them with non-digit input images — these images would contain distinctions that the network deemphasizes. For example, if we presented images of letters to this network, we would not expect to get a very sensible hidden layer representation. Figure 3.10 illustrates this phenomenon, showing that the digit hidden layer almost always collapses across the distinctions present in the letter inputs. In this case the collapsing happened because the hidden units simply did not respond to the letters (with the exception of

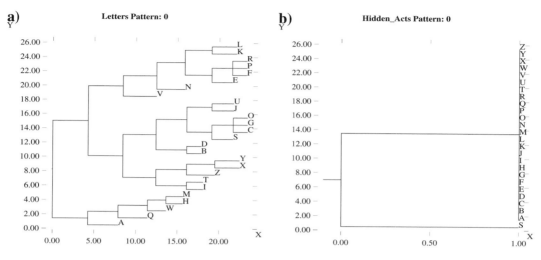

Figure 3.10: Cluster plots for letters in the digit network. **a)** Shows cluster plot of input letter images. **b)** Shows cluster plot of hidden layer digit detectors when shown these images. The hidden layer units were not activated by the majority of the letter inputs, so the representations overlap by 100 percent, meaning that the hidden layer makes no distinction between these patterns.

the hidden unit for the digit "8" responding to the sufficiently similar letter "S", resulting in a single cluster for that hidden unit activity). However, even if things are done to remedy this problem (e.g., lowering the unit's leak currents so that they respond more easily), many distinctions remain collapsed due to the fact that the weights are not specifically tuned for letter patterns, and thus do not distinguish among them.

In summary, we have seen that collections of detectors operating on the feedforward flow of information from the input to the hidden layer can transform the similarity structure of the representations. This process of transformation is central to all of cognition — when we categorize a range of different objects with the same name (e.g., "chair"), or simply recognize an abstract pattern as the same regardless of the exact location or size we view this pattern in, we are transforming input signals to emphasize some distinctions and deemphasize others. We will see in subsequent chapters that by chaining together multiple stages (layers) of such transformations (as we expect happens in the cortex based on the connectivity structure discussed in the previous section), very powerful and substantial overall transformations can be produced.

3.3.1 Exploration of Transformations

Now, we will explore the ideas just presented.

↪ Open the project `transform.proj.gz` in `chapter_3` to begin.

You will see a network (the digits network), the `xform_ctrl` overall control panel, and the standard PDP++ Root window (see appendix A for more information).

Let's first examine the network, which looks just like figure 3.6. It has a 5x7 `Input` layer for the digit images, and a $2x5$ `Hidden` layer, with each of the 10 hidden units representing a digit.

↪ Select the `r.wt` button (lower left of the window — you may need to scroll), and then click on each of the different hidden units.

You will see that the weights exactly match the images of the digits the units represent, just as our single 8 detector from the previous chapter did.

Although it should be pretty obvious from these weights how each unit will respond to the set of digit input patterns that exactly match the weight patterns, let's explore this nonetheless.

↪ Select the `act` button to view the unit activities in the network, and hit the `Step` button in the control panel.

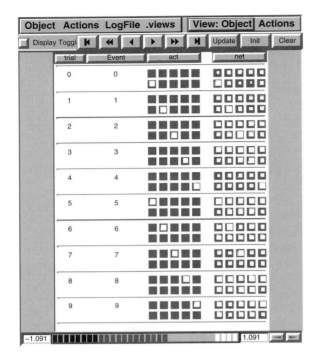

Figure 3.11: The GridLog display of hidden unit activations in response to the 10 digit inputs. Level of activity is encoded as the size of the white square within each grey unit grid box.

As before, this presents the first input pattern (0) to the network, and updates the activations in the network over a series of cycles until equilibrium activations have effectively been reached for all units (see section 2.4.5). Note that we are using the noisy XX1 rate coded activation function, as with most of our simulations.

↪ Proceed to Step through the entire sequence of digits.

You should have observed that each unit was activated when its matching digit was presented, and not when any of the other digits were presented.

To record this pattern of hidden unit activations over the different inputs, we will use a window called a **GridLog**. This window displays the activity states of the network over time as rows of colored squares (figure 3.11).

↪ Press View on the control panel and select GRID_LOG. When the window appears, press the full-

forward button at the top of the log (right-most VCR-style button, >|), to move to the end of the data that was recorded during the previous stepping.

You should see that the GridLog has recorded the activities (and net inputs) of the hidden units for each of the digits, so you can easily see the overall pattern of activation across all the inputs.

Bias Weights

Before we continue, it is important to understand the role of the *bias weights* in this simulation (see section 2.5.1 from the previous chapter for the definition of bias weights). The digit images used as input patterns have somewhat different numbers of active units (as you might have observed in the detector exercise in the previous chapter).

↪ Press View in the control panel and select EVENTS to see all of the digit input patterns.

You might have expected these differences in the number of active input units to result in different net input and activation levels for the corresponding hidden units. Instead, all the activations shown in the Grid-Log appear roughly similar. The discrepancy here is attributable to the use of bias weights, which compensate for these differences in overall activity level coming from the inputs.

↪ Iconify (minimize) the events window, and select bias.wt in the NetView window.

You should see a pattern of different valued bias weights on the hidden units. Let's evaluate the contributions of these bias weights by running the network without them.

↪ On the xform_ctrl, select BIASES_OFF for the biases field, hit Apply, and then Run.

This will run through all of the digits, and you can view the GridLog to see the resulting activities and net inputs.

Question 3.1 *How did the lack of bias weights affect the hidden unit activities, and their relation to the number of active units in the input patterns?*

↪ Turn the bias weights back on (BIASES_ON and Apply), and select bias.wt to view in the Network window if it isn't already selected (you may need to hit `Update` in this window if `bias.wt` was already selected, to update the display).

Question 3.2 *Explain how these bias weights contribute to producing the originally observed hidden unit activities.*

Cluster Plots

Next we will produce some cluster plots like those shown previously.

↪ `Run` the network with the biases on again. Hit the `Cluster` button in the `xform_ctrl` control panel, and select `CLUSTER_DIGITS`.

You should get a window containing the cluster plot for the similarity relationships among the digit images.

↪ For comparison, click on `View` in the control panel and select `EVENTS`).

Compare the amount of overlap between activated pixels in the digit images with the cluster plot results.

↪ Iconify the events window when done.

Next let's look at the similarity relationships among the hidden unit representations of the digits.

↪ Do `Cluster` again, selecting `CLUSTER_HIDDEN` this time.

You should get a cluster plot that looks much like that shown in figure 3.8b, except there is just one label for each digit category. This shows that the network has transformed the complex patterns of input similarity into equally distinct hidden representations of the digit categories.

Note that we have *binarized* the hidden unit activation values (i.e., changed values greater than .5 to 1, and those less than .5 to 0) for the purposes of clustering. Otherwise, small differences in the activation values of the units would distract from the main structure of the cluster plot (which is actually the same regardless of whether the activations are binarized or not). For the present purposes, we are more interested in whether a detector has fired or not, and not in the specific activation value of that detector, though in general the graded values can play a useful role in representations, as we will discuss later.

↪ Do `Object/Close` to remove the cluster plot windows (cluster plots are the only windows that you should close in this way, because they are temporary).

The next step is to run the case where there are multiple instances of each digit (the `NOISY_DIGITS` case).

↪ Set `env_type` to `NOISY_DIGITS`, `Apply` and then do `View`, `EVENTS` to see the different noisy versions of the digit images. Press `Run` to present these to the network.

You should see that the appropriate hidden unit is active for each version of the digits (although small levels of activity in other units should also be observed in some cases).

↪ Now do `CLUSTER_HIDDEN`.

You should see the same plot as shown in figure 3.8b. You can compare this with the `CLUSTER_NOISY_DIGITS` cluster plot of the input digit images (same as figure 3.8a). This clearly shows that the network has collapsed across distinctions between different noisy versions of the same digits, while emphasizing the distinctions between different digit categories.

Selectivity and Leak

In the detector exploration from the previous chapter (section 2.6.3), we saw that manipulating the amount of leak conductance altered the selectivity of the unit's response. By lowering the leak, the unit responded in a graded fashion to the similarity of the different digit images to the detector's weight pattern. Let's see what kinds of effects this parameter has on the behavior of the present network. The control panel shows that the leak conductance (`g_bar_l`) for the hidden units has been set to a value of 6.

↪ Reduce the (`g_bar_l`) for the hidden units from 6 to 5 and `Run` (still using `NOISY_DIGITS`).

Question 3.3 **(a)** *What happens generally to the hidden activations with this reduction in leak value?* **(b)** *How does this affect the cluster plot of hidden unit activities?* **(c)** *How about for a* `g_bar_l` *of 4?* **(d)** *If the goal of this network was to have the same hidden representation for each version of the same digit, and different representations for different digits, how does* *changing the units' excitability (via the leak current) affect the success of the network, and why?*

Letter Inputs

Now, we will see how the network responds to letter inputs instead of digits.

↪ First, set the `g_bar_l` leak conductance back to 6 (or `Defaults`) and make sure `act` is selected in the NetView window. Then set `env_type` to `LETTERS` (`Apply`) and press `Run`.

Notice the letters being presented over the input layer on the network.

↪ Use the VCR-like controls at the top of the Grid-Log to scroll the display back to the start of the letter presentations, because these have scrolled off the "top" of the display (the single < button is a good choice for fine-grained scrolling).

The only significant response came to the "S" letter input from the "8" hidden unit — note that "S" is very similar to the "8".

↪ Press the fast-forward-to-the-end button (>|) on the grid log, so that it will continue to scroll when you next `Run` it. Press `Cluster`, `CLUSTER_LETTERS`. Next, press `Cluster` and `CLUSTER_HIDDEN`.

The first cluster plot should look like figure 3.10a, and the second should look like figure 3.10b. You should be able to see in these cluster plots that these digit units do not respond very informatively to the letter stimuli.

Question 3.4 (a) *Based on your experiences in the previous question, what would you expect to happen to the cluster plot of hidden responses to letter inputs as you lowered the* `g_bar_l` *leak current to a value of 4? Do this — were you right?* **(b)** *Would you say that this hidden representation is a good one for conveying letter identity information? Why or why not? (Hint: Pay particular attention to whether any letters are collapsed in the cluster plot — i.e., having no distance at all between them.)* **(c)** *Can you find any setting of* `g_bar_l` *that gives you a satisfactory hidden representation of letter information? Explain.*

↪ Go to the `PDP++Root` window. To continue on to the next simulation, close this project first by selecting

`.projects/Remove/Project_0`. Or, if you wish to stop now, quit by selecting `Object/Quit`.

3.3.2 Localist versus Distributed Representations

The digit network we explored in the previous section used very simple detectors with weight patterns that directly matched the input patterns they were intended to detect, often referred to as **template matching** representations. Another aspect of these units was that only one unit represented each input pattern, referred to as a **local** or **localist** representation, which often goes hand in hand with template matching ideas. Such representations are also often referred to as **grandmother cell** representations, because their use must imply that somewhere in the brain is a neuron that (uniquely) represents one's grandmother.

Though useful for demonstration purposes, localist representations are not particularly realistic or powerful. Thus, it is unfortunate that the detector model of the neuron is often associated with this type of representation — as we made clear in the previous chapter, the detector *function* can apply to very complex and difficult to describe nonlocalist *contents* or representations.

Recordings of cortical neurons have consistently shown that the brain uses **distributed** representations, where each neuron responds to a variety of different input stimuli, and that many neurons are active for each input stimulus. For example, researchers have presented visual stimuli that are systematically varied along a number of different dimensions (size, shape, color, etc.), and recorded the activities of neurons in the areas of the cortex that process visual inputs (see Desimone & Ungerleider, 1989; Tanaka, 1996, for reviews). In all cases that we know, these studies have shown that cortical neurons exhibit measurable **tuning curves**, which means that they respond in a graded fashion to stimuli within a range of different parameter values (figure 3.12). Furthermore, it is clear both from the overlap in these tuning curves and from multiple parallel recording that many neurons are simultaneously encoding the same input stimuli.

It is often useful to think about distributed units as representing *features* of input stimuli, where a given stimulus is represented by a collection of units that each

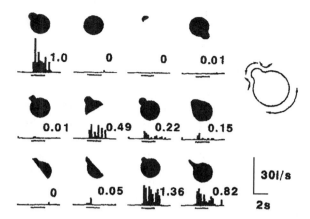

Figure 3.12: Tuning functions of a cortical neuron in response to visual shapes, showing the distributed nature of these representations — the neuron responds to a range of different shapes (and multiple neurons respond to the same shape, though this is not represented here). The neural response is shown below the corresponding visual image that was presented to a monkey. The neuron was located in cortical area IT (specifically TE). Reproduced from Tanaka (1996).

represent a subcomponent or feature of the stimulus, known as a **feature-based** representation. Of course, as with the notion of detectors, a distributed representation can be effective without needing clearly defined or easily described featural representations. Indeed, in the case of **coarse coded** representations of continuous dimensions (see section 1.6.2), the "features" are just arbitrary ranges of the underlying dimension over which the unit gives a graded response.

It is important to emphasize that the issue of whether one can provide some kind of simple interpretation of what a given unit seems to encode is in principle unrelated to the distinction between localist versus distributed representations. Thus, it is possible to have feature-based distributed representations with easily described featural encodings, or localist representations where it is difficult to describe the representations. Nevertheless, localist representations are most useful (and typically used) in cases where one can easily label the units, and often it is difficult to determine exactly what individual units in a distributed representation encode.

Although we used localist units in our digit network example, we will see in a moment that distributed representations have the same capacity to implement transformations of the input pattern, where these transformations emphasize some distinctions and deemphasize others. Using a feature-based notion of distributed representations, we can imagine that by detecting some features and not others, the resulting activity pattern over the hidden layer will emphasize distinctions based on these features, and it will deemphasize distinctions based on features that were not encoded.

The main advantages of distributed representations over localist ones are as follows (Hinton et al., 1986):

Efficiency: Fewer total units are required to represent a given number of input stimuli if the representation is shared across units, because individual stimuli can be represented as different combinations of unit activities, of which there are a very large number for even modest numbers of units. In contrast, one unit per pattern is required for localist representations.

Similarity: Distributed representations provide a natural means of encoding the similarity relationships among different patterns as a function of the number of units in common (*pattern overlap*).

Generalization: A network with distributed representations can often respond appropriately to novel input patterns by using appropriate (novel) combinations of hidden units. This type of generalization is impossible for localist networks, because they require the use of an entirely new unit to represent a novel input pattern.

Robustness: Having multiple units participating in each representation makes it more robust against damage, since there is some redundancy.

Accuracy: In representing continuous dimensions, distributed (*coarse coded*) representations are much more accurate than the equivalent number of localist representations, because a lot of information is contained in the relative activities of the set of active units. Even in the binary case, a distributed representation over n units can encode as many as 2^n different values, whereas localist units can only represent n different values (at an accuracy of $1/n$).

Learning: Distributed representations allow for the bootstrapping of small changes that is critical for learning (see section 1.6.5 and chapters 4–6). Furthermore, learning tends not to result in perfectly interpretable representations at the single unit level (i.e., not template matching units).

As should be clear, distributed representations are critical for many of the key properties of neural networks described in the introductory chapter. Despite this, some researchers maintain that localist representations are preferable, in part for their simplicity, which was admittedly useful in the previous section. Nevertheless, most of the remaining models in this book employ distributed representations. In section 3.5 we also discuss the important difference between **sparse distributed** representations and generic distributed representations.

3.3.3 *Exploration of Distributed Representations*

Now, we will explore the difference between localist and distributed representations.

↪   Open the project `loc_dist.proj.gz` in `chapter_3` to begin.

This project looks very similar to the previous one — it is in fact a superset of it, having both the previous localist network, and a new distributed one. To begin, we will first replicate the results we obtained before using the localist network.

↪ Press `View` on the overall control panel (now called `loc_dist_ctrl`) and select `GRID_LOG`. Then do `Run`.

You should see the responses of the same localist network just as before.

↪ Set `network` to `DISTRIBUTED_NETWORK` instead of `LOCALIST_NETWORK`, and hit `Apply`.

You will now see the distributed network take the place of the localist one. This network contains only 5 hidden units. Let's explore this network by examining the weights into these hidden units.

↪ Select `r.wt` in the network window, and click on each of the units.

You will notice that these units are configured to detect parts or *features* of digit images, not entire digits as in the localist network. Thus, you can imagine that

these units will be active whenever one of these features is present in the input.

↪ Press `Run`. Do `View`, `EVENTS` to see the input patterns.

Now verify for yourself in the GridLog that the firing patterns of the hidden units make sense given the features present in the different digits. The only case that is somewhat strange is the third hidden unit firing for the digit "0" — it fires because the left and right sides match the weight pattern. There is an important lesson here — just because you might have visually encoded the third hidden unit as the "middle horizontal line" detector, it can actually serve *multiple roles*. This is just a simple case of the kind of complexity that surrounds the attempt to describe the *content* of what is being detected by neurons. Imagine if there were 5,000 weights, with a much more complicated pattern of values, and you can start to get a feel for how complicated a neuron's responses can be.

Now, let's see what a cluster plot of the hidden unit representations tells us about the properties of the transformation performed by this distributed network.

↪   Select `NOISY_DIGITS` for the `env_type` (`Apply`), and `Run`. Then, do `Cluster` and choose `CLUSTER_HIDDEN`.

This should produce a cluster plot like that shown in figure 3.13. Although there are a couple of obvious differences between this plot and the one for the localist network shown in figure 3.8b, it should be clear that the distributed network is also generally emphasizing the distinctions between different digits while deemphasizing (collapsing) distinctions among noisy versions of the same digit.

One difference in the distributed network is that it sometimes collapsed noisy versions of *different* digits together (a 2 with the 5's, and a 0 with the 4's), even though in most cases the different versions of the same digit were properly collapsed together. It also did not always collapse all of the different images of a digit together, sometimes only getting 2 out of 3. The reason for these problems is that the noisy versions actually shared more features with a different digit representation. In most cases where we use distributed representations, we use a learning mechanism to discover the individual feature detectors, and learning will usually

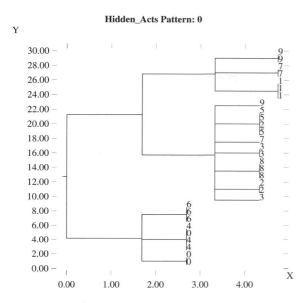

Figure 3.13: Cluster plot of the distributed representations of the noisy digit inputs. Some "errors" are made where different digits are collapsed together, and not all versions of the same digit are in a single cluster. Nevertheless, it does a pretty good job of emphasizing the distinctions between digits and deemphasizing those among different versions of the same digit.

do a better job than our simple hand-set weight values at emphasizing and deemphasizing the appropriate distinctions as a function of the task we train it on.

Another aspect of the distributed cluster plot is that the digit categories are not equally separate elements of a single cluster group, as with the localist representation. Thus, there is some residual similarity structure between different digits reflected in the hidden units, though less than in the input images, as one can tell because of the "flatter" cluster structure (i.e., the clusters are less deeply nested within each other, suggesting more overall equality in similarity differences). Of course, this residual similarity might be a good thing in some situations, as long as a clear distinction between different digits is made. Again, we typically rely on learning to ensure that the representations capture the appropriate transformations.

Another test we can perform is to test this network on the letter input stimuli.

↪ Set env_type to LETTERS and Run. Then do a cluster plot on the resulting hidden units.

Although this network clearly does a better job of distinguishing between the different letters than the localist network, it still collapses many letters into the same hidden representation. Thus, we have evidence that these distributed feature detectors are appropriate for representing distinctions among digits, but not letters.

Question 3.5 *The distributed network achieves a useful representation of the digits using half the number of hidden units as the localist network (and this number of hidden units is 1/7th the number of input units, greatly compressing the input representation) — explain how this efficiency is achieved.*

↪ Go to the PDP++Root window. To continue on to the next simulation, close this project first by selecting .projects/Remove/Project_0. Or, if you wish to stop now, quit by selecting Object/Quit.

3.4 Bidirectional Excitatory Interactions

In many ways, bidirectional excitatory connectivity (also known as **interactivity** or **recurrence**) behaves in just the same way as feedforward or unidirectional excitatory connectivity in producing transformations of the input patterns, except that the transformation can go both ways. Thus, in addition to having the ability to activate a digit category unit from an image of a digit (as in the feedforward networks explored above), a bidirectionally connected network can also produce an image of a digit given the digit category. This is like *mental imagery* where you produce an image based on a conception (e.g., "visualize the digit 8"), which involves processing going **top-down** instead of the **bottom-up** direction explored previously.

With **lateral** connectivity (i.e., connections among units within the same layer), one part of a pattern can be used to activate other parts. This process goes by the name of **pattern completion**, because the pattern is being completed (made full) by processing a part of it. Some closely related phenomena are **mutual support**, **resonance** (Grossberg, 1976), and **amplification**, where either lateral connectivity or bidirectional bottom-up and top-down connectivity (or both) can enhance the activations of interconnected units, making them more strongly activated.

Many phenomena associated with bidirectionally connected networks can be described in terms of **attractor dynamics**, where the network appears to be *attracted* to a particular final activity state given a range of initial activity patterns. This range of initial configurations that lead to the same final pattern is called the **attractor basin** for that attractor. Although we can describe the terminology of the attractor in this section, a full exploration of this phenomenon awaits the introduction of inhibitory mechanisms, and is thus postponed until section 3.6.

3.4.1 Bidirectional Transformations

We begin our introduction to the bidirectional case by exploring a bidirectional version of the the localist digit network. We will see that this network can perform the same kinds of transformations as the unidirectional one, but in both directions.

↪   Open the project `bidir_xform.proj.gz` in `chapter_3` to begin.

Note that this project looks very similar to the previous digit networks, having the same windows, etc. The main control panel for this one is called `bd_xform_ctrl`.

We first examine the network. Note that there are two arrows connecting the `Input` and `Hidden` layers — one going up and the other coming back down. This indicates bidirectional connectivity. We can view this connectivity as before.

↪   Select the `r.wt` button in the network window and click on the hidden units and the input units.

When you click on the hidden units, you will see the now-familiar digit image templates. When you click on the input units, you will see that they now receive from the hidden units as well. Note that different input units receive from different numbers of sending units — this reflects the different types of pattern overlap among the digit images.

A more direct way to see what would happen if you activated a hidden unit is to view its **sending weights**.

↪   Select the `s.wt` button, and then select various hidden units.

These sending weights look just like the receiving ones — templates of appropriate digit image. We next verify that in fact these weights are **symmetric** (the same in both directions).

↪   Alternately click on `r.wt` and `s.wt` while a given hidden unit is selected.

You should notice no difference in the display. The interesting thing about symmetric weights is that, as you can see, *a given unit activates the same things that activate it*. This guarantees a kind of *consistency* in what things get activated in bidirectional networks. We will discuss the biological basis of weight symmetry in detail in chapter 5, where it plays an important role in the mathematical derivation of our error-driven learning mechanism.

Now we can run the network and see what these weights produce. First, let's replicate the previous feedforward results.

↪   First, open the GridLog by doing `View` and selecting `GRID_LOG`. Then, select the `act` button to view the unit activities in the network, and press `Run`.

This will present the images to the input layer for all of the digits. You may notice that the network displays the activations during the *settling* process (as they are being updated on their way to equilibrium) instead of just at the final equilibrium state as before. This will come in handy later. Note also that the grid log shows both the input and hidden activation states now. The results for this run should be exactly the same as for the feedforward network — the bidirectionality of the weights has no additional effect here because the input units are *clamped* (fixed) to the pattern in the event, and are not actually computing their activations or otherwise paying any attention to their weights.

Now let's go in the opposite direction.

↪   Set `env_type` to `CATEGS` (`Apply`) and `Run`.

This will run the network by clamping the digit category units in the hidden layer, instead of the digit images in the input. The resulting input patterns are those driven by the top-down weights from these units, as you might have noticed if you saw the dynamics of activation updating in the network window during the settling for each pattern. Otherwise, it is somewhat difficult

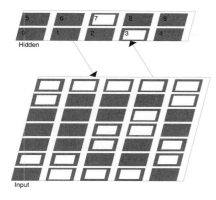

Figure 3.14: Results of top-down activation of both the 3 and 7 digit categories.

to tell any difference between the two runs, since they both produce basically the same patterns of activity on both layers. However, you can tell that the hidden units are clamped during CATEGS because they are all at the same activation value, whereas this value varies when the input images are presented. The images also have a slightly lower activity value when driven from the digit category units. Furthermore, you can always click on the ext button in the network window to see which units are being driven by external inputs (i.e., clamped).

↪ Click on the ext button in the network window.

You should see that the hidden units, not the input units, are being driven by external input.

This simple exercise demonstrates how bidirectional connectivity enables information to flow, and transformations to be computed, in both bottom-up and top-down directions. There are a number of other important issues surrounding this phenomenon. For example, what happens when there are different digit images that correspond to the same categorical hidden unit? With just a localist hidden representation, only the *prototypical* input (i.e., the one described exactly by the weights) will be activated in a top-down fashion. However, in the more realistic case of a distributed representation, lots of different input images can be produced by activating different combinations of hidden units.

We can get a sense of the effects of activating multiple combinations of hidden units in the localist network.

↪ Set env_type to COMBOS (Apply), and then do View EVENTS.

You will see an EnviroView with one event and its pattern displayed. This pattern contains the input that will be presented to the hidden layer units. Let's first run the default case where the 3 and 7 units are activated.

↪ Press Run.

Figure 3.14 shows the results you should see.

Question 3.6 (a) *Describe what happens to the input layer activations when digit categories 7 and 3 are activated (be sure to note even subtle differences in activation).* **(b)** *How do you account for this result?* **(c)** *Can you change the value of* g_bar_l *to enhance any differences between the levels of activation of the active units? Explain why this helps.* **(d)** *How might this kind of enhancement of differences be generally useful in cognition?*

You can now observe the effects of activating your own combinations of digit categories.

↪ Click with the left mouse button on any of the digit categories to toggle the input on or off. Be sure to press the Apply button in the environment window, which will be highlighted, so that your changes take effect. Have fun trying different combinations!

↪ Go to the PDP++Root window. To continue on to the next simulation, close this project first by selecting .projects/Remove/Project_0. Or, if you wish to stop now, quit by selecting Object/Quit.

3.4.2 Bidirectional Pattern Completion

Now we will explore *pattern completion* in a network with bidirectional connections within a single layer of units. Thus, instead of top-down and bottom-up processing, this network exhibits *lateral* processing. The difference is somewhat evanescent, because the same underlying processing mechanisms are at work in both cases. However, laterality implies that the units involved are somehow more like *peers*, whereas top-down bottom-up implies that they have a hierarchical relationship.

We will see in this exploration that by activating a subset of a "known" pattern in the network (i.e., one that is consistent with the network's weights), the bidirectional connectivity will fill in or complete the remaining portion of the pattern. This is the pattern completion phenomenon.

↪ **Open the project** `pat_complete.proj.gz` **in** `chapter_3` **to begin.**

You should see a network window displaying a single-layered network. As usual, we begin by examining the weights of the network.

↪ **Select** `r.wt` **and click on different units.**

You can see that all the units that belong to the image of the digit 8 are interconnected with weights of value 1, while all other units have weights of 0. Thus, it would appear that presenting any part of the image of the 8 would result in the activation of the remaining parts. We will first test the network's ability to complete the pattern from the initial subset of half of the image of the digit 8.

↪ **To view this test case, do** `View`, `EVENTS` **on the main control panel** (`pat_comp_ctrl`). **Then, select the** `act` **button to view the unit activities in the network. Next, press the** `Run` **button.**

This presents the input to some of the units (as determined by the event pattern shown in the environment window), and the others become activated. Notice that we are viewing the activations being updated during *settling*, so that you can tell which ones were clamped from the environment and which are being *completed* as a result.

There is no fundamental difference between this pattern completion phenomenon and any of the other types of excitatory processing examined so far — it is simply a result of the unclamped units detecting a pattern of activity among their neighbors and becoming activated when this pattern sufficiently matches the pattern encoded in the weights. However, pattern completion as a concept is particularly useful for thinking about *cued recall* in memory, where some cue (e.g., a distinctive smell, an image, a phrase, a song) triggers one's memory and results in the recall of a related episode or event. This will be discussed further in chapter 9.

Note that unlike previous simulations, this one employs something called **soft clamping**, where the inputs from the event pattern are presented as additional excitatory input to the neurons instead of directly setting the activations to the corresponding values. This latter form of clamping (which we have been using previously) is called **hard clamping**, and it results in faster processing than soft clamping. However, soft clamping is necessary in this case because some of the units in the layer need to update their activation values as a function of their weights to produce pattern completion.

Question 3.7 (a) *Given the pattern of weights, what is the minimal number of units that need to be clamped to produce pattern completion to the full 8? You can determine your answer by toggling off the units in the event pattern one-by-one until the network no longer produces the complete pattern when it is* `Run` *(don't forget to press* `Apply` *in the environment window after clicking).* **(b)** *The* `g_bar_l` *parameter can be altered to lower this minimal number. What value of this parameter allows completion with only one input active?*

↪ **Hit** `Defaults` **to restore the original** `g_bar_l` **value.**

Question 3.8 (a) *What happens if you activate only inputs which are not part of the 8 pattern? Why?* **(b)** *Could the weights in this layer be configured to support the representation of another pattern in addition to the 8 (such that this new pattern could be distinctly activated by a partial input), and do you think it would make a difference how similar this new pattern was to the 8 pattern? Explain your answer.*

A phenomenon closely related to pattern completion is *mutual support* or *resonance*, which happens when the activity from a set of units that have excitatory interconnections produces extra activation in all of these units. The amount of this extra activation provides a useful indication of how strongly interconnected these units are, and also enables them to better resist interference from noise or inhibition. We next observe this effect in the simulation.

↪ **Click the entire pattern of the 8 to be input to the network, together with one other unit which is not part of the 8. Then, change the leak current** (`g_bar_l`) **from 3 to 7.5, and hit** `Run`.

Note that the units which are part of the interconnected 8 pattern experience mutual support, and are thus able to overcome the relatively strong level of leak current, whereas the unit that does not have these weights suffers significantly from it.

Finally, note that this (and the preceding simulations) are highly simplified, to make the basic phenomena and underlying mechanisms clear. As we will see when we start using learning algorithms in chapters 4–6, these networks will become more complex and can deal with a large number of intertwined patterns encoded over the same units. This makes the resulting behavior much more powerful, but also somewhat more difficult to understand in detail. Nevertheless, the same basic principles are at work.

↪ Go to the PDP++Root window. To continue on to the next simulation, close this project first by selecting .projects/Remove/Project_0. Or, if you wish to stop now, quit by selecting Object/Quit.

3.4.3 Bidirectional Amplification

The above examples involving bidirectional connectivity have been carefully controlled to avoid what can be one of the biggest problems of bidirectional connectivity: *uncontrolled positive feedback*. However, this positive feedback also gives rise to the useful phenomenon of **amplification**, where excitatory signals reverberating between neurons result in dramatically enhanced activation strengths. One can think of amplification as just a more extreme example of the kind of mutual support or resonance explored in the previous simulation.

Amplification is critical for explaining many aspects of cognition, including the word-superiority effect discussed in the introduction (section 1.6.3), and others that we encounter later. Positive feedback becomes a problem when it results in the uncontrolled spread of excitation throughout the entire network, producing what is effectively an epileptic seizure with virtually every unit becoming activated. The inhibitory mechanisms described in the next section are necessary to take full advantage of bidirectional amplification without suffering from these consequences.

In this section, we will explore a couple of simple demonstrations of amplification in action, and see how it can lead to the ability to **bootstrap** from weak initial activation to a fully active pattern (the term *boot-*

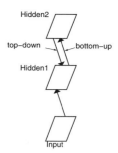

Figure 3.15: Bidirectionally connected network with bottom-up and top-down connections between the two hidden layers.

strap comes from the notion of pulling oneself up by one's own bootstraps — making something from nothing). We will also see how amplification can cause uncontrolled spread of activation throughout the network.

Exploration of Simple Top-Down Amplification

We begin by exploring the simple case of the top-down amplification of a weak bottom-up input via bidirectional excitatory connections.

↪ Open the project amp_top_down.proj.gz in chapter_3 to begin.

You will see a network with 3 layers: an input, and 2 bidirectionally connected hidden layers (hidden1 and hidden2), with 1 unit in each layer (figure 3.15).

↪ You can explore the weights using r.wt as before. Return to act when done.

Now, we can pull up a graph log to plot the activations of the two hidden-layer units over time as the network settles in response to the input.

↪ Press View in the amp_td_ctrl control panel and select GRAPH_LOG. Then, hit Run.

You should see something like figure 3.16 in your graph window. The activation coming top-down from the hidden2 unit is *amplifying* the relatively weak initial activation of the hidden1 unit, resulting in the strong activation of both units. This is an excellent example of *bootstrapping*, because the hidden1 unit has to activate the hidden2 unit in the first place before it can receive the additional top-down excitation from it. Let's test the effects of the leak current.

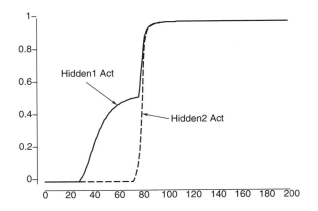

Figure 3.16: Bootstrapping phenomenon where the activation of the *hidden1* unit is just strong enough to start activating *hidden2*, which then comes back and reinforces hidden1 producing strong activation in both.

↪ Increase the strength of the leak current `g_bar_l` from 3.4 to 3.5, and press `Run`. Next decrease the strength of the leak current and observe the effects.

You should see that with a higher leak current (3.5), the resulting `hidden1` activation is now insufficient to activate `hidden2`, and no bootstrapping or amplification occurs. With decreases to the leak current, the bottom-up activation of `hidden1` is relatively strong, so that the bootstrapping and amplification from `hidden2` are less noticeable.

This simple case of bootstrapping and amplification provides some insight into the word-superiority effect studied by McClelland and Rumelhart (1981) and summarized in the introductory chapter. Recall that the basic effect is that people can recognize letters in the context of words better than letters in the context of nonwords. The puzzle is how word-level information can affect letter-level processing, when the letters presumably must be recognized before words can be activated in the first place. Based on this exploration, we can see how initially weak activation of letters (i.e., the hidden 1 unit) can go up to the word-level representations (i.e., the hidden 2 unit), and come back down to bootstrap and amplify corresponding letter-level representations.

Note that although this example is organized according to bottom-up and top-down processing, the same principles apply to lateral connectivity. Indeed, one could simply move the `hidden2` unit down into the same layer as `hidden1`, where they would be just like two parts of one interconnected pattern, and if one were activated, it would be bootstrapped and amplified by the other.

↪ Go to the `PDP++Root` window. To continue on to the next simulation, close this project first by selecting `.projects/Remove/Project_0`. Or, if you wish to stop now, quit by selecting `Object/Quit`.

Exploration of Amplification with Distributed Representations

The previous example illustrated the benefits of bidirectional excitatory amplification, and how bootstrapping can occur. However, when distributed representations are used, such amplification can lead to the activation of inappropriate units. In particular, the overlapping connections required to implement distributed representations can allow excitation to spread overzealously. We will see below how this spread can be checked by inhibition, but without that, we must resort to increasing the leak current to prevent activation spread. The problem here is, as you saw with the above example, if there is too much leak current, then it is impossible to bootstrap the representations into activation in the first place, so that the benefits of bidirectional excitatory amplification are not available. Thus, this example provides some strong motivation for the next section on inhibitory interactions.

↪ Open the project `amp_top_down_dist.proj.gz` in `chapter_3` to begin.

The network here is like that in the previous example, except that now there are multiple units per layer.

↪ Click on the `r.wt` button, and then click on the 3 `hidden1` units.

Notice that they each receive one corresponding input from the input units (this is called **one-to-one** connectivity). Notice also that the left and right `hidden1` units receive uniquely from the left and right `hidden2` units, while the center `hidden1` unit receives from *both* `hidden2` units.

↪ Now click on the the left and right `hidden2` units.

Observe that the connectivity is symmetric, so that the left unit receives from the left and center `hidden1` units, while the right one receives from the center and right `hidden1` units.

Thus, the connectivity pattern can be interpreted as representing 3 separable features in the input and `hidden1` units, with the `hidden2` units representing 2 "objects" each consisting of 2 out of these 3 features. As labeled in the simulation, you can think of the first object as a *TV*, which has the two features of a *CRT* and *speakers*, while the other is a *synthesizer*, which has *speakers* and a *keyboard*. Thus, there is a one-feature overlap between these objects, and it is this shared feature that will cause the network trouble.

Now we will present activity to only the left input unit, which is unique to the *TV* object, and observe the network's response. To see the trajectory of settling in the network, we will open a grid log.

↪ Press `View` in the `amp_td_dist_ctrl` control panel, and select `GRID_LOG`. Then, select the `act` button to view the unit activities in the network, and then press `RunUniq` in the control panel.

As you can see by watching the network settle, and by looking at a trace of it in the grid log to the right (showing the activations for the `hidden1` and `hidden2` units every 10 updates (cycles) of settling, see figure 3.17), the `CRT` hidden unit (on the left) first activates the `TV` unit, and then this comes back down to activate the `Speakers` feature. This is a good example of a *pattern completion*-like phenomenon that uses top-down activation instead of lateral activation. However, once the `Speakers` unit becomes activated, it then activates the `Synth` unit in the `hidden2` layer, which then does the same kind of top-down activation of the `Keyboard` unit. The result is the uninterpretable activation of all 3 hidden units.

↪ Try increasing the leak current (search with larger steps first and then narrow your way down, and don't search in finer steps than .001) to see if you can get the network to just activate the features associated with TV (left and center hidden features, `CRT` and `Speakers`).

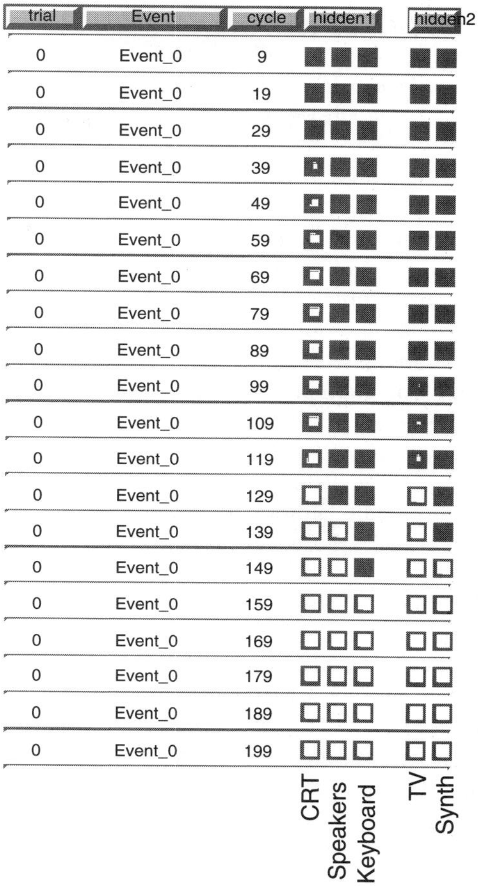

Figure 3.17: The GridLog display of the two layers of hidden unit activations in response to the unique input (left-most input unit, CRT). Activity inevitably spreads over to the other feature units via top-down activation from the TV unit and Synth units in the second hidden layer.

Question 3.9 (a) *List the values of* `g_bar_l` *where the network's behavior exhibited a qualitative transition in what was activated at the end of settling, and describe these network states.* (b) *Using the value of* `g_bar_l` *that activated only the desired two hidden units at the end of settling, try increasing the* `dt_vm` *parameter from .03 to .04, which will cause the network to settle faster in the same number of cycles by increas-*

ing the rate at which the membrane potential is updated on each cycle — are you still able to activate only the left two hidden feature units? What does this tell you about your previous results?

↪   Next try to activate the ambiguous (center) input feature, `Speakers`, by pressing the `RunAmbig` button.

One reasonable response of the network to this input would be to weakly activate the other features associated with this ambiguous input in `Hidden1`, indicating that it cannot choose between these two possibilities. This is impossible to achieve, however, because of the spreading activation phenomenon.

↪   `RunAmbig` first with a leak value of 1.737, and then with a leak value of 1.736.

You can see that the network does not activate the other feature units at all with a leak of 1.737, whereas a value of 1.736 causes all of the units in the network to become strongly activated. The network exhibits strongly bimodal behavior, and with only a constant leak current to control the excitation, does not allow for graded levels of activation that would otherwise communicate useful information about things like ambiguity.

↪   Next, set the leak current to 1.79 and press the `RunFull` button.

This activates both the `CRT` and `Speakers` inputs. You should see that the activation overflows to the third feature unit.

↪   Finally, increase the leak from 1.79 to 1.8 and `RunFull`.

Two inputs get weakly activated, but the `TV` unit in the `hidden2` layer does not. Thus, even with complete and unambiguous input for the `TV` features, activation either spreads unacceptably, or the network fails to get appropriately activated.

You should have observed from these explorations that bidirectional excitatory connectivity is a double-edged sword; although it can do some interesting amplification and pattern completion processing, it can also easily get carried away. In short, this type of connectivity acts like a microphone next to the speaker that it is driving (or a video camera pointed at its own monitor output) — you get too much *positive feedback*.

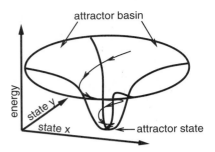

Figure 3.18: Diagram of attractor dynamics, where the activation state of the network converges over settling onto a given attractor state from any of a range of initial starting states (the attractor basin). The points in this space correspond (metaphorically) to different activation states in the network.

It is useful to note that these bidirectional networks tend to be strongly bimodal and *nonlinear* with respect to small parameter changes (i.e., they either get activated or not, with little grey area in between). This is an important property of such networks — one that will have implications in later chapters. This bimodal non-linear network behavior is supported (and encouraged) by the nonlinearities present in the point neuron activation function (see section 2.5.4). In particular, the saturating nonlinearity property of the *sigmoidal* noisy X-over-X-plus-1 function provides a necessary upper limit to the positive feedback loop. Also important is the effect of the gain parameter γ, which magnifies changes around the threshold value and contributes to the all-or-nothing character of these units.

↪   Go to the `PDP++Root` window. To continue on to the next simulation, close this project first by selecting `.projects/Remove/Project_0`. Or, if you wish to stop now, quit by selecting `Object/Quit`.

3.4.4   Attractor Dynamics

The notion of an *attractor* provides a unifying framework for understanding the effects of bidirectional excitatory connectivity. As we stated previously, an attractor is a stable activation state that the network settles into from a range of different starting states (think of one of those "gravity wells" at the science museum that sucks in your coins, as depicted in figure 3.18). The range of initial states that lead to the same final attractor state comprise the *attractor basin* for the attractor (think of a wash basin or sink).

In part for the reasons we just encountered in the previous exploration, a fuller treatment and exploration of attractors awaits the incorporation of inhibitory dynamics and the more general constraint satisfaction framework described later in section 3.6. Nevertheless, it is useful to redescribe some of the effects of bidirectional excitatory connectivity that we just explored in terms of attractor dynamics.

For example, one can think of pattern completion as the process of the network being attracted toward the stable state of the complete pattern from any of a number of different partial initial states. Thus, the set of partial initial states that lead to the complete state constitute the basin of attraction for this attractor.

Similarly, the bootstrapping effects of bidirectional amplification can be seen as reflecting a starting point out in the shallow slope of the farthest reaches of the attractor basin. As the activation strength slowly builds, the network gets more and more strongly pulled in toward the attractor, and the rate of activation change increases dramatically. Furthermore, the problematic case where the activation spreads to all units in the network can be viewed as a kind of superattractor that virtually any initial starting state is drawn into.

In section 3.6, we will see that the notion of an attractor actually has a solid mathematical basis not so far removed from the metaphor of a gravity well depicted in figure 3.18. Further, we will see that this mathematical basis depends critically on having symmetric bidirectional excitatory connections, along with inhibition to prevent the network from being overcome by a single superattractor.

3.5 Inhibitory Interactions

In virtually every simulation encountered so far, the leak current has played a central role in determining the network's behavior, because the leak current has been the only *counterweight* to the excitatory input coming from other neurons. However, as we discussed in the previous chapter (section 2.4.6), the neuron actually has two such counterweights, leak and inhibition (which can be

viewed as representing the likelihoods of two different kinds of *null hypotheses* in the Bayesian hypothesis testing framework analysis of detector function, see section 2.7). In this section, we will explore the unique contribution of the inhibitory counterweight.

As we saw in previous explorations, an important limitation of the leak current as a counterweight is that it is a *constant*. Thus, it cannot easily respond to dynamic changes in activation within the network (which is why you have had to manipulate it so frequently). In contrast, inhibition can play the role of a *dynamic* counterweight to excitatory input, as a function of the inhibitory input provided by the *inhibitory interneurons* known to exist in the cortex (section 3.2). These neurons appear to sample the general level of activation in the network, and send a dynamically adjusted amount of inhibition based on this activation level to nearby excitatory neurons.

The role of the inhibitory interneurons can be viewed like that of a thermostat-controlled air conditioner that prevents the network from getting too "hot" (active). Just as a thermostat samples the temperature in the air, the inhibitory neurons sample the activity of the network. When these inhibitory neurons detect that the network is getting too active, they produce more inhibition to counterbalance the increased activity, just as a thermostat will turn on the AC when the room gets too hot. Conversely, when they don't detect much activity, inhibitory neurons don't provide as much inhibition.

Thermostats typically have a **set point** behavior, where they maintain a roughly constant indoor temperature despite varying levels of heat influx from the external environment. The set point is achieved through the kind of **negative feedback** mechanism just described — the amount of AC output is proportional to the excess level of heat above the set point.

In the cortex there are two forms of connectivity involving the inhibitory neurons and their connections with the principal excitatory neurons, which give rise to **feedforward** and **feedback** inhibition (figure 3.19). As we will see in the following explorations, both types of inhibition are necessary. Note also that the inhibitory neurons inhibit themselves, providing a negative feedback loop to control their own activity levels, which will turn out to be important.

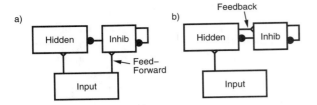

Figure 3.19: Two basic types of inhibitory connectivity (excitation is shown with the open triangular connections, and inhibition with the filled circular ones). **a)** Shows *feedforward* inhibition driven by the input layer activity, which *anticipates* and compensates for excitation coming into the layer. **b)** Shows *feedback* inhibition driven by the same layer that is being inhibited, which *reacts* to excitation within the layer. Inhibitory interneurons typically inhibit themselves as well.

Feedforward inhibition occurs when the inhibitory interneurons in a hidden layer are driven directly by the inputs to that layer, and then send inhibition to the principal (excitatory) hidden layer neurons (figure 3.19a). Thus, these hidden layer neurons receive an amount of inhibition that is a function of the level of activity in the input layer (which also projects excitatory connections into the hidden layer). This form of inhibition *anticipates* and *counterbalances* the excitation coming into a given layer from other layers. The anticipation effect is like having your thermostat take into account the temperature *outside* in deciding how much AC to provide *inside*. As a result, a hidden layer excitatory neuron will receive roughly proportional and offsetting amounts of excitation and inhibition. You might think this would prevent the neurons from ever getting active in the first place — instead, it acts as a kind of *filter*, because only those neurons that have particularly strong excitatory weights for the current input pattern will be able to overcome the feedforward inhibition.

Feedback inhibition occurs when the same layer that is being inhibited excites the inhibitory neurons, producing a *negative feedback loop* (figure 3.19b). Thus, feedback inhibition *reacts* to the level of excitation within the layer itself, and prevents the excitation from *exploding* (spreading uncontrollably to all units) as was observed in the previous section. This is like the usual thermostat that samples the same indoor air it regulates.

To speed up and simplify our simulations, we can summarize the effects of inhibitory interneurons by computing an **inhibition function** directly as a function of the amount of excitation in a layer, without the need to explicitly simulate the inhibitory interneurons themselves. The simplest and most effective inhibition functions are two forms of a **k-winners-take-all** (kWTA) function, described later. These functions impose a thermostat-like *set point* type of inhibition by ensuring that only k (or less) out of n total units in a layer are allowed to be strongly active.

We next discuss some of the particularly useful functional properties of inhibition, then explore the inhibitory dynamics of a cortical-like network with feedforward and feedback inhibition, and then introduce and explore the kWTA inhibition functions.

3.5.1 General Functional Benefits of Inhibition

There are several important general functional consequences of inhibition. First, inhibition leads to a form of **competition** between neurons. In the case of feedforward inhibition, only the most strongly activated neurons are able to overcome the inhibition, and in the case of feedback inhibition, these strongly active neurons are better able to withstand the inhibitory feedback, and their activity contributes to the inhibition of the other neurons. This competition is a very healthy thing for the network — it provides a mechanism for **selection**: finding the most appropriate representations for the current input pattern. This selection process is akin to *natural selection*, also based on competition (for natural resources), which results in the evolution of life itself! The selection process in a network occurs both on a moment-by-moment *on-line* basis, and over longer time periods through interaction with the learning mechanisms described in the next chapter. It is in this learning context that competition produces something akin to the evolution of representations.

The value of competition has long been recognized in artificial neural network models (Kohonen, 1984; McClelland & Rumelhart, 1981; Rumelhart & Zipser, 1986; Grossberg, 1976). Also, McNaughton and Morris (1987) showed how feedforward inhibition can result in a form of feedforward *pattern completion* — we will return to this in chapter 9. Furthermore, some have tried to make a very strong mapping between evolutionary selection and that which takes place in a neural network (e.g., Edelman, 1987), but we are inclined to rely on more basic competition and learning mechanisms in our understanding of this process.

Inhibition can lead to **sparse distributed** representations, which are distributed representations having a relatively small percentage of active units (e.g., 10–25%). Such representations achieve a balance between the benefits of distributed representations (section 3.3.2) and the benefits of inhibitory competition, which makes the representations *sparse* (i.e., having a relatively small percentage of active units).

Several theorists (e.g., Barlow, 1989; Field, 1994) have argued that the use of sparse distributed representations is particularly appropriate given the general structure of the natural environment. For example, in visual processing, a given object can be defined along a set of feature dimensions (e.g., shape, size, color, texture), with a large number of different values along each dimension (i.e., many different possible shapes, sizes, colors, textures, etc.). Assuming that the individual units in a distributed representation encode these feature values, a representation of a given object will only activate a small subset of units (i.e., the representations will be sparse). More generally, it seems as though the world can be usefully represented in terms of a large number of categories with a large number of exemplars per category (animals, furniture, trees, etc.). If we again assume that only a relatively few such exemplars are processed at a given time, a bias favoring sparse representations is appropriate.

Inhibition provides a built-in propensity or *bias* to produce sparse distributed representations, which can greatly benefit the development (learning) of useful representations of a world like ours where such representations are appropriate (of course, one could imagine hypothetical alternate universes where such a bias would be inappropriate). We will pick up on this theme again in chapter 4.

Finally, another way of viewing inhibition and sparse distributed representations is in terms of a balance between *competition* and the **cooperation** that needs to

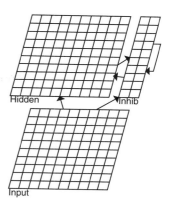

Figure 3.20: Network for exploring inhibition, with feedforward and feedback connections as in the previous figure.

take place in a distributed representation where multiple units contribute to represent a given thing. The extremes of complete competition (e.g., a localist representation with only one unit active) or complete cooperation (e.g., a fully distributed representation where each unit participates in virtually every pattern) are generally not as good as having a balance between the two (e.g., Dayan & Zemel, 1995; Hinton & Ghahramani, 1997).

3.5.2 Exploration of Feedforward and Feedback Inhibition

↪ Open the project `inhib.proj.gz` in `chapter_3` to begin.

You will see the usual three windows, including a `inhib_ctrl` overall control panel. The network contains a $10x10$ input layer, which projects to both the $10x10$ hidden layer of excitatory units, and a layer of 20 inhibitory neurons (figure 3.20). These inhibitory neurons will regulate the activation level of the hidden layer units, and should be thought of as the inhibitory units for the hidden layer (even though they are in their own layer for the purposes of this simulation). The ratio of 20 inhibitory units to 120 total hidden units (17 percent) is like that found in the cortex, which is commonly cited as roughly 15 percent (White, 1989a; Zilles, 1990). The inhibitory neurons are just like the excitatory neurons, except that their outputs contribute to the inhibitory conductance of a neuron instead of its excitatory conductance. We have also set one of the activation parameters to be different for these inhibitory neurons, as discussed below.

Let's begin as usual by viewing the weights of the network.

↪ Select r.wt and click on some of the hidden layer and inhib layer units.

Most of the weights are random, except for those from the inhibitory units, which are fixed at a constant value of .5. Notice also that the hidden layer excitatory units receive from the input and inhibitory units, while the inhibitory units receive feedforward connections from the input layer, and feedback connections from the excitatory hidden units, as well as inhibitory connections from themselves.

Now, we will run the network. First, we can open a graph log that will record the overall levels of activation (average activation) in the hidden and inhibitory units.

↪ Hit View in the control panel and select GRAPH_LOG.

The avg_act_Hidd line (in red) plots the average hidden activations, and the avg_act_Inhi line (in orange) plots the average inhibitory activations.

↪ Now, select act to view activations in the network window, and press Run in the control panel.

You will see the input units activated by a random activity pattern, and after several cycles of activation updating, the hidden and inhibitory units will become active. The activation appears quite controlled, as the inhibition counterbalances the excitation from the input layer. Note that the level of the leak current g_bar_l is very small at .01, so that virtually all of the counterbalancing of excitation is being performed by the inhibition, not by the leak current. From the average activity plotted in the graph window (figure 3.21), you should see that the hidden layer (red line) has around 10 percent activation.

In the next sections, we manipulate some of the parameters in the control panel to get a better sense of the principles underlying the inhibitory dynamics in the network. Because we will be running the network many times, you may want to toggle the network display off to speed up the settling process (the graph log contains the relevant information anyway).

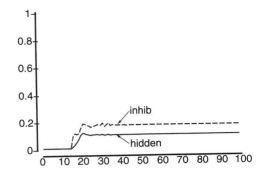

Figure 3.21: Plot of average hidden (excitatory — red line in the actual simulation) and inhibitory (orange line) unit activities, showing how inhibition anticipates excitation.

↪ To toggle the display off, click on the Display button in the upper left-hand corner of the NetView window.

Strength of Inhibitory Conductances

Let's start by manipulating the maximal conductance for the inhibitory current into the excitatory units, g_bar_i.hidden (note that the . means that hidden is a subfield of the overall g_bar_i field that occupies one line in the control panel), which multiplies the level of inhibition (considered to be a proportion of the maximal value) coming into the hidden layer (excitatory) neurons. Clearly, one would predict that this plays an important role.

↪ Decrease g_bar_i.hidden from 5 to 3 and press Run. Then increase g_bar_i.hidden to 7 and press Run.

Question 3.10 (a) *What effect does decreasing* g_bar_i.hidden *have on the average level of excitation of the hidden units and of the inhibitory units?* **(b)** *What effect does increasing* g_bar_i.hidden *have on the average level of excitation of the hidden units and of the inhibitory units?* **(c)** *Explain this pattern of results.*

↪ Set g_bar_i.hidden back to 5.

Now, let's see what happens when we manipulate the corresponding parameter for the inhibition coming into the inhibitory neurons, g_bar_i.inhib. You might expect to get results similar to those just obtained for `g_bar_i.hidden`, but be careful — inhibition upon inhibitory neurons could have interesting consequences.

↪ First Run with a `g_bar_i.inhib` of 4 for comparison. Then decrease `g_bar_i.inhib` to 3 and Run, and next increase `g_bar_i.inhib` to 5 and Run.

With a `g_bar_i.inhib` of 3, you should see that the excitatory activation drops, but the inhibitory level stays roughly the same! With a value of 5, the excitatory activation level increases, but the inhibition again remains the same. This is a difficult phenomenon to understand, but the following provide a few ways of thinking about what is going on.

First, it seems straightforward that reducing the amount of inhibition on the inhibitory neurons should result in more activation of the inhibitory neurons. If you just look at the very first blip of activity for the inhibitory neurons, this is true (as is the converse that increasing the inhibition results in lower activation). However, once the feedback inhibition starts to kick in as the hidden units become active, the inhibitory activity returns to the same level for all runs. This makes sense if the greater activation of the inhibitory units for the `g_bar_i.inhib` = 3 case then inhibits the hidden units more (which it does, causing them to have lower activation), which then would result in *less* activation of the inhibitory units coming from the feedback from the hidden units. This reduced activation of the inhibitory neurons cancels out the increased activation from the lower `g_bar_i.inhib` value, resulting in the same inhibitory activation level. The mystery is why the hidden units remain at their lower activation levels once the inhibition goes back to its original activation level.

One way we can explain this is by noting that this is a *dynamic* system, not a static balance of excitation and inhibition. Every time the excitatory hidden units start to get a little bit more active, they in turn activate the inhibitory units more easily (because they are less apt to inhibit themselves), which in turn provides just enough extra inhibition to offset the advance of the hidden units. This battle is effectively played out at the level of the *derivatives* (changes) in activations in the two pools of units, not their absolute levels, which would explain why we cannot really see much evidence of it by looking at only these absolute levels.

A more intuitive (but somewhat inaccurate in the details) way of understanding the effect of inhibition on inhibitory neurons is in terms of the location of the thermostat relative to the AC output vent — if you place the thermostat very close to the AC vent (while you are sitting some constant distance away from the vent), you will be warmer than if the thermostat was far away from the AC output. Thus, how strongly the thermostat is driven by the AC output vent is analogous to the `g_bar_i.inhib` parameter — larger values of `g_bar_i.inhib` are like having the thermostat closer to the vent, and will result in higher levels of activation (greater warmth) in the hidden layer, and the converse for smaller values.

↪ Set `g_bar_i.inhib` back to 4 before continuing (or hit `Defaults`).

Roles of Feedforward and Feedback Inhibition

Next we assess the importance and properties of the feedforward versus feedback inhibitory projections by manipulating their relative strengths. The `inhib_ctrl` control panel has two parameters that determine the relative contribution of the feedforward and feedback inhibitory pathways: `scale.ff` applies to the feedforward weights from the input to the inhibitory units, and `scale.fb` applies to the feedback weights from the hidden layer to the inhibitory units. These parameters uniformly scale the strengths of an entire projection of connections from one layer to another, and are the arbitrary `wt_scale.rel` (r_k) relative scaling parameters described in section 2.5.1.

↪ Set `scale.ff` to 0, effectively eliminating the feedforward excitatory inputs to the inhibitory neurons from the input layer.

Question 3.11 (a) *How does this affect the behavior of the excitatory and inhibitory average activity levels?* (b) *Explain this result. (Hint: think about the anticipatory effects of feedforward inhibition.) Next, set* `scale.ff` *back to .35 and* `scale.fb` *to 0 to turn off the feedback inhibition.* (c) *Now what happens?* (d) *Try finding a value of* `scale.ff` *(in increments of .05) that gives roughly the same activity level as the initial default system — how does this differ from the initial* *system? Explain this pattern of results.* **(e)** *Explain why both kinds of inhibition are useful for producing a system that responds in a rapid but controlled way to excitatory inputs.*

Time Constants and Feedforward Anticipation

We just saw that feedforward inhibition is important for anticipating and offsetting the excitation coming from the inputs to the hidden layer. In addition to this feedforward inhibitory connectivity, the anticipatory effect depends on a difference between excitatory and inhibitory neurons in their rate of updating, which is controlled by the vm_dt parameters dt.hidden and dt.inhib in the control panel (cf. section 2.4.5, equation 2.7). As you can see, the excitatory neurons are updated at .04 (slower), while the inhibitory are at .15 (faster). The faster updating of the inhibitory neurons allows them to more quickly become activated by the feedforward input, and send anticipatory inhibition to the excitatory hidden units before they actually get activated.

↪ To verify this, click on Defaults, set dt.inhib to .04, and then Run.

The faster time constant also enables inhibition to more rapidly adapt to changes in the overall excitation level. There is ample evidence that cortical inhibitory neurons respond faster to inputs than pyramidal neurons (e.g., Douglas & Martin, 1990).

One other important practical point about these update rate constants will prove to be an important advantage of the simplified inhibitory functions described in the next section. These rate constants must be set to be relatively slow to prevent oscillatory behavior.

↪ To see this, press Defaults, and then set dt.inhib to .2, and dt.hidden to .1 and Run.

These oscillations are largely prevented with finer time scale upgrading, because the excitatory neurons update their activity in smaller steps, to which the inhibitory neurons are better able to smoothly react.

Effects of Learning

One of the important things that inhibition must do is to compensate adequately for the changes in weight values that accompany learning. Typically, as units learn,

they develop greater levels of variance in the amount of excitatory input received from the input patterns, with some patterns providing strong excitation to a given unit and others producing less. This is a natural result of the specialization of units for representing (detecting) some things and not others. We can test whether the current inhibitory mechanism adequately handles these changes by simulating the effects of learning, by giving units excitatory weight values with a higher level of variance.

↪ First, press Defaults to return to the default parameters. Run this case to get a baseline for comparison.

In this case, the network's weights are produced by generating random numbers with a mean of .25, and a uniform variance around that mean of .2.

↪ Next set the wt_type field in the control panel to TRAINED instead of the default UNTRAINED.

The weights are then initialized with the same mean but a variance of .7 using Gaussian (normally) distributed values. This produces a much higher variance of excitatory net inputs for units in the hidden layer. There is also an increase in the total overall weight strength with the increase in variance because there is more room for larger weights above the .25 mean, but not much more below it.

↪ Press Run to see what difference this makes for the overall excitatory level.

You should observe a greater level of excitation using the TRAINED weights compared to the UNTRAINED weights.

↪ You can verify that the system can compensate for this change by increasing the g_bar_i.hidden to 8.

Bidirectional Excitation

To make things simpler at the outset, we have so far been exploring a relatively easy case for inhibition where the network does not have the bidirectional excitatory connectivity that overwhelmed the constant leak counterweight in section 3.4.3. Now, let's try running a network with two bidirectionally connected hidden layers (figure 3.22).

↪ First, select Defaults to get back the default parameters, do a Run for comparison, and then set network to BIDIR_EXCITE instead of FF_EXCITE.

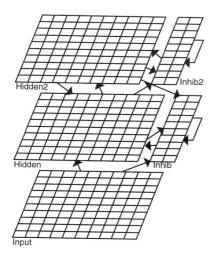

Figure 3.22: Inhibition network with bidirectional excitatory connectivity.

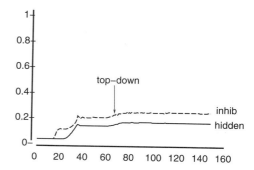

Figure 3.23: Plot of average hidden (excitatory) and inhibitory unit activities for the first hidden layer, showing where the top-down excitation comes in. Although detectable, the extra excitation is well controlled by the inhibition.

In extending the network to the bidirectional case, we also have to extend our notions of what feedforward inhibition is. In general, the role of feedforward inhibition is to anticipate and counterbalance the level of excitatory input coming into a layer. Thus, in a network with bidirectional excitatory connectivity, the inhibitory neurons for a given layer also have to receive the top-down excitatory connections, which play the role of "feedforward" inhibition.

↪ Verify that this network has both bidirectional excitatory connectivity and the "feedforward" inhibition coming back from the second hidden layer by examining the r.wt weights as usual.

↪ Now Run this network.

The graph log (figure 3.23) shows the average activity for only the first hidden and inhibitory layers (as before). Note that the initial part up until the point where the second hidden layer begins to be active is the same as before, but as the second layer activates, it feeds back to the first layer inhibitory neurons, which become more active, as do the excitatory neurons. However, the overall activity level remains quite under control and not substantially different than before, which is in distinct contrast to the earlier simulations with just a leak current operating.

Next, we will see that inhibition is differentially important for bidirectionally connected networks.

↪ Set the g_bar_i.hidden parameter to 3, and Run.

This reduces the amount of inhibition on the excitatory neurons. Note that this has a relatively small impact on the initial, feedforward portion of the activity curve, but when the second hidden layer becomes active, the network becomes catastrophically over activated — an epileptic fit!

↪ Set the g_bar_i.hidden parameter back to 5.

Set Point Behavior

Our final exploration of inhibition provides some motivation for the summary inhibition functions presented in the next section. Here, we explore what happens to the activity levels when different overall levels of excitatory input are presented to the network.

↪ First, Clear the graph log and Run the network for purposes of comparison.

The input pattern is set to have the default of 20 (out of 100) units active, which is what we have been using all along.

↪ Change the input_pct field in the control panel to 15 instead of 20, Apply, and then hit the NewInput button to make a new input pattern with this new percentage activity. Then do Run.

This changes the input pattern to have 15 units active. When you Run now, the activity level is not substantially different from the previous case (a difference of 1–2%).

↪ Next, set `input_pct` to 25, `Apply`, `NewInput`, and `Run`.

Again, you should observe only modest increases in activity level.

Thus, the network appears to be relatively robust to changes in overall input excitation, though it does show some effect. Perhaps a more dramatic demonstration comes from the relatively small differences between the initial activity level in the hidden units compared to the subsequent level after the input from the second hidden layer has kicked in. It is this approximate *set point* behavior, where the system tends to produce a relatively fixed level of activity regardless of the magnitude of the excitatory input, that is captured by the inhibition functions described in the next section.

Question 3.12 *Explain in general terms why the system exhibits this set point behavior.*

↪ Last, you can also change the activation function, using the `ActFun` button.

You should see that the same basic principles apply when the units use a spiking activation function.

↪ To continue on to the next simulation, you can leave this project open because we will use it again. Or, if you wish to stop now, quit by selecting `Object/Quit` in the `PDP++Root` window.

3.5.3 The k-Winners-Take-All Inhibitory Functions

We saw in the previous section that the appropriate combination of feedforward and feedback inhibition gives rise to the controlled activation of excitatory neurons, even when they are bidirectionally connected. Because the inhibitory interneurons are essentially just sensing the overall level of excitation coming into a layer and delivering some roughly proportional level of inhibition, it would seem plausible that the general effects of these inhibitory neurons could be summarized by directly computing the inhibitory current into the excitatory neurons using an *inhibitory function* that takes into account this overall level of excitation. Doing so would avoid the need to explicitly simulate the inhibitory neurons and all of their connectivity, which

adds significantly to the amount of computation required for a given simulation. In addition, we might be able to do this in such a way as to avoid the need to use slow time constants in updating the units, which would save even more processing resources.

The class of inhibitory functions that we adopt here are known as *k-winners-take-all* (kWTA) functions (Majani, Erlarson, & Abu-Mostafa, 1989), of which we develop two different versions (**basic kWTA** and **average-based kWTA**). A kWTA function ensures that no more than k units out of n total in a layer are active at any given time. From a biological perspective, a kWTA function is attractive because it captures the *set point* property of the inhibitory interneurons, where the activity level is maintained through negative feedback at a roughly constant level (i.e., k). From a functional perspective, a kWTA function is beneficial in that it enforces the development of sparse distributed representations, whose benefits were discussed previously.

There is an important tension that arises in the kWTA function between the need to apply a firm set point constraint on the one hand, and the need for flexibility in this constraint on the other. We know that a firm activation constraint is needed to prevent runaway excitation in a bidirectionally connected network. We will also see in the next chapter that a strong inhibitory constraint is important for learning. Nevertheless, it also seems reasonable that the network would benefit from some flexibility in determining how many units should be active to represent a given input pattern.

One general solution to this firmness/flexibility tradeoff that is implemented to varying extents by both versions of kWTA functions is to make the k parameter an *upper limit*, allowing some flexibility in the range between 0 and k units, and in the graded activation values of the k active units. This upper limit quality results from the impact of the leak current, which can be set to be strong enough to filter out weakly excited units that might nevertheless be in the top k of the units. Thus, perhaps a more accurate name for these functions would be *k-or-less* WTA. In addition, the two different versions of kWTA functions represent different tradeoffs in this balance between a firm constraint and flexibility, with the basic kWTA function being more firm and the average-based kWTA function being more flexible.

Our primary interest in constructing an inhibition function is to achieve a simple and computationally effective approximation to the *behavior* of an actual cortical network, specifically its set point nature as represented by the kWTA function. Thus, as long as our function captures this target behavior, the details of how we implement it need not be particularly biologically plausible themselves. Indeed, as will be clear in the next section, the implementation is not particularly biologically plausible, but it is efficient, and directly implements the kWTA objective. We can only tolerate this kind of implausibility by knowing that the resulting function approximates a much more plausible network based directly on the inhibitory interneurons known to exist in the cortex — we assume that all of our kWTA models could be reimplemented using this much more realistic form of inhibition and function in qualitatively the same way (only they would take a lot longer to run!).

kWTA Function Implementation

First, it should be clear that the k units active in a kWTA function are the ones that are receiving the most excitatory input (g_e). Thus, the first step in computing both versions of the kWTA functions is to sort the units according to g_e (note that in practice a complete sort is not necessary, as will become clear, so the computation can be optimized considerably). Then, a layer-wide level of inhibitory conductance (g_i) is computed such that the top k units will (usually) have above-threshold equilibrium membrane potentials with that value of g_i, while the rest will remain below firing threshold. This inhibitory conductance is then used by each unit in the layer when updating their membrane potentials.

Thus, to implement kWTA we need to be able to compute the amount of inhibitory current that would put a unit just at threshold given its present level of excitatory input, which we write as g_i^Θ, where Θ is the threshold membrane potential value. The necessary equation should be familiar to you from the exercises in chapter 2, where you used the equilibrium membrane potential equation (2.9) to compute the threshold level of leak current. Thus, the specific form of the point neuron activation function is important for enabling the appropriate amount of inhibition to be easily computed. Doing

this computation for the inhibitory conductance at the threshold (g_i^Θ), we get:

$$g_i^\Theta = \frac{g_e^* \bar{g}_e(E_e - \Theta) + g_l \bar{g}_l(E_l - \Theta)}{\Theta - E_i} \quad (3.2)$$

where g_e^* represents the excitatory input minus the contribution from the bias weight. Networks learn much better using this g_e^* value here, presumably because it allows the bias weights to override the kWTA constraint, thereby introducing an important source of flexibility.

In the basic version of the kWTA algorithm (KWTA in the simulator), we simply compute g_i as a value intermediate between the g_i^Θ values for the k and $k+1th$ units as sorted by level of excitatory conductance (g_e). This ensures that the $k+1th$ unit remains below threshold, while the kth unit is above it. Expressed as a formula, this is:

$$g_i = g_i^\Theta(k+1) + q(g_i^\Theta(k) - g_i^\Theta(k+1)) \quad (3.3)$$

where the constant $0 < q < 1$ determines where exactly to place the inhibition between the k and $k+1th$ units. A value of $q = .25$ is typically used, which enables the kth unit to be reasonably far above the inhibitory threshold depending on how the g_i^Θ terms are distributed.

To see the importance of the shape of the distribution, we have plotted in figure 3.24 several different possible such distributions. These plots show the values of g_i^Θ (which are monotonically related to g_e) for the rank ordered units. Thus, the g_i value computed by equation 3.3 can be plotted directly on these graphs, and it is easy to see how far the upper k units are above this inhibitory value. The greater this distance (shown by the bracket on the Y axis in the graphs), the more strongly activated these units will be.

As you can see, the strongest activity (greatest distance above g_i) is produced when there is a clear separation between the most active units and those that are less active. This is a desirable functional property for the inhibition function, because the activation then reflects something like the "confidence" in the active units being definitively more excited. Furthermore, those units that are just above the g_i will have weak or no activation values, even if they are at a rank position above the

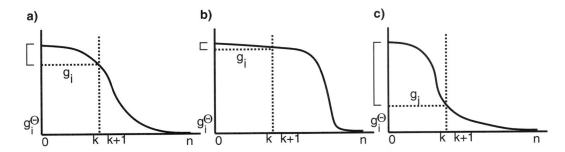

Figure 3.24: Possible distributions of level of excitation across units in a layer, plotted on the Y axis by g_i^Θ (which is monotonically related to excitatory net input g_e), and rank order index on the X axis. The basic kWTA function places the layer-wide inhibitory current value g_i between the k and $k+1th$ most active units, as shown by the dotted lines. The shape of the distribution significantly affects the extent to which the most highly activated units can rise above the threshold, as is highlighted by the brackets on the Y axis, which indicate the distance between the most active unit and the inhibitory threshold. **a)** Shows a standard kind of distribution, where the most active units are reasonably above the inhibition. **b)** Has many strongly activated units below the threshold, resulting in a small excitatory-inhibitory differential for the most activated units. **c)** Has few strongly active units, resulting in a very large differential for the most activated units.

k threshold, depending on the strength of the leak current and/or their bias weights. Thus, there is some room for flexibility in the kWTA constraint.

The second version of the kWTA function, the *average-based kWTA* function (KWTA_AVG in the simulator), provides still greater flexibility regarding the precise activity level in the layer, while still providing a relatively firm upper limit. The tradeoff in lack of precision about the exact activity level is often worth the advantages to the network in having a bit more flexibility in its representations. In this version, the layer-wide inhibitory conductance g_i is placed in between the average g_i^Θ values for the top k units and the average g_i^Θ values for the remaining n-k units. This averaging makes the level of inhibition a function of the distribution of excitation across the entire layer, instead of a function of only two units (k and $k + 1$) as was the case with the basic WTA function (equation 3.3). We will see in a moment that this imparts a greater degree of flexibility in the overall activity level.

The expression for the average of g_i^Θ for the top k units is:

$$\langle g_i^\Theta \rangle_k = \frac{1}{k} \sum_{i=1}^{k} g_i^\Theta(i) \qquad (3.4)$$

and for the remaining $n - k$ units:

$$\langle g_i^\Theta \rangle_{n-k} = \frac{1}{n - k} \sum_{i=k+1}^{n} g_i^\Theta(i) \qquad (3.5)$$

Then we can just plug these averages into the same basic formula as used before for placing the inhibitory conductance somewhere in between these two values:

$$g_i = \langle g_i^\Theta \rangle_{n-k} + q(\langle g_i^\Theta \rangle_k - \langle g_i^\Theta \rangle_{n-k}) \qquad (3.6)$$

The q value in this case is a much more important variable than in the basic kWTA function, because the two averaged inhibitory conductances typically have a greater spread and the resulting g_i value is not specifically guaranteed to be between the k and $k + 1$th units. Thus, it is typically important to adjust this parameter based on the overall activity level of a layer (α), with a value of .5 being appropriate for activity levels of around 25 percent, and higher values for lower (sparser) levels of activity (e.g., .6 for 15%).

Depending on the distribution of excitation (and therefore g_i^Θ) over the layer, there can be more or less than k units active under the average-based kWTA function (figure 3.25). For example, when there are some strongly active units just below the k rank order level, they will tend to be above threshold for the computed

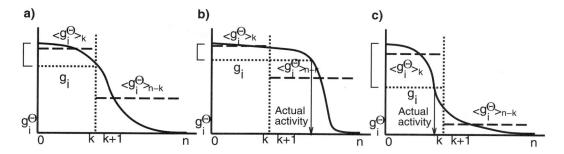

Figure 3.25: Plots of the average-based kWTA inhibitory function for the same distributions of excitatory input as the previous figure. The dashed lines represent the average g_i^Θ values for the top k units ($\langle g_i^\Theta \rangle_k$) and the remaining $n - k$ values ($\langle g_i^\Theta \rangle_{n-k}$). Although case **a)** has the inhibition in a similar place as the basic kWTA function (between k and $k + 1$), **b)** results in a *lower* level of inhibition than basic kWTA with more than k units becoming active (shown by the actual activity arrow), and **c)** results in a *higher* level of inhibition than basic kWTA with fewer than k units becoming active (again shown by actual activity arrow).

inhibition, resulting in more than k total units active (figure 3.25b). In contrast, when the lower portion of the top k units are not strongly excited, they will tend to be below threshold with the computed g_i value, resulting in fewer than k units active.

Thus, when the learning algorithm is shaping the representations in the network, it has a little bit more flexibility in choosing appropriate overall levels of activation for different cases. The downside of this flexibility is that activation levels are less tightly controlled, which can be a problem, especially in layers having very sparse activity levels. Thus, we typically use the average-based kWTA function for layers with 15 or more percent activity, and the basic kWTA function for sparser layers (especially localist layers having only one active unit).

Finally, we know from our previous explorations that the inhibitory-interneuron based inhibition that more closely reflects the kind of inhibition actually present in the cortex is a complex function of a number of parameters. The cortex has likely evolved appropriate parameters for achieving a reasonable balance between flexibility and firmness in activation control. Therefore, we are not too concerned with the extra degree of freedom afforded to the modeler in selecting an appropriate version of the kWTA function. Ideally, as computational resources get more powerful, it will become feasible to use more biologically plausible forms of inhibition.

3.5.4 Exploration of kWTA Inhibition

Now, let's explore the kWTA inhibition functions and compare their behavior with that of the previous networks.

↪ Open the project `inhib.proj.gz` in `chapter_3` to begin. (Or, if you already have this project open from the previous exercise, reset the parameters to their default values using the `Defaults` button.) Make sure the graph log is open (`View`, `GRAPH_LOG`). Set `network` to `BIDIR_EXCITE` to select the bidirectionally connected network, and `Run`.

This should reproduce the standard activation graph for the case with actual inhibitory neurons.

↪ Now, set the `inhib_type` to `KWTA_INHIB` instead of the default `UNIT_INHIB` to use the basic kWTA function described above. Hit `Apply`.

The k value of this function is set according to the `kwta_pct` value in the `inhib_ctrl` control panel (this percentage is automatically translated into a corresponding k value, 15 in this case, by the software).

↪ Press `Run`.

Notice that roughly the same level of activity results (the inhibitory activity is at zero, because these units are not used for this function). Also, the activity function is somewhat smoother, because the kWTA function effectively does a perfect job of anticipating the appropriate level of inhibition required. Further, the activation of the hidden layer starts much earlier because we can use a faster `dt.hidden` parameter (.2 instead of .04 — more on this below).

↪ Now select `KWTA_AVG_INHIB` for the `inhib_type` to use the average-based kWTA function (`Apply`), and `Run` again.

You should observe that the hidden layer activation stabilizes on the target activation level of 15 percent.

↪ To test the set point behavior of the kWTA functions, run the network with `input_pct` levels of 10 and 30 (do not forget to hit `NewInput`) in addition to the standard 20 (you can do this for both types of kWTA function).

Notice that these functions exhibit stronger set point behavior than the inhibitory unit based inhibition (with the average-based kWTA showing just slightly more variability in overall activity level). This is because the kWTA functions are designed explicitly to have a set point, whereas the inhibitory units only roughly produce set-point behavior. Thus, we must always remember that the kWTA functions are merely an *idealized approximation* of the effects of inhibitory neurons, and do not behave in an identical fashion.

Next we will see one of the main advantages of the kWTA functions.

↪ Set the `input_pct` back to the default 20 (and `NewInput`). Set `inhib_type` to `KWTA_INHIB` and try to find the fastest update parameter `dt.hidden` (in increments of .1, to a maximum of 1) that does not result in significant oscillatory behavior.

Question 3.13 (a) *What was the highest value of* `dt.hidden` *that you found? How does this compare with the value of this parameter for unit-based inhibition (.04)?* **(b)** *Why do you think kWTA can use such a fast update rate where unit-based inhibition cannot?*

↪ Return the `dt.hidden` parameter to .2 before continuing.

For the *k-or-less* property of the basic kWTA function to apply, you have to set a leak current value `g_bar_l` that prevents weak excitation from activating the units, but allows strong excitation to produce activation.

↪ To see this k-or-less property, increase `g_bar_l` (in .1 increments) to find a value that prevents excitation from an `input_pct` of 10 or less from activating any of the hidden units, but allows excitation of 20 or more to activate both layers.

↪ Go to the `PDP++Root` window. To continue on to the next simulation, close this project first by selecting `.projects/Remove/Project_0`. Or, if you wish to stop now, quit by selecting `Object/Quit`.

3.5.5 Digits Revisited with kWTA Inhibition

To cap off our explorations of inhibition, we return to the digits example and revisit some of the issues we originally explored without the benefits of inhibition. This will give you a better sense of how inhibition, specifically the basic kWTA function, performs in a case where the representations are more than just random activation patterns.

↪ Open the project `inhib_digits.proj.gz` in `chapter_3` to begin.

This is essentially identical to the `loc_dist.proj.gz` project you explored in section 3.3.3, except that basic kWTA inhibition is in effect, and is controlled by the `hidden_k` parameter that specifies the maximum number of hidden units that can be strongly active. The bias weights have also been turned off by default for the localist network, for reasons that will become clear below.

↪ View the `GRID_LOG`, then `Run` with the default `hidden_k` parameter of 1.

You should get the expected localist result that a single hidden unit is strongly active for each input. Note that the leak current `g_bar_l` is relatively weak at 1.5, so it is not contributing to the selection of the active unit (you can prove this to yourself by setting it to 0 and re-running — be sure to set it back to 1.5 if you do this).

↪ Now, increase the `hidden_k` parameter to 2, and `Run` again.

Notice that in several cases, only 1 unit is strongly activated. This is because the second and third (*k* and *k+1th*) units had identical excitatory net input values, meaning that when the inhibition was placed right between them, it was placed right at their threshold levels of inhibition. Thus, both of these units were just at threshold (which results in the weak activation shown due to the effects of the noise in the noisy XX1 activation function as described in section 2.5.4). This is like the situation shown in figure 3.24b, except that the most active unit is well above the *k* and *k+1th* ones.

↪ Continue to increase the `hidden_k` parameter, and `Run`.

You should observe that this provides increasingly distributed patterns in the hidden layer (with some variation in the total number of active units due to the effects of ties as just discussed). The advantage of controlling the number of active units through the kWTA inhibition function instead of the trial-and-error manipulation of the `g_bar_l` parameter is that you have precise and direct control over the outcome. Once this parameter is set, it will also apply regardless of changes in many network parameters that would affect the `g_bar_l` parameter.

Now, let's explore the use of kWTA inhibition in the distributed, feature-based network.

↪ Set `network` to `DISTRIBUTED_NETWORK` instead of `LOCALIST_NETWORK`. Set `hidden_k` back to 1, `Apply`, and press `Run`.

Notice how, except when there were ties, we were able to force this distributed network to have a single hidden unit active — this would have been very difficult to achieve by setting the `g_bar_l` parameter due to the fine tolerances involved in separating units with very similar levels of excitation.

↪ Do a `Cluster` on the `CLUSTER_HIDDEN` unit activities.

Question 3.14 (a) *How well does one feature do at representing the similarity structure of the digits?* (b) *What value of the* `hidden_k` *parameter produces a cluster without any collapsed distinctions?* (c) *How many of the hidden patterns actually have that many units active?* (d) *What mechanism explains why not every pattern had* `hidden_k` *units active?* (e) *Keeping the* `hidden_k` *value you just found, what happens to the activity levels and clustering when you reduce the leak current to 1? 0?*

↪ Go to the `PDP++Root` window. To continue on to the next simulation, close this project first by selecting `.projects/Remove/Project_0`. Or, if you wish to stop now, quit by selecting `Object/Quit`.

3.5.6 Other Simple Inhibition Functions

Historically speaking, the predecessor to the kWTA inhibition function was the single winner-takes-all (WTA) function. A simple case of WTA was used in the **competitive learning** algorithm (Rumelhart & Zipser, 1986; Grossberg, 1976), in which the most excited unit's activity is set to 1, and the rest to zero. A "softer" version of this idea was developed by Nowlan (1990) using some of the same kinds of Bayesian mathematics discussed in section 2.7. In this case, units were activated to the extent that their likelihood of generating (predicting) the input pattern was larger than that of other units. Thus the activity of each unit had the form:

$$y_j = \frac{l_j}{\sum_k l_k} \qquad (3.7)$$

where l_j is the likelihood measure ($P(data|h)$) for each unit, and the denominator comes from replacing $P(data)$ with a sum over the conditional probabilities for all the mutually exclusive and exhaustive hypotheses (as represented by the different units).

This mutual exclusivity assumption constitutes a significant limitation of this type of model. As we saw above, distributed representations obtain their considerable power by enabling things to be represented by multiple cooperating units. The exclusivity assumption is inconsistent with the use of such distributed representations, relegating the single WTA models to using localist representations (even when the units have graded "soft" activation values). Nevertheless, these simpler models are important because they admit to a firm mathematical understanding at the level of the entire network, which is not generally possible for the kWTA function.

A related form of activation function to the simple WTA function is the **Kohonen network** (Kohonen, 1984), which builds on ideas that were also proposed by von der Malsburg (1973). Here, a single "winner" is chosen as before, but now a *neighborhood* of units around this winner also gets to be active, with the activation trailing off as a function of distance from the winner. When used with learning, such networks exhibit many interesting properties deriving from their built-in tendency to treat neighboring items in similar ways. We will revisit these ideas in chapter 8, in a model of early visual processing and learning.

An important limitation of the Kohonen network derives from the rigidity of its representation — it does not possess the full power of distributed representations because it cannot "mix and match" different units to represent different combinations of features. However, we will see later how we can build a neighborhood bias into the lateral connectivity between units, which accomplishes effectively the same thing as the Kohonen network, but does so within the more flexible kWTA framework described above. Such an approach is more similar to that of von der Malsburg (1973), which also used explicit lateral connectivity.

Finally, a number of models have been constructed using units that communicate both excitation and inhibition directly to other units (McClelland & Rumelhart, 1981; Grossberg, 1976, 1978). The McClelland and Rumelhart (1981) model goes by the name of *interactive activation and competition* (IAC), and was one of the first to bring a number of the principles discussed in this chapter to bear on cognitive phenomena (namely the word superiority effect described previously). Interactive activation is the same as bidirectional excitatory connectivity, which provided top-down and bottom-up processing in their model. Grossberg (1976, 1978) was a pioneer in the development of these kinds of bidirectionally connected networks, and was one of the first to document many of the properties discussed above.

These models have some important limitations, however. First, the fact that special inhibitory neurons were not used is clearly at odds with the separation of excitation and inhibition found in the brain. Second, this kind of direct inhibition among units is not very good at sustaining distributed representations where multiple units are active and yet competing with each other. The case where one unit is active and inhibiting all the others is stable, but a delicate balance of excitation and inhibition is required to keep two or more units active at the same time without either one of them dominating the others or too many units getting active. With separate inhibitory neurons, the inhibition is summed and "broadcast" to all the units within the layer, instead of being transmitted point-to-point among excitatory neurons. This summed inhibition results in smoother, more

consistent activation dynamics with distributed representations, as we saw in the earlier explorations.

3.6   Constraint Satisfaction

Having explored the distinct effects of excitation and inhibition, we can now undertake a more global level of analysis where bidirectional excitation and inhibition can be seen as part of a larger computational goal. This more global level of analysis incorporates many of the more specific phenomena explored previously, and consolidates them under a unified conceptual and mathematical framework.

The overall perspective is called **constraint satisfaction**, where the network can be seen as simultaneously trying to satisfy a number of different constraints imposed on it via the external inputs from the environment, and the weights and activation states of the network itself. Mathematically, it can be shown that symmetrically connected bidirectional networks with sigmoidal activation functions are maximizing the extent to which they satisfy these constraints. The original demonstration of this point was due to Hopfield (1982, 1984), who applied some ideas from physics toward the understanding of network behavior. These **Hopfield networks** were extended with more powerful learning mechanisms by in the **Boltzmann machine** (Ackley, Hinton, & Sejnowski, 1985).

The crucial concept borrowed from physics is that of an **energy function**. A physical system (e.g., a crystal) has an energy function associated with it that provides a global measure of energy of the system, which depends on its temperature and the strength of the interactions or connections between the particles (atoms) in the system. A system with a higher temperature has particles moving at faster velocities, and thus higher energy. The interactions between particles impose the constraints on this system, and part of the energy of the system is a function of how strong these constraints are and to what extent the system is obeying them or not — a system that is not obeying the constraints has higher energy, because it takes energy to violate the constraints. Think of the constraints as gravity — it takes energy to oppose gravity, so that a system at a higher elevation above the ground has violated these constraints to a greater extent and has higher energy. A system that has satisfied the constraints is at a lower state of energy, and nature always tries to settle into a lower energy state by satisfying more constraints.

A simple example of an energy function is a Euclidean (sum of squares) distance function between two objects (a and b) that don't like to be separated (e.g., two magnets with opposite poles facing each other). An energy function for such a system would be:

$$E = (x_a - x_b)^2 + (y_a - y_b)^2 \qquad (3.8)$$

in two dimensions with x and y coordinates. As the two objects get closer together, the distance value obviously gets smaller, meaning that the constraint of having the objects closer together gets more satisfied according to this energy function. As we will see, energy functions often have this "squared" form of the distance function.

In a network of neurons, a state that has satisfied more constraints can also be thought of as having a lower energy. When we apply the mathematics of these energy functions to networks, we find that the simple act of updating the activations of the units in the network results in the same kind of settling into a lower energy state by satisfying more constraints. The standard form of the network energy function is as follows:

$$E = -\frac{1}{2} \sum_j \sum_i x_i w_{ij} x_j \qquad (3.9)$$

where x_i and x_j represent the sending and receiving unit activations, respectively, and w_{ij} is the weight connecting them. Note that each unit in the network appears as both a sender and a receiver in the double-sum term — it is this double-counting that motivates the $\frac{1}{2}$ factor in the equation, as we will see.

It is important that the weights connecting two units be at least roughly *symmetric*, so that the influences of one unit are reciprocated by those of the other unit. This symmetry enables the network to find a single *consistent* state that satisfies all of the units — if the weights were not symmetric, then one unit could be "satisfied" but the other "unsatisfied" with the same state, which would obviously not lead to a consistent global state. We will discuss the biological basis for weight symmetry in chapter 5, where it plays an important role in

mathematically deriving a biologically plausible form of error-driven learning. As we will see, only a very rough, not exact, form of symmetry is required.

The constraints are represented in this function as the extent to which the *activations are consistent with the weights*. Thus, if there is a large weight between two units, and these units are strongly active, they will contribute to a *smaller* energy value (because of the minus sign). This opposition of the magnitude and the sign of the energy term is confusing, so we will use the negative value of the energy function, which is called **harmony** (Smolensky, 1986):

$$H = \frac{1}{2} \sum_j \sum_i x_i w_{ij} x_j \qquad (3.10)$$

Here, two units are said to contribute to greater *harmony* (also known as lower energy) if they are strongly active and connected by a large weight. In this terminology, the network settling acts to increase the overall harmony of the activation states.

To see how this occurs, let's take the simplest case of a linear unit that computes its activation as follows:

$$x_j = \sum_i x_i w_{ij} \qquad (3.11)$$

What we want to do is to show that updating the activation according to this equation is equivalent to maximizing harmony in the network. One standard way to maximize an equation is to figure out how its value changes as a result of changes to the constituent variables. This requires taking the *derivative* of the function with respect to the variable in question (activation x_j in this case). We will discuss this process of maximizing or minimizing functions using derivatives in greater detail in chapter 5, so if you don't understand it, take it on faith now, and you can come back to this point after you have read that chapter (where it plays a very central role in developing one of our learning mechanisms).

If we take the derivative of the harmony equation (3.10) with respect to one unit's activation value (x_j), we get:

$$\frac{\partial H}{\partial x_j} = \sum_i x_i w_{ij} \qquad (3.12)$$

Note that as we mentioned previously, $x_i w_{ij} x_j$ and $x_j w_{ji} x_i$ both appear in the double-sum term in the harmony equation, and we assume that $w_{ij} = w_{ji}$ due to symmetry, so this cancels out the $\frac{1}{2}$ term. The result is just the same as equation 3.11, meaning that updating the activations of a network of these units is indeed the same as maximizing the harmony in the network.

The preceding analysis can also be made for a network using sigmoidal units, which are more similar to the point neuron activation function we have been using (see section 2.5.4). For this to work out mathematically, the harmony/energy equation needs to be augmented with a **stress** or **entropy** term, which reflects the extent to which the activation states of units in the network are "undecided" (e.g., in the middle of their range of values). The resulting overall equation is called **goodness** in harmony-based parlance, and **free energy** in physics-based lingo. However, the results of adding this additional term do not typically affect the ordinal relationship between the harmonies of different states — in other words, harmony and goodness are usually fairly redundant measures. Thus, we will restrict our focus to the simpler harmony term.

Given that the point neuron activation function used in Leabra will result in the increased activity of units connected by strong weights, just like the simpler cases above, it is not surprising that the use of this function will tend to increase the overall harmony of the network. Thus, we can understand the general processing in these networks as performing constraint satisfaction by working to maximize the overall harmony. The exercises that follow explore this idea.

3.6.1 Attractors Again

In section 3.4.4, we introduced the notion of an *attractor*, which is a stable activation state that the network will tend to settle into from a range of different starting states (the attractor basin). We can now relate the notion of an attractor to the constraint-satisfaction ideas presented above. Specifically, the tendency of the activation updates to maximize the harmony of the network means that the network will tend to converge on the most harmonious states possible given a particular set of input constraints. These most harmonious states

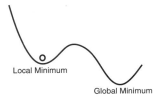

Figure 3.26: A local minimum in the energy function. Noise can shake the system (represented by the ball) so that it finds the global minimum (or at least a better local minimum).

are referred to as **maxima** of the harmony function (or **minima** of the energy function), and they correspond to attractor states.

The process of converging on an attractor over settling (e.g., as represented by figure 3.18) is thus isomorphic to the process of updating the activations and improving the harmony of the network's states. Thus, constraint satisfaction and the associated mathematics of the harmony or energy function provides a nice formalization of the notion of an attractor. In the next section, we will see how noise and inhibition interact with this constraint satisfaction/attractor process.

3.6.2 The Role of Noise

Noise (e.g., in the membrane potential or activation values) can play an important role in constraint satisfaction. Basically, noise helps to keep things from getting *stuck*. Think about how you get ketchup or Parmesan cheese out of their containers — you shake them. This shaking is a form of noise, and it keeps the system (ketchup) from getting stuck in a suboptimal state. Similarly, noise added to the activations of units can prevent the network from getting stuck in a suboptimal state that fails to satisfy as many of the constraints as other, more optimal states (figure 3.26). These suboptimal states are called **local maxima** or **local minima** (depending on whether you're using harmony or energy, respectively), as compared to the (somewhat mythical) **global maxima** (or minima), which is the most optimal of all possible states (i.e., having the maximum harmony value possible). In all but the simplest networks, we must typically accept only local maxima. However, by using noise, we are more likely to find *better* local maxima.

In actual neurons, there is plenty of naturally occurring noise in the precise timing of output spikes. However, when we use the rate-code functions instead of discrete spikes, we lose this source of noise (even in the noisy XX1 function, which builds the noise into the shape of the function — see section 2.5.4). Thus, in the relatively rare cases where we have a network that is suffering from excessive local maxima problems, we can add some additional noise back into the activation function (or we can switch to spikes). However, when dealing with *ambiguous* stimuli with truly equal possible interpretations (see the Necker cube example below), noise is also necessary to "break the tie."

In especially tough constraint satisfaction problems, we may need to resort to a special technique called **simulated annealing** (Kirkpatrick, Gelatt, & Vecchi, 1983), which simulates the slow cooling methods used to create high-quality metals. In a neural network, this can be simulated by gradually reducing the level of noise as the network settles. The idea is that early on in processing, you want to explore a wide range of different activation states in search of better maxima, which is facilitated by relatively high levels of noise. Then, as you home in on a good state, you want to reduce the noise level and ease your way into the maximum. There is a facility for specifying an **annealing schedule** in the simulator that controls the noise level as a function of the number of processing cycles performed during settling, but we do not use this in any of the simulations for this text.

3.6.3 The Role of Inhibition

The set point-like kWTA inhibitory function has an important impact on the constraint satisfaction performance of the network. Basically, constraint satisfaction is a form of **parallel search**, where the network searches through a number of different possible states before finding one that satisfies the constraints fairly optimally. Because each unit is updating in parallel, the search proceeds in parallel instead of sequentially visiting a huge number of distinct states in sequence. Viewed in this way, the role of kWTA inhibition is to restrict the search space dramatically. Thus, instead of having the possibility of going into states with a

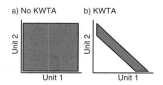

Figure 3.27: Illustration in two dimensions (units) of how kWTA inhibition can restrict the search space to a smaller subset of possible patterns. **a)** represents a network without kWTA inhibition, which can explore all possible combinations of activation states. **b)** shows the effect of kWTA inhibition in restricting the activation states that can be explored, leading to faster and more effective constraint satisfaction.

wide range of different overall activity levels, a network with kWTA inhibition can only produce states with a relatively narrow range of overall activity levels (figure 3.27).

The advantages of so restricting the search space is that the network will settle faster and more reliably into good states, *assuming that these good states are among those allowed by the kWTA algorithm*. Thus, one has to adopt the idea of *sparse distributed representations* and, through learning or other means, have a network where all the important possible representations are within the range of activities allowed by the kWTA function. We will see that such sparse distributed representations are quite useful for the cognitive tasks studied in later chapters, and that the network with kWTA inhibition does indeed settle faster and more reliably into good constraint satisfaction solutions (see Vecera & O'Reilly, 1998 for a comparison between networks with and without kWTA constraints).

3.6.4 Explorations of Constraint Satisfaction: Cats and Dogs

We will begin our exploration with a simple **semantic network** intended to represent a (very small) set of relationships among different features used to represent a set of entities in the world. In our case, we represent some features of cats and dogs: their color, size, favorite food, and favorite toy. The network contains information about a number of individual cats and dogs, and is able to use this information to make *generaliza-*

tions about what cats and dogs in general have in common, and what is unique about them. It can also tell you about the *consistency* of a given feature with either cats or dogs — this is where the harmony function can be useful in assessing the total constraint satisfaction level of the network with a particular configuration of feature inputs. The network can also be used to perform *pattern completion* as a way of retrieving information about a particular individual or individuals. Thus, this simple network summarizes many of the topics covered in this chapter.

The knowledge embedded in the network is summarized in table 3.1. This knowledge is encoded by simply setting a weight of 1 between an *instance* node representing an individual cat or dog and the corresponding feature value that this individual possesses (c.f., the Jets and Sharks model from McClelland & Rumelhart, 1988). Each of the groups of features (i.e., values within one column of the table) are represented within distinct layers that have their own within-layer inhibition. In addition, all of the identity units and the name units are within their own separate layers as well. We use the KWTA_AVG inhibitory function here, because it will be important for the network to have some flexibility in the actual number of active units per layer. The *k* parameter is set to 3 for most layers, except Species where it is 1, and Size where it is 2.

↪   Open project cats_and_dogs.proj.gz in (in chapter_3) to begin.

As usual, take some time to examine the weights in the network, and verify that the weights implement the knowledge shown in the table.

↪   Now, press View in the cat_dog_ctrl overall control panel and select EVENTS to open the EnviroView window.

You will see a replica of the network displayed in the environment window — these are the inputs that will be *soft clamped* into the corresponding network units when the Run button is pressed.

Let's first verify that when we present an individual's name as input, it will recall all of the information about that individual. This is a form of pattern completion with a single unique input cue. You should see that Morris in the Name layer units of the EnviroView is already on by default — we will use this.

↪   Press Run in the control panel.

You should see that the network activates the appropriate features for Morris. You can think about this process as finding the most harmonious activation state given the input constraint of Morris, and the constraints in the network's weights. Equivalently, you can think about it as settling into the Morris attractor.

↪   Go ahead and try a few other name activations (be sure to press the highlighted Apply button in the EnviroView to make your changes stick). Also be sure to click the previous one off by just clicking on it again (this toggles the activity of that input).

Now, let's see how this network can give us general information about cats versus dogs, even though at some level it just has information about a set of individuals.

↪   Select only the Cat Species input in the EnviroView, and press Apply and then Run.

You should find that the network activates all those features that are typical of cats. You can repeat this for dogs.

Question 3.15 **(a)** *Explain the reason for the different levels of activation for the different features of cats when just* Cat *was activated.* **(b)** *How might this be useful information?*

Now let's make use of some of the constraint satisfaction ideas. We can view the *harmony* of the network over cycles of settling using a graph log.

↪   Press View and select GRAPH_LOG. Clear the log, and run the network again with just the Cat input selected.

Notice that, as we expected, this value appears to monotonically increase over settling, indicating that the network is increasingly satisfying the constraints as the activations are updated.

Now, let's make a more *specific* query for the network.

↪   Activate the Orange color input in addition to Cat, and press Run.

You should see that although the initial harmony value was slightly larger (reflecting the greater excitation present from the input), the final harmony value was significantly lower that that for just Cat alone.

Species	Name	Color	Size	Food	Toy
Cat	Morris	Orange	Small	Grass	String
	Socks	Black & White	Small	Bugs	Feather
	Sylvester	Black & White	Small	Grass	String
	Garfield	Orange	Medium	Scraps	String
	Fuzzy	White	Medium	Grass	Feather
Dog	Rex	Black	Large	Scraps	Bone
	Fido	Brown	Medium	Shoe	Shoe
	Spot	Black & White	Medium	Scraps	Bone
	Snoopy	Black & White	Medium	Scraps	Bone
	Butch	Brown	Large	Shoe	Shoe

Table 3.1: Feature values for the individual cats and dogs used in this exploration.

This lower harmony reflects the fact that the more constraints you impose externally, the less likely the network will be able to satisfy them as well. Put another way, Cat is an easy constraint to satisfy, so the resulting harmony is large. Cat plus Orange is harder to satisfy because it applies to fewer things, so the harmony is lower.

There are a seemingly infinite number of different ways that you can query the network — go ahead and present different input patterns and see what kinds of responses the network gives you. Most of them will we hope be recognizable as a reasonable response to the set of constraints provided by the input pattern.

It is sometimes interesting to try to figure out how the activation spreads through the network as it settles. You can open up a GridLog for this purpose. It shows the state of the network every grid_interval (default = 5) cycles of updating.

↪ Press View and select GRID_LOG to open the grid log.

Have fun experimenting!

↪ Go to the PDP++Root window. To continue on to the next simulation, close this project first by selecting .projects/Remove/Project_0. Or, if you wish to stop now, quit by selecting Object/Quit.

3.6.5 Explorations of Constraint Satisfaction: Necker Cube

Now, lets explore the use of constraint satisfaction in processing ambiguous stimuli. The example we will

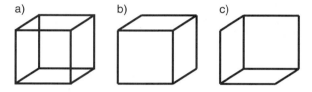

Figure 3.28: Necker cube **a)**, which can be seen as looking down on it **b)** or looking up at it **c)**.

use is the *Necker cube*, which is shown in figure 3.28, and can be viewed as a cube in one of two orientations. People tend to oscillate back and forth between viewing it one way versus the other. However, it is very rare that they view it as both at the same time — in other words, they tend to form a *consistent* overall interpretation of the ambiguous stimulus. This consistency reflects the action of a constraint satisfaction system that favors interpretations that maximize the constraints imposed by the possible interpretations. Alternatively, we can say that there are two stable attractors, one for each interpretation of the cube, and that the network will be drawn into one or the other of these attractor states.

↪ Open the project necker_cube.proj.gz in chapter_3 to begin. Press the Init button in the network window (located in the group of buttons on the left of the window).

This should update the display (figure 3.29) so that you can see two "cubes" with units at each vertex, with each cube representing one of the two possible interpre-

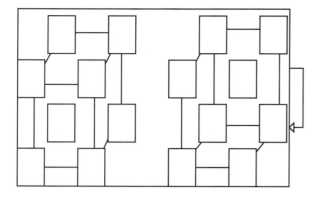

Figure 3.29: Necker cube network, with the group of units on the left representing the vertices of the downwards looking view (**b**) in previous figure), and the group on the right representing the vertices of the upward-looking view (**c**) in previous figure).

tations (the left cube corresponding to figure 3.28b, and the right to figure 3.28c). All of the units are within one layer, which has the basic kWTA inhibition operating with a k parameter of 8. Thus, only one of the two cubes can be active at any given time under these constraints. As usual, let's examine the weights. Notice that each unit is connected to its local neighborhood of vertices. Thus, when one vertex gets active, it will tend to activate the others, leading to the activation of a consistent interpretation of the entire cube. However, at the same time, the other interpretation of the cube is also activating its vertices, and, via the inhibition, competing to get active.

↪ Return to viewing `act` in the network. To view the harmony, do `View` and select `GRAPH_LOG`. Then, press `Run` to view the competition process in action.

During running, both interpretations receive equal but weak amounts of excitatory input. You should see that as the network settles there is a point where some units in both cubes are active, with some wavering of strength back and forth until one cube eventually wins out and is fully active while the other remains inactive.

↪ Try `Run`ning many times.

You should note that which cube wins is random. If you are persistent, you should eventually observe a case where part of each cube is activated, instead of one en-

tire cube being active and the other not (warning, this could take hundreds of tries, depending on how fortuitous your random seeds are). When this happens, note the plot of the harmony value in the graph log. It should be substantially below all the other traces that correspond to a consistent solution on one cube. Thus, an inconsistent partial satisfaction of the weight constraints has lower harmony than full satisfaction of the constraints in one cube.

Noise added to the membrane potential is playing an important role in this simulation — without it, there is nothing to "break the tie" between the two cube interpretations. To see this, let's manipulate the level of noise.

↪ Try the following values of `noise_var`: 0, .1, .01, .000001.

Question 3.16 (a) *Report what differences you observed in the settling behavior of the network for these different values.* **(b)** *What does this tell you about how noise is affecting the process?*

You might also try playing with different activation functions by setting the `act_fun` parameter.

Finally, one of the important psychological aspects of the Necker cube stimulus is that people tend to oscillate between the two possible interpretations. This probably occurs because the neurons that are activated for one interpretation get *tired* eventually, allowing the other competing units to become active. This process of neurons getting tired is called **accommodation**, and is a well established property of neurons that was covered in section 2.9.

↪ Use the `accommodation` field to turn this property on or off (`ACCOMMODATE` or `DONT_ACCOMMODATE`).

When it is on, the network runs for 500 cycles instead of 60, and you should observe at least two oscillations from one cube to the next as the neurons get tired.

↪ To stop now, quit by selecting `Object/Quit` in the `PDP++Root` window.

3.7 Summary

We now have a number of important principles of network function at our disposal. These principles provide an important new language for describing the dynamics of cognition — including transforming patterns to emphasize and deemphasize distinctions, settling into an attractor, bootstrapping, inhibitory competition, and constraint satisfaction. We will see in the next chapter that by combining this language with principles of learning, we have a very powerful toolkit for both understanding why networks of neurons (and by extension the brains of animals and people) behave in the ways they do, and for getting them to behave in the ways we want them to.

General Structure of Cortical Networks

The cortex is typically described as having six different layers of neurons, but these can be categorized into three primary groups or **functional layers** (figure 3.3), the: **input** (cortical layer 4), **hidden** (cortical layers 2 and 3), and **output** layers (cortical layers 5 and 6). The input layer receives information from the senses via the **thalamus**, and the output neurons send motor and other control outputs to a wide range of **subcortical** areas. The hidden layer serves to mediate the output of the network in response to the input signal by means of **transformations** that provide a useful and typically more elaborated or processed basis for driving the outputs of the network. There is a large amount of interconnectivity between the layers, but various forms of data support the idea that information flows primarily from *input to hidden to output* via excitatory neurons. Further, these excitatory neurons are **bidirectionally connected**, so that information can also flow backwards along these pathways. Inhibitory neurons exist in all of the cortical layers, and they receive the same types of excitatory inputs as the excitatory neurons in these layers. However, they do not send their outputs very far — they typically inhibit a number of excitatory neurons within a relatively close proximity to themselves. Thus, inhibition appears to provide a kind of **local feedback** or regulatory mechanism.

Excitatory Interactions

Excitatory neurons can connect with other excitatory neurons in several distinct ways. A **unidirectional** or **feedforward** connectivity pattern is where one set of neurons connects with another set, but not vice versa. This is not typically found in the cortex, but many properties of feedforward processing generalize to the more common bidirectional case. Unidirectional excitatory connectivity can **transform** input activity patterns in a way that **emphasizes** some distinctions, while at the same time **deemphasizing** or **collapsing** across other possible distinctions. Much of cognition can be understood in terms of this process of developing representations that emphasize relevant distinctions and collapse across irrelevant ones. **Distributed** representations, where each unit participates in the representation of multiple inputs, and each input is represented by multiple units, have a number of desirable properties, making them predominant in our models and apparently in the cortex. **Localist** representations, where a single unit represents a given input, are less powerful, but can be useful for demonstration purposes.

Bidirectional (a.k.a. **recurrent** or **interactive**) connectivity is predominant in the cortex, and has several important functional properties not found in simple unidirectional connectivity. We emphasize the **symmetric** case (i.e., where both directions have the same weight value), which is relatively simple to understand compared to the asymmetric case. First, it is capable of performing unidirectional-like transformations, but in both directions, which enables **top-down** processing similar to *mental imagery*. It can also propagate information **laterally** among units within a layer, which leads to **pattern completion** when a partial input pattern is presented to the network and the excitatory connections activate the missing pieces of the pattern. Bidirectional activation propagation typically leads to the **amplification** of activity patterns over time due to mutual excitation between neurons. There are several other important subtypes of amplifying effects due to bidirectional excitatory connections, including: **mutual support**, **top-down** support or biasing, and **bootstrapping**. Many of these phenomena are described under the general term of **attractor dynamics**, because the network appears to be attracted to a particular activation state.

Inhibitory Interactions

Bidirectional excitatory connectivity is like having a microphone next to the speaker that it is driving (or pointing a video camera at its own monitor output) — you get **feedback**. To control runaway positive excitation, the cortex has inhibitory neurons that activate inhibitory synaptic channels on the excitatory neurons. Two forms of inhibition are present in the cortex: **feedforward** (driven by the level of excitation coming into a layer) and **feedback** (driven by the level of excitation within the layer itself). The combination of these forms of inhibition results in **set point** behavior, which occurs around a point where more excitation leads to more inhibition, resulting in less excitation, but less excitation leads to less inhibition, resulting in more excitation. Thus, the system has a preferred level of excitation. Instead of explicitly simulating all of the inhibitory neurons, we can use a summary function that imposes set point inhibition directly, resulting in greater efficiency and simplicity. We use two forms of **k winners take all** (kWTA) functions, where the set point is specified as a parameter k neurons (out of n total neurons) that are to be active at any given time. In addition to controlling excitation, inhibition results in a form of **competition** between neurons. This competition is a healthy one, and it produces a **selection** pressure in activation dynamics and learning that results in an evolution-like *survival (and adaptation) of the fittest* representations. Finally, it produces **sparse distributed** representations, which make sense in terms of several aspects of the general structure of our world.

Constraint Satisfaction

The combined effect of excitatory and inhibitory interactions can be understood in terms of **constraint satisfaction**, where the activity patterns in the network evolve or **settle** over time in a way that maximizes the satisfaction of constraints internal and external to the network. This process can be understood mathematically by using an **energy function**, which summarizes the overall level of satisfaction or **harmony** in the network. We can show that the net effect of activation propagation is always to increase the overall harmony measure. Inhibition can improve the reliability and min-

imize the settling time associated with large constraint satisfaction problems.

3.8 Further Reading

Textbooks on neuropsychology or cognitive neuroscience will provide a wealth of information about the basic structure of the cortex and cognitive functions of the different cortical areas. Bear, Conners, and Paradiso (1996) and Kalat (1995) are good for the basics, and Banich (1997) is good for cognitive functions (as are the later chapters of this text). Also, Kandel et al. (1991) is an often-used reference, though it is more medically oriented.

White (1989a) provides a wealth of information about the anatomical and physiological properties of the cortex, and Shepherd (1990) contains a number of useful chapters on the anatomy and physiology of a variety of brain areas including the cortex and hippocampus.

Rakic (1994) provides an overview of the developmental construction of the cortex.

Abbott and Sejnowski (1999) is a collection of papers on detailed computational models on *Neural codes and distributed representations*.

Hertz et al. (1991) provides a detailed introductory treatment of constraint satisfaction, energy functions, and the like.

Chapter 4

Hebbian Model Learning

Contents

4.1   **Overview** **115**
4.2   **Biological Mechanisms of Learning** **116**
4.3   **Computational Objectives of Learning** **118**
    4.3.1   Simple Exploration of Correlational Model Learning *121*
4.4   **Principal Components Analysis** **122**
    4.4.1   Simple Hebbian PCA in One Linear Unit . . *122*
    4.4.2   Oja's Normalized Hebbian PCA *124*
4.5   **Conditional Principal Components Analysis** . . . **125**
    4.5.1   The CPCA Learning Rule *127*
    4.5.2   Derivation of CPCA Learning Rule *128*
    4.5.3   Biological Implementation of CPCA Hebbian Learning *129*
4.6   **Exploration of Hebbian Model Learning** **130**
4.7   **Renormalization and Contrast Enhancement** . . **132**
    4.7.1   Renormalization *133*
    4.7.2   Contrast Enhancement *134*
    4.7.3   Exploration of Renormalization and Contrast Enhancement in CPCA *135*
4.8   **Self-Organizing Model Learning** **137**
    4.8.1   Exploration of Self-Organizing Learning . . *138*
    4.8.2   Summary and Discussion *142*
4.9   **Other Approaches to Model Learning** **142**
    4.9.1   Algorithms That Use CPCA-Style Hebbian Learning *143*
    4.9.2   Clustering *143*
    4.9.3   Topography *143*
    4.9.4   Information Maximization and MDL *144*
    4.9.5   Learning Based Primarily on Hidden Layer Constraints *144*
    4.9.6   Generative Models *145*
4.10 **Summary** **145**
4.11 **Further Reading** **146**

4.1   Overview

Learning is perhaps the single most important mechanism in a neural network, because it provides the primary means of setting the weight parameters, of which there are often thousands in a model and trillions in the brain. Learning depends on both individual neuron-level mechanisms and network-level principles (developed in the previous chapter) to produce an overall network that behaves appropriately given its environment. The importance of a mathematically rigorous treatment of learning mechanisms (also called *algorithms* or *rules*) was driven home by the critical analyses of Minsky and Papert (1969), and such mathematical analyses have played a key role in most learning algorithms developed since. These mathematical analyses must be complemented with biological, psychological, and more pragmatic constraints in achieving a useful learning mechanism for cognitive neuroscience modeling. Thus, we use many levels of analysis in developing ideas about how learning should and does occur in the human cortex.

We begin with the biological mechanisms that underlie learning, *long-term potentiation (LTP)* and *long-term depression (LTD)*, which refer to the strengthening (potentiation) and weakening (depression) of weights in a nontransient (long term) manner. The form of LTP/D found in the cortex has an *associative* or *Hebbian* form, which depends on both presynaptic and postsynaptic neural activity. Hebbian learning can be viewed as performing *model learning*, where the objective is to develop a good internal model of the important (statistical) structure of the environment. This type of learning is often called *self-organizing* because it can be used without any explicit feedback from the environment.

This chapter is the first of three chapters on learning mechanisms. It focuses on Hebbian model learning. In the next chapter, we develop an alternative form of learning called error-driven task learning, which does a much better job at learning to solve tasks. The third chapter then explores the combination of Hebbian and error-driven learning, along with other more specialized mechanisms necessary to address the important and difficult forms of task learning known as *sequence* and *temporally delayed* learning.

This chapter begins with a simple Hebbian learning algorithm that captures basic aspects of biological learning and picks up on correlational information in the environment by performing a version of *principal components analysis* (PCA). This simple form of Hebbian learning is then elaborated in an algorithm that performs *conditional principal components analysis* (CPCA), motivated by both computational and biological considerations. Finally, two correction factors are introduced that preserve the essential aspects of Hebbian learning while making the algorithm more effective.

4.2 Biological Mechanisms of Learning

The modern era of the study of the biology of learning at a cellular level began with the discovery of **long-term potentiation (LTP)** (Bliss & Lomo, 1973). This term contrasts with the many other transient forms of *potentiation* that were known at the time, but that were not suitable for the permanent storage of knowledge. Potentiation refers to an increase in the measured *depolarization* or excitation delivered by a controlled stimulus onto a receiving neuron. Bliss and Lomo discovered that high-frequency stimulation (typically 100Hz

for 1 second) will cause a long-lasting potentiation effect, with increases in synaptic efficacy of 50 to 100 percent or more. We now know a considerable amount about the biological mechanisms underlying LTP, and the related phenomenon of LTD, which is a long-lasting depression (weakening) of synaptic efficacy.

The most common form of LTP/D in the cortex is known as **NMDA-mediated LTP/D**. There is a very nice connection between the way the **NMDA receptor** works and the functional characteristics of this form of LTP/D. These functional characteristics are generally summarized by the term **associative** or **Hebbian**, which means that the activity states of both the presynaptic and postsynaptic neurons are important for enabling potentiation (or depression) to occur (i.e., there is an *association* between these neurons). Hebb (1949) introduced the idea that co-active representations should become more strongly linked: if a given neuron consistently participates in the firing of another neuron, then the connection between the two neurons should be strengthened.

Focusing on the LTP case for the moment, the observed associativity can be explained by the fact that the NMDA receptor depends on both presynaptic and postsynaptic activity before it will open. Presynaptic activity is required because the NMDA channel will not open unless the excitatory neurotransmitter glutamate, released when the presynaptic neuron is active, is bound to the receptor. Postsynaptic activity is required because the postsynaptic membrane potential must be sufficiently elevated (excited) to cause magnesium ions (Mg^+) to move out of the opening of the NMDA receptor channel, which they would otherwise block.

Once the NMDA channels do open, they allow calcium ions (Ca^{++}) to enter the postsynaptic neuron. As we noted in chapter 2, there is usually an extremely low base concentration of calcium inside the neuron. Thus, an influx of calcium can make a big difference, in this case by triggering a complex cascade of chemical processes, ultimately resulting in the modification of the synaptic efficacy (weight) of the primary excitatory input receptors, the AMPA receptors (figure 4.1). As discussed in section 2.3.2, there are a number of factors, both presynaptic and postsynaptic, which can lead to the modification of overall synaptic efficacy. The debate as

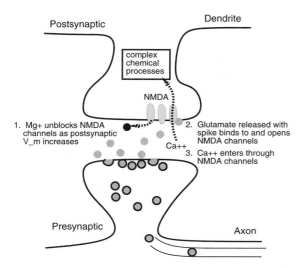

Figure 4.1: Sketch of biological mechanisms that lead to LTP/D. NMDA channels open when the postsynaptic membrane potential (V_m) is sufficiently elevated and glutamate is being released by the presynaptic neuron. This allows calcium ions into the postsynaptic neuron, which triggers a cascade of complex chemical processes that ultimately result in the modification of synaptic efficacy.

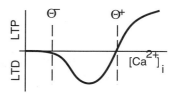

Figure 4.2: Relationship between LTP and LTD, where a moderate amount of increased intracellular calcium ($[Ca^{++}]_i$) leads to LTD, but a larger amount leads to LTP.

to which factors are important is far from resolved, but it does appear that both presynaptic and postsynaptic factors could be involved in LTP/D. However, our computational learning mechanisms depend more on the nature of the events that trigger this synaptic modification than on the mechanisms that actually implement it.

LTD is somewhat less well understood. One prominent idea is that LTD occurs when the synapse is active at a somewhat lower level than that required to trigger LTP (Artola, Brocher, & Singer, 1990). Thus, one explanation of this finding would be that the less effective opening of the NMDA channels (e.g., fewer channels opened or opened for a shorter time) results in a lower concentration of calcium ions, which triggers a different cascade of chemical processes that ultimately end up *reducing* synaptic efficacy instead of enhancing it. Figure 4.2 shows an illustration of this relationship between LTP and LTD, where the threshold for LTD is given by Θ^-, and the higher LTP threshold is Θ^+. This relationship is consistent with one hypothesis about the

nature of these complex chemical cascades (Lisman, 1989, 1994; Bear & Malenka, 1994). Further, this form of LTD is consistent both with the LTD necessary for model learning, and with that necessary for task learning, as will be explained below in section 5.8.3.

Although the NMDA-mediated LTP/D mechanism is relatively simple and consistent with a large amount of data, the biological picture may be somewhat more complicated, for a number of reasons:

- Other receptors, channels, and neurotransmitters may play a role in LTP/D. For example: (a) there is evidence for the involvement of the metabotropic glutamate (mGlu) receptors in LTP (Bashir, Bortolotto, & Davies, 1993; Bear & Malenka, 1994), (b) there are a number of other ways in which calcium can enter the postsynaptic neuron (e.g., non NMDA voltage-dependent calcium channels), and (c) LTP/D may be regulated by a number of other modulatory neurotransmitters (dopamine, serotonin, etc.) in ways that are not understood or appropriately manipulated in experiments (see section 6.7 for a more detailed discussion of the role of dopamine in learning).

- There is little evidence that the standard 100Hz for 1 second's activity required for LTP induction occurs with any reliability in the natural activation patterns of the cortex. More generally, LTP/D may be sensitive to particular combinations of inducing activation signal properties (timing, intensity, frequency, duration, etc.) in ways that have not been explored empirically (indeed, this kind of timing sensitivity is important for achieving biologically plausible error-driven learning, as we will see later).

- Some studies assessing the impact of NMDA receptor blockade show preserved behaviorally measured learning despite NMDA blockade. Such studies are generally difficult to interpret, however, because NMDA-blocking drugs have significant other effects on behavior (Keith & Rudy, 1990). In addition, any preserved learning observed in these studies can be accounted for by many of the above complications to the simple NMDA story (e.g., by the role of non-NMDA factors like voltage-gated calcium channels or mGlu receptors).

Thus, the story, at least at the level of biological mechanisms, may end up being somewhat more involved than the elegant NMDA-mediated associativity described above.

Nevertheless, despite a number of unresolved complications, the biological data suggests that associative learning is probably occurring in the cortex. The generally uncertain state of this data only serves to highlight the need for computational models to explore what kind of synaptic modification rules lead to effective overall learning, because these details appear to be difficult to extract from the biology.

4.3 Computational Objectives of Learning

In this section, we develop a computational-level motivation for one general goal of learning and see how this goal can be accomplished using some of the biological mechanisms discussed in the previous section. We call this goal **model learning** to emphasize the idea that learning is directed toward developing **internal models** of the world. Figure 4.3 shows an illustration of how an internal model captures some of the important features of the world, and also why this is a difficult thing to do. The basic idea is that there is some kind of underlying **structure** or regularities (e.g., natural laws, constants, general characteristics) of the world, and that this should somehow be represented to function properly.

From our subjective experience of having a relatively "transparent" knowledge of the physical structure of the world, one might think that model learning is easy and automatic, but there are two fundamental and difficult problems faced by model learning. One has to do with

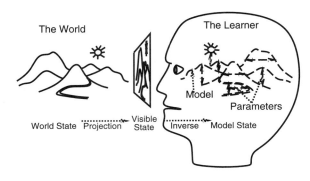

Figure 4.3: Sketch of the objective of model learning — to produce an internal model that represents the "important" features of the world: structural regularities, natural laws, constants, general characteristics (not the literal copy of the world that might otherwise be suggested by the figure). This is complicated because the true state of the world is "hidden" from us — we only see a sequence of piecemeal collapsed projections of the world state, which we have to somehow invert to produce the corresponding state in our model.

the impoverished nature of our sensory access to the underlying structure of the world, and the other has to do with the overwhelming amount of information delivered by our senses. These may seem at first glance to be contradictory, but they are not — our senses deliver a large quantity of low-quality information that must be highly processed to produce the apparently transparent access to the world that we experience.

We will see that the quality problem can be remedied by introducing appropriate a priori (i.e., built in from the start) **biases** that supplement and organize the incoming information. The information overload problem can be addressed by *biasing* learning in favor of simpler or **parsimonious** models that end up ignoring some kinds of information in favor of representing enough relevant information in a manageable form. As we will elaborate, both of these techniques can be recognized in the methods of scientific research, which can be viewed as an explicit and deliberate extension of the model learning process, and has many of the same problems.

The problem with our access to the world via our senses is that we only receive a series of relatively limited two-dimensional snapshots (and sound bites, etc.), which can be thought of as **projections** of the very high-dimensional world onto a much lower-dimensional sensory organ. A projection is a mathematical term for transforming a higher-dimensional matrix onto a lower dimensional one — think of Plato's cave and the real world projecting shadows on the wall.

Inverting these projected world states back into something resembling the world is difficult because so much information is lost in this projection down onto our senses. Marr (1982) characterized this situation by saying that vision is an **ill-posed** problem, in that the input data do not sufficiently constrain our interpretation of it — it is difficult to decide among the large number of possible internal models that could fit the sensory input data equally well. Put another way, it is difficult to know what the real underlying causes of our perceptions are, and what are mere coincidences or appearances (i.e., noise).

The model learning problem can be made easier by **integrating** across many individual experiences. Thus, although any single observation may be ambiguous and noisy, over time, the truth will eventually shine through! In science, this is known as *reproducibility* — we only believe in phenomena that can be reliably demonstrated across many different individual experiments in different labs. The law of large numbers also says that noise can be averaged away by integrating statistics over a large sample. We will see that this integration process is critical to successful model learning, and that it is naturally performed by slowly adding up small weight changes so that the resulting weights represent *aggregate statistics* over a large sample of experiences. Thus, the network ends up representing the stable patterns that emerge over a wide range of experiences with the world.

However, just aggregating over many experiences is not enough to enable the development of a good internal model. For example, if you just averaged over all the pixel intensities of the images experienced by the retina, you would just get a big gray wash. Thus, one also needs to have some *prior expectations* or *biases* about what kinds of patterns are particularly informative, and how to organize and structure representations in a way that makes sense given the general structure of the world. If these biases provide a reasonable fit to the properties of the actual world, then model learning becomes easier and more reliable across individuals.

For example, let's imagine that you were faced with the task of learning to control a complex new video game using the keyboard, with no explicit help available. If you had grown up playing video games, you would know in advance what kinds of actions a video game protagonist generally makes, and which sets of keys are likely to control these actions. In other words, you would have a set of appropriate a priori biases to structure your internal model of video games. You might have some uncertainty about some of the details, but a few quick experiments will have you playing in no time. In contrast, a complete video game novice will have to resort to trying all the keys on the keyboard, observing the corresponding responses of the protagonist, and slowly compiling an inventory. If there are any interdependencies between these actions (e.g., you can only "kick" after the "jump" button was pressed), then the task becomes that much more difficult, because the space of possible such contingencies is even greater. Thus, appropriate biases can make model learning much easier. However, it is essential to keep in mind that if your biases are *wrong* (e.g., the video game is completely unlike any other), then learning can take even longer than without these biases (e.g., you persist in trying a subset of keys, while the really important ones are never tried).

In this video game example, the biases came from prior experience and can be attributed to the same kinds of learning processes as the novice would use. Although this type of biasing happens in our networks too, understanding the kinds of biases that are present *from the very start of learning* presents more of a challenge. We assume that evolution has built up over millions of years a good set of biases for the human brain that facilitate its ability to learn about the world. This essential role for genetic predispositions in learning is often under-emphasized by both proponents and critics of neural network learning algorithms, which are too often characterized as completely tabula rasa (blank slate) learning systems. Instead, these learning mechanisms reflect a dynamic interplay between genetic biases and experience-based learning. The difficulty is that the genetic-level biases are not typically very obvious or easily describable, and so are often overlooked.

It is useful to contrast the kinds of genetic predispositions that can be important for biasing neural network learning with those that are typically discussed by *nativists* (psychologists who emphasize the genetic contributions to behavior). As emphasized by Elman et al. (1996), most nativists think in terms of people being born with *specific knowledge* or representations (e.g., the knowledge that solid things are generally impenetrable; Spelke, Breinlinger, Macomber, & Jacobson, 1992). In neural network terms, building in this kind of specific knowledge would require a very detailed pattern of weights, and is relatively implausible given how much information the genome would have to contain and how difficult it would be for this to be expressed biologically using known developmental mechanisms such as concentration gradients of various growth and cellular adhesion factors.

In contrast, architectural biases (e.g., which areas are generally connected with which other areas) and parametric biases (e.g., how fast one area learns compared to another, or how much inhibition there is in different areas) can presumably be relatively easily encoded in the genome and expressed through the actions of regulatory factors during development. Because even subtle differences in these biases can lead to important differences in learning, it is often not easy to characterize the exact nature of the biological biases that shape learning. Nevertheless, we will see that more general aspects of the biology of networks (specifically the role of inhibition) and the biology of learning (specifically its associative or Hebbian character) serve as important biases in model learning.

A more pragmatic issue that arises in the context of introducing biases into learning is that it requires more work from the modeler. Essentially, modelers have to replace the powerful parameter selection process of natural selection and evolution with their own hunches and trial-and-error experience. For this reason, many people have shied away from using more strongly biased models, favoring the use of very general purpose learning principles instead. Unfortunately, there is a basic underlying tradeoff in the use of biases in learning, so there is "no free lunch" — no way to achieve the benefits of appropriate biases without paying the price of finding good ones for a given task (Wolpert, 1996b, 1996a).

This tradeoff in the role of biases in learning has long been appreciated in the statistics community, where it goes by the name of the **bias-variance dilemma** (Geman, Bienenstock, & Doursat, 1992). It is a dilemma because if learners rely on their biases too strongly, they will not learn enough from their actual experiences, and will thus end up getting the wrong model (think of the experienced video game player who misses the important new keys in favor of using only the familiar ones). On the other hand, if learners rely on their experiences too strongly, then, assuming each learner has somewhat idiosyncratic experiences, they will all end up with different models that reflect these idiosyncrasies. Hence, there will be a lot of model *variance*, which, assuming there is one real underlying state of the world, also means a lot of wrong models. Thus, the proper weighting of biases versus experience is a true dilemma (tradeoff), and there really are no generally optimal solutions.

The history of scientific research contains many examples where biases were critical for seeking out and making sense of phenomena that would have otherwise remained incomprehensible. However, some of the best-known examples of bias in science are negative ones, where religious or other beliefs interfered with the ability to understand our world as it truly is. Thus, science provides an excellent example of the double-edged nature of biases.

One of the most pervasive biases in science is that favoring parsimonious explanations. We will see that model learning can also be biased in favor of developing relatively simple, general models of the world in several ways. The parsimony bias was espoused most famously by William of Occam in the 1300s, for whom the phrase *Occam's razor*, which cuts in favor of the simplest explanation for a phenomenon, was named. One of the primary practical advantages of developing parsimonious models of the world is that this often results in greater success in **generalization**, which is the application of models to novel situations. Think of it this way: if you just memorized a bunch of specific facts about the world instead of trying to extract the simpler essential regularity underlying these facts, then you would be in trouble when dealing with a novel situation where none of these specifics were relevant. For example, if you encode a situation where a tiger leaps

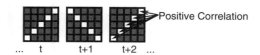

Figure 4.4: Positive correlations exist between elements of a feature such as a line that reliably exists in the environment (i.e., it repeats at different times, intermixed among other such correlated features). Model learning should represent such correlations.

out and tries to attack you (but you narrowly escape) as "stay away from tigers in this part of the woods," then you'll probably be in trouble when you go to another part of the woods, or encounter a lion.

4.3.1 Simple Exploration of Correlational Model Learning

Our approach toward model learning is based on **correlations** in the environment. These correlations are important, because in general it seems that the world is inhabited by things with relatively stable features (e.g., a tree with branches, mammals with legs, an individual's face with eyes, nose, and mouth, and so on), and these features will be manifest as reliable correlations in the patterns of activity in our sensory inputs.

Figure 4.4 shows a simple example of the correlations between the individual pixels (picture elements) that make up the image of a line. These pixels will all be active together when the line is present in the input, producing a positive correlation in their activities. This correlation will be reliable (present across many different input images) to the extent that there is something reliable *in the world* that tends to produce such lines (e.g., edges of objects). Further, the parsimony of our model can be enhanced if only the strongest (most reliable) features or components of the correlational structure are extracted. We will see in the next section how Hebbian learning will cause units to represent the strongest correlations in the environment.

Before delving into a more detailed analysis of Hebbian learning, we will first explore a simplified example of the case shown in figure 4.4 in a simulation. In this exploration, we will see how a single unit (using a Hebbian learning mechanism that will be explained in

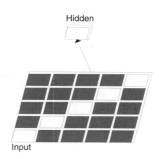

Figure 4.5: Network for the demonstration of Hebbian correlational model learning of the environmental regularity of a line.

detail below) learns to represent the correlations present between the pixels in a line.

↪   Open the project `hebb_correl.proj.gz` in `chapter_4` to begin.

You will see a network with a $5x5$ input layer and a single receiving hidden unit (figure 4.5), in addition to the usual other windows. To make things as simple as possible, we will just present a single rightward leaning diagonal line and see what effect the Hebbian learning has on this hidden unit's weights. Thus, the environment will have these units 100 percent correlated with each other and the firing of the hidden unit, and this extreme strong correlation should be encoded by the effects of the Hebbian learning mechanism on the weights.

First, let's look at the initial weights of this hidden unit.

↪   Select `r.wt` in the network window, and then click on the hidden unit.

You should see a uniform set of .5 weight values, which provide an "blank page" starting point for observing the effects of subsequent learning.

↪   Then, click back on `act`, and then do `Run` in the `hebb_correl_ctrl` control panel.

You will just see the activation of the right-leaning diagonal line.

↪   Then, click back on `r.wt`.

You will see that the unit's weights have learned to represent this line in the environment.

↪   Click on `Run` again.

You can now see the entire progression from the initial weights to the line representation while looking at the weights.

The simple point of this exploration is that Hebbian learning will tend to cause units to represent stable things in the environment. This is a particularly simple case where there was just a single thing in the environment, but it serves to convey the point. We will explore more interesting cases later. But first, let's try to understand the mathematical and conceptual basis of Hebbian learning.

↪ Go to the `PDP++Root` window. To continue on to the next simulation, close this project first by selecting `.projects/Remove/Project_0`. Or, if you wish to stop now, quit by selecting `Object/Quit`.

4.4 Principal Components Analysis

The general mathematical framework that we use to understand why Hebbian learning causes units to represent correlations in the environment is called **principal components analysis** (PCA). As the name suggests, PCA is all about representing the major (principal) structural elements (components) of the correlational structure of an environment.[1] By focusing on the principal components of correlational structure, this framework holds out the promise of developing a reasonably *parsimonious* model. Thus, it provides a useful, mathematical, overall level of analysis within which to understand the effects of learning. Further, we will see that PCA can be implemented using a simple *associative* or *Hebbian* learning mechanism like the NMDA-mediated synaptic modification described earlier.

In what follows, we develop a particularly useful form of Hebbian learning that performs a version of PCA. We will rely on a combination of top-down mathematical derivations and bottom-up intuitions about how weights should be adapted, and we will find that there is a nice convergence between these levels of analysis. To make the fundamental computations clear, we will start with the simplest form of Hebbian learning,

---

[1]Note that although PCA technically refers to the extraction of *all* of the principal components of correlation (which can be arranged in sequential order from first (strongest) to last (weakest)), we will use the term to refer only to the strongest such components.

and then incrementally fix various problems until we arrive at the algorithm that we can actually use in our simulations. The objective of this presentation is to show how the main theme of extracting and representing the principal components of correlational structure from the environment using Hebbian learning can be implemented in a simple, biologically plausible, and computationally effective manner.

The culmination of this effort comes in the use of this Hebbian learning in a *self-organizing* network that achieves the model learning objective of representing the general statistical structure of the environment, as we will explore in a simple and easily comprehensible case. Chapter 8 provides a more impressive demonstration of the capabilities of this type of model learning in replicating the way that the visual system represents the statistical structure contained in actual visual scenes of the natural environment.

4.4.1 Simple Hebbian PCA in One Linear Unit

To capture the simplest version of Hebbian correlational learning, we focus first on the case of a single linear receiving unit that receives input from a set of input units. We will see that a simple Hebbian learning equation will result in the unit extracting the first principle component of correlation in the patterns of activity over the input units.

Imagine that there is an *environment* that produces activity patterns over the input units, such that there are certain correlations among these input units. For concreteness, let's consider the simple case where the environment is just the one line shown in figure 4.4, which is repeatedly presented to a set of 25 input units. Because it is linear, the receiving unit's activation function is just the weighted sum of its inputs (figure 4.6):

$$y_j = \sum_k x_k w_{kj} \qquad (4.1)$$

where k (rather than the usual i) indexes over input units, for reasons that will become clear. Also in this and all subsequent equations in this chapter, all of the variables are a function of the current time step t, normally designated by the (t) notation after every variable; however, we drop the (t)'s to make things easier to read. Furthermore, we assume that each time step corresponds to a different pattern of activity over the inputs.

Let's assume that the weights into the receiving unit learn on each time step (input pattern) t according to a very simple Hebbian **learning rule** (formula for changing the weights) where the weight change for that pattern ($\Delta_t w_{ij}$, denoted `dwt` in the simulator) depends associatively on the activities of both presynaptic and postsynaptic units as follows:

$$\Delta_t w_{ij} = \epsilon x_i y_j \qquad (4.2)$$

where ϵ is the **learning rate** parameter (`lrate` in the simulator) and i is the index of a particular input unit. The learning rate ϵ is an arbitrary constant that determines how rapidly the weights are updated as a function of each experience — we will see in chapter 9 that this is an important parameter for understanding the nature of memory. The weight change expression in equation 4.2 (and all the others developed subsequently) is used to update the weights using the following **weight update** equation:

$$w_{ij}(t+1) = w_{ij}(t) + \Delta_t w_{ij} \qquad (4.3)$$

To understand the overall effect of the weight change rule in equation 4.2, we want to know what is going to happen to the weights as a result of learning over all of the input patterns. This is easily expressed as just the sum of equation 4.2 over time (where again time t indexes the different input patterns):

$$\Delta w_{ij} = \epsilon \sum_t x_i y_j \qquad (4.4)$$

We can analyze this sum of weight changes more easily if we assume that the arbitrary learning rate constant ϵ is equal to $\frac{1}{N}$, where N is the total number of patterns in the input. This turns the sum into an *average*:

$$\Delta w_{ij} = \langle x_i y_j \rangle_t \qquad (4.5)$$

(where the $\langle x \rangle_t$ notation indicates the average or *expected value* of variable x over patterns t).

If we substitute into this equation the formula for y_j (equation 4.1, using the index k to sum over the inputs),

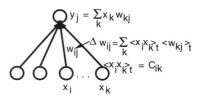

Figure 4.6: Schematic for how the correlations are computed via the simple Hebbian learning algorithm.

which is just a linear function of the activities of all the other input units, we find that, after a little bit of algebra, the weight changes are a function of the *correlations* between the input units:

$$\begin{aligned}
\Delta w_{ij} &= \langle x_i \sum_k x_k w_{kj} \rangle_t \\
&= \sum_k \langle x_i x_k \rangle_t \langle w_{kj} \rangle_t \\
&= \sum_k \mathbf{C}_{ik} \langle w_{kj} \rangle_t \qquad (4.6)
\end{aligned}$$

This new variable $\mathbf{C}_{ik}$ is an element of the **correlation matrix** between the two input units i and k, where correlation is defined here as the expected value (average) of the product of their activity values over time ($\mathbf{C}_{ik} = \langle x_i x_k \rangle_t$). You might be familiar with the more standard correlation measure:

$$\mathbf{C}_{ik} = \frac{\langle (x_i - \mu_i)(x_k - \mu_k) \rangle_t}{\sqrt{\sigma_i^2 \sigma_k^2}} \qquad (4.7)$$

which subtracts away the mean values (μ) of the variables before taking their product, and normalizes the result by their variances (σ^2). Thus, an important simplification in this form of Hebbian correlational learning is that it assumes that the activation variables have zero mean and unit variance. We will see later that we can do away with this assumption for the form of Hebbian learning that we actually use.

The main result in equation 4.6 is that the changes to the weight from input unit i are a weighted average over the different input units (indexed by k) of the correlation between these other input units and the particular input unit i (figure 4.6). Thus, where strong correlations exist across input units, the weights for those units

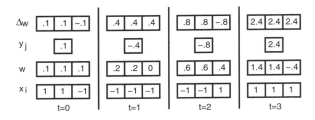

Figure 4.7: Demonstration of the simple Hebbian algorithm, where the first two units are perfectly correlated with each other, and the third is completely uncorrelated. For each input pattern x_i, y_j is computed as $\sum_i x_i w_{ij}$, and then the change in weights Δw_{ij} (which is added in at the next time step) is computed as $x_i y_j$.

will increase because this average correlation value will be relatively large. Interestingly, if we run this learning rule long enough, the weights will become dominated by the strongest set of correlations present in the input, with the gap between the strongest set and the next strongest becoming increasingly large. Thus, this simple Hebbian rule learns the *first* (strongest) principal component of the input data.

A simple, concrete demonstration of this learning rule is shown in figure 4.7, where there are 3 input units and the single linear output unit. Over the 4 different input patterns, the first two units are perfectly correlated with each other, while the third is perfectly uncorrelated (and all units have zero mean, as we assumed). Notice how the two correlated units "gang up" against the uncorrelated one by determining the sign (and magnitude) of the hidden unit activation y_j, which then ensures that their weights just keep increasing, while the uncorrelated one's weights "thrash" up and down. If you run through another iteration of these patterns, you will notice that the weights for the two correlated ones increase rapidly (indeed, exponentially), but the uncorrelated one remains small due to the thrashing.

For the more mathematically inclined, we can say that the simple Hebbian learning rule adapts the weights toward the **principal eigenvector** (i.e., the one with the largest *eigenvalue*) of the correlation matrix $\mathbf{C}$. This can be seen by rewriting equation 4.6 in vector notation:

$$\Delta \mathbf{w_j} = \mathbf{C} \mathbf{w_j} \qquad (4.8)$$

Note that this analysis adopts the simplification of multiplying $\mathbf{C}$ by the weight vector itself instead of its expected value, assuming that it is changing relatively slowly. Thus, the matrix $\mathbf{C}$ serves as the update function for a simple linear system over the state variables represented by the weight vector $\mathbf{w_j}$. It is well known that this results in the state variables being dominated by the strongest eigenvector (component) of the update matrix.

4.4.2 Oja's Normalized Hebbian PCA

One problem with the simple Hebbian learning rule is that the weights become infinitely large as learning continues. This is obviously not a good thing. Fortunately, it is relatively simple to *normalize* the weight updating so that the weights remain bounded. Although we will not end up using exactly this algorithm (but something rather similar), we will explain how a very influential version of Hebbian learning achieves this weight normalization. This algorithm was proposed by Oja (1982), who developed the following modified Hebbian learning rule, which subtracts away a portion of the weight value to keep it from growing infinitely large:

$$\Delta w_{ij} = \epsilon(x_i y_j - y_j^2 w_{ij}) \qquad (4.9)$$

To understand how this learning rule keeps the weights from growing without bound, we can consider the simple case where there is just one input pattern (so we can avoid the need to average over multiple patterns) and look for a stable value of the weight after learning for a long time on this one pattern. We simply need to set the above equation equal to zero, which will tell us when the *equilibrium* or *asymptotic* weight values have been reached (note that this is the same trick we used in chapter 2 to find the equilibrium membrane potential):

$$
\begin{aligned}
0 &= \epsilon(x_i y_j - y_j^2 w_{ij}) \\
w_{ij} &= \frac{x_i}{y_j} \\
w_{ij} &= \frac{x_i}{\sum_k x_k w_{kj}} \qquad (4.10)
\end{aligned}
$$

Thus, the weight from a given input unit will end up representing the proportion of that input's activation relative to the total weighted activation over all the other inputs. This will keep the weights from growing without bound. Finally, because it is primarily based on the same correlation terms $\mathbf{C}_{ik}$ as the previous simple Hebbian learning rule, this Oja rule still computes the first principal component of the input data (though the proof of this is somewhat more involved, see Hertz et al., 1991 for a nice treatment).

4.5 Conditional Principal Components Analysis

To this point, we have considered only a single receiving unit and seen how it can represent the principal component of the correlations in the inputs. In this section, we explore ways in which this simple form of PCA can be extended to the case where there is an entire layer of receiving (hidden) units. To see that the simple PCA rule will not directly work in this context, consider what would happen if we just added multiple hidden units using the same activation function and learning rule as the unit we analyzed above. They would all end up learning the exact same pattern of weights, because there is usually only one strongest (first) principal component to the input correlation matrix, and these algorithms are guaranteed to find it.

There are two general ways of dealing with this problem, both of which involve introducing some kind of interaction between the hidden units to make them do different things. Thus, the problem here is not so much in the form of the weight update rule *per se,* but rather in the overall activation dynamics of the hidden units. It is important to appreciate that there is such an intimate relationship between activation dynamics and learning. Indeed, we will repeatedly see that how a unit behaves (i.e., its activation dynamics) determines to a great extent what it learns.

One solution to the problem of redundant hidden units is to introduce specialized lateral connectivity between units configured to ensure that subsequent units end up representing the sequentially weaker components of the input correlation matrix (Sanger, 1989; Oja, 1989). Thus, an explicit ordering is imposed on the hidden units, such that the first unit ends up representing the principal component with the strongest correlations, the next unit gets the next strongest, and so on. We will call this **sequential principal components analy-**

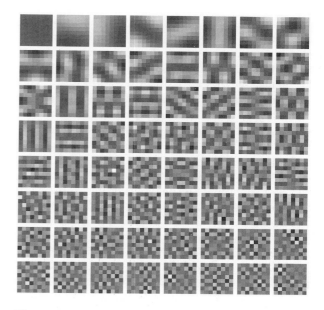

Figure 4.8: Sequential PCA (SPCA) performed on small patches drawn from images of natural scenes, with the first principal component (the "blob") in the upper left, and subsequent components following to the right and down. Each square in the large grid shows a grid of receiving weights for one of 64 hidden units, from a common layer of input units. Figure reproduced from Olshausen and Field (1996).

sis (SPCA). This solution is unsatisfactory for several reasons, from computational-level principles to available data about how populations of neurons encode information.

For example, SPCA assumes that all input patterns share some common set of correlations (which would be represented by the first principal component), and that individual patterns can be differentiated by sequentially finer and finer distinctions represented by the subsequent components. This amounts to an assumption of *hierarchical structure*, where there is some central overarching tendency shared by everything in the environment, with individuals being special cases of this overall principal component. In contrast, the world may be more of a *heterarchy*, with lots of separate categories of things that exist at roughly the same level.

Support for the heterarchical view over the hierarchical one comes from a comparison between the representations produced by various learning mechanisms and primary visual cortex representations. To show that the hierarchical view is inconsistent with these visual cortex representations, Olshausen and Field (1996) ran the SPCA algorithm on randomly placed windows onto natural visual scenes (e.g., as might be produced by fixating randomly at different locations within the scenes), with the resulting principal components shown in figure 4.8. As you can see, the first principal component in the upper left of the figure is just a big blob, because SPCA averages over all the different images, and the only thing that is left after this averaging is a general correlation between close-by pixels, which tend to have similar values. Thus, each individual image pixel has participated in so many different image features that the correlations present in any given feature are washed away completely. This gives a blob as the most basic thing shared by every image. Then, subsequent components essentially just divide this blob shape into finer and finer sub-blobs, representing the residual average correlations that exist after subtracting away the big blob.

In contrast, models that produce heterarchical representations trained on the same natural scenes produce weight patterns that much more closely fit those of primary visual cortex (figure 4.9 — we will explore the network that produced these weight patterns in chapter 8). This figure captures the fact that the visual system uses a large, heterogeneous collection of feature detectors that divide images up into line segments of different orientations, sizes, widths etc., with each neuron responding preferentially to a small coherent category of such line properties (e.g., one neuron might fire strongly to thin short lines at a 45-degree angle, with activity falling off in a graded fashion as lines differ from this "preferred" or prototypical line).

As Olshausen and Field (1996) have argued, a representation employing a large collection of roughly equivalent feature detectors enables a small subset of neurons to efficiently represent a given image by encoding the features present therein. This is the essence of the argument for *sparse distributed representations* discussed in chapter 3. A further benefit is that each feature will tend

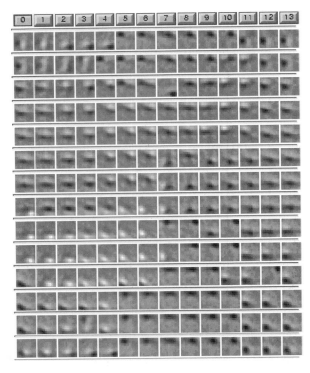

Figure 4.9: Example of heterarchical feature coding by simple cells in the early visual cortex, where each unit has a preferred tuning for bars of light in a particular orientation, width, location, and so on, and these tunings are evenly distributed over the space of all possible values along these feature dimensions. This figure is from a simulation described in chapter 8.

to be activated about as often as any other, providing a more equally distributed representational burden across the neurons. In contrast, the units in the SPCA representation will be activated in proportion to their ordering, with the first component active for most images, and so on.

One way of stating the problem with SPCA is that it computes correlations *over the entire space of input patterns*, when many of the meaningful correlations exist only *in particular subsets of input patterns*. For example, if you could somehow restrict the application of the PCA-like Hebbian learning rule to those images where lines of roughly a particular orientation, size, width,

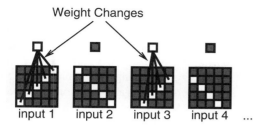

Weight Changes

input 1   input 2   input 3   input 4   ...

Figure 4.10: Conditionalizing the PCA computation — the receiving unit only learns about those inputs that it happens to be active for, effectively restricting the PCA computation to a subset of the inputs (typically those that share a relevant feature, here rightward-leaning diagonal lines).

length, or the like were present, then you would end up with units that encode information in essentially the same way the brain does, because the units would then represent the correlations among the pixels in this particular subset of images. One way of expressing this idea is that units should represent the **conditional** principal components, where the conditionality restricts the PCA computation to only a subset of input cases (figure 4.10).

In the remainder of this section, we develop a version of Hebbian learning that is specifically designed for the purpose of performing **conditional PCA (CPCA)** learning. As you will see, the resulting form of the learning rule for updating the weights is quite similar to Oja's normalized PCA learning rule presented above. Thus, as we emphasized above, the critical difference is not so much in the learning rule itself but rather in the accompanying activation dynamics that determine when individual units will participate in learning about different aspects of the environment.

The heart of CPCA is in specifying the conditions under which a given unit should perform its PCA computation — in other words, the *conditionalizing function*. Mechanistically, this conditionalizing function amounts to whatever forces determine when a receiving unit is active, because this is when PCA learning occurs. We adopt two main approaches toward the conditionalizing function. Later in this chapter we will use inhibitory competition together with the tuning properties of Hebbian learning to implement a *self-organizing* conditionalizing function. Thus, the units themselves evolve their own conditionalizing function as a result of a complex interaction between their own learning experience, and competition with other units in the network. In the next chapter, we will see that error-driven task learning can provide a conditionalizing function based on the patterns of activation necessary to solve tasks. In chapter 6, we explore the combination of both types of conditionalizing functions.

Before we proceed to explore these conditionalizing functions, we need to develop a learning rule based specifically on the principles of CPCA. To develop this rule, we initially assume the existence of a conditionalizing function that turns the units on when the input contains things they should be representing, and turns them off when it doesn't. This assumption enables us to determine that the learning rule will do the appropriate things to the weights given a known conditionalizing function. Then we can go on to explore self-organizing learning.

By developing this CPCA learning rule, we develop a slightly different way of framing the *objective* of Hebbian learning that is better suited to the idea that the relevant environmental structure is only conditionally present in subsets of input patterns, and not unconditionally present in every input pattern. We will see that this framing also avoids the problematic assumption of a linear activation function in previous versions of PCA. The CPCA rule is more consistent with the notion of individual units as hypothesis detectors whose activation states can be understood as reflecting the underlying probability of something existing in the environment (or not).

4.5.1 The CPCA Learning Rule

The CPCA learning rule takes the conditionalizing idea literally. It assumes that we want the weights for a given input unit to represent the conditional probability that the input unit (x_i) was active given that the receiving unit (y_j) was also active. We can write this as:

$$\begin{aligned} w_{ij} &= P(x_i = 1 | y_j = 1) \\ &= P(x_i | y_j) \end{aligned} \tag{4.11}$$

where the second form uses simplified notation that will continue to be used below. We will call the learning rule that achieves such weight values the CPCA algorithm.

The important characteristic of CPCA represented by equation 4.11 is that the weights will reflect the extent to which a given input unit is active across the subset of input patterns represented by the receiving unit (i.e., conditioned on this receiving unit). If an input pattern is a very typical aspect of such inputs, then the weights from it will be large (near 1), and if it is not so typical, they will be small (near 0).

It is useful to relate the conditional probabilities computed by CPCA to the correlations computed by PCA. A conditional probability of .5 means zero correlation (i.e., the input is equally likely to be on as off when the receiving unit is active), and values larger than .5 indicate positive correlation (input more likely to be on than off when the receiving unit is on), while values less than .5 indicate negative correlation (input more likely to be off than on when the receiving unit is on). Note that there is at least one important difference between conditional probabilities and correlations: conditional probabilities depend on the direction you compute them (i.e., $P(a|b) \neq P(b|a)$ in general), whereas correlations come out the same way regardless of which way you compute them.

One further intuition regarding the relationship between CPCA and PCA is that the receiver's activation y_j, which serves as the conditionalizing factor in CPCA, is a function of the other inputs to the unit, and thus serves to make the weights from a given sending unit dependent on the extent of its correlation with other units, as reflected in y_j. Thus, the same basic mechanism is at work here in CPCA as we saw in PCA. However, we will see later that CPCA is also capable of reflecting other important conditionalizing factors that determine when the receiving unit is active (e.g., competition amongst the hidden units).

Following the analysis of Rumelhart and Zipser (1986), we show below that the following weight update rule achieves the CPCA conditional probability objective represented in equation 4.11:

$$\Delta w_{ij} = \epsilon[y_j x_i - y_j w_{ij}]$$
$$= \epsilon y_j (x_i - w_{ij}) \tag{4.12}$$

where ϵ is again the learning rate parameter (`lrate` in the simulator). The two equivalent forms of this equation are shown to emphasize the similarity of this learning rule to Oja's normalized PCA learning rule (equation 4.9), while also showing its simpler form. The main difference between this and equation 4.9 is that the Oja's rule subtracts off the square of the activation times the weight, while equation 4.12 just subtracts off the activation times the weight. Thus we would expect that the CPCA will produce roughly similar weight changes as the Oja rule, with a difference in the way that normalization works (also note that because the activations in CPCA are all positive probability-like values, the difference in squaring the activation does not affect the sign of the weight change).

The second form of equation 4.12 emphasizes the following interpretation of what this form of learning is accomplishing: the weights are adjusted to match the value of the sending unit activation x_i (i.e., minimizing the difference between x_i and w_{ij}), weighted in proportion to the activation of the receiving unit (y_j). Thus, if the receiving unit is not active, no weight adjustment will occur (effectively, the receiving unit doesn't care what happens to the input unit when it is not itself active). If the receiving unit is very active (near 1), it cares a lot about what the input unit's activation is, and tries to set the weight to match it. As these individual weight changes are accumulated together with a slow learning rate, the weight will come to approximate the expected value of the sending unit when the receiver is active (in other words, equation 4.11).

The next section shows formally how the weight update rule in equation 4.12 implements the conditional probability objective in equation 4.11. For those who are less mathematically inclined, this analysis can be skipped without significantly impacting the ability to understand what follows.

4.5.2 Derivation of CPCA Learning Rule

This analysis, based on that of Rumelhart and Zipser (1986), uses the same technique we used above to understand Oja's normalized PCA learning rule. Thus, we will work backward from the weight update equation (equation 4.12), and, by setting this to zero and thus solving for the equilibrium weight value, show that the weights converge in the asymptotic case to the conditional probability of equation 4.11.

First, we need to re-express the relevant variables in probabilistic terms. Thus, the activations of the sending and receiving units will be assumed to represent *probabilities* that the corresponding units are active, which is consistent with the analysis of the point neuron function in terms of Bayesian hypothesis testing presented in chapter 2. We use the expression $P(y_j|t)$ to represent the probability that the receiving unit y_j is active given that some particular input pattern t was presented. $P(x_i|t)$ represents the corresponding thing for the sending unit x_i. Thus, substituting these into equation 4.12, the total weight update computed over all the possible patterns t (and multiplying by the probability that each pattern occurs, $P(t)$) is:

$$\Delta w_{ij} = \epsilon \sum_t [P(y_j|t)P(x_i|t) - P(y_j|t)w_{ij}]P(t)$$

$$= \epsilon \left(\sum_t P(y_j|t)P(x_i|t)P(t) - \right.$$

$$\left. \sum_t P(y_j|t)P(t)w_{ij} \right) \quad (4.13)$$

As before, we set Δw_{ij} to zero to find the equilibrium weight value, and then we solve the resulting equation for the value of w_{ij}. This results in the following:

$$0 = \epsilon \left(\sum_t P(y_j|t)P(x_i|t)P(t) - \right.$$

$$\left. \sum_t P(y_j|t)P(t)w_{ij} \right)$$

$$w_{ij} = \frac{\sum_t P(y_j|t)P(x_i|t)P(t)}{\sum_t P(y_j|t)P(t)} \quad (4.14)$$

Now, the interesting thing to note here is that the numerator $\sum_t P(y_j|t)P(x_i|t)P(t)$ is actually the definition of the joint probability of the sending and receiving units both being active together across all the patterns t, which is just $P(y_j, x_i)$. Similarly, the denominator $\sum_t P(y_j|t)P(t)$ gives the probability of the receiving unit being active over all the patterns, or $P(y_j)$. Thus,

we can rewrite the preceding equation as:

$$w_{ij} = \frac{P(y_j, x_i)}{P(y_j)}$$

$$= P(x_i|y_j) \quad (4.15)$$

at which point it becomes clear that this fraction of the joint probability over the probability of the receiver is just the definition of the conditional probability of the sender given the receiver. This is just equation 4.11, which is right where we wanted to end up.

4.5.3 Biological Implementation of CPCA Hebbian Learning

At the beginning of this chapter, we described the biological mechanisms thought to underlie weight changes in the cortex, and showed how these generally support a Hebbian or associative type of learning. However, the CPCA learning rule is slightly more complex than a simple product of sending and receiving unit activations, and thus requires a little further explanation. We will see that we can account for the general characteristics of weight changes as prescribed by the CPCA learning rule (equation 4.12) using the same basic NMDA-mediated LTP/D mechanisms that were described previously. For reference, the CPCA equation is:

$$\Delta w_{ij} = \epsilon y_j (x_i - w_{ij}) \quad (4.16)$$

For our first pass at seeing how the biology could implement this equation, let's assume that the weight is at some middling value (e.g., around .5) — we will consider the effects of different weight values in a moment. With this assumption, there are three general categories of weight changes produced by CPCA:

1. When the sending and receiving units are both strongly active (and thus $x_i > w_{ij}$), the weight should increase (LTP). We can easily account for this case by the associative nature of NMDA-mediated LTP.

2. When the receiving unit is active, but the sending unit not (i.e., $x_i < w_{ij}$), then LTD will occur. This case can be explained by the NMDA channels being open (as a function of postsynaptic activity unblocking the Mg^+), and the small amount of presynaptic activity causing a small but above zero level

of calcium influx, which should lead to LTD. It is also possible that postsynaptic activity will activate other voltage-gated calcium channels, which could provide the weak concentrations of calcium necessary to induce LTD without any presynaptic activity at all.

3. When the receiving unit is not active, the likelihood (and/or magnitude) of any weight change goes to zero. This can be explained by the Mg^+ blocking of the NMDA channels, and also by the lack of activation of voltage-gated calcium channels, both of which lead to no influx of postsynaptic calcium, and thus no weight changes.

Finally, the effect of CPCA learning with different values of weights can be summarized as follows: when the weight is large (near 1), further increases will happen less frequently (as it becomes less likely that x_i is larger than the weight) and will be smaller in magnitude, while decreases will show the opposite pattern. Conversely, when the weight is small, increases become more likely and larger in magnitude and the opposite holds for decreases. This general pattern is exactly what is observed empirically in LTP/LTD studies, and amounts to the observation that both LTP and LTD *saturate* at upper and lower bounds, respectively. This can be thought of as a form of **soft weight bounding**, where the upper and lower bounds (1 and 0 in this case) are enforced in a "soft" manner by slowing the weight changes exponentially as the bounds are approached. We will return to this issue in the context of task learning in a later section.

4.6 Exploration of Hebbian Model Learning

We now revisit the simulation we ran at the beginning of this chapter, and see how a single unit learns in response to different patterns of correlation between its activity and a set of input patterns. This exploration will illustrate how conditionalizing the activity of the receiving unit can shape the resulting weights to emphasize a feature present in only a subset of input patterns. However, we will find that we need to introduce some additional factors in the learning rule to make this emphasis really effective. These factors will be even more important for

the self-organizing case that is explored in a subsequent section.

↪ Open the project `hebb_correl.proj.gz` in `chapter_4` to begin (if it is still open from the previous exercises, you will want to close and reopen it to start with a clean slate).

As before, we will want to watch the weights of the hidden unit as it learns.

↪ Select `r.wt` as the variable to view in the network window, and click on the hidden unit. Now, select `View` and `EVENTS` in the `hebb_correl_ctrl` control panel.

You should see an environment window with 2 events, one having a right-leaning diagonal line, and the other having a left leaning one. These are the two sets of correlations that exist in this simple environment.

To keep things simple in this simulation, we will manipulate the percentage of time that the receiving unit is active in conjunction with each of these events to alter the conditional probabilities that drive learning in the CPCA algorithm. Thus, we are only simulating those events that happen when the receiver is active — when the receiver is not active, no learning occurs, so we can just ignore all these other events for the present purposes. As a result, what we think of as conditional probabilities actually appear in the simulation as just plain unconditional probabilities —- we are ignoring everything outside the conditional (where the unit is inactive). In later simulations, we will explore the more realistic case of multiple receiving units that are activated by different events, and we will see how more plausible ways of conditional probability learning can arise through self-organizing learning.

We will next view the probabilities or *frequencies* associated with each event.

↪ Locate the `Evt Label` parameter in the environment window (upper left hand side), and select `FreqEvent::freq` to be displayed as the label below each event in the display on the right side of the window.

You should see `frequency: 1` below the `Right` event, and 0 below the `Left` one, indicating that the receiving unit will be active all of the time in conjunction with the right-leaning diagonal line, and none of the time with the left-leaning one (this was the default for the initial exploration from before).

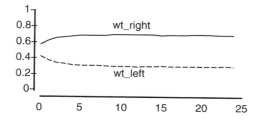

Figure 4.11: Plot of the weights from the rightward line (wt_right) and the leftward line (wt_left).

Again, these absolute probabilities of presenting these lines actually correspond to conditional probabilities, because we are ignoring all the other possible cases where the receiving unit is inactive — we are implicitly conditioning the entire simulation on the receiving unit being active (so that it is indeed always active for every input pattern).

The parameter p_right in the control panel determines the frequencies of the events in the environment, with the Right event being set to p_right and Left to 1-p_right.

↳ Set p_right to .7, and hit Apply — you will see the FreqEvent::freq values updated to .7 and .3. Then, go ahead and iconify the environment window before continuing.

Keep in mind as we do these exercises that this single receiving unit will ordinarily just be one of multiple such receiving units looking at the same input patterns. Thus, we want this unit to specialize on representing one of the correlated features in the environment (i.e., 1 of the 2 lines in this case). We can manipulate this specialization by making the conditional probabilities weighted more toward one event over the other.

↳ Now, press the Run button in the control panel.

This will run the network through 20 sets (epochs) of 100 randomly ordered event presentations, with 70 of these presentations being the Right event, and 30 being the Left event given a p_right value of .7. The CPCA Hebbian learning rule (equation 4.12) is applied after each event presentation and the weights updated accordingly. You will see the display of the weights in the network window being updated after each of these 20 epochs.

Another way to look at the development of the weights over learning is to use a graph log.

↳ Do View, GRAPH_LOG to pull up the graph log, then do Run again.

The graph log (figure 4.11) displays the value of one of the weights from a unit in the right-leaning diagonal line (wt_right, in red), and from a unit in the left-leaning diagonal line (wt_left, in orange). You should notice that as learning proceeds, the weights from the units active in the Right event will hover right around .7 (with the exception of the central unit, which is present in both events and will have a weight of around 1), while the weights for the Left event will hover around .3. Thus, as expected, the CPCA learning rule causes the weights to reflect the conditional probability that the input unit is active given that the receiver was active. Experiment with different values of p_right, and verify that this holds for all sorts of different probabilities.

The parameter lrate in the control panel, which corresponds to ϵ in the CPCA learning rule (equation 4.12), determines how rapidly the weights are updated after each event.

↳ Change lrate to .1 and Run.

Question 4.1 (a) *How does this change in the learning rate affect the general character of the weight updates as displayed in the network window?* (b) *Explain why this happens.* (c) *Explain the relevance (if any) this might have for the importance of integrating over multiple experiences (events) in learning.*

↳ Set the lrate parameter back to .005.

When you explored different values of p_right previously, you were effectively manipulating how *selective* the receiving unit was for one type of event over another. Thus, you were taking advantage of the conditional aspect of CPCA Hebbian learning by effectively conditionalizing its representation of the input environment. As we stated earlier, instead of manipulating the frequency with which the two events occurred in the environment, you should think of this as manipulating the frequency with which the receiving unit was co-active with these events, because the receiving unit is always active for these inputs.

Now we want to compare the conditionalizing aspect of CPCA with the unconditional PCA algorithm. Let's assume that each event (`Right` and `Left`) has an equal probability of appearing in the environment.

↪ Set `p_right` to .5, `Apply`, and `Run`.

This will simulate the effects of a standard (unconditional) form of PCA, where the receiving unit is effectively always on for the entire environment (unlike CPCA which can have the receiving unit active when only one of the lines is present in the environment).

Question 4.2 (a) *What result does* `p_right`=*.5 lead to for the weights?* **(b)** *Does this weight pattern suggest the existence of two separate diagonal line features existing in the environment? Explain your answer.* **(c)** *How does this compare with the "blob" solution for the natural scene images as discussed above and shown in figure 4.8?*

Question 4.3 (a) *How would you set* `p_right` *to simulate the hidden unit controlled in such a way as to come on only when there is a right-leaning diagonal line in the input, and never for the left one?* **(b)** *What result does this lead to for the weights?* **(c)** *Explain why this result might be more informative than the case explored in the previous question.* **(d)** *How would you extend the architecture and training of the network to represent this environment of two diagonal lines in a fully satisfactory way? Explain your answer.*

The simple environment we have been using so far is not very realistic, because it assumes a one-to-one mapping between input patterns and the categories of features that we would typically want to represent.

↪ Switch the `env_type` from `ONE_LINE` to the `THREE_LINES` environment in the control panel (and `Apply`). Then, do `View`, `EVENTS` to see this environment.

Notice that there are now three different versions of both the left and right diagonal lines, with "upper" and "lower" diagonals in addition to the original two "center" lines. In this environment, `p_right` is spread among all three types of right lines, which are conceived of as mere subtypes of the more general category of right lines (and likewise for `1-p_right` and the left lines).

↪   Set `Evt Label` in the environment to `FreqEvent::freq`, and set `p_right` to .7, (and `Apply`) — you should see the frequencies of .7/3(= .2333) for the right lines and .3/3(= .1) for the left ones. Then, `Run`.

You should see that the right lines all have weights of around .2333 and the left lines have weights around .1. Although this is the correct result for representing the conditional probabilities, this result illustrates a couple of problems with the CPCA learning algorithm. First, when units represent categories of features instead of single instances, the weights end up being *diluted* because the receiving unit is active for several different input patterns, so the conditional probabilities for each individual pattern can be relatively small. Second, this dilution can be compounded by a receiving unit that has somewhat less than perfect selectivity for one category of features (right) over others (left), resulting in relatively small differences in weight magnitude (e.g., .233 for right versus .1 for left). This is a real problem because units are generally not very selective during the crucial early phases of learning for reasons that will become clear later.

Thus, in some sense, the CPCA algorithm is *too faithful* to the actual conditional probabilities, and does not do enough to emphasize the selectivity of the receiving unit. Also, these small overall weight values reduce the *dynamic range* of the weights, and end up being inconsistent with the weight values produced by the task learning algorithm described in chapter 5. The next section shows how we can deal with these limitations of the basic CPCA rule. After that, we will revisit this simulation.

↪ Go to the `PDP++Root` window. To continue on to the next simulation, close this project first by selecting `.projects/Remove/Project_0`. Or, if you wish to stop now, quit by selecting `Object/Quit`.

4.7   Renormalization and Contrast Enhancement

The CPCA algorithm results in normalized (0–1) weight values, which, as we saw in the previous section, tend to not have much *dynamic range* or *selectivity*, limiting the effectiveness of this form of the learning algorithm. These problems can be remedied by introducing two correction factors that make the algorithm more effective, while preserving the basic underlying computation performed by it to stay true to its biological and computational motivations. The first correction factor is a way of *renormalizing* the weights by taking into account the expected activity level over the sending layer (which is typically sparse). This resolves the dynamic range problem. The second correction factor is a way of *enhancing the contrast* between weak and strong weights (correlations) by applying a nonlinear sigmoidal function to the weights. This resolves the selectivity problem.

It is important to note how these correction factors fit within our framework of mechanisms with a clear biological basis. As described in section 4.5, the CPCA algorithm captures the essential aspects of model learning subserved by the biological mechanisms of LTP and LTD. The correction factors introduced in this section represent quantitative adjustments to this CPCA algorithm (i.e., they affect only the magnitude, not the sign, of weight changes) that retain the qualitative features of the basic CPCA algorithm that are motivated by the biological and computational considerations. The resulting algorithm performs efficient model learning.

Note that the explorations should make very clear the effects of these correction factors. Thus, do not despair if you do not fully understand this section — a rereading of this section following the explorations should make more sense.

4.7.1 Renormalization

When the sending layer has a low expected activity level, any given sending unit is not very active on average. Thus, when we consider the conditional probability computed by the CPCA learning rule (equation 4.11), we would expect a similarly low average probability of a given sending unit x_i being active given that the receiver is active. Indeed, if there is really no correlation between the activity of the sender and the receiver, then we expect the conditional probability to be around α, where α is the expected activity level of the sending layer (typically between .10 and .25 in our simulations). This violates the notion that a probability of .5 should represent a lack of correlation, while smaller

values represent negative correlation, and larger values represent positive correlation.

Renormalization simply restores the idea that a conditional probability of .5 indicates a lack of correlation, in effect *renormalizing* the weights to the standard 0-1 range. The best way to accomplish this renormalization is simply to increase the upper-bound for weight increases in an expanded form of the CPCA weight-update equation:

$$\begin{aligned} \Delta w_{ij} &= \epsilon[y_j x_i - y_j w_{ij}] \\ &= \epsilon[y_j x_i (1 - w_{ij}) + \\ &\quad y_j (1 - x_i)(0 - w_{ij})] \end{aligned} \quad (4.17)$$

(you can use simple algebra to verify that the second form of the equation is equivalent to the first).

This expanded form can be understood by analogy to the membrane potential update equation from chapter 2. The $y_j x_i$ term is like an excitatory "conductance" that drives the weights upward toward a "reversal potential" of 1, while the $y_j(1 - x_i)$ term is an inhibitory "conductance" that drives the weights downward toward a "reversal potential" of 0. Thus, to correct for the sparse activations, we can make this "excitatory reversal potential" greater than 1, which will increase the range of the weight values produced:

$$\Delta w_{ij} = \epsilon[y_j x_i (m - w_{ij}) + y_j (1 - x_i)(0 - w_{ij})] \quad (4.18)$$

where $m > 1$ is the new maximum weight value for the purposes of learning. The weights are still clipped to the standard 0-1 range, resulting in a potential loss of resolution above some value of the conditional probability — this rarely happens in practice, however. Equation 4.18 preserves a linear relationship between the true underlying conditional probability and the equilibrium weight value, which is very important.[2] We set the correction factor m using the following equation:

$$m = \frac{.5}{\alpha} \quad (4.19)$$

---

[2] Another obvious way of compensating for expected activity levels is to multiply the increase and decrease terms by appropriate complementary factors. However, doing so produces a convex relationship between the weight and the actual conditional probability, which distorts learning by making things appear more correlated than they actually are.

so that an expected activity level α of .5 will be the same as standard CPCA, but smaller values will produce relatively larger weights.

Finally, to establish a continuum between the basic CPCA learning rule without renormalization and the version with it, we introduce a parameter q_m (savg_cor in the simulator, which stands for "sending average (activation) correction") which is between 0 and 1 and specifies how close to the actual α we should go (starting at .5) in compensating for the expected activity level. Thus, we compute the effective activity level that we will use in equation 4.19 as follows:

$$\alpha_m = .5 - q_m(.5 - \alpha) \qquad (4.20)$$

and then compute m as $m = \frac{.5}{\alpha_m}$. So, when $q_m = 0$, no renormalization occurs, and when $q_m = 1$, the weights are maximally renormalized to fit the 0–1 range.

4.7.2 Contrast Enhancement

Whereas renormalization addresses the dynamic range issue, contrast enhancement addresses the selectivity problem with the basic CPCA algorithm. The idea is to enhance the contrast between the stronger and weaker correlations, such that the weights predominantly reflect the contribution of the stronger correlations, while the weaker correlations are ignored or minimized. This further accentuates the existing tendency of CPCA to represent the principal component of the correlations. Thus, contrast enhancement can be seen as accentuating the extent to which the transformations learned by the hidden units emphasize some aspects of the input pattern and deemphasize others, which we discussed in chapter 3 as one of the most important functions that hidden units perform.

Contrast enhancement constitutes an important source of bias in favor of a simpler (more parsimonious) representation of the strongest, most basic structure of the environment over its weaker and more subtle aspects. Clearly, an appropriate balance between simplicity and fidelity needs to be struck (as we will discuss at greater length), but the basic CPCA equation tends to be too heavily weighted toward fidelity, so that there is a benefit to imposing an additional simplicity bias.

Contrast enhancement can also be understood in the context of the effects of *soft weight bounding*, which is a property of the CPCA algorithm. Because the weights are constrained to live within the 0–1 range, and they approach these extremes exponentially slowly, this makes it difficult for units to develop highly selective representations that produce strong activation for some input patterns and weak activation for others. Thus, contrast enhancement counteracts these limitations by expanding the rate of change of weight values around the intermediate range, while still retaining the advantages of soft weight bounding.

We implement contrast enhancement using a sigmoidal function, which provides an obvious mechanism for contrast enhancement as a function of the *gain* parameter that determines how sharp or gradual the function is. This function can enhance the contrast between weight values by transforming the linear relationship between weight values (which in turn are conditional probabilities computed by the CPCA algorithm) into a sigmoidal nonlinear relationship mediated by a gain parameter. Biologically, this would amount to a differential sensitivity to weight changes for weight values in the middle range as opposed to the extremes, which is plausible but not established.

Note that this kind of contrast enhancement on the weights is not equivalent to the effects of the more standard gain parameter on the activation values. Changing the activation gain can make the unit more or less sensitive to differences in the total net input (the sending activations times the weights). In contrast, changing the contrast enhancement of the weights affects each weight value separately, and allows the unit to be more sensitive *at the level of each individual input* instead of at the level of the total input. Put another way, weight contrast enhancement gives a unit a more sensitive filter or template for detecting patterns over its inputs, whereas activation contrast enhancement just makes the net response more sensitive around the threshold, but does not increase the contrast of the signal coming into the unit.

In the simulator, we implement weight contrast enhancement by introducing an *effective weight* $\hat{w}_{ij}$ which is computed from the underlying *linear weight* using the following sigmoidal function:

$$\hat{w}_{ij} = \frac{1}{1 + \left(\frac{w_{ij}}{1 - w_{ij}}\right)^{-\gamma}} \qquad (4.21)$$

where γ is the *weight gain* parameter (`wt_gain` in the simulator, stored in the `wt_sig` field) that controls the extent of contrast enhancement performed. Note that this function can be derived from the same $\frac{a}{a+b}$ form that has been used repeatedly throughout the text:

$$\hat{w}_{ij} = \frac{w_{ij}}{w_{ij} + (1 - w_{ij})} \qquad (4.22)$$

(though it is more difficult to have a gain parameter for the equation in this latter form). See figure 4.12 for a plot of this function for the standard `wt_gain` parameter of 6.

The effective weight value $\hat{w}$ is used for computing the net inputs to units and is the standard `wt` value in the simulator. The original linear weight value is only used as an internal variable for computing weight changes (it basically makes sure that the averaging over events results in the appropriate conditional probability values). Thus, it would probably be very difficult to measure something that reflects the linear weight value biologically, as it could just be subsumed into the dynamics of the synaptic modification process. Implementationally, we get the original linear weight value from the effective weight value by applying the inverse of the sigmoidal function.

One can add an additional parameter to the sigmoid function that controls its *offset*. This offset acts much like a *threshold* and can be useful for imposing a higher threshold for correlation to further enhance the contrast between the different features present in the input. This offset parameter θ (`wt_off` in the simulator, also stored in the `wt_sig` field) is introduced into the effective weight value equation as follows:

$$\hat{w}_{ij} = \frac{1}{1 + \left(\theta \frac{w_{ij}}{1 - w_{ij}}\right)^{-\gamma}} \qquad (4.23)$$

with values of θ greater than 1 imposing a higher threshold on the underlying linear correlation values

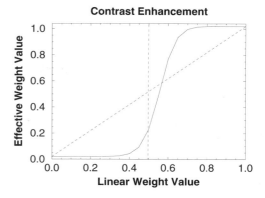

Figure 4.12: Effective weight value as a function of underlying linear weight value, showing contrast enhancement of correlations around the middle values of the conditional probability as represented by the linear weight value. Note that the midpoint of the function is shifted upward by the offset parameter `wt_off`.

for a given weight value. The results for the standard `wt_off` value of 1.25 are shown in figure 4.12.

Note that the point around threshold (nominally .5, but this is affected by `wt_off`) becomes a dividing line in the contrast enhancement process — values above are enhanced, while those below are weakened. Thus, when the sigmoidal nonlinearity is introduced, it suddenly becomes much more important where numerically different conditional probability values fall relative to this contrast enhancement threshold. The `savg_cor` renormalization parameter plays an important role in determining this point, in addition to the obvious importance of the `wt_off` parameter. We will see this in the following simulations.

4.7.3 Exploration of Renormalization and Contrast Enhancement in CPCA

↪ Open the project `hebb_correl.proj.gz` in `chapter_4` to begin (if it is still open from the previous exercises, you will want to close and reopen it to start with a clean slate). View the `r.wt` weights of the hidden unit as before. View the GRAPH_LOG.

We are first going to explore the renormalization of the weights by taking into account the α expected activity level over the input layer. Because most of our line stimuli have 5 units active, and there are 25 units in the input layer, this α value is set to .2. Let's explore this issue using an environment where the features have zero correlation with the receiving unit, and see how the renormalization results in weight values of .5 for this case.

↪   Set env_type in the control panel to the FIVE_HORIZ lines environment (Apply). Do View and EVENTS to see this environment.

You should see that the environment contains 5 horizontal lines, each of which is presented with equal probability (i.e., 1/5 or .2). Thus, these line features represent the zero correlation case, because they each co-occur with the receiving unit with the same probability as the expected activity level over the input layer (.2). In other words, you would expect this same level of co-occurrence if you simply activated input units at random such that the overall activity level on the input was at .2.

↪   Click on r.wt in the network window (and select the hidden unit), and then Run the network.

You will see that because of the very literal behavior of the unmodified CPCA algorithm in reflecting the conditional probabilities, the weights are all around .2 at the end of learning. Thus, if we were interpreting these weights in terms of the standard meaning of conditional probabilities (i.e., where .5 represents zero correlation), we would conclude that the input units are anticorrelated with the receiving unit. However, we know that this is not correct given the sparse activity levels in the input.

↪   Now, set savg_cor (which is the q_m parameter in equation 4.20) in the control panel to a value of 1 instead of 0.

This means that we will now be applying the full correction for the average activity level in the sending (input) layer.

↪   Run the network again.

You should observe that the weights now hover around .5, which is the correct value for expressing the lack of correlation.

Although the ability to fully correct for sparse sending activations is useful, one does not always want to do this. In particular, if we have any prior expectation about how many individual input patterns should

be represented by a given hidden unit, then we can set savg_cor appropriately so that the .5 level corresponds roughly to this prior expectation. For example, if we know that the units should have relatively *selective* representations (e.g., one or two input features per unit), then we might want to set savg_cor to .5 or even less, because the full correction for the input layer α will result in larger weights for features that are relatively weakly correlated compared to this expected level of selectivity. If units are expected to represent a number of input features, then a value of savg_cor closer to 1 is more appropriate. We will revisit this issue.

Now, let's explore the contrast enhancement sigmoid function of the effective weights. The parameters wt_gain and wt_off in the control panel control the gain and offset of the sigmoid function. First, we will plot the shape of the contrast enhancement function for different values of these parameters.

↪   First set wt_gain to 6 instead of 1. Click the PlotEffWt button in the control panel, which will bring up a graph log.

You should see a sigmoidal function (the shape of the resulting effective weights function) plotted in a graph log window at the bottom of your screen. The horizontal axis represents the raw linear weight value, and the vertical axis represents the contrast enhanced weight value. The increase in wt_gain results in substantial contrast enhancement.

↪   Try setting wt_gain to various different values, and then clicking the PlotEffWt button to observe the effect on the shape of this function.

We next see the effects of wt_gain on learning.

↪   First, select Defaults, change savg_cor to 1, SelectEnv the THREE_LINES environment, and Run.

This run provides a baseline for comparison. You should see a somewhat bloblike representation in the weights, where the right lines are a bit more strong than the left lines, but not dramatically so.

↪   Now increase wt_gain from 1 to 6, and Run again.

You should very clearly see that only the right lines are represented, and with relatively strong weights. Thus, the contrast enhancement allows the network to represent the reality of the distinct underlying left and right categories of features even when it is imperfectly selective (.7) to these features. This effect will be especially important for self-organizing learning, as we will see in the next section.

Now, let's use the `wt_off` parameter to encourage the network to pay attention to only the *strongest* of correlations in the input.

↪ Leaving `wt_gain` at 6, change `wt_off` to 1.25, and do `PlotEffWt` to see how this affects the effective weight function. You may have to go back and forth between 1 and 1.25 a couple of times to be able to see the difference.

↪ With `wt_off` set to 1.25, `Run` the network.

Question 4.4 (a) *How does this change the results compared to the case where* `wt_off` *is 1?* **(b)** *Explain why this occurs.* **(c)** *Find a value of* `wt_off` *that makes the non-central (non-overlapping) units of the right lines (i.e., the 4 units in the lower left corner and the 4 units in the upper right corner) have weights around .1 or less.* **(d)** *Do the resulting weights accurately reflect the correlations present in any single input pattern? Explain your answer.* **(e)** *Can you imagine why this representation might be useful in some cases?*

An alternative way to accomplish some of the effects of the `wt_off` parameter is to set the `savg_cor` parameter to a value of less than 1. As described above, this will make the units more *selective* because weak correlations will not be renormalized to as high a weight value.

↪ Set `wt_off` back to 1, and set `savg_cor` to .7.

Question 4.5 (a) *What effect does this have on the learned weight values?* **(b)** *How does this compare with the* `wt_off` *parameter you found in the previous question?*

This last question shows that because the contrast enhancement from `wt_gain` magnifies differences around .5 (with `wt_off=1`), the `savg_cor` can have a big effect by changing the amount of correlated activity necessary to achieve this .5 value. A lower `savg_cor` will result in smaller weight values for more weakly correlated inputs — when the `wt_gain` parameter is large, then these smaller values get pushed down toward zero, causing the unit to essentially ignore these inputs. Thus, these interactions between contrast enhancement

and renormalization can play an important role in determining what the unit tends to detect.

These simulations demonstrate how the correction factors of renormalization and contrast enhancement can increase the effectiveness of the CPCA algorithm. These correction factors represent quantitative adjustments to the CPCA algorithm to address its limitations of dynamic range and selectivity, while preserving the basic computation performed by the algorithm to stay true to its biological and computational motivations.

↪ Go to the `PDP++Root` window. To continue on to the next simulation, close this project first by selecting `.projects/Remove/Project_0`. Or, if you wish to stop now, quit by selecting `Object/Quit`.

4.8 Self-Organizing Model Learning

Up to this point, we have focused on a single receiving unit with artificially specified activations to more clearly understand how the weights are adjusted in the CPCA Hebbian learning rule. However, this is obviously not a very realistic model of learning in the cortex. In this section, we move beyond these more limited demonstrations by exploring a network having multiple receiving units that compete with each other under the kWTA inhibitory function. The result is self-organizing model learning, where the interaction between activation dynamics (especially inhibitory competition) and Hebbian learning result in the development of representations that capture important aspects of the environmental structure.

In the context of the CPCA learning algorithm, self-organization amounts to the use of competition between a set of receiving units as a way of conditionalizing the responses of these units. Thus, a given unit will become active to the extent that it is more strongly activated by the current input pattern than other units are — this can only happen if the weights into this unit are sufficiently well tuned to that input pattern. Thus, because the CPCA learning algorithm causes tuning of the weights to those input units that are co-active with the receiving unit, there is effectively a positive feedback system here — any initial selectivity for a set of input patterns will become reinforced by the learning algorithm, producing even greater selectivity.

As with all such positive feedback systems, there is a potential for *runaway positive feedback* (e.g., like we saw with bidirectional excitatory connectivity in the previous chapter). This phenomenon is manifest in the self-organizing learning case as individual receiving units that end up representing a disproportionate number of input features, while other receiving units represent very few or no such features. One important check against this "hogging" phenomenon happens when learning causes units to become more *selectively* tuned to a subset of input patterns — thus, as a unit ends up representing one set of patterns, this causes the unit to become less likely to be activated for other ones.

For example, consider the case of the unit that selectively represented the right diagonal line in the above explorations. With the appropriate contrast enhancement parameters, learning for this unit caused its weights to *decrease* for the left diagonal line even as they increased for the right diagonal line. Thus, this unit would have been much less likely to respond to left diagonal lines, which would allow another unit to "win" the competition for that case, resulting in good representations of both types of lines.

4.8.1 Exploration of Self-Organizing Learning

We will continue with the "lines" theme in this exploration, by exposing a set of hidden units to an environment consisting of horizontal and vertical lines on a $5x5$ input "retina."

↪   Open the project self_org.proj.gz in chapter_4 to begin.

We focus first on the network. The $5x5$ input projects to a hidden layer of 20 units, which are all fully connected to the input with random initial weights.

↪ As usual, select r.wt and view the weights for these units.

Because viewing the pattern of weights over all the hidden units will be of primary concern as the network learns, we have a special grid log window that displays the weights for all hidden units.

↪   To see this, press View in the self_org_ctrl control panel, and select WT_MAT_LOG.

This will display all of the weights in the grid log window that comes up (figure 4.13 shows this display

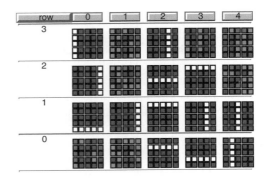

Figure 4.13: Grid log view of all the weights for the hidden units after 30 epochs of learning. The larger-scale grid represents the layout of the hidden units, with the smaller grid within each of the larger grid elements showing the weights from the input for the corresponding hidden unit. This network has learned to represent the correlations present in the individual lines, even though every input has two lines present.

for a trained network — your grid log window will eventually look like this one.). The larger-scale $5x4$ grid is topographically arranged in the same layout as the network. Within each of these 20 grid elements is a smaller $5x5$ grid representing the input units, showing the weights for each unit. By clicking on the hidden units in the network window, you should be able to verify this correspondence.

Now, let's see the environment the network will be experiencing.

↪ Press View and select EVENTS in the control panel.

This will bring up a window showing 45 events representing different combinations of vertical and horizontal lines. This is all unique pairwise combinations of each type of line. Thus, there are no real correlations between the lines, with the only reliable correlations being between the pixels that make up a particular line. To put this another way, each line can be thought of as appearing in a number of different randomly related contexts (i.e., with other lines).

It should be clear that if we computed the correlations between individual pixels across all of these images, everything would be equally (weakly) correlated with everything else. Thus, learning must be conditional on the particular type of line for any meaningful correlations to be extracted. We will see that this conditionality will simply self-organize through the interactions of the learning rule and the kWTA inhibitory competition. Note also that because two lines are present in every image, the network will require at least two active hidden units per input, assuming each unit is representing a particular line.

↪   Iconify the environment window when you are done examining the patterns, and return to viewing `activations` in the network window. Now hit `Step` in the control panel to present a single pattern to the network.

You should see one of the event patterns containing two lines in the input of the network, and a pattern of roughly two active hidden units.

The hidden layer is using the average-based kWTA inhibition function, with the k parameter set to 2 as you can see in the `hidden_kwta_k` parameter in the control panel. This function allows for some variability of actual activation level depending on the actual distribution of excitation across units in the hidden layer. Thus, when more than two units are active, these units are being fairly equally activated by the input pattern due to the random initial weights not being very selective. This is an important effect, because these weaker additional activations may enable these units to bootstrap into stronger activations through gradual learning, should they end up being reliably active in conjunction with a particular input feature (i.e., a particular line in this case).

↪   You can `Step` some more. When you tire of single stepping, just press the `Run` button on the process control panel. You will want to turn off the `Display` in the network, to make things run faster.

After 30 *epochs* (passes through all 45 different events in the environment) of learning, the network will stop. You should have noticed that the weights grid log was updated after every 5 epochs, and that the weights came to more and more clearly reflect the lines present in the environment (figure 4.13). Thus, individual units developed *selective* representations of the correlations present within individual lines, while ignoring the random context of the other lines.

These individual line representations developed as a result of the interaction between learning and inhibitory

competition as follows. Early on, the units that won the inhibitory competition were those that happened to have larger random weights for the input pattern. CPCA learning then tuned these weights to be more selective for that input pattern, causing them to be more likely to respond to that pattern and others that overlap with it (i.e., other patterns sharing one of the two lines). To the extent that the weights are stronger for one of the two lines in the input, the unit will be more likely to respond to inputs having this line, and thus the conditional probability for the input units in this line will be stronger than for the other units, and the weights will continue to increase. This is where the contrast enhancement bias plays an important role, because it emphasizes the strongest of the unit's correlations and deemphasizes the weaker ones. This will make it much more likely that the strongest correlation in the environment — the single lines — end up getting represented.

You might have noticed in the weights displayed in the grid log during learning that some units initially seemed to be becoming selective for multiple lines, but then as other units were better able to represent one of those lines, they started to lose that competition and fall back to representing only one line. Thus, the dynamics of the inhibitory competition are critical for the self-organizing effect, and it should be clear that a firm inhibitory constraint is important for this kind of learning (otherwise units will just end up being active a lot, and representing a mish-mash of line features). Nevertheless, the average-based kWTA function is sufficiently flexible that it can allow more than two units to become active, so you will probably see that sometimes multiple hidden units end up encoding the same line feature.

The net result of this self-organizing learning is a nice *combinatorial* distributed representation, where each input pattern is represented as the combination of the two line features present therein. This is the "obvious" way to represent such inputs, but you should appreciate that the network nevertheless had to discover this representation through the somewhat complex self-organizing learning procedure.

↪   To see this representation in action, turn the network `Display` back on, and `Step` through a few more events.

Notice that in general two or more units are strongly activated by each input pattern, with the extra activation reflecting the fact that some lines are coded by multiple units.

Another thing to notice in the weights shown in the grid log (figure 4.13) is that some units are obviously not selective for anything. These "loser" units (also known as "dead" units) were never reliably activated by any input feature, and thus did not experience much learning. It is typically quite important to have such units lying around, because self-organization requires some "elbow room" during learning to sort out the allocation of units to stable correlational features. Having more hidden units also increases the chances of having a large enough range of initial random selectivities to seed the self-organization process. The consequence is that you need to have more units than is minimally necessary, and that you will often end up with leftovers (plus the redundant units mentioned previously).

From a biological perspective, we know that the cortex does not produce new neurons in adults, so we conclude that in general there is probably an excess of neural capacity relative to the demands of any given learning context. Thus, it is useful to have these leftover and redundant units, because they constitute a *reserve* that could presumably get activated if new features were later presented to the network (e.g., diagonal lines). We are much more suspicious of algorithms that require precisely tuned quantities of hidden units to work properly (more on this later).

Unique Pattern Statistic

Although looking at the weights is informative, we could use a more concise measure of how well the network's internal model matches the underlying structure of the environment. We can plot one such measure in a graph log as the network learns.

↪ Do `View` on the control panel and select `TRAIN_GRAPH_LOG`. Turn the network `Display` back off, and `Run` again.

This log shows the results of a **unique pattern statistic** (`UniquePatStat` in simulator parlance, shown as `unq_pats` in the log), which records the number of unique hidden unit activity patterns that were produced as a result of probing the network with all 10 different types of horizontal and vertical lines (presented individ-

ually). Thus, there is a separate testing process which, after each epoch of learning, tests the network on all 10 lines, records the resulting hidden unit activity patterns (with the kWTA parameter set to 1, though this is not critical due to the flexibility of the average-based kWTA function), and then counts up the number of unique such patterns.

The logic behind this measure is that if each line is encoded by (at least) one distinct hidden unit, then this will show up as a unique pattern. If, however, there are units that encode two or more lines together (which is not a good model of this environment), then this will not result in a unique representation for these lines, and the resulting measure will be lower. Thus, to the extent that this statistic is less than 10, the internal model produced by the network does not fully capture the underlying independence of each line from the other lines. Note, however, that the unique pattern statistic does not care if *multiple* hidden units encode the same line (i.e., if there is redundancy across different hidden units) — it only cares that the *same* hidden unit not encode *two different* lines.

You should have seen on this run that the model produced a perfect internal model according to this statistic, which accords well with our analysis of the weight patterns. To get a better sense of how well the network learns in general, you can run a *batch* of 8 training runs starting with a different set of random initial weights each time.

↪ Do `View`, `BATCH_LOG` to open up a text log to record a summary of the training runs. Then press the `Batch` button.

Instead of updating every 5 epochs, the weight display updates at the end of every training run, and the graph log is not updated at all. Instead, after the 8 training runs, the batch text log window will show summary statistics about the average, maximum, and minimum of the unique pattern statistic. The last column contains a count of the number of times that a "perfect 10" on the unique pattern statistic was recorded. You should get a perfect score for all 8 runs.

Parameter Manipulations

Now, let's explore the effects of some of the parameters in the control panel. First, let's manipulate the `wt_gain` parameter, which should affect the contrast (and therefore selectivity) of the unit's weights.

↪ Set `wt_gain` to 1 instead of 6, `Apply`, and `Batch` run the network.

Question 4.6 **(a)** *What statistics for the number of uniquely represented lines did you obtain?* **(b)** *In what ways were the final weight patterns shown in the weight grid log different from the default case?* **(c)** *Explain how these two findings of hidden unit activity and weight patterns are related, making specific reference to the role of selectivity in self-organizing learning.*

↪ Set `wt_gain` back to 6, change `wt_off` from 1.25 to 1, `Apply`, and run a `Batch`. To make the effects of this parameter more dramatic, lower `wt_off` to .75 and `Batch` again.

Question 4.7 **(a)** *What statistics did you obtain for these two cases (1 and .75)?* **(b)** *Was there a noticeable change in the weight patterns compared to the default case? (Hint: Consider what the unique pattern statistic is looking for.)* **(c)** *Explain these results in terms of the effects of* `wt_off` *as adjusting the threshold for where correlations are enhanced or decreased as a function of the* `wt_gain` *contrast enhancement mechanism.* **(d)** *Again, explain why this is important for self-organizing learning.*

↪ Set `wt_off` back to 1.25 (or hit `Defaults`).

Now, let's consider the `savg_cor` parameter, which controls the amount of renormalization of the weight values based on the expected activity level in the sending layer. A value of 1 in this parameter will make the weights increase more rapidly, as they are driven to a larger maximum value (equation 4.18). A value of 0 will result in smaller weight increases. As described before, smaller values of `savg_cor` are appropriate when we want the units to have more selective representations, while larger values are more appropriate for more general or categorical representations. Thus, using a smaller value of this parameter should help to prevent units from developing less selective representations of multiple lines. This is why we have a default value of .5 for this parameter.

↪ Switch to using a `savg_cor` value of 1, and then `Batch` run the network.

You should observe results very similar to those when you decreased `wt_off` — both of these manipulations reduce the level of correlation that is necessary to produce strong weights.

↪ Set `savg_cor` back to .5, and then set `wt_mean` to .5.

This sets the initial random weight values to have a mean value of .5 instead of .25.

↪ Batch run the network, and pay particular attention to the weights.

You should see that this ended up eliminating the loser units, so that every unit now codes for a line. This result illustrates one of the interesting details about self-organizing learning. In general, the CPCA rule causes weights to increase for those input units that are active, and decrease for those that are not. However, this qualitative pattern is modulated by the soft weight bounding property discussed earlier — larger weights increase less rapidly and decrease more rapidly, and vice versa for smaller weights.

When we start off with larger weight values, the amount of weight decrease will be large relative to the amount of increase. Thus, hidden units that were active for a given pattern will subsequently receive *less* net input for a similar but not identical pattern (i.e., a pattern containing 1 of the 2 lines in common with the previous pattern), because the weights will have decreased substantially to those units that were off in the original pattern but on in the subsequent one. This decreased probability of reactivation means that other, previously inactive units will be more likely to be activated, with the result that all of the units end up participating. This can sometimes be a useful effect if the network is not drawing in sufficient numbers of units, and just a few units are "hogging" all of the input patterns.

Finally, let's manipulate the learning rate parameter `lrate`.

↪ First, set `wt_mean` back to .25, and then set `lrate` to .1 instead of .01 and do a `Batch` run.

Question 4.8 **(a)** *Does this tenfold increase in learning rate have any noticeable effect on the network, as measured by the unique pattern statistics and the weight patterns shown in the grid log?* **(b)** *Explain why this might be the case, comparing these results to the effects of learning rate that you observed in question 4.1.*

This exercise should give you a feel for the dynamics that underlie self-organizing learning, and also for the importance of contrast enhancement for the CPCA algorithm to be effective. More generally, you should now appreciate the extent to which various parameters can provide appropriate (or not) a priori biases on the learning process, and the benefit (or harm) that this can produce.

↪ To stop now, quit by selecting `Object/Quit` in the `PDP++Root` window.

4.8.2   Summary and Discussion

This exploration demonstrates that the combination of CPCA Hebbian learning and the kWTA competitive activation function does produce a useful model of the correlational structure of a simple input domain. We will see several other similarly successful demonstrations in later chapters, with environments that are much more complex and based directly on real-world data. Despite these successes, it is important to note that we have not provided an overarching mathematical analysis that proves that CPCA + kWTA will do something sensible.

Unfortunately, such an analysis remains essentially impossible as long as anything resembling the kWTA activation function is involved, because any analytical treatment would quickly come up against the intractable combinatorial explosion caused by the complex interdependencies among hidden units imposed by this function. For example, we saw in the previous exploration that these interdependencies (e.g., a balance of competition and cooperation) were essential for successful learning, so we are not inclined to abandon the general kWTA approach.

Thus, in this particular instance, we have opted for relying on a conceptual-level understanding of the learning algorithm instead of resorting to a more mathematically analyzable, but less powerful framework. It is important to appreciate that although summary mathematical analyses can be useful (and are very strongly emphasized by the neural network community), they are by no means a good predictor of what actually works in practice, and vice versa — many algorithms that have no corresponding concise mathematical analysis work quite well, and many that do have such an analysis do not work well at all. Because we have found that CPCA + kWTA does indeed work very well across a wide range of cognitively relevant tasks, the need for additional mathematical confirmation of this fact remains somewhat diminished (though we are by no means saying that such an analysis, if possible, would not be extremely welcome).

In the next section, we discuss a number of important points of contact with more easily analyzed frameworks that further our basis for understanding the essential principles behind CPCA + kWTA. Finally, we will see in the next chapter that error-driven learning does admit to a more complete overall analysis, so that if we use CPCA + kWTA in the context of this form of learning, we can have a reasonable mathematical assurance that something useful will result.

4.9   Other Approaches to Model Learning

CPCA Hebbian learning used together with the competitive kWTA activation function is but one of many possible instantiations of the general objectives of model learning. Its advantages are its relative simplicity and consistency with the network properties developed in chapter 3, the biological plausibility of Hebbian learning, and, perhaps most importantly, its ability to develop sparse distributed representations (the virtues of which were evident in the preceding exploration). In this section, we will summarize a number of other important approaches to model learning. This should provide a broader perspective on the field, and a better appreciation for the relative properties of CPCA + kWTA and where they came from.

We begin with model learning algorithms that are very similar to CPCA + kWTA, and discuss some alternative ways of viewing the objectives of this type of learning. Then, we cover some other approaches that use very different mechanisms, but still achieve a model learning objective.

4.9.1 Algorithms That Use CPCA-Style Hebbian Learning

There are several different Hebbian learning algorithms that use a learning rule that is either identical or very similar to CPCA (equation 4.12). We have already mentioned the one that provided the basis for our analysis of CPCA, the *competitive learning* algorithm of Rumelhart and Zipser (1986). We have also discussed the other algorithms in our discussion of inhibitory competition functions in chapter 3. These include the "soft" competitive learning algorithm of Nowlan (1990) and the *Kohonen network* of Kohonen (1984). The primary difference between these other algorithms and CPCA + kWTA is in the nature of the kWTA activation dynamics, not in the way that the weights are adjusted. These activation dynamics are a very important part of the overall learning algorithm, because the activations determine the limits of what kinds of representations can be learned, and shape the process of learning.

As we discussed in chapter 3, the kWTA inhibitory function results in a sparse distributed representation, whereas the activation functions used in these other learning algorithms do not. Both competitive learning and its softer version assume only one unit is active at a time (i.e., a localist representation), and although the Kohonen network does have multiple units active, the activations of all the units are tied directly to a single winner, and it lacks the kind of combinatorial flexibility that we saw was important in our exploration of self-organizing learning.

4.9.2 Clustering

The competitive learning algorithm provides an interesting interpretation of the objective of self-organizing learning in terms of *clustering* (Rumelhart & Zipser, 1986; Duda & Hart, 1973; Nowlan, 1990). Figure 4.14 shows how competitive learning moves the weights toward the centers of the *clusters* or natural groupings in the input data. It is easy to see that strongly correlated input patterns will tend to form such clusters, so

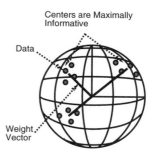

Figure 4.14: The competitive learning algorithm causes the weight vectors to move toward the centers of input data clusters (adapted from Rumelhart & Zipser, 1986). Linsker (1988) showed that these centers are maximally informative.

in some sense this is really just another way of looking at the PCA idea. Importantly, it goes beyond simple PCA by incorporating the additional assumption that there are multiple separate clusters, and that different hidden units should specialize on representing different clusters. This is the essence of the conditionalizing idea in CPCA, where a given unit only learns on those patterns that are somehow relevant to its cluster. If you recall the digit network from the previous chapter, it should be clear that this kind of clustering would tend to produce representations of the tightest clusters in the inputs, which corresponded to the noisy versions of the same digits.[3]

However, when one moves beyond the single active unit case by using something like the kWTA function, clustering becomes a somewhat less apt metaphor. Nevertheless, it is possible to think in terms of multiple clusters being active simultaneously (represented by the k active units).

4.9.3 Topography

The Kohonen network provides another interpretation of self-organizing learning in terms of the formation of *topographic maps*. The idea here is to not only represent the basic correlational structure of the environment, but also to represent the neighborhood relation-

---

[3]Note also that this kind of clustering has been used in a similar way as the cluster plots from the previous chapter for condensing and analyzing high-dimensional data.

ships among different input patterns. The neighborhood of activity around the single winner in a Kohonen network causes the hidden units to represent similar things as their neighbors, resulting in topographic maps over learning.

The networks studied by Miller and colleagues (Miller et al., 1989; Miller, 1994) have also focused on the development of topography, and can be seen as more biologically based versions of the same basic principles embodied in the Kohonen network. We explore these issues in more detail in chapter 8 in the context of a simple CPCA + kWTA model that also has lateral excitatory connections that induce a topographic representation much like that observed in primary visual cortex.

4.9.4 Information Maximization and MDL

Yet another important approach toward understanding the effects of Hebbian learning was developed by Linsker (1988) in terms of *information maximization*. The idea here is that model learning should develop representations that maximize the amount of information conveyed about the input patterns. The first principal component of the correlation matrix conveys the most information possible for a single unit, because it causes the unit's output to have the greatest amount of *variance* over all the input patterns, and variance is tantamount to information.

However, this idea of maximizing information must be placed into the context of other constraints on the representations, because if taken to an extreme, it would result in the development of representations that capture all of the information present in the input. This is both unrealistic and undesirable, because it would result in relatively unparsimonious representations.

Thus, it is more useful to consider the role of Hebbian learning in the context of a *tradeoff* between maximizing information, and minimizing the complexity of the representations (i.e., parsimony). This fidelity/simplicity tradeoff (which we alluded to previously) is elegantly represented in a framework known as *minimum description length* (MDL; Zemel, 1993; Rissanen, 1986). The MDL framework makes it clear that kWTA inhibitory competition leads to more parsimonious models. By lowering the overall information

capacity of the hidden layer, inhibition works to balance the information maximization objective. This is understood in MDL by measuring the information in the hidden layer relative to a set of *prior* assumptions (e.g., that only a few units should be active), so that less information is required to specify a representation that closely fits these assumptions.

It should also be emphasized in this context that the form of Hebbian learning used in CPCA is always extracting only the first principal component from the subset of input patterns where the receiving unit is active. Thus, the learning rule itself, in addition to the inhibitory competition, imposes a pressure to develop a relatively parsimonious model of those input patterns (note that although the first principal component is the most informative, it is typically far from capable of representing all the information present in the set of input patterns). Furthermore, the contrast enhancement function imposes an even greater parsimony bias, as discussed previously.

4.9.5 Learning Based Primarily on Hidden Layer Constraints

As discussed previously, model learning tends to work better with appropriate constraints or biases, but inappropriate constraints can be a bad thing. A number of self-organizing models depend very heavily on constraints imposed on the hidden layer representations that exhibit just this kind of tradeoff. Perhaps the prototypical example of this type is the BCM algorithm (Bienenstock, Cooper, & Munro, 1982), which has the strong constraint that each hidden unit is active for essentially the same percentage of time as every other hidden unit. This is effective when the relevant features are uniformly distributed in the environment, and when you have a good match between the number of units in the hidden layer and the number of features. However, when these constraints do not match the environment, the algorithm's performance suffers.

As we discussed previously, we are particularly concerned about making assumptions on the precise number of hidden units, because there are many reasons to believe that the cortex has an overabundance of neurons relative to the demands of any given learning task. Also, in the case of BCM, the notion that everything occurs in the environment with the same basic frequency seems problematic.

The popular independent components analysis (ICA) algorithm (Bell & Sejnowski, 1995) takes an approach to model learning that is similar in many ways to BCM. ICA was designed to do blind source separation — separating a set of independent signals that have been mixed together, as in a cocktail party of voices recorded by a set of microphones. ICA requires that the number of hidden units be equal to the number of underlying sources (features) in the environment (as in BCM), and it also requires that this number be equal to the number of input units (i.e., the input-hidden weight matrix must be square). Furthermore, ICA learns by making the hidden units maximally independent from each other (as defined by mutual information), so that what a given unit learns is highly dependent on what the other units have learned. Under appropriate conditions, ICA can do an excellent job of picking out independent components in the inputs. However, like BCM, ICA suffers when its constraints do not fit the environment.

In contrast with BCM and ICA, the CPCA + kWTA algorithm distributes its constraints more evenly between those that apply at the individual unit level, and those that depend on the interactions between the units. Specifically, CPCA plus the contrast enhancement bias encourages the individual unit to specialize in what it represents, and to emphasize the strongest correlations (principal component) while deemphasizing weaker ones. The kWTA function then interacts with these unit-level constraints in shaping the overall development of representations. This more balanced distribution of constraints makes CPCA + kWTA much less dependent on the precise numbers of hidden units, for example.

4.9.6 Generative Models

Generative models are an important class of self-organizing learning models based on the idea of *recognition by synthesis* (Dayan et al., 1995; Saul et al., 1996; Carpenter & Grossberg, 1987; Ullman, 1994). The idea is to generate some top-down image of what you are perceiving based on your internal model of the world, and then learn based on the difference between what was generated and what is actually being perceived. One advantage of this learning mechanism is that it requires the internal model to fit as precisely as possible the actual input patterns. Thus, it should in principle lead to fewer representations of spurious correlations, and "hog" units may not be as much of a problem because they will produce a worse fit to the details of specific patterns. Further, generative models can be easily understood in terms of the Bayesian statistical framework, because the likelihood term that plays an important role in this framework is essentially like a generative model in that it expresses the extent to which the hypothesis (i.e., internal model) would have produced the data (i.e., the actual perceptual input).

Although appealing in many respects, there are some problems with generative models. For example, generative models require that there be a clear directionality and hierarchy to processing. Thus, a given layer in the network must be considered a internal model of the layer below it, and as something to be modeled by the layer above it. The processing associated with these different relationships is different, so the kind of interactive, bidirectional constraint satisfaction processing that we explored in chapter 3 is not really feasible in generative models (at least not current versions). Not only is this at odds with the known biology, but we will also see in the second part of the book that many cognitive phenomena depend on bidirectional constraint satisfaction processing and do not easily admit to the more rigid hierarchical structuring required by generative models. Despite these current limitations, it may be possible that more cognitively and biologically plausible generative models will be developed in the future.

4.10 Summary

In this chapter we explored in detail one approach based on **Hebbian learning** that achieves the **model learning** objective of developing an **internal model** of the important structural features of the environment (i.e., things that are strongly **correlated**). Because Hebbian learning is also biologically plausible, it satisfies both computational and biological constraints for a learning mechanism useful for cognitive neuroscience modeling.

Biological Mechanisms of Learning

The biological basis of learning is thought to be **long-term potentiation (LTP)** and **long-term depression (LTD)**. These mechanisms are **associative** or **Hebbian** in nature, meaning that they depend on both presynaptic and postsynaptic activation. The associative nature of LTP/D can be understood in terms of two requirements for opening the **NMDA receptor**: presynaptic neural activity (i.e., the secretion of the excitatory neurotransmitter glutamate) and postsynaptic activity (i.e., a sufficiently excited or depolarized membrane potential to unblock the magnesium ions from the channel). The NMDA channel allows **calcium ions** (Ca^{++}) to enter the synapse, which triggers a complex sequence of chemical events that ultimately results in the modification of synaptic efficacy (weight). The available data suggests that when both presynaptic and postsynaptic neurons are strongly active, the weight increases (LTP) due to a relatively high concentration of calcium, but weaker activity results in weight decrease (LTD) due to an elevated but lower concentration of calcium.

Hebbian Model Learning

Model learning is difficult because we get a large amount of low quality information from our senses. The use of appropriate a priori **biases** about what the world is like is important to supplement and organize our experiences. A bias favoring simple or **parsimonious** models is particularly useful. The objective of representing **correlations** is appropriate because these reflect reliable, stable features of the world. A parsimonious representation of such correlations involves extracting the **principal components** (features, dimensions) of these correlations. A simple form of Hebbian learning will perform this **principal components analysis (PCA)**, but it must be modified to be fully useful. Most importantly, it must be **conditionalized (CPCA)**, so that individual units represent the principal components of only a *subset* of all input patterns. The basic CPCA algorithm can be augmented with **renormalization** and **contrast enhancement**, which improve the dynamic range of the weights and the selectivity of the units to the strongest correlations in the input. **Self-organizing** learning can be accomplished by the interaction between CPCA Hebbian learning together with the network property of **inhibitory competition** as described in the previous chapter, and results in distributed representations of statistically informative principal **features** of the input.

4.11   Further Reading

The last few chapters of Hertz et al. (1991) on competitive learning provide a clear and more mathematically detailed introduction to unsupervised/self-organizing learning.

Hinton and Sejnowski (1999) is a collection of influential papers on *Unsupervised learning* (model learning).

Much of Kohonen's pioneering work in unsupervised learning is covered in Kohonen (1984), though the treatment is somewhat mathematically oriented and can be difficult to understand.

The paper by Linsker (1988) is probably the most comprehensible by this influential self-organizing learning researcher.

Probably the most influential biologically oriented application of unsupervised model learning has been in understanding the development of ocular dominance columns, as pioneered by Miller et al. (1989).

The journal *Neural Computation* and the *NIPS* conference proceedings (*Advances in Neural Information Processing*) always have a large number of high-quality articles on computational and biological approaches to learning.

Chapter 5

Error-Driven Task Learning

Contents

5.1   **Overview** **147**
5.2   **Exploration of Hebbian Task Learning** **148**
5.3   **Using Error to Learn: The Delta Rule** **150**
     5.3.1   Deriving the Delta Rule *152*
     5.3.2   Learning Bias Weights *152*
5.4   **Error Functions, Weight Bounding, and Activation Phases** **154**
     5.4.1   Cross Entropy Error *154*
     5.4.2   Soft Weight Bounding *155*
     5.4.3   Activation Phases in Learning *156*
5.5   **Exploration of Delta Rule Task Learning** **156**
5.6   **The Generalized Delta Rule: Backpropagation** . . **158**
     5.6.1   Derivation of Backpropagation *160*
     5.6.2   Generic Recursive Formulation *161*
     5.6.3   The Biological Implausibility of Backpropagation *162*
5.7   **The Generalized Recirculation Algorithm** **162**
     5.7.1   Derivation of GeneRec *163*
     5.7.2   Symmetry, Midpoint, and CHL *165*
5.8   **Biological Considerations for GeneRec** **166**
     5.8.1   Weight Symmetry in the Cortex *166*
     5.8.2   Phase-Based Activations in the Cortex . . . *167*
     5.8.3   Synaptic Modification Mechanisms *168*
5.9   **Exploration of GeneRec-Based Task Learning** . . **170**
5.10   **Summary** **171**
5.11   **Further Reading** **172**

5.1   Overview

An important component of human learning is focused on solving specific tasks (e.g., using a given tool or piece of software, reading, game playing). The objective of learning to solve specific tasks is complementary to the model learning objective from the previous chapter, where the goal was to represent the general statistical structure of the environment apart from specific tasks. In this chapter, we focus on *task learning* in neural networks. A simple but quite general conception of what it means to solve a task is to produce a specific output pattern for a given input pattern. The input specifies the context, contingencies, or demands of the task, and the output is the appropriate response. Reading text aloud or giving the correct answer for an addition problem are two straightforward examples of input-output *mappings* that are learned in school. We will see that there are many other more subtle ways in which tasks can be learned.

It would be ideal if the CPCA Hebbian learning rule developed for model learning was also good at learning to solve tasks, because we would then only need one learning algorithm to perform both of these important kinds of learning. Thus, we begin the chapter by seeing how well it does on some simple input-output mappings. Unfortunately, it does not perform well.

To develop a learning mechanism that will perform well on task learning, we derive an *error-driven* learning algorithm called the *delta rule* that makes direct use of discrepancies or *errors* in task performance to ad-

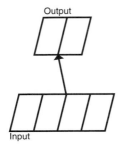

Figure 5.1: Pattern associator network, where the task is to learn a mapping between the input and output units.

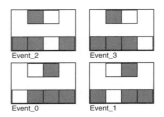

Figure 5.2: The easy pattern associator task mapping, which can be thought of as categorizing the first two inputs as "left" with the left hidden unit, and the next two inputs as "right" with the right hidden unit.

just the weights. This kind of learning has also been labeled as *supervised* learning, but we will see that there are a multitude of ecologically valid sources of such "supervision" that do not require the constant presence of a omniscient teacher. The multilayer generalization of the delta rule is called *backpropagation*, which allows errors occurring in a distant layer to be propagated backwards to earlier layers, enabling the development of multiple layers of transformations that make the overall task easier to solve.

Although the original, mathematically direct mechanism for implementing the backpropagation algorithm is biologically implausible, a formulation that uses bidirectional activation propagation to communicate error signals, called *GeneRec*, is consistent with known properties of LTP/D reviewed in the previous chapter, and is generally quite compatible with the biology of the cortex. It allows error signals occurring anywhere to affect learning everywhere.

5.2 Exploration of Hebbian Task Learning

This exploration is based on a very simple form of task learning, where a set of 4 input units project to 2 output units. The "task" is specified in terms of the relationships between patterns of activation over the input units, and the corresponding desired or **target** values of the output units. This type of network is often called a **pattern associator**, because the objective is to associate patterns of activity on the input with those on the output.

↪ Open the project `pat_assoc.proj.gz` in `chapter_5` to begin.

You should see in the network window that there are 2 output units receiving inputs from 4 input units through a set of feedforward weights (figure 5.1).

↪ Locate the `pat_assoc_ctrl` control panel, press the `View` button, and select `EVENTS`.

As you can see in the environment window that pops up (figure 5.2), the input-output relationships to be learned in this "task" are simply that the leftmost two input units should make the left output unit active, while the rightmost units should make the right output unit active. This is a relatively easy task to learn because the left output unit just has to develop strong weights to these leftmost units and ignore the ones to the right, while the right output unit does the opposite. Note that we use kWTA inhibition within the output layer, with a k parameter of 1.

The network is trained on this task by simply clamping both the input and output units to their corresponding values from the events in the environment, and performing CPCA Hebbian learning on the resulting activations.

↪ Iconify the network window, and do `View`, `TEST_GRID_LOG`. Then, press `Step` in the control panel 4 times.

You should see all 4 events from the environment presented in a random order. At the end of this *epoch* of 4 events, you will see the activations updated in a quick blur — this is the result of the testing phase, which is run after every epoch of training. During this testing phase, all 4 events are presented to the network, except this time, the output units are not clamped, but are instead updated according to their weights from the input units (which are clamped as before). Thus, the testing phase records the *actual* performance of the network on this task, when it is not being "coached" (that is why it's a test).

The results of testing are displayed in the test grid log that was just opened. Each row represents one of the 4 events, with the input pattern and the actual output activations shown on the right. The `sum_se` column reports the **summed squared error** (SSE), which is simply the summed difference between the actual output activation during testing (o_k) and the *target* value (t_k) that was clamped during training:

$$SSE = \sum_k (t_k - o_k)^2 \qquad (5.1)$$

where the sum is over the 2 output units. We are actually computing the *thresholded* SSE, where absolute differences of less than .5 are treated as zero, so the unit just has to get the activation on the correct side of .5 to get zero error. We thus treat the units as representing underlying binary quantities (i.e., whether the pattern that the unit detects is present or not), with the graded activation value expressing something like the likelihood of the underlying binary hypothesis being true. All of our tasks specify binary input/output patterns.

With only a single training epoch, the output unit is likely making some errors.

↪ Now, turn off the `Display` button in the upper left hand side of the network window, then open a graph log of the error over epochs using `View`, `TRAIN_GRAPH_LOG`. Then press the `Run` button.

You will see the grid log update after each epoch, showing the pattern of outputs and the individual SSE (`sum_se`) errors. Also, the train graph log provides a summary plot across epochs of the sum of the thresholded SSE measure across all the events in the epoch. This shows what is often referred to as the **learning curve** for the network, and it should have rapidly gone to zero, indicating that the network has learned the task. Training will stop automatically after the network has exhibited 5 correct epochs in a row (just to make sure it has really learned the problem), or it stops after 30 epochs if it fails to learn.

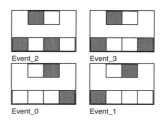

Figure 5.3: The hard pattern associator task mapping, where there is overlap among the patterns that activate the different output units.

Let's see what the network has learned.

↪ Turn the network `Display` back on, and press the `TestStep` button 4 times.

This will step through each of the training patterns and update the test grid log. You should see that the network has learned this easy task, turning on the left output for the first two patterns, and the right one for the next two. Now, let's take a look at the weights for the output unit to see exactly how this happened.

↪ Click on `r.wt` in the network window, and then on the left output unit.

You should see that, as expected, the weights from the left 2 units are strong (near 1), and those from the right 2 units are weak (near 0). The complementary pattern should hold for the right output unit.

Question 5.1 *Explain why this pattern of strong and weak weights resulted from the CPCA Hebbian learning algorithm.*

Now, let's try a more difficult task.

↪ Set `env_type` on the `pat_assoc_ctrl` control panel to `HARD`, and `Apply`. Then, do `View`, `EVENTS`.

In this harder environment (figure 5.3), there is overlap among the input patterns for cases where the left output should be on, and where it should be off (and the right output on). This overlap makes the task hard because the unit has to somehow figure out what the most distinguishing or *task relevant* input units are, and set its weights accordingly.

This task reveals a problem with Hebbian learning. It is only concerned with the correlation (conditional probability) between the output and input units, so it cannot learn to be sensitive to which inputs are more task relevant than others (unless this happens to be the same as the input-output correlations, as in the easy task). This hard task has a complicated pattern of overlap among the different input patterns. For the two cases where the left output should be on, the middle two input units are very strongly correlated with the output activity (conditional probability $P(x_i|y_j) = 1$), while the outside two inputs are only half-correlated ($P(x_i|y_j) = .5$). The two cases where the left output should be off (and the right one on) overlap considerably with those where it should be on, with the last event containing both of the highly correlated inputs. Thus, if the network just pays attention to correlations, it will tend to respond to this last case when it shouldn't.

Let's see what happens when we run the network on this task.

↪ Press the `Run` button in the `pat_assoc_ctrl`, which does a `New Init` to produce a new set of random starting weights, and then does a `Run`. You should be viewing the weights of the left output unit in the network window, with the `Display` turned on so you can see them being updated as the network learns.

You should see from these weights that the network has learned that the middle two units are highly correlated with the left output unit, as we expected.

↪ Do `TestStep` 4 times.

You should see that the network is not getting the right answers. Different runs will produce slightly different results, but the middle two events should turn the right output unit on, while the first and last either turn on the left output, or produce weaker activation across both output units (i.e., they are relatively equally excited).

The weights for the right output unit show that it has strongly represented its correlation with the second input unit, which explains the pattern of output responses. This weight for the right output unit is stronger than those for the left output unit from the two middle inputs because of the different overall activity levels in the different input patterns — this difference in α affects the renormalization correction for the CPCA Hebbian learning rule as described earlier (note that even if this renormalization is set to a constant across the different events, the network still fails to learn).

↪ Do several more `Run`s on this HARD task.

Question 5.2 (a) *Does the network ever solve the task?* **(b)** *Report the final* `sum_se` *at the end of training for each run.*

↪ Experiment with the parameters that control the contrast enhancement of the CPCA Hebbian learning rule (`wt_gain` and `wt_off`), to see if these are playing an important role in the network's behavior.

You should see that changes to these parameters do not lead to any substantial improvements. Hebbian learning does not seem to be able to solve tasks where the correlations do not provide the appropriate weight values. It seems unlikely that there will generally be a coincidence between correlational structure and the task solution. Thus, we must conclude that Hebbian learning is of limited use for task learning. In contrast, we will see in the next section that an algorithm specifically designed for task learning can learn this task without much difficulty.

↪ To continue on to the next simulation, you can leave this project open because we will use it again. Or, if you wish to stop now, quit by selecting `Object/Quit` in the `PDP++Root` window.

5.3 Using Error to Learn: The Delta Rule

In this section we develop a task-based learning algorithm from first principles, and continue to refine this algorithm in the remainder of this chapter. In the next chapter, we will compare this new task-based learning mechanism with Hebbian learning, and provide a framework for understanding their relative advantages and disadvantages.

An obvious objective for task learning is to adapt the weights to produce the correct output pattern for each input pattern. To do this, we need a measure of how closely our network is producing the correct outputs, and then some way of improving this measure by adjusting the weights. We can use the *summed squared error* (SSE) statistic described previously to measure how close to correct the network is. First, we will want to extend this measure to the sum of SSE over all events, indexed by t, resulting in:

$$SSE = \sum_t \sum_k (t_k - o_k)^2 \qquad (5.2)$$

where t_k is again the target value (not to be confused with the event index t), and o_k is the actual output activation, and both are implicitly functions of time (event) t.

Equation 5.2 will be zero when the outputs exactly match the targets for all events in the environment or **training set**, and larger values will reflect worse performance. The goal of task learning can thus be cast as that of *minimizing* this error measure (also known as **gradient descent** in error). We refer to this as **error-driven** learning. In this context, SSE (equation 5.2) serves as an **objective function** for error-driven learning, in that it specifies the objective of learning.

One standard and rather direct way to minimize any function is to first take its *derivative* with respect to the free parameters. The derivative gives you the slope of the function, or how the function changes with changes to the free parameters. For example:

- The derivative of a network's error with respect to its weights indicates how the error changes as the weights change.

Once this derivative has been computed, the network's weights can then be adjusted to minimize the network's errors. The derivative thus provides the basis for our learning rule. We will work through exactly how to take this derivative in a moment, but first we will present the results to provide a sense of what the resulting learning rule looks and acts like.

Taking the negative of the derivative of SSE with respect to the weights, we get a weight update or learning rule called the **delta rule**:

$$\Delta w_{ik} = \epsilon(t_k - o_k)s_i \qquad (5.3)$$

where s_i is the input (stimulus) unit activation, and ϵ is the learning rate as usual. This is also known as *least mean squares* (LMS), and it has been around for some time (Widrow & Hoff, 1960). Essentially the same equation is used in the *Rescorla-Wagner* rule for classical (Pavlovian) conditioning (Rescorla & Wagner, 1972).

It should make sense that this learning rule will adjust the weights to reduce the error. Basically, it says that the weights should change as a function of the *local error*

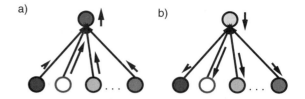

Figure 5.4: Illustration of the credit assignment process, where the activity of a unit is represented by how bright it is. **a)** If the output unit was not very active and it should have been more so (i.e., $t_k - o_k$ is positive), then the weights will all increase, but in proportion to the activity of the sending units (because the most active sending units can do the most good). **b)** The same principle holds when the output unit was too active.

for the individual output unit $(t_k - o_k)$ and the activation of the sending unit s_i. Thus, those sending units that are more active when a big error is made will receive most of the *blame* for this error. For example, if the output unit was active and it shouldn't have been (i.e., $(t_k - o_k)$ is negative), then weights will be decreased from those input units which were active. On the other hand, if the output unit *wasn't* active when it should have been, then the weights will increase from those input units that were active. Thus, the next time around, the unit's activation should be closer to the target value, and hence the error will be reduced.

This process of adjusting weights in proportion to the sending unit activations is called **credit assignment** (though a more appropriate name might be *blame* assignment), illustrated in figure 5.4. Credit assignment is perhaps the most important computational property of error-driven learning rules (i.e., on a similar level as correlational learning for Hebbian learning rules).

One can view the representations formed by error-driven learning as the result of a *multiple credit satisfaction* mechanism — an integration of the synergies and conflicts of the credit assignment process on each input-output pattern over the entire training set. Thus, instead of reflecting the strongest correlations, as Hebbian learning does, the weights here reflect the strongest *solutions* to the task at hand (i.e., those solutions that satisfy the most input-output mappings).

5.3.1 Deriving the Delta Rule

Now that we can see how the delta rule works, we will show how it can be derived directly from the derivative of the sum-squared error measure in equation 5.2 with respect to the weights from the input units. Box 5.1 provides a primer on derivatives for readers unfamiliar with the mathematical details of derivatives. The most important thing is to understand the effects of these derivatives in terms of credit assignment as explained above.

The mathematical expression of the derivative of the error in terms of its components is written as follows:

$$\frac{\partial SSE}{\partial w_{ik}} = \frac{\partial SSE}{\partial o_k} \frac{\partial o_k}{\partial w_{ik}} \qquad (5.4)$$

which is simply to say that the derivative of the error with respect to the weights is the product of two terms: the derivative of the error with respect to the output, and the derivative of the output with respect to the weights. In other words, we can understand how the error changes as the weights change in terms of how the error changes as the output changes, together with how the output changes as the weights change. We can break down derivatives in this way ad infinitum (as we will see later in the chapter in the derivation of backpropagation) according to the **chain rule** from calculus, in which the value in the denominator in one term must be the numerator in the next term. Then we can consider each term separately.

We first consider $\frac{\partial SSE}{\partial o_k}$, where $SSE = \sum_t \sum_k (t_k - o_k)^2$. To break this more complicated function into more tractable parts, we use the fact that the derivative of a function $h(x)$ that can be written in terms of two component functions, $h(x) = f(g(x))$, is the product of the derivatives of the two component functions: $h'(x) = f'(g(x))g'(x)$ (which is actually just another instantiation of the chain rule). In the case of SSE, using o_k as the variable instead of x, $f(g(o_k)) = g(o_k)^2$ and $g(o_k) = t_k - o_k$, and $f'(g(o_k)) = 2g(o_k)$ (because the derivative of x^2 is $2x$) and $g'(o_k) = -1$ (because t_k is a constant with respect to changes in o_k, its derivative is 0, so it disappears, and then the derivative of $-1x$ with respect to x is $-1x^0 = -1$). Multiplying these terms gives us:

$$\frac{\partial SSE}{\partial o_k} = -2(t_k - o_k) \qquad (5.5)$$

Notice that the sums over events and different output units drop out when considering how to change the weights for a particular output unit for a particular event. The learning rule is thus "local" in the sense that it only depends on the single output unit and a single input/output pattern.

Now we can consider the second term, $\frac{\partial o_k}{\partial w_{ik}}$. Although we will subsequently be able to accommodate more complex activation functions, we start with a linear activation function to make the derivation simpler:

$$o_k = \sum_i s_i w_{ik} \qquad (5.6)$$

The derivative of the linear activation function is simply:

$$\frac{\partial o_k}{\partial w_{ik}} = s_i \qquad (5.7)$$

In other words, the input signal indicates how the output changes with changes in the weights. Notice again that all the elements of the sum that do not involve the particular weight drop out.

Putting the two terms together, the full derivative for the case with linear activations is:

$$\frac{\partial SSE}{\partial w_{ik}} = -2(t_k - o_k)s_i \qquad (5.8)$$

We can use the negative of this derivative for our learning rule, because we minimize functions (e.g., error) by moving the relevant variable (e.g., the weight) opposite the direction of the derivative. Also, we can either absorb the factor of 2 into the arbitrary learning rate constant ϵ, or introduce a factor of $\frac{1}{2}$ in the error measure (as is often done), canceling it out. This gives us the delta rule shown previously:

$$\Delta w_{ik} = \epsilon(t_k - o_k)s_i \qquad (5.9)$$

5.3.2 Learning Bias Weights

One issue we have not focused on yet is how the *bias weights* learn. Recall that the bias weights provide a constant additional input to the neuron (section 2.5.1), and that proper bias weight values can be essential for

Box 5.1: How to Compute a Derivative

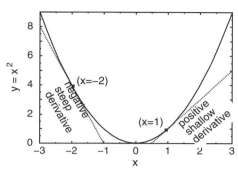

To see how derivatives work, we will first consider a very simple function, $y = x^2$, shown in the above figure, with the goal of minimizing this function. Remember that eventually we will want to minimize the more complex function that relates a network's error and weights. In this simple case of $y = x^2$, it is clear that to minimize y, we want x to be 0, because y goes to 0 as x goes to 0. However, it is not always so apparent how to minimize a function, so we will go through the more formal process of doing so.

To minimize $y = x^2$, we need to understand how y changes with changes to x. In other words, we need the derivative of y with respect to x. It turns out that the derivative of x^2 is $2x$ (and more generally, the derivative of bx^a is $bax^{(a-1)}$). This means that the slope of the function $y = x^2$ at any given point equals $2x$. The above figure shows the slope of the function $y = x^2$ at two points, where $x = 1$ (so the slope equals 2) and where $x = -2$ (so the slope = -4). It should be clear from the figure and the formula for the derivative that when x is positive the slope is positive, indicating that y increases as x increases; and, when x is negative the slope is negative, indicating that y decreases as x increases. Moreover, the further x is from 0, the further we are from minimizing y, and the larger the derivative. To minimize y, we thus want to change x in the direction opposite the derivative, and in step sizes according to the absolute magnitude of the derivative. Doing this for any value of x will eventually take x to 0, thereby minimizing y.

The logic behind minimizing the network's error with respect to its weights is identical, but the process is complicated by the fact that the relationship between error and weights is not as simple as $y = x^2$. More specifically, the weights do not appear directly in the error equation 5.2 in the way that x appears in the equation for y in our simple $y = x^2$ example. To deal with this complexity, we can break the relationship between error and weights into its components. Rather than determining in a single step how the error changes as the weights change, we can determine in separate steps how the error changes as the network output changes (because the output does appear directly in the error equation), and how the network output changes as the weights change (because the weights appear directly in the equation for the network output, simplified for the present as described below). Then we can put these terms together to determine how the error changes as the weights change.

producing useful representations, for example by allowing units to represent weaker inputs (e.g., section 3.3.1). There really is no straightforward way to train bias weights in the Hebbian model-learning paradigm, because they do not reflect any correlational information (i.e., the correlation between a unit and itself, which is the only kind of correlational information a bias weight could represent, is uninformative). However, error-driven task learning using the delta rule algorithm can put the bias weights to good use.

The standard way to train bias weights is to treat them as weights coming from a unit that is always active (i.e., $s_i = 1$). If we substitute this 1 into equation 5.9, the bias weight (β_k) change is just:

$$\Delta\beta_k = \epsilon(t_k - o_k) \qquad (5.10)$$

Thus, the bias weight will always adjust to directly decrease the error. For example, to the extent that a unit is often active when it shouldn't be, the bias weight change will be more negative than positive, causing the bias weight to decrease, and the unit to be less active. Thus, the bias weight learns to correct any relatively *constant* errors caused by the unit being generally too active or too inactive.

From a biological perspective, there is some evidence that the general level of excitability of cortical neurons is plastic (e.g., Desai et al., 1999), though this data does not specifically address the kind of error-driven mechanism used here.

5.4 Error Functions, Weight Bounding, and Activation Phases

Three immediate problems prevent us from using the delta rule as our task-based learning mechanism; (1) The delta rule was derived using a linear activation function, but our units use the point-neuron activation function; (2) The delta rule fails to enforce the biological constraints that weights can be only either positive or negative (see chapters 2 and 3), allowing weights to switch signs and take on any value; (3) The target output values are of questionable biological and psychological reality. Fortunately, reasonable solutions to these problems exist, and are discussed in the following sections.

5.4.1 Cross Entropy Error

At this point, we provide only an approximate solution to the problem of deriving the delta rule for the point-neuron activation function. Later in the chapter, a more satisfying solution will be provided. The approximate solution involves two steps. First, we approximate the point neuron function with a sigmoidal function, which we argued in chapter 2 is a reasonable thing to do. Second, we use a different error function that results in the cancellation of the derivative for the sigmoidal activation function, yielding the same delta rule formulation derived for linear units (equation 5.9). The logic behind this result is that this new error function takes into account the saturating nature of the sigmoidal function, so that the weight changes remain linear (for the mathematically disinclined, this is all you need to know about this problem).

The new error function is called **cross entropy** (abbreviated CE; Hinton, 1989a), and is a distancelike

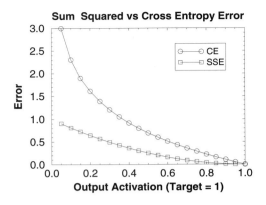

Figure 5.5: Comparison of the cross entropy (CE) and sum-squared error (SSE) for a single output with a target value of 1. CE is larger, especially when the output is near 0.

measure for probability distributions. It is defined as:

$$CE = -\sum_t \sum_k t_k \log o_k + (1 - t_k) \log(1 - o_k)$$

(5.11)

where the actual output activation o_k and the target activation t_k must be probability-like variables in the 0–1 range (and the target t_k is either a 0 or a 1). The *entropy* of a variable x is defined as $x \log x$, so CE represents a cross entropy measure because it is the entropy *across* the two variables of t_k and o_k, considered as both the probability of the units being on (in the first term) and their probabilities of being off (in the second term involving $1 - t_k$ and $1 - o_k$).

Like the SSE function, CE is zero if the actual activation is equal to the target, and increasingly larger as the two are more different. However, unlike squared error, CE does not treat the entire 0-1 range uniformly. If one value is near 1 and the other is near 0, this incurs an especially large penalty, whereas more "uncertain" values around .5 produce less of an error (figure 5.5). Thus, CE takes into account the underlying binary true/false aspect of the units-as-detectors by placing special emphasis on the 0 and 1 extremes.

For convenience, we reproduce the net input and sigmoid functions from chapter 2 here. Recall that the *net input* term η_k accumulates the weighted activations of the sending units:

$$\eta_k = \sum_i s_i w_{ik} \qquad (5.12)$$

It is sometimes convenient to write the sigmoid function as $\sigma(\eta_k)$, where the σ is intended to evoke the sigmoidal character of the function:

$$o_k = \sigma(\eta_k) = \frac{1}{1 + e^{-\eta_k}} \qquad (5.13)$$

Now, we can take the derivative of the CE error function with respect to the weight, again using the chain rule. To deal with the more complex sigmoidal activation function, we have to extend the chain rule to include a separate step for the derivative of the activation function with respect to its net input $\frac{do_k}{d\eta_k}$, and then the net input with respect to the weight $\frac{\partial \eta_k}{\partial w_{ik}}$:

$$\frac{\partial CE}{\partial w_{ik}} = \frac{\partial CE}{\partial o_k} \frac{do_k}{d\eta_k} \frac{\partial \eta_k}{\partial w_{ik}} \qquad (5.14)$$

Again, we will break this out into the component terms:

$$\frac{\partial CE}{\partial o_k} = \frac{t_k}{o_k} - \frac{(1 - t_k)}{(1 - o_k)} = \frac{t_k - o_k}{o_k(1 - o_k)} \qquad (5.15)$$

and[1]

$$\frac{do_k}{d\eta_k} = \sigma'(\eta_k) = o_k(1 - o_k) \qquad (5.16)$$

Most readers need not derive this derivative themselves; it is somewhat involved. Finally, the derivative of the net input term is just like that of the linear activation from before:

$$\frac{\partial \eta_k}{\partial w_{ik}} = s_i \qquad (5.17)$$

When we put these terms all together, the denominator of the first term cancels with the derivative of the sigmoid function, resulting in exactly the same delta rule we had before:

$$\frac{\partial CE}{\partial w_{ik}} = -(t_k - o_k)s_i \qquad (5.18)$$

---

[1]Note here that we can use the ′ (prime) notation to indicate the derivative of the sigmoid function. We use d to indicate a simple derivative, because this equation has a single variable (η_k), in contrast with most other cases where we use ∂ to indicate a *partial* derivative (i.e., with respect to only one of multiple variables).

Thus, the introduction of the sigmoid is offset by the use of the CE error function, so that the weights are adapted in the same way as when a linear activation function is used.

5.4.2 Soft Weight Bounding

The second problem, the unbounded nature of the error-driven weights, is incompatible with both the facts of biology and the point-neuron activation function, which requires a separation between excitation and inhibition. Therefore, we use the following mechanism for bounding the error-driven weights (note that this does not apply to the bias weights, which have no such sign constraints):

$$\Delta w_{ik} = [\Delta_{ik}]_+ (1 - w_{ik}) + [\Delta_{ik}]_- w_{ik} \qquad (5.19)$$

where Δ_{ik} is the weight change computed by the error-driven algorithm (e.g., equation 5.9), and the $[x]_+$ operator returns x if $x > 0$ and 0 otherwise, while $[x]_-$ does the opposite, returning x if $x < 0$, and 0 otherwise.

Equation 5.19 imposes the same kind of soft weight bounding that the CPCA algorithm has naturally, where the weights approach the bounds of 1 and 0 exponentially slowly (softly). Note that this equation has the same general form as the expanded form of the CPCA Hebbian weight update rule (equation 4.17), and also the equation for updating the membrane potential from chapter 2. Thus, like these other functions, it provides a natural interpretation of weight values centered on the middle value of .5.

For example, when there is a series of individual weight changes of equal magnitude but opposite sign, the weight will hover around .5, which corresponds well with the Hebbian interpretation of .5 as reflecting lack of positive or negative correlation. Similarly, as positive weight increases outweigh negative ones, the weight value increases proportionally, and likewise decreases proportionally for more negative changes than positive.

Weight bounding is appealing from a biological perspective because it is clear that synaptic efficacy has limits. We know that synapses do not change their sign, so they must be bounded at the lower end by zero. The upper bound is probably determined by such things as the maximal amount of neurotransmitter that can be released and the maximal density and alignment of postsynaptic receptors. What the soft weight bounding mechanism does is to assume that these natural bounds are approached exponentially slowly — such exponential curves are often found in natural systems. However, we do not know of any specific empirical evidence regarding the nature of the synaptic bounding function.

5.4.3 Activation Phases in Learning

Finally, we need to address the third problem concerning the plausibility and nature of the target signal. Perhaps the simplest interpretation would be to think of the target as just another activation state, but one that corresponds to the experience of either an explicit instructional signal from some external source, or an actual observed **outcome** of some event in the world. In this context, the activation state o_k produced by the network can be thought of as either an overt response, or an internal **expectation** or prediction of an outcome. Thus, two activation states may follow from a given input, an expectation followed by an actual outcome, or an overt response followed by feedback to that response. We will discuss these and other scenarios in more detail in section 5.8 once we have developed a more complete picture of the biological mechanisms that could implement error driven learning.

Figure 5.6 shows how the expectation and outcome activation states can be implemented as two different **phases** of activation. For reasons that will become clear, we call the expectation-like phase the **minus phase**, and the outcome-like target phase the **plus phase**. In this phase-based framework, delta rule learning involves taking the difference between the plus and minus phases of the output activation states. One way of thinking about the names of these phases is that the minus phase is *subtracted* from the plus phase. We can translate the equation for the delta rule to refer to the different phases of the output activation, using the plus and minus superscripts to denote phase:

$$\Delta w_{ik} = \epsilon(o_k^+ - o_k^-)s_i \qquad (5.20)$$

In the simulator, these phase variables are stored as act_m (minus phase) and act_p (plus phase).

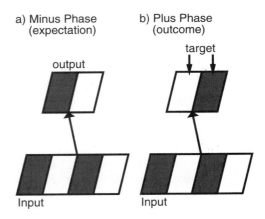

Figure 5.6: Phases of activation (minus and plus) in error-driven learning. In the minus phase, the input activates the output pattern according to the weights, producing something like an expectation or response. In the plus phase, the actual outcome or correct response (target) is clamped onto the output units. In this example, the expectation was incorrect, as you can tell from the difference in output layer activation state between the two phases.

For this phase-based learning to work, some record of both phases of activation must be available at the time of learning. These two states likely occur in rapid succession, going from expectation to subsequent outcome, so that the necessary record is plausible. We will explore specific biological mechanisms later, and proceed now to explore the properties of the delta rule in the next section.

5.5 Exploration of Delta Rule Task Learning

↪   Open the project pat_assoc.proj.gz in chapter_5 to begin. (Or, if you already have this project open from the previous exercise, reset the parameters to their default values using the Defaults button.) View the TRAIN_GRAPH_LOG and the TEST_GRID_LOG. Then, select DELTA instead of HEBB for the learn_rule in the pat_assoc_ctrl control panel, and Apply.

This will switch weight updating from the default CPCA Hebbian rule explored previously to the delta rule. The effects of this switch can be seen in the lrn field, which shows the learning rate for the weights (lrate, always .01) and for the bias weights (bias_lrate, which is 0 for Hebbian learning because it has no way of training the bias weights, and is equal to lrate for delta rule), and the proportion of Hebbian learning (hebb, 1 or 0 — we will see in the next chapter that intermediate values of this parameter can be used as well).

Before training the network, we will explore how the minus-plus activation phases work in the simulator.

↪ Make sure that you are monitoring activations in the network, and set step_level to STEP_SETTLE instead of STEP_TRIAL in the control panel.

This will increase the resolution of the stepping so that each press of the Step button will perform the settling (iterative activation updating) process associated with each phase of processing.

↪ Next hit the Step button.

You will see in the network the actual activation produced in response to the input pattern (also known as the *expectation,* or *response,* or *minus phase* activation).

↪ Now, hit Step again.

You will see the target (also known as the *outcome,* or *instruction,* or *plus phase*) activation. Learning occurs after this second, plus phase of activation. You can recognize targets because their activations are exactly .95 or 0 — note that we are clamping activations to .95 and 0 because units cannot easily produce activations above .95 with typical net input values due to the saturating nonlinearity of the rate code activation function. You can also switch to viewing the targ in the network, which will show you the target inputs prior to the activation clamping. In addition, the minus phase activation is always viewable as act_m and the plus phase as act_p.

Now, let's monitor the weights.

↪ Click on r.wt, and then on the left output unit. Then Run the process control panel to complete the training on this EASY task.

The network has no trouble learning this task. However, if you perform multiple Run's, you might notice that the final weight values are quite variable relative to the Hebbian case (you can always switch the LearnRule back to HEBB in the control panel to compare between the two learning algorithms).

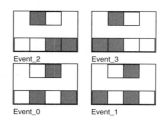

Figure 5.7: The impossible pattern associator task mapping, where there is complete overlap among the patterns that activate the different output units.

This variability in the weights reflects a critical weakness of error-driven learning — it's *lazy*. Basically, once the output unit is performing the task correctly, learning effectively stops, with whatever weight values that happened to do the trick. In contrast, Hebbian learning keeps adapting the weights to reflect the conditional probabilities, which, in this task, results in roughly the same final weight values regardless of what the initial random weights were. We will return to this issue later, when we discuss the benefits of using a combination of Hebbian and error-driven learning.

Now for the real test.

↪ Set env_type to HARD. Then, press Run.

You should see that the network learns this task without apparently much difficulty. Thus, because the delta rule performs learning as a function of how well the network is actually doing, it can adapt the weights specifically to solve the task.

Question 5.3 (a) *Compare and contrast in a qualitative manner the nature of the weights learned by the delta rule on this HARD task with those learned by the Hebbian rule (e.g., note where the largest weights tend to be) — be sure to do multiple runs to get a general sense of what tends to be learned.* (b) *Using your answer to the first part, explain why the delta rule weights solve the problem, but the Hebbian ones do not (don't forget to include the bias weights* bias.wt *in your analysis of the delta rule case).*

After this experience, you may think that the delta rule is all powerful, but we can temper this enthusiasm and motivate the next section.

↪ Set `env_type` to `IMPOSSIBLE`. Then do `View`, `EVENTS`.

Notice that each input unit in this environment (figure 5.7) is active equally often when the output is active as when it is inactive. These kinds of problems are called *ambiguous cue* problems, or *nonlinear discrimination* problems (Sutherland & Rudy, 1989; O'Reilly & Rudy, in press). This kind of problem might prove difficult, because every input unit will end up being equivocal about what the output should do. Nevertheless, the input patterns are not all the same — people could learn to solve this task fairly trivially by just paying attention to the overall patterns of activation. Let's see if the network can do this.

↪ Press `Run` on the general control panel.

Do it again. And again. Any luck?

Because the delta rule cannot learn what appears to be a relatively simple task, we conclude that something more powerful is necessary. Unfortunately, that is not the conclusion that Minsky and Papert (1969) reached in their highly influential book, *Perceptrons*. Instead, they concluded that neural networks were hopelessly inadequate because they could not solve problems like the one we just explored (specifically, they focused on the exclusive-or (XOR) task)! This conclusion played a large role in the waning of the early interest in neural network models of the 1960s. Interestingly, we will see that only a few more applications of the chain rule are necessary to remedy the problem, but this fact took a while to be appreciated by most people (roughly fifteen years, in fact).

↪ Go to the `PDP++Root` window. To continue on to the next simulation, close this project first by selecting `.projects/Remove/Project_0`. Or, if you wish to stop now, quit by selecting `Object/Quit`.

5.6 The Generalized Delta Rule: Backpropagation

As we saw, the delta rule, though much better than Hebbian learning for task-based learning, also has its limits. What took people roughly fifteen years to really appreciate was that this limitation only applies to networks with only two layers (an input and output layer, as in the above pattern associator models). The delta rule can be relatively directly extended or *generalized* for networks

with *hidden* layers between the input and output layers, resulting in an algorithm commonly called **backpropagation** that can learn even the "impossible" shown in figure 5.7. Indeed, with enough hidden units, this algorithm can learn any function that uniquely maps input patterns to output patterns. Thus, backpropagation is a truly powerful mechanism for task-based learning.

In chapter 3, we discussed the advantages of hidden units in mediating *transformations* of the input patterns. These transformations emphasize some aspects of the input patterns and deemphasize others, and we argued that by chaining together multiple stages of such transformations, one could achieve more powerful and complex mappings between input patterns and output patterns. Now, we are in a position to formalize some of these ideas by showing how a backpropagation network with hidden units can transform the input patterns in the `IMPOSSIBLE` pattern associator task, so that a subsequent stage of transformation from the hidden layer to the output layer can produce the desired mapping.

Another way to think about these transformations is in terms of *re-representing* the problem. Students of psychology may be familiar with *insight problems* that require one to re-represent problems to find their then relatively easy solutions. For example, try to figure out how the following statement makes sense: "A man wants to go home, but he can't because a man with a mask is there." The words here have been chosen so that, out of context, they don't really make sense. However, if you are able to re-represent these words in the context of "baseball," then you will see that it all makes perfect sense.

Another example comes from simple tool use — a stick can be turned into a club by re-representing it as something other than a part of a tree. Indeed, much of cognition is based on the development of appropriate re-representations (transformations) of input patterns. From a computational perspective, computer scientists have long appreciated that selecting an appropriate representation is perhaps the most important step in designing an algorithm. Thus, the importance of developing learning mechanisms like backpropagation that can produce such re-representations in a series of hidden layers can hardly be overstated. We will return to this issue repeatedly throughout the text.

a)

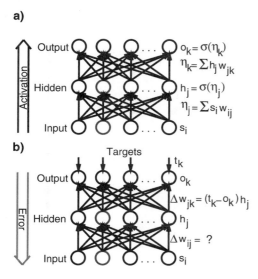

Figure 5.8: Illustration of the basic processes in the standard backpropagation algorithm. **a)** Shows the feedforward propagation of activations, with each layer using the same sigmoidal logistic activation function $\sigma(\eta)$. **b)** Shows the error backpropagation step, where the challenge is to figure out how to update the weights from the input units to the hidden units, because we already know how to adjust the hidden to output weights using the delta rule.

Though it took some time before backpropagation was rediscovered by Rumelhart, Hinton, and Williams (1986a) (the idea had been independently discovered several times before: Bryson & Ho, 1969; Werbos, 1974; Parker, 1985), this algorithm is really just a simple extension of the delta rule that continues the *chain rule* down into the hidden units and their weights. To see how this works, let's take the standard case of a three-layered network (input, hidden, and output) with feedforward connectivity and sigmoidal activation functions, shown in figure 5.8. We will write the activation of an output unit as o_k, that of a hidden unit as h_j, and that of an input (or stimulus) unit as s_i.

The first thing to note is that the weights from the hidden units into the output units can be trained using the simple delta rule as derived previously, because this part of the network is just like a single layer network. Thus, the real challenge solved by backpropagation is

training the weights from the input to the hidden layer.

As usual, we will first present the net result of the backpropagation algorithm — the actual learning rule equations that are used to change the weights. Then we will present the sequence of mathematical steps that led to the learning rule in the next section. Thus, those who lack the patience or mathematical background to explore the derivation in the next section can nevertheless achieve some level of understanding of how the algorithm works in this section. We do caution, however, that much of the interesting material in this and subsequent sections hinges on some of the details of the derivation, so you will miss quite a bit if you skip it.

The weights at every layer in the network are adjusted in backpropagation according to the following learning rule:

$$\Delta w_{ij} = -\epsilon \delta_j x_i \qquad (5.21)$$

where x_i represents the activation of the sending unit associated with the weight w_{ij} being changed, δ_j is the contribution of the receiving unit j toward the overall error at the output layer (which we will define in a moment), and ϵ is the learning rate as usual. Perhaps the most important thing to notice about this learning rule is that it captures the basic credit assignment property of the delta rule, by virtue of adjusting the weights in proportion to the activation of the sending unit.

The weight update rule for bias weights can be derived as usual by just setting the sending activation x_j to 1, so that equation 5.21 becomes:

$$\Delta \beta_j = -\epsilon \delta_j \qquad (5.22)$$

Now, let's try to understand δ. First, for the output units, we know from the delta rule that:

$$\delta_k = -(t_k - o_k) \qquad (5.23)$$

and this accords well with the idea that δ_k is the contribution of the output unit k to the overall error of the network. The crux of backpropagation is computing δ_j, the contribution of the hidden unit j to the overall network error. We will see that this contribution can be computed as:

$$\delta_j = \left(\sum_k \delta_k w_{jk} \right) (h_j(1 - h_j)) \qquad (5.24)$$

This equation shows that the backpropagation of error involves two terms. The first term passes back the δ terms from the output layer in much the same way that the activation values are passed forward in the network: by computing a weighted sum of $\delta_k w_{jk}$ over the output units. This weighted sum is then multiplied by the second term, $h_j(1 - h_j)$, which is the derivative of the activation function $\sigma'(\eta_j)$. This multiplication by the derivative is analogous to passing the net input through the activation function in the forward propagation of activation. Thus, it is useful to think of error backpropagation as roughly the *inverse* of forward activation propagation.

The multiplication by the derivative of the activation function in equation 5.24 has some important implications for the qualitative behavior of learning. Specifically, this derivative can be understood in terms of how much difference a given amount of weight change is actually going to make on the activation value of the unit — if the unit is in the sensitive middle range of the sigmoid function, then a weight change will make a big difference. This is where the activation derivative is at its maximum (e.g., $.5(1 - .5) = .25$). Conversely, when a unit is "pegged" against one of the two extremes (0 or 1), then a weight change will make relatively little difference, which is consistent with the derivative being very small (e.g., $.99(1 - .99) = .0099$). Thus, the learning rule will effectively focus learning on those units which are more labile (think of lobbying undecided senators versus those who are steadfast in their opinions — you want to focus your efforts where they have a chance of paying off).

One final note before we proceed with the details of the derivation is that one can iteratively apply equation 5.24 for as many hidden layers as there are in the network, and all the math works out correctly. Thus, backpropagation allows many hidden layers to be used. Box 5.2 summarizes the backpropagation algorithm.

5.6.1 Derivation of Backpropagation

For this derivation, we again need the net input and sigmoidal activation equations. $\eta_j = \sum_i s_i w_{ij}$ is the net input for unit j. The sigmoidal activation function is $h_j = \sigma(\eta_j)$, and its derivative is written as $\sigma'(\eta_j)$, and

Box 5.2: The Backpropagation Algorithm

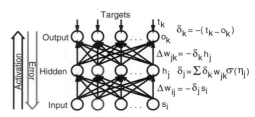

Activations are computed using a standard sigmoidal activation function (see box 2.1 in chapter 2). We use the cross entropy error function (though sum-squared error, SSE, is also commonly used):

$$CE = -\sum_t \sum_k t_k \log o_k + (1 - t_k) \log(1 - o_k)$$

where t_k is the target value, and o_k is the actual output activation. Minimizing this error is the objective of backpropagation.

Error backpropagation takes place via the same kinds of weighted-sum equations that produce the activation, except everything happens in reverse, so it is like the inverse of the activation propagation. For the output units, the delta (δ) error term is:

$$\delta_k = -(t_k - o_k)$$

which is backpropagated down to the hidden units using the following equation (which can be iteratively applied for as many hidden layers as exist in the network):

$$\delta_j = \left(\sum_k \delta_k w_{jk}\right)(h_j(1 - h_j))$$

where $h_j(1-h_j)$ is the derivative of the sigmoidal activation function for hidden unit activation h_j, also written as $\sigma'(\eta_j)$ where η_j is the net input for unit j.

The weights are then updated to minimize this error (by taking the negative of it):

$$\Delta w_{ij} = -\epsilon \delta_j x_i$$

where ϵ is the learning rate parameter (lrate), and x_i is the sending unit activation.

is equal to $h_j(1 - h_j)$. We also continue to use the cross entropy error function.

The main idea behind backpropagation is that we can train the weights from the input to the hidden layer by applying the chain rule all the way down through the network to this point. This chain of derivatives is:

$$\frac{\partial CE}{\partial w_{ij}} = \sum_k \frac{dCE}{do_k} \frac{do_k}{d\eta_k} \frac{\partial \eta_k}{\partial h_j} \frac{dh_j}{d\eta_j} \frac{\partial \eta_j}{\partial w_{ij}} \qquad (5.25)$$

Because this is quite a mouthful, let's break it up into smaller bites. First, let's look at the first three derivative terms:

$$\frac{\partial CE}{\partial h_j} = \sum_k \frac{dCE}{do_k} \frac{do_k}{d\eta_k} \frac{\partial \eta_k}{\partial h_j} \qquad (5.26)$$

This expression tells us how much a change in the activation of this hidden unit would affect the resulting error value *on the output layer*. Thus, you might imagine that this expression has something to do with the weights from this hidden unit to the output units, because it is through these weights that the hidden unit influences the outputs.

Indeed, as you might have already noticed, this expression is very similar to the chain rule that gave us the delta rule, because it shares the first two steps with it. The only difference is that the final term in the delta rule is the derivative of the net input into the output unit with respect to the *weights* (which is equal to the sending unit activation), whereas the final term here is the derivative of this same net input with respect to the *sending unit activation h_j* (which is equal to the weight w_{jk}). In other words, the derivative of $h_j w_{jk}$ with respect to w_{jk} is h_j, and its derivative with respect to h_j is w_{jk}.

Thus the expression for the derivative in equation 5.26 is just like the delta rule, except with a weight at the end instead of an activation:

$$\frac{\partial CE}{\partial h_j} = \sum_k \frac{dCE}{do_k} \frac{do_k}{d\eta_k} \frac{\partial \eta_k}{\partial h_j} = -\sum_k (t_k - o_k) w_{jk} \qquad (5.27)$$

This computation is very interesting, because it suggests that hidden units can compute their contribution to the overall output error by just summing over the errors of all the output units that they project to, and weighting

these errors by the strength of that unit's contribution to the output units. You might recognize that this is the first term in the computation of δ_j from equation 5.24.

For now, we continue the great chain of backpropagation and compute the remaining derivatives. These are actually quite similar to those we have already computed, consisting just of the derivative of the sigmoidal activation function itself, and the derivative of the net input (to the hidden unit) with respect to the weights (which you know to be the sending activation):

$$\frac{dh_j}{d\eta_j} \frac{\partial \eta_j}{\partial w_{ij}} = h_j(1 - h_j) s_i \qquad (5.28)$$

so the overall result of the entire chain of derivatives is:

$$\frac{\partial CE}{\partial w_{ij}} = \frac{\partial CE}{\partial h_j} \frac{\partial h_j}{\partial w_{ij}} = -\sum_k (t_k - o_k) w_{jk} h_j (1 - h_j) s_i \qquad (5.29)$$

As before, we can use the negative of equation 5.29 to adjust the weights in such a way as to minimize the overall error. Thus, in a three-layer network, backpropagation is just the delta rule for the output unit's weights, and equation 5.29 for the hidden unit's weights.

5.6.2 Generic Recursive Formulation

If we just use the chain rule, we miss out on the elegant recursiveness of backpropagation expressed in equations 5.21 and 5.24. Thus, we need to introduce the δ term to achieve this more elegant formulation. As we mentioned previously, equation 5.27 only contains the first term in the expression for δ. Thus, δ_j is equal to $\frac{\partial CE}{\partial \eta_k}$, and not $\frac{\partial CE}{\partial h_j}$. The reason is simply that the computation breaks up more cleanly if we formalize δ in this way. Thus, for the hidden units, δ_j is:

$$\delta_j = \frac{\partial CE}{\partial \eta_j} = \sum_k \frac{dCE}{do_k} \frac{do_k}{d\eta_k} \frac{\partial \eta_k}{\partial h_j} \frac{dh_j}{d\eta_j}$$

$$= -\sum_k (t_k - o_k) w_{jk} h_j (1 - h_j) \qquad (5.30)$$

where it then becomes apparent that we can express δ_j in terms of the δ_k variables on the layer above it (the output layer in this case, but it could be another hidden layer):

$$\delta_j = \sum_k \delta_k w_{jk} h_j (1 - h_j) \qquad (5.31)$$

5.6.3 The Biological Implausibility of Backpropagation

Unfortunately, despite the apparent simplicity and elegance of the backpropagation learning rule, it seems quite implausible that something like equations 5.21 and 5.24 are computed in the cortex. Perhaps the biggest problem is equation 5.24, which would require in biological terms that the δ value be propagated *backward* from the dendrite of the receiving neuron, across the synapse, into the axon terminal of the sending neuron, down the axon of this neuron, and then integrated and multiplied by both the strength of that synapse and some kind of derivative, and then propagated back out its dendrites, and so on. As if this were not problematic enough, nobody has ever recorded anything that resembles δ in terms of the electrical or chemical properties of the neuron.

As we noted in the introduction, many modelers have chosen to ignore the biological implausibility of backpropagation, simply because it is so essential for achieving task learning, as suggested by our explorations of the difference between Hebbian and delta rule learning. What we will see in the next section is that we can rewrite the backpropagation equations so that error propagation between neurons takes place using standard activation signals. This approach takes advantage of the notion of activation phases that we introduced previously, so that it also ties into the psychological interpretation of the teaching signal as an actual state of experience that reflects something like an outcome or corrected response. The result is a very powerful task-based learning mechanism that need not ignore issues of biological plausibility.

5.7 The Generalized Recirculation Algorithm

An algorithm called **recirculation** (Hinton & McClelland, 1988) provided two important ideas that enabled

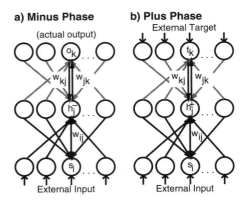

Figure 5.9: Illustration of the GeneRec algorithm, with bidirectional symmetric connectivity as shown. **a)** In the minus phase, external input is provided to the input units, and the network settles, with some record of the resulting minus phase activation states kept. **b)** In the plus phase, external input (target) is also applied to the output units in addition to the input units, and the network again settles.

backpropagation to be implemented in a more biologically plausible manner. The recirculation algorithm was subsequently generalized from the somewhat restricted case it could handle, resulting in the *generalized recirculation* algorithm or **GeneRec** (O'Reilly, 1996a), which serves as our task-based learning algorithm in the rest of the text.

GeneRec adopts the activation *phases* introduced previously in our implementation of the delta rule. In the *minus phase*, the outputs of the network represent the *expectation* or *response* of the network, as a function of the standard activation settling process in response to a given input pattern. Then, in the *plus phase*, the environment is responsible for providing the *outcome* or *target* output activations (figure 5.9). As before, we use the $^+$ superscript to indicate plus-phase variables, and $^-$ to indicate minus-phase variables in the equations below.

It is important to emphasize that the full bidirectional propagation of information (bottom-up and top-down) occurs during the settling in each of these phases, with the only difference being whether the output units are updated from the network (in the minus phase) or are set to the external outcome/target values (in the plus

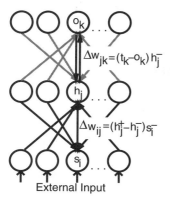

Figure 5.10: Weight updates computed for the GeneRec algorithm.

phase). In particular, the hidden units need to receive the top-down activation from both the minus and plus phase output states to determine their contribution to the output error, as we will see in a moment.

As usual, we will first discuss the final learning rule that the GeneRec derivation produces before deriving the mathematical details. Conveniently, the learning rule is the same for all units in the network, and is essentially just the delta rule:

$$\Delta w_{ij} = \epsilon(y_j^+ - y_j^-)x_i^- \qquad (5.32)$$

for a receiving unit with activation y_j and sending unit with activation x_i in the phases as indicated (figure 5.10). As usual, the rule for adjusting the bias weights is just the same as for the regular weights, but with the sending unit activation set to 1:

$$\Delta \beta_j = \epsilon(y_j^+ - y_j^-) \qquad (5.33)$$

If you compare equation 5.32 with equation 5.21 from backpropagation ($\Delta w_{ij} = -\epsilon \delta_j x_i$), it should be clear that the phase-based difference in activation states of the receiving unit ($y_j^+ - y_j^-$) is equivalent to $-\delta$ in backpropagation. Thus, the difference between the two phases of activation states is an indication of the unit's contribution to the overall error signal. Interestingly, bidirectional connectivity ends up naturally propagating both parts of this signal throughout the network, so that just computing the difference can drive learning.

These activation states are local to the synapse where the weight changes must occur, and we will see below how such weight changes can happen in a biological synapse.

There are a number of important properties of the GeneRec learning rule. First, GeneRec allows an error signal occurring anywhere in the network to be used to drive learning everywhere, which enables many different sources of error signals to be used. In addition, this form of learning is compatible with — and, moreover, requires — the bidirectional connectivity known to exist throughout the cortex, and which is responsible for a number of important computational properties such as constraint satisfaction, pattern completion, and attractor dynamics (chapter 3). Furthermore, the subtraction of activations in GeneRec ends up implicitly computing the derivative of the activation function, which appears explicitly in the original backpropagation equations (in equation 5.24 as $h_j(1 - h_j)$). In addition to a small gain in biological plausibility, this allows us to use any arbitrary activation function (e.g., the point neuron function with kWTA inhibition) without having to explicitly take its derivative. Thus, the same GeneRec learning rule works for virtually any activation function.

The next section presents the derivation of equation 5.32, and the subsequent section introduces a couple of simple improvements to this equation.

5.7.1 Derivation of GeneRec

Two important ideas from the recirculation algorithm allow us to implement backpropagation learning in a more biologically plausible manner. First, as we discussed above, recirculation showed that bidirectional connectivity allows output error to be communicated to a hidden unit in terms of the difference in its activation states during the plus and minus activation phases ($y_j^+ - y_j^-$), rather than in terms of the δ's multiplied by the synaptic weights in the other direction. Bidirectional connectivity thus avoids the problems with backpropagation of computing error information in terms of δ, sending this information backward from dendrites, across synapses, and into axons, and multiplying this information with the strength of that synapse.

Second, recirculation showed that this difference in the *activation* of a hidden unit during plus and minus phases $(y_j^+ - y_j^-)$ is a good approximation for the difference in the *net input* to a hidden unit during plus and minus phases, multiplied by the derivative of the activation function. By using the difference-of-activation-states approximation, we implicitly compute the activation function derivative, which avoids the problem in backpropagation where the derivative of the activation function must be explicitly computed. The mathematical derivation of GeneRec begins with the net inputs and explicit derivative formulation, because this can be directly related to backpropagation, and then applies the difference-of-activation-states approximation to achieve the final form of the algorithm (equation 5.32).

Let's first reconsider the equation for the δ_j variable on the hidden unit in backpropagation (equation 5.30):

$$\delta_j = -\sum_k (t_k - o_k) w_{jk} h_j (1 - h_j)$$

Recall the primary aspects of biological implausibility in this equation: the passing of the error information on the outputs backward, and the multiplying of this information by the feedforward weights and by the derivative of the activation function.

We avoid the implausible error propagation procedure by converting the computation of error information multiplied by the weights into a computation of the net input to the hidden units. For mathematical purposes, we assume for the moment that our bidirectional connections are symmetric, or $w_{jk} = w_{kj}$. We will see later that the argument below holds even if we do not assume exact symmetry. With $w_{jk} = w_{kj}$:

$$\delta_j = -\sum_k (t_k - o_k) w_{jk} h_j (1 - h_j)$$

$$= -\sum_k (t_k - o_k) w_{kj} h_j (1 - h_j)$$

$$= -\left(\sum_k (t_k w_{kj}) - \sum_k (o_k w_{kj}) \right) h_j (1 - h_j)$$

$$= -(\eta_j^+ - \eta_j^-) h_j (1 - h_j) \qquad (5.34)$$

That is, w_{kj} can be substituted for w_{jk} and then this

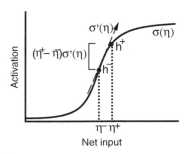

Figure 5.11: The difference in activation states approximates the difference in net input states times the derivative of the activation function: $(h_j^+ - h_j^-) \approx (\eta_j^+ - \eta_j^-)\sigma'(\eta_j)$.

term can be multiplied through $(t_k - o_k)$ to get the difference between the net inputs to the hidden units (from the output units) in the two phases. Bidirectional connectivity thus allows error information to be communicated in terms of net input to the hidden units, rather than in terms of δs propagated backward and multiplied by the strength of the feedforward synapse.

Next, we can deal with the remaining $h_j(1 - h_j)$ in equation 5.34 by applying the difference-of-activation-states approximation. Recall that $h_j(1 - h_j)$ can be expressed as $\sigma'(\eta_j)$, the derivative of the activation function, so:

$$\delta_j = -(\eta_j^+ - \eta_j^-)\sigma'(\eta_j) \qquad (5.35)$$

This product can be approximated by just the difference of the two sigmoidal activation values computed on these net inputs:

$$\delta_j \approx -(h_j^+ - h_j^-) \qquad (5.36)$$

That is, the difference in a hidden unit's activation values is approximately equivalent to the difference in net inputs times the slope of the activation function. This is illustrated in figure 5.11, where it should be clear that differences in the Y axis are approximately equal to differences in the X axis times the slope of the function that maps X to Y.

As noted previously, this simplification of using differences in activation states has one major advantage (in addition to being somewhat simpler) — it eliminates the need to explicitly compute the derivative of the activation function. Instead, this derivative is *implicitly* computed in the difference of the activation states.

Once we have the δ terms for the hidden units computed as the difference in activation across the two phases, we end up with equation 5.32:

$$\Delta w_{ij} = -\epsilon \delta_j s_i = \epsilon (h_j^+ - h_j^-) s_i^- \quad (5.37)$$

Thus, through bidirectional connectivity and the approximation of the product of net input differences and the derivative of the activation function, hidden units implicitly compute the information needed to minimize error as in backpropagation, but using only locally available activity signals.

Finally, it should be noted that GeneRec is only an approximation to the actual backpropagation procedure. In a bidirectional network with potentially complex settling dynamics, the propagation of the two phases of activation values separately and the calculation of their difference (GeneRec) is not guaranteed to be the same as directly propagating the difference itself (backpropagation). However, the approximation holds up quite well even in deep multilayered networks performing complicated learning tasks (O'Reilly, 1996a).

5.7.2 Symmetry, Midpoint, and CHL

As we mentioned, we can improve upon equation 5.32 ($\Delta w_{ij} = \epsilon (y_j^+ - y_j^-) x_i^-$) in two small but significant ways. First, there is a more sophisticated way of updating weights, known as the *midpoint method*, that uses the average of both the minus and plus phase activation of the sending unit x_i, instead of just the minus phase alone (O'Reilly, 1996a):

$$\Delta w_{ij} = \epsilon (y_j^+ - y_j^-) \frac{x_i^- + x_i^+}{2} \quad (5.38)$$

Second, the mathematical derivation of the learning rule depends on the weights being symmetric, and yet the basic GeneRec equation is not symmetric (i.e., the weight changes computed by unit j from unit i are not the same as those computed by unit i from unit j). So, even if the weights started out symmetric, they would not likely remain that way under the basic GeneRec equation. Making the weight changes symmetric (the

same in both directions) both preserves any existing weight symmetry, and, when combined with a small amount of weight decay (Hinton, 1989b) and/or soft weight bounding, actually works to symmetrize initially asymmetric weights. A simple way of preserving symmetry is to take the average of the weight updates for the different weight directions:

$$\begin{aligned} \Delta w_{ij} &= \epsilon \frac{1}{2} \left[(y_j^+ - y_j^-) \frac{(x_i^+ + x_i^-)}{2} + \right. \\ &\quad \left. (x_i^+ - x_i^-) \frac{(y_j^+ + y_j^-)}{2} \right] \\ &= \epsilon \left[x_i^+ y_j^+ - x_i^- y_j^- \right] \quad (5.39) \end{aligned}$$

(where the $\frac{1}{2}$ for averaging the weight updates in the two different directions gets folded into the arbitrary learning rate constant ϵ). Because many terms end up canceling, the weight change rule that results is a simple function of the coproduct of the sending and receiving activations in the plus phase, minus this coproduct in the minus phase. The simplicity of this rule makes it more plausible that the brain might have adopted such a symmetry producing mechanism.

To summarize the mathematical side of things before providing further biological, ecological, and psychological support for something like the GeneRec algorithm in the human cortex (which we address in the next section): we use equation 5.39 to adjust the weights in the network, subject additionally to the *soft weight bounding* procedure described previously. The bias weight update remains unaffected by the symmetry and midpoint modifications, and is thus given by equation 5.33.

The learning rule in equation 5.39 provides an interesting bridge to a set of other learning algorithms in the field. Specifically, it is identical to the **contrastive Hebbian learning (CHL)** algorithm, which is so named because it is the contrast (difference) between two Hebbian-like terms (the sender-receiver coproducts). We will therefore refer to equation 5.39 as the CHL learning rule. In the following subsection, we discuss the original derivation of CHL and other similar algorithms.

GeneRec, CHL and other Algorithms

The CHL algorithm traces its roots to the **mean field** (Peterson & Anderson, 1987) or **deterministic Boltzmann machine (DBM)** (Hinton, 1989b) learning algorithms, which also use locally available activation variables to perform error-driven learning in recurrently connected networks. The DBM algorithm was derived originally for networks called **Boltzmann machines** that have noisy units whose activation states can be described by a probability distribution known as the Boltzmann distribution (Ackley et al., 1985). In this probabilistic framework, learning amounts to reducing the distance between the two probability distributions that arise in the minus and plus phases of settling in the network.

The CHL/DBM algorithm has been derived from the Boltzmann machine learning algorithm through the use of approximations or restricted cases of the probabilistic network (Hinton, 1989b; Peterson & Anderson, 1987), and derived without the use of the Boltzmann distribution by using the continuous Hopfield energy function (Movellan, 1990). However, all of these derivations require problematic assumptions or approximations, which led some to conclude that CHL was fundamentally flawed for deterministic (non-noisy) networks (Galland, 1993; Galland & Hinton, 1990). Furthermore, the use of the original (noisy) Boltzmann machine has been limited by the extreme amounts of computation required, requiring many runs of many cycles to obtain the averaged probability estimates needed for learning.

Thus, the derivation of CHL directly from the backpropagation algorithm for completely deterministic (non-noisy) units (via GeneRec) restores some basis for optimism in its ability to learn difficult problems. Further, although the generic form of CHL/GeneRec does have some remaining performance limitations, these are largely eliminated by the use of this learning rule in the context of a kWTA inhibition function and in conjunction with the CPCA Hebbian learning rule. Most of the problems with plain CHL/GeneRec can be traced to the consequences of using purely error-driven learning in a unconstrained bidirectionally connected network (O'Reilly, 1996b, in press). We will explore some of these issues in chapter 6.

5.8 Biological Considerations for GeneRec

We have seen that GeneRec can implement error backpropagation using locally available activation variables, making it more plausible that such a learning rule could be employed by real neurons. Also, the use of activation-based signals (as opposed to error or other variables) increases plausibility because it is relatively straightforward to map unit activation onto neural variables such as time-averaged membrane potential or spiking rate (chapter 2). However, three main features of the GeneRec algorithm could potentially be problematic from a biological perspective: 1) weight symmetry, 2) the origin of plus and minus phase activation states, and 3) the ability of these activation states to influence synaptic modification according to the learning rule.

5.8.1 Weight Symmetry in the Cortex

Recall that the mathematical derivation of GeneRec depends on symmetric weights for units to compute their sending error contribution based on what they receive back from other units. Three points address the biological plausibility of the weight symmetry requirement in GeneRec:

- As mentioned above, a symmetry preserving learning algorithm like the CHL version of GeneRec, when combined with either soft weight bounding or small amounts of weight decay, will automatically lead to symmetric weights even if they did not start out that way. Thus, if the brain is using something like CHL, then as long as there is bidirectional *connectivity*, the weight values on these connections will naturally take on symmetric values. The next two points address this much weaker constraint of bidirectional connectivity.

- The biological evidence strongly suggests that the cortex is bidirectionally connected at the level of cortical areas (e.g., Felleman & Van Essen, 1991; White, 1989a). The existence of this larger-scale bidirectional connectivity suggests that the cortex may have come under some kind of evolutionary pressure to produce reciprocal bidirectional connectivity — the use of such connectivity to perform a particularly powerful form of error-driven learning would certainly constitute one such evolutionary pressure.

- Individual unit bidirectional connectivity (for which we are not aware of any specific biological evidence) is not critical to the proper functioning of CHL, as long as there are other pathways for error signals to propagate along (Galland & Hinton, 1991). Specifically, Galland and Hinton (1991) showed that CHL was still effective even when all of the connectivity was asymmetric (i.e., for each pair of hidden and output units, only one of the two possible connections between them existed). This robustness can be attributed to redundancy in the ways that error signal information can be obtained; a given hidden unit could obtain the error signal directly from the output units, or indirectly through connections to other hidden units.

Thus, GeneRec actually requires only rough bidirectional connectivity, the existence of which is supported by biological evidence. Also, the Hebbian learning mechanism that we will use in conjunction with GeneRec in Leabra (the next chapter discusses this combination in detail) is only approximately symmetric, but the use of this form of learning generally improves learning, so it is clear that the symmetry requirement is only approximate.

5.8.2 Phase-Based Activations in the Cortex

The phase-based activations that are central to the GeneRec algorithm raise perhaps the most controversial aspect of error-driven learning in the cortex: Where does the teaching signal come from? As discussed previously, we view the teaching signal as just another state of experience (i.e., an activation state in the network) that results from the actual *outcome* of some previous conditions. Thus, the minus phase can be viewed as the *expectation* of the outcome given these conditions.

For example, after hearing the first few words of a sentence, you will develop an expectation of which word is likely to come next. The state of the neurons upon generating this expectation is the minus phase. The experience of the actual word that comes next es-

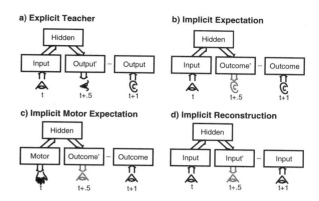

Figure 5.12: Origin of different forms of error signals, for a simple three-layer network. The right-most layer in each figure represents the state of the adjacent layer (to the left) at subsequent time step, not an additional layer. **a)** Explicit teaching signal, where an overt output is made, and then corrected. **b)** Implicit expectation-based error signal where an input triggers a subsequent expectation, which is then experienced. **c)** Implicit expectation based on motor output, where the consequences of the motor action are expected and then experienced. **d)** Implicit reconstruction of a single input layer, like an auto-encoder (note that here there are just two layers, with the different input boxes representing different states over time).

tablishes a subsequent state of activation, which serves as the plus locomotive phase.[2] This idea that the brain is constantly generating expectations, and that the discrepancies between these expectations and subsequent outcomes can be used for error-driven learning, has been suggested by McClelland (1994) as a psychological interpretation of the backpropagation learning procedure. It is particularly attractive for the GeneRec/CHL version of backpropagation, which uses only activation states, because it requires no additional mechanisms for providing specific teaching signals other than the effects of experience on neural activation states via standard activation propagation mechanisms.

Figure 5.12 provides some illustrations of how these kinds of expectation-based signals could arise under various conditions. Figure 5.12a shows the case that

---

[2]The word "locomotive" here is just to demonstrate that such expectations are being generated and it is salient when they are violated.

people typically assume when they think of error-driven learning, where a teaching signal is explicitly provided (e.g., a student misreads a word, and the teacher explicitly corrects the student). Figure 5.12b shows how similar kinds of error signals can arise as a result of making an implicit expectation (e.g., about how a word should be pronounced), followed by the actual experience of hearing the word pronounced (e.g., by one's parent during bedtime reading). Figures 5.12c and d show different contexts in which these implicit expectations can be generated, including expecting the outcome of motor output, and then experiencing the actual outcome, or even "expecting" the actual input that one just received, which amounts to a kind of generative model (cf. Dayan et al., 1995).

Another form of implicit error signal (not shown in the figure) can be produced by the mismatch between different sensory representations of the same underlying event (Becker, 1996; de Sa & Ballard, 1998; Kay, Floreano, & Phillips, 1998). Thus, each modality creates an expectation about how the other modality will represent the event, and the difference between this expectation and how the modality actually represents the event is an error signal for training both modalities.

In addition to the multitude of ways that error signals could be based on expectation-outcome differences, ERP recordings of electrical activity over the scalp during behavioral tasks indicate that cortical activation states reflect expectations and are sensitive to differential outcomes. For example, the widely-studied *P300* wave, a positive-going wave that occurs around 300 msec after stimulus onset, is considered to measure a violation of subjective expectancy determined by preceding experience over both the short and long term (Hillyard & Picton, 1987). Thus, one could interpret the P300 as reflecting a plus phase wave of activation following in a relatively short time-frame the activation of minus phase expectations. Although the specific properties of the P300 itself might be due to specialized neural mechanisms for monitoring discrepancies between expectations and outcomes, its presence suggests the possibility that neurons in the mammalian neocortex experience two states of activation in relatively rapid succession, one corresponding to expectation and the other corresponding to outcome.

Further evidence for expectation-outcome states in the cortex comes from the updating of spatial representations in the parietal cortex as a function of eye movements (saccades) — neurons actually first anticipate what their new input coding will be as a function of the motor plan, and then the same neurons update to reflect their actual input coding as a result of executing the motor plan (Colby, Duhamel, & Goldberg, 1996). Specifically, these parietal neurons first represent what they will "see" after an eye movement *before the eye movement is executed*, and then update to reflect what they actually see after the eye movement. When these anticipatory and actual representations are discrepant, there would be just the kind of expectation–outcome difference that could be used for learning.

Although these ideas and data support the idea that the brain can learn from error signals using phase-like differences that occur naturally in many situations, a number of details remain to be resolved. For example, our models assume that the input and output layers are physically distinct, and that the output undergoes a minus–plus phase transition while the input remains constant. Although this is reasonable for many types of error signals (e.g., reading a word, forming an auditory expectation of its pronunciation, followed by hearing the actual pronunciation), other types of error signals require an expectation to be formed within the same modality as the input that triggered the expectation (e.g., seeing a block about to fall off a ledge, and forming the expectation of what will happen next). In this case, the same set of perceptual units need to serve as both input and "output" (i.e., expectation) units. Preliminary explorations of this kind of learning suggest that the same learning mechanism apply (O'Reilly, 1996b), but such issues remain to be systematically addressed. See chapter 12 for more discussion.

5.8.3 Synaptic Modification Mechanisms

Having suggested that the minus and plus phase activations follow each other in rapid succession, it remains to be shown how these two activation states could influence synaptic modification in a manner largely consistent with the CHL version of GeneRec (equation 5.39). We will see that the biological mechanisms for LTP/D

Minus Phase	Plus Phase					
	$x_i^+ y_j^+ \approx 0$			$x_i^+ y_j^+ \approx 1$		
	CHL	CPCA	Combo	CHL	CPCA	Combo
$x_i^- y_j^- \approx 0$	0	0	0	+	+	+
$x_i^- y_j^- \approx 1$	−	0	−	0	+	+

Table 5.1: Directions of weight change according to the CHL and CPCA Hebbian learning rules for four qualitative conditions of minus and plus phase activation coproduct values. CPCA, which doesn't care about phases, is assumed to take place in the plus phase. A plausible biological mechanism produces the combination of the two rules, shown in the Combo column.

that were discussed in section 4.2 are capable of implementing the critical aspect of CHL. However, recall that we already showed in section 4.5.3 that these biological mechanisms were consistent with the CPCA Hebbian learning rule. Thus, to the extent that CHL is inconsistent with CPCA, we cannot possibly argue that the biology supports both. However, what we can (and will) argue is that the biology is consistent with the *combination* of CPCA and CHL.

Table 5.1 shows how the CHL and CPCA learning rules agree and differ on the direction of weight change for four different qualitative values of the minus and plus phase coproducts of sending unit x_i and receiving unit y_j. Note that CPCA does not have phase-based variables, so we further specify that it occurs in the plus phase, because it makes sense to learn the correlation structure of the plus phase, not the minus phase. As you can see, the two learning rules agree for the first row of the table, corresponding to the case where there was no activity in the expectation (minus) phase. In the second row, the rules differ, but the conflict is not as bad as it could be, because they do not predict different signs of weight change — one rule predicts no weight change while the other predicts a weight change. Thus, the combination of the two rules is not so drastically in conflict with either one. Further, we will see in chapter 6 that the combination of error-driven and Hebbian associative learning can be generally beneficial for solving many different kinds of tasks.

Three of the four cells in table 5.1 are consistent with the CPCA Hebbian learning rule, which we have already shown can be accounted for by the biology of LTP/D (section 4.5.3). Thus, what remains to be explained is the lower left-hand cell of the table, where the coproduct was active in the minus phase, but inactive in the plus phase. CHL requires a weight decrease here (i.e., LTD). We refer to this cell as the *error correction* case, because it represents an incorrect expectation that should be suppressed through error-driven learning. In other words, this cell represents the situation where there was a strong expectation associated with these units (in the minus phase) that was not actually experienced in the outcome (plus phase). This is the most important contribution of error-driven learning, because it enables the network to correct a faulty expectation or output. Otherwise, Hebbian learning is capable of doing the right things.

To explain this error correction case, we appeal to the relationship between intracellular calcium ion concentration and the direction of synaptic modification proposed by Artola et al. (1990), which was discussed in section 4.2 and shown in figure 4.2. To refresh, the idea is that there are two thresholds for synaptic modification, Θ^+ and Θ^-. A level of intracellular calcium ($[Ca^{++}]_i$) that is higher than the high threshold Θ^+ leads to LTP, while one lower than this high threshold but above the lower Θ^- threshold leads to LTD.

Under this two-threshold mechanism, it seems plausible that minus phase synaptic activity ($x_i^- y_j^-$) that is not followed by similar or greater levels of plus phase synaptic activity ($x_i^+ y_j^+$) will lead to a level of $[Ca^{++}]_i$ that is above the Θ^- threshold but below the Θ^+ threshold, thus resulting in the LTD required for error correction. In short, minus phase activations are not persistent enough on their own to build up the LTP level of calcium, and thus only lead to LTD if not maintained into the plus phase, which is presumably longer-lasting and thus capable of accumulating LTP-levels of calcium.

In light of this proposed mechanism, one can interpret the findings that repeated trains of low-frequency pulses (e.g., 1 Hz) of activation produce LTD (Bear & Malenka, 1994) as constituting a series of minus phase level activations that are not persistent enough to produce LTP, and thus result in just the kind of LTD that is predicted by the error correction case.

The proposed mechanism may also interact with an additional mechanism that indicates when activations should be considered to be in the plus phase, and thus when learning should occur based on the level of calcium at that point. This would reduce the need for the assumption that the minus phase is relatively transient compared to the plus phase. It seems plausible that such a plus-phase signal could be produced by the same kinds of dopamine-releasing mechanisms that have been described by Schultz, Apicella, and Ljungberg (1993) and modeled by Montague, Dayan, and Sejnowski (1996) (we will discuss this more in section 6.7 in the next chapter). These midbrain dopamine systems apparently fire whenever there is a mismatch between expectation and outcome (specifically in the case of reward, which is what has been studied, but it might be more general than that). It is also known that dopamine can modulate the efficacy of LTP, which is appropriate for a plus-phase like "learn now" signal.

In summary, the available data are consistent with a biological mechanism that would enable error-driven task learning, but much more work would need to be done to establish this fact conclusively and to illuminate its nature and dynamics more precisely.

5.9 Exploration of GeneRec-Based Task Learning

Now, let's put some of this theory to work and see how GeneRec does on some small-scale task learning problems. We will use the same problems used in the pattern associator case, but we add an extra hidden layer of units between the inputs and outputs. This should in theory enable the network to solve the "impossible" task from before.

↪   Open the project `generec.proj.gz` in `chapter_5` to begin.

This project is identical to the pattern associator one, with one major and one minor exception. The major ex-

ception is that we have introduced a hidden layer of 3 units. Note that there are only feedforward connections from the input to this hidden layer, because the input is clamped in both minus and plus phases and so would not be affected by feedback connections anyway, but that there are bidirectional connections between the hidden and output layers, as required by the GeneRec algorithm. The minor exception is that we have increased the learning rate from .01 to .05 so that it takes less time to solve the "impossible" problem. Let's start by giving the network the hardest problem. By default, the `learn_rule` is set to GENEREC, and `env_type` is IMPOSSIBLE.

↪   View the `TRAIN_GRAPH_LOG` and the `TEST_GRID_LOG`, and then press Run.

As before, the train graph log displays the SSE error measure over epochs of training. The testing grid log is now updated only after every 10 epochs of training, and it also shows the states of the 3 hidden units.

As before, the training of the network stops automatically after it gets the entire training set correct 5 epochs in a row. Note that this 5 correct repetitions criterion filters out the occasional spurious solutions that can happen due to the somewhat noisy behavior of the network during learning, as evidenced by the jagged shape of the learning curve. The reason for this noisy behavior is that a relatively small change in the weight can lead to large overall changes in the network's behavior due to the bidirectional activation dynamics, which produces a range of different responses to the input patterns.

This sensitivity of the network is a property of all *attractor* networks (i.e., networks having bidirectional connectivity), but is not typical of feedforward networks. Thus, a feedforward backpropagation network learning this same task will have a smooth, monotonically decreasing learning curve. Some people have criticized the nature of learning in attractor networks because they do not share the smoothness of backpropagation. However, we find the benefits of bidirectional connectivity and attractor dynamics to far outweigh the aesthetics of the learning curve. Furthermore, larger networks exhibit smoother learning, because they have more "mass" and are thus less sensitive to small weight changes.

↪ Press `Run` several times to get a sense of how fast the network learns in general.

Question 5.4 *Provide a general characterization of how many epochs it took for your network to learn (e.g., slowest, fastest, rough average).*

↪ Press `TestStep` 4 times to refresh the testing grid log after learning is done.

Question 5.5 (a) *Explain what the hidden units represent to enable the network to solve this "impossible" task (make specific reference to this problem, but describe the general nature of the hidden unit contributions across multiple runs).* **(b)** *Use the weight values as revealed in the network display (including the bias weights) to explain why each hidden unit is activated as it is. Be sure to do multiple runs, and extract the general nature of the network's solution. Your answer should just discuss qualitative weight values, e.g., "one hidden unit detects the left two inputs being active, and sends a strong weight to the right output unit."* **(c)** *Extrapolating from this specific example, explain in more general terms why hidden units can let networks solve difficult problems that could not otherwise be solved directly.*

Just to confirm that merely adding hidden units and increasing the learning rate does not enable the network to solve this problem, let's try running this network with Hebbian learning.

↪ Set the `learn_rule` to `HEBB` (i.e., CPCA), `Apply`, and then `Run` a couple more times. Note that changing `learn_rule` affects the `lrn` values as described earlier.

You should observe complete failure. However, Hebbian learning can work quite well with hidden units in simple tasks.

↪ To see this, set `env_type` to `EASY`, and `Apply`. `Run` several times.

The network should learn within a couple of epochs (with 5 more added at the end to make sure).

↪ Now, set `learn_rule` to `GENEREC`, and `Run` several times.

Question 5.6 *How fast does GeneRec learn this* `EASY` *task compared to the Hebbian rule? Be sure to run several times in both, to get a good sample.*

This last exercise should leave an important impression on you — sometimes Hebbian learning can be much faster and more reliable than error-driven learning. The reasons for this speedup will be explored in greater depth later, but clearly it interacts with the nature of the task. Thus, if we knew that the tasks faced by the network were typically going to be "easy," then it might make sense to use Hebbian instead of error-driven learning. We will see that in fact a combination of both types of learning usually works best.

↪ To stop now, quit by selecting `Object/Quit` in the `PDP++Root` window.

5.10 Summary

Task learning is a complementary learning objective to model learning — it can be formalized in terms of learning an **input-output mapping**. A simple such **pattern associator** task reveals the limitations of Hebbian learning for task learning. If the discrepancy or **error** between the desired or **target** output pattern and the **actual** output pattern is used to drive learning, then networks can learn much more successfully. This is the idea behind the **delta rule**, which minimizes error by adapting weights as a function of the **derivative** of the error. To learn more complicated input/output relationships, networks with at least one intermediate *hidden* layer are necessary. These **multilayer** networks require a generalized form of the delta rule which **backpropagates** error signals by using the **chain rule** to propagate the error derivative back through multiple layers of units.

Although there is scant evidence that cortical neurons communicate such error signals directly, it is possible to use the difference between two activation states or **phases** to compute essentially the same error derivative. The first of these activation phases corresponds to an **expectation** or **production** of a particular output pattern, while the second corresponds to the experience of the actual desired **outcome**. As long as the network has symmetric bidirectional weights, the difference between these two activation states for a unit anywhere in the network reflects that unit's contribution to the overall error. This is the idea behind the **GeneRec** algorithm, which is a generalization of the earlier **recir-**

culation algorithm. An improved form of GeneRec is equivalent to the **contrastive Hebbian learning (CHL)** algorithm, which we use in our networks.

For biological synapses to compute the weight changes necessary for the CHL algorithm, they would have to perform LTD when the expectation state for a unit exceeded its outcome state, and LTP otherwise. Assuming a relatively rapid transition between the expectation and outcome activation phases, one would expect LTD with a transient (erroneous) expectation, as is consistent with the biology of LTD. The GeneRec algorithm thus provides a biologically plausible yet powerful form of learning that can learn arbitrary input/output mappings (tasks).

5.11   Further Reading

The Chauvin and Rumelhart (1995) book on backpropagation is a good source for basic ideas and further developments in backpropagation learning.

Crick (1989) provides an influential critique about the biological plausibility of backpropagation.

For further details on the GeneRec algorithm, consult O'Reilly (1996a) and O'Reilly (in press).

The journal *Neural Computation* and the *NIPS* conference proceedings (*Advances in Neural Information Processing*) always have a large number of high-quality articles on computational and biological approaches to learning.

Chapter 6

Combined Model and Task Learning, and Other Mechanisms

Contents

6.1   **Overview** 173

6.2   **Combined Hebbian and Error-driven Learning** . 173

     6.2.1   *Pros and Cons of Hebbian and Error-Driven Learning* 174

     6.2.2   *Advantages to Combining Hebbian and Error-Driven Learning* 175

     6.2.3   *Inhibitory Competition as a Model-Learning Constraint* 175

     6.2.4   *Implementation of Combined Model and Task Learning* 176

     6.2.5   *Summary* 177

6.3   **Generalization in Bidirectional Networks** 178

     6.3.1   *Exploration of Generalization* 179

6.4   **Learning to Re-represent in Deep Networks** . . . 181

     6.4.1   *Exploration of a Deep Network* 183

6.5   **Sequence and Temporally Delayed Learning** . . . 186

6.6   **Context Representations and Sequential Learning** 187

     6.6.1   *Computational Considerations for Context Representations* 188

     6.6.2   *Possible Biological Bases for Context Representations* 189

     6.6.3   *Exploration: Learning the Reber Grammar* . 189

     6.6.4   *Summary* 193

6.7   **Reinforcement Learning for Temporally Delayed Outcomes** 193

     6.7.1   *The Temporal Differences Algorithm* 195

     6.7.2   *Phase-Based Temporal Differences* 198

     6.7.3   *Exploration of TD: Classical Conditioning* . 199

6.8   **Summary** 202

6.9   **Further Reading** 202

6.1 Overview

Having developed and explored two different kinds of learning in the previous two chapters (Hebbian model learning in chapter 4 and error-driven task learning in chapter 5), we now explore their combination into one unified learning model. This model provides the advantages of both forms of learning, and it demonstrates some important synergies that arise from their combination.

We also explore two other kinds of learning mechanisms that are necessary to deal with tasks that: (1) involve temporally extended *sequential* processing, and (2) have temporally delayed contingencies. Both of these mechanisms can be implemented with simple extensions of our basic model and task learning framework, and both have a clear biological basis.

6.2 Combined Hebbian and Error-driven Learning

In this section, we address two important and related questions: (1) What are the relative advantages and disadvantages of Hebbian and error-driven learning, and

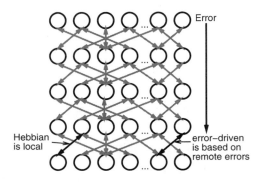

Figure 6.1: Illustration of the different fates of weights within a deep (many-layered) network under Hebbian versus error-driven learning. Hebbian learning is completely local — it is only a function of local activation correlations. In contrast, error-driven learning is ultimately a function of possibly remote error signals on other layers. This difference explains many of their relative advantages and disadvantages, as explained in the text and table 6.1.

	Pro	Con
Hebbian	autonomous,	myopic,
(local)	reliable	greedy
Error-driven	task-driven,	co-dependent,
(remote)	cooperative	lazy

Table 6.1: Summary of the pros and cons of Hebbian and error-driven learning, which can be attributed to the fact that Hebbian learning operates locally, whereas error-driven learning depends on remote error signals.

(2) How might these two forms of learning be used in the cortex? Then, we explore the combined use of Hebbian and error-driven learning in two simulations that highlight the advantages of their combination.

6.2.1 Pros and Cons of Hebbian and Error-Driven Learning

One can understand a number of the relative advantages and disadvantages of Hebbian and error-driven learning in terms of a single underlying property (figure 6.1 and table 6.1). This property is the *locality* of the learning algorithms — whether the changes to a given weight depend only on the immediate activations surrounding that weight (*local*), or the changes depend on more remote signals (*nonlocal*). Although both Hebbian and GeneRec error-driven learning can be *computed* locally as a function of activation signals, error-driven learning really depends on nonlocal error signals to drive weight changes, while Hebbian learning has no such remote dependence.

We can understand the superior task-learning performance of error-driven learning in terms of this locality difference. It is precisely because error-driven learning has this remote dependence on error signals elsewhere in the network that it is successful at learning tasks, because weights throughout the network (even in very early layers as pictured in figure 6.1) can be adjusted to solve a task that is only manifest in terms of error signals over a possibly quite distant output layer. Thus, all of the weights in the network can work together toward the common goal of solving the task. In contrast, Hebbian learning is so local as to be myopic and incapable of adjusting weights to serve the greater good of correct task performance — all Hebbian learning cares about is the local correlational structure over the inputs to a unit.

The locality of Hebbian learning mechanisms has its own advantages, however. In many situations, Hebbian learning can directly and immediately begin to develop useful representations by representing the principal correlational structure, without being dependent on possibly remote error signals that have to filter their way back through many layers of representations. With error-driven learning, the problem with all the weights trying to work together is that they often have a hard time sorting out who is going to do what, so that there is too much *interdependency*. This interdependency can result in very slow learning as these interdependencies work themselves out, especially in networks with many hidden layers (e.g., figure 6.1). Also, error-driven units tend to be somewhat "lazy" and just do whatever little bit that it takes to solve a problem, and nothing more.

A potentially useful metaphor for the contrast between error-driven and Hebbian learning comes from traditional left-wing versus right-wing approaches to governance. Error-driven learning is like left-wing politics (e.g., socialism) in that it seeks cooperative, organized solutions to overall problems, but it can get bogged down with bureaucracy in trying to ensure that everyone is working together for the common good. Also, by stifling individual motivation, socialism can induce a similar kind of laziness. In contrast, Hebbian learning is like right-wing politics in that it encourages rapid and decisive progress as motivated ("greedy") individuals do whatever they can in their local environment unfettered by government intervention, but with only some vague hope that things might eventually work out for the common good. All too often, local greed ends up impeding overall progress.

6.2.2 Advantages to Combining Hebbian and Error-Driven Learning

The second question posed earlier asks how Hebbian and error-driven learning might be used in the cortex. Does one part of the cortex perform Hebbian model learning, while another does error-driven task learning? Many practitioners in the field would probably assume that something like this is the case, with sensory processing proceeding largely, if not entirely, on the basis of model learning, while higher, more output oriented areas use task learning. Although there may be some general appeal to this division, we favor a more *centrist* view, where learning throughout the cortex is driven by a *balance* between error-driven and Hebbian factors operating at each synapse.

From a purely computational perspective, it seems likely that the most optimal learning will result from a combination of both error-driven and Hebbian learning, so that the advantages of one can counteract the disadvantages of the other. Specifically, the "motivated" local Hebbian learning can help to kickstart and shape the ongoing development of representations when the interdependencies of error-driven learning would otherwise lead to slow and lazy learning. At the same time, the power of error-driven learning can ensure that the weights are adjusted throughout the network to solve tasks.

In combining these two forms of learning, we have found it useful to remain somewhat "left of center," in the terms of the political metaphor — we consider error-driven task-based learning to be the primary form of learning, with Hebbian model learning playing an important but secondary role. This emphasis on task-based

learning provides assurances that tasks will get learned, but the addition of model learning provides some important *biases* that should facilitate learning in many ways.

In the field of machine learning, the use of such biases is often discussed in terms of **regularization**, where an otherwise underconstrained type of learning can benefit from the additional constraints imposed by these biases. A commonly used form of regularization in neural networks is **weight decay**, where a small portion of each weight value is subtracted when the weights are updated — this encourages the network to use only those weights that are reliably contributing something to the solution, because otherwise they will just decay to zero.

Hebbian learning can be a much better regularizer than weight decay because it actually makes a positive contribution to the development of representations instead of just subtracting away excess degrees of freedom in the weights. Of course, the types of representations formed by Hebbian learning must be at least somewhat appropriate for the task at hand for this to be a benefit, but we have argued that the representational biases imposed by Hebbian learning should be generally useful given the structure of our world (chapter 4). We will see many examples throughout the remainder of the text where Hebbian model learning plays a critical role in biasing error-driven learning, and we will explore these issues further in two simple demonstration tasks in subsequent sections.

Finally, we remind the reader that another good reason for combining error-driven and Hebbian learning is that the biological mechanism for synaptic modification discussed in section 5.8.3 suggests that both Hebbian and error-driven contributions are present at the synapse.

6.2.3 Inhibitory Competition as a Model-Learning Constraint

Inhibitory competition (e.g., with one of the kWTA functions) represents an important additional constraint on the learning process that can substantially improve the performance of the network. We think of this inhibitory competition as another kind of model-learning constraint (in addition to Hebbian learning), because it

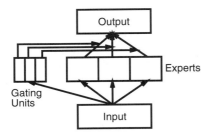

Figure 6.2: The mixtures-of-experts architecture, where the gating units undergo a soft WTA competition (aka softmax), and their output gates (multiplies) the contribution of their corresponding expert to the problem.

imposes a bias toward forming sparse distributed representations (models) of the environment, and is an essential aspect of the Hebbian model-learning framework, as we saw in the self-organizing exploration in chapter 4.

Although inhibitory competition of one form or another has long been used in a model learning context, it has not been used much in a task learning context. This is in part because a form of competition that allows distributed representations to develop (e.g., kWTA), which is essential for solving most interesting tasks, has not been widely used. The error derivatives of a competitive activation function, especially one that allows for distributed representations, can be also difficult to compute. As we saw in chapter 5, these derivatives are important for error-driven learning. We can avoid the derivative problem by using the GeneRec algorithm, because it computes the derivatives implicitly.

One context where something like inhibitory competition has been used in a task learning situation is in the **mixtures of experts** framework (Jacobs, Jordan, Nowlan, & Hinton, 1991), illustrated in figure 6.2. Here, a "soft" WTA (winner-take-all) competition takes place among a special group of units called the *gating* units, which then provide a multiplicative modulation of the outputs of corresponding groups of other units (the *experts*), which can specialize on solving different parts of the overall task.

Although each expert group can have distributed representations, many of the same limitations of WTA algorithms that operate on individual units apply here as well. For example, the extreme nature of the WTA competition encourages only one expert network to be active at a time, which limits the extent that different experts can cooperate to solve problems. Thus, the mixtures of experts algorithm just makes the individual "units" more powerful, but has the same limited overall dynamics as other WTA systems. In contrast, one can think of the effect of using a kWTA algorithm in a task-learning context as a better kind of fine-grained mixtures of experts mechanism, in that it encourages the specialization of different units to different aspects of the task but also allows cooperation and powerful distributed representations.

6.2.4 Implementation of Combined Model and Task Learning

The implementation of combined model and task learning is quite straightforward. It amounts to simply adding together the weight changes computed by Hebbian model learning with those computed by error-driven task learning. There is an additional parameter k_{hebb} (hebb in the simulator, which is a component of the lmix field that has err that is automatically set to 1-hebb) that controls the relative proportion or weighting of these two types of learning, according to the following function:

$$\Delta w_{ij} = k_{hebb}(\Delta_{hebb}) + (1 - k_{hebb})(\Delta_{err}) \quad (6.1)$$

where the two learning components Δ_{hebb} and Δ_{err} are given by the CPCA Hebbian rule (equation 4.12) and the CHL GeneRec error-driven rule (equation 5.39), respectively.

The hebb parameter is typically .01 or smaller (ranging down to .0005), and values larger than .05 are rarely used. This small magnitude reflects our emphasis on error-driven learning, and also some inherent differences in the magnitudes of the two different learning components. For example, error signals are typically much smaller in magnitude (especially after a bit of training) than Hebbian weight changes. Hebbian learning is also constantly imposing the same kind of pressure throughout learning, whereas error signals change often depending on what the network is getting right and wrong. Thus, the relative consistency of Hebbian learning makes it have a larger effective impact as well.

A relatively small value of `hebb` compensates for these inequalities in the magnitudes of the error-driven and Hebbian components.

It is important to note that the k_{hebb} parameter is mostly useful as a means of measuring the relative importance of Hebbian versus error-driven learning in different simulations — it is possible that a single value of this parameter would suffice for modeling all the different areas of the cortex. On the other hand, different areas could differ in this parameter, which might be one way in which genetic biological biases can influence the development and specialization of different areas (chapter 4).

Note that the Hebbian rule is computed using the plus-phase activation states, which makes sense both computationally (you want to move toward these activation states; there is not much sense in learning the statistical structure of mistakes), and biologically given the evidence that learning happens in the plus phase (section 5.8.3).

6.2.5 Summary

By combining error-driven and Hebbian learning with the unit and network properties discussed in previous chapters, we have developed a comprehensive set of principles for understanding how learning might work in the cortex, and explored both the biological and functional consequences of these principles. A summary illustration of these principles is provided in box 6.1, which captures the essential properties of the *Leabra* algorithm. These properties can be summarized according to six core principles (O'Reilly, 1998):

1. biological realism
2. distributed representations
3. inhibitory competition (kWTA)
4. bidirectional activation propagation
5. error-driven learning (GeneRec)
6. Hebbian learning (CPCA).

We have seen how these six principles have shaped our thinking about learning in the cortex, and we have also seen a glimpse of how these principles can have complex and interesting interactions. We have emphasized how error-driven and Hebbian learning can inter-

Box 6.1: Summary of Leabra Mechanisms

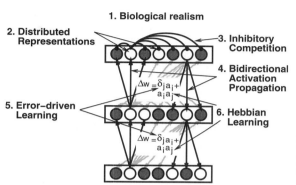

This figure provides an illustration of the six core principles behind Leabra. Biological realism (1) is an overarching constraint. Distributed representations (2) have multiple units active, while inhibitory competition (3, implemented in principle via inhibitory connectivity) ensures that relatively few such units are active. Bidirectional activation propagation (4, implemented by bidirectional connectivity) enables both bottom-up and top-down constraints to simultaneously shape the internal representation, and allows error signals to be propagated in a biologically plausible fashion. Error-driven learning (5) shapes representations according to differences between expected outputs and actual ones (represented by the error term δ_j). Hebbian learning (6) shapes representations according to the co-occurrence (correlation) statistics of items in the environment (represented by the product of the sending and receiving unit activations).

The activation function for Leabra was summarized in box 2.2 in chapter 2. The learning mechanism is a combination of Hebbian model learning via the CPCA Hebbian learning mechanism and error-driven task learning via the CHL version of GeneRec, as follows:

$$\Delta w_{ij} = \epsilon \left[k_{hebb} \left(y_j^+ (x_i^+ - w_{ij}) \right) \right.$$
$$\left. + (1 - k_{hebb}) \left(x_i^+ y_j^+ - x_i^- y_j^- \right) \right]$$

act in a positive way to produce better overall learning. In the next section, we will see that although bidirectional connectivity can sometimes cause problems, for example with generalization, these problems can be remedied by using the other principles (especially Hebbian learning and inhibitory competition). The subsequent section explores the interactions of error-driven and Hebbian learning in deep networks. The explorations of cognitive phenomena in the second part of the book build upon these basic foundations, and provide a richer understanding of the various implications of these core principles.

6.3 Generalization in Bidirectional Networks

One benefit of combining task and model learning in bidirectionally connected networks comes in *generalization*. Generalization is the ability to treat novel items systematically based on prior learning involving similar items. For example, people can pronounce the nonword "nust," which they've presumably never heard before, by analogy with familiar words like "must," "nun," and so on. This ability is central to an important function of the cortex — encoding the structure of the world so that an organism can act appropriately in novel situations. Generalization has played an important role in the debate about the extent to which neural networks can capture the regularities of the linguistic environment, as we will discuss in chapter 10. Generalization has also been a major focus in the study of machine learning (e.g., Weigend, Rumelhart, & Huberman, 1991; Wolpert, 1996b, 1996a; Vapnik & Chervonenkis, 1971).

In chapter 3, we briefly discussed how networks typically generalize in the context of distributed representations. The central idea is that if a network forms distributed internal representations that encode the compositional features of the environment in a combinatorial fashion, then novel stimuli can be processed successfully by activating the appropriate novel combination of representational (hidden) units. Although the combination is novel, the constituent features are familiar and have been trained to produce or influence appropriate outputs, such that the novel combination of features should also produce a reasonable result. In the domain of reading, a network can pronounce nonwords

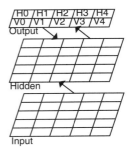

Figure 6.3: Network for the model-and-task exploration. The output units are trained to represent the existence of a line of a particular orientation in a given location, as indicated by the labels (e.g., H0 means horizontal in position 0 (bottom)).

correctly because it represents the pronunciation consequences of each letter using different units that can easily be recombined in novel ways for nonwords (as we will see in chapter 10).

We will see in the next exploration that the basic GeneRec network, as derived in chapter 5, does not generalize very well. Interactive networks like GeneRec are dynamic systems, with activation dynamics (e.g., *attractors* as discussed in chapter 3) that can interfere with the ability to form novel combinatorial representations. The units interact with each other too much to retain the kind of independence necessary for novel recombination (O'Reilly, in press, 1996b).

A solution to these problems of too much interactivity is more systematic attractor structures, for example *articulated* or *componential* attractors (Noelle & Cottrell, 1996; Plaut & McClelland, 1993). Purely error-driven GeneRec does not produce such clean, systematic representations, and therefore the attractor dynamics significantly interfere with generalization. As discussed previously, units in an error-driven network tend to be lazy, and just make the minimal contribution necessary to solve the problem. We will see that the addition of Hebbian learning and kWTA inhibitory competition improves generalization by placing important constraints on learning and the development of systematic representations.

6.3.1 Exploration of Generalization

Let's explore some of these ideas regarding the importance of Hebbian learning and inhibitory competition for generalization performance. We will explore one simple example that uses the oriented lines environment explored previously in the model learning chapter.

↪ Open project `model_and_task.proj.gz` in `chapter_6`.

Notice that the network now has an output layer — each of the ten output units corresponds with a horizontal or vertical line in one of the five different positions (figure 6.3).

The task to be learned by this network is quite simple — activate the appropriate output units for the combination of lines present in the input layer. This task provides a particularly clear demonstration of the generalization benefits of adding Hebbian learning to otherwise purely error-driven learning. However, because the task is so simple it does not provide a very good demonstration of the weaknesses of pure Hebbian learning, which is actually capable of learning this task most of the time. The next section includes demonstrations of the limitations of Hebbian learning.

The `model_task_ctrl` control panel contains three learning parameters in the `lrn` field. The first two subfields of `lrn` control the learning rate of the network weights (`lrate`) and the bias weights (`bias_lrate`). The `bias_lrate` is 0 for pure Hebbian learning because it has no way of training the bias weights, and is equal to `lrate` for error-driven learning. The third subfield is the parameter `hebb`, which determines the relative weighting of Hebbian learning compared to error-driven learning (equation 6.1). This is the main parameter we will investigate to compare purely Hebbian (model) learning (hebb=1), purely error-driven (task) learning (hebb=0), and their combination (hebb between 0 and 1). Because we have to turn off the learning in the bias weights when doing pure Hebbian learning, we will use the `learn_rule` field to select the learning rule, which sets all of the parameters appropriately. Let's begin with pure error-driven (task) learning.

↪ Set `learn_rule` to `PURE_ERR`, and `Apply`.

Let's see how the network is trained.

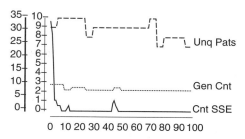

Figure 6.4: Graph log, showing count of trials with training errors (Cnt SSE, solid line, red in actual network), number of lines distinctly represented (Unq Pats, dashed, yellow), and generalization error (Gen Cnt, dotted, green — note that this is on the same scale as the training SSE).

↪ Press `Step` in the control panel.

This is the minus phase of processing for the first event, showing two lines presented in the input, and undoubtedly the wrong output units activated. Now let's see the plus phase.

↪ Press `Step` again.

The output units should now reflect the 2 lines present in the input (position 0 is bottom/left).

↪ You can continue to `Step` through more trials.

The network is only being trained on 35 out of the 45 total patterns, with the remaining 10 reserved for testing generalization. Because each of the individual lines is presented during training, the network should be able to recognize them in the novel combinations of the testing set. In other words, the network should be able to generalize to the testing items by processing the novel patterns in terms of novel combinations of existing hidden representations, which have appropriate associations to the output units.

↪ After you tire of `Stepping`, open up a training graph log using `View`, `TRAIN_GRAPH_LOG`, and then press `Run`. You should turn off the `Display` button on the network, and watch the graph log.

As the network trains, the graph log is updated every epoch with the training error statistic, and every 5 epochs with two important test statistics (figure 6.4). Instead of using raw SSE for the training error statistic, we will often use a count of the number of events for which there is any error at all (again using the .5 threshold on

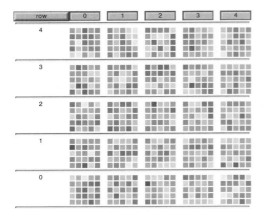

Figure 6.5: Final weights after training with pure error-driven learning. Note how random they look compared to the weights learned when Hebbian learning is used (cf. figure 4.13).

each unit), so that each unit has to have its activation on the right side of .5 for the event not to be counted in this measure. This is plotted in the red line in the graph log, and the simulator labels it as `cnt_sum_se` in the log.

One of the test statistics, plotted in green, measures the *generalization* performance of the network (`gen_cnt`). The green line plots this generalization performance in terms of the number of testing events that the network gets *wrong* (out of the 10 testing items), so the smaller this value, the better the generalization performance. This network appears to be quite bad at generalizing, with 9 of the 10 novel testing patterns having errors.

The other test statistic, plotted in yellow (`unq_pats`), is the same unique pattern statistic as used before (section 4.8.1), which measures the extent to which the hidden units represent the lines distinctly (from 0 meaning no lines distinctly represented to 10 meaning all lines distinctly represented). This unique pattern statistic shows that the hidden units do not uniquely represent all of the lines distinctly, though this statistic does not seem nearly as bad as either the generalization error or the weights that we consider next.

↪ Do `View`, `WT_MAT_LOG` in the control panel, to display the weight values for each of the hidden units.

You should see that the weights look relatively random (figure 6.5) and clearly do not reflect the linear structure of the underlying environment. To see how much these weights change over learning from the truly random initial weights, we can run again and watch the weight log, which is updated every 5 epochs as before.
↪ Press `Run`.

The generalization error measure, the hidden unit weights, and the unique pattern statistic all provide converging evidence for a coherent story about why generalization is poor in a purely error-driven network. As we said, generalization here depends on being able to recombine representations that systematically encode the individual line elements independent of their specific training contexts. In contrast, error-driven weights are generally relatively underconstrained by learning tasks, and thus reflect a large contribution from the initial random values, rather than the kind of systematicity needed for good generalization. This lack of constraint prevents the units from systematically carving up the input/output mapping into separable subsets that can be independently combined for the novel testing items — instead, each unit participates haphazardly in many different aspects of the mapping. The attractor dynamics in the network then impair generalization performance. Thus, the poor generalization arises due to the effects of the partially-random weights on the attractor dynamics of the network, preventing it from combining novel line patterns in a systematic fashion.

To determine how representative this particular result is, we can run a batch of 5 training runs. To record the results of these training runs, we need to open up a few logs.
↪   Do `View`, `TRAIN_TEXT_LOG`, and `View`, `BATCH_TEXT_LOG`, and then press the `Batch` button on the control panel.

The batch text log will present summary statistics from the 5 training runs, and the train text log shows the final results after each training run.

Question 6.1 *Report the summary statistics from the batch text log (`Batch_1_Textlog` for your batch run. Does this indicate that your earlier observations were generally applicable?*

Given the explanation above about the network's poor generalization, it should be clear why both Hebbian learning and kWTA inhibitory competition can improve generalization performance. At the most general level, they constitute additional *biases* that place important constraints on learning and the development of representations. More specifically, Hebbian learning constrains the weights to represent the correlational structure of the inputs to a given unit, producing systematic weight patterns (e.g., cleanly separated *clusters* of strong correlations; chapter 4).

Inhibitory competition helps in two ways. First, it encourages individual units to specialize on representing a subset of items, thus parceling up the task in a much cleaner and more systematic way than would occur in an otherwise unconstrained network. Second, as discussed in chapter 3 (section 3.6.3), inhibitory competition restricts the settling dynamics of the network, greatly constraining the number of states that the network can settle into, and thus eliminating a large proportion of the attractors that can hijack generalization.

Let's see if we can improve the network's generalization performance by adding some Hebbian learning. We cannot easily test the effects of kWTA inhibition in our simulation framework, because removing inhibitory competition necessitates other problematic compensatory manipulations such as the use of positive/negative valued weights; however, clear advantages for inhibitory competition in generalization have been demonstrated elsewhere (O'Reilly, in press).

↪ Set `learn_rule` on the control panel to `HEBB_AND_ERR`, and `Apply`.

You should see a `lrn.hebb` value of .05 in the control panel now.

↪ Do a `Run` in the control panel (you may want to do a `View` of the `TRAIN_GRAPH_LOG` if that window was iconified or is otherwise no longer visible). After this, do a `Batch` run to collect more data.

Question 6.2 (a) *How did this .05 of additional Hebbian learning change the results compared to purely error-driven learning?* (b) *Report the results from the batch text log (`Batch_1_Textlog`) for the batch run.* (c) *Explain these results in terms of the weight patterns, the unique pattern statistic, and the general ef-*

fects of Hebbian learning in representing the correlational structure of the input.

You should have seen a substantial improvement from adding the Hebbian learning. Now, let's see how well pure Hebbian learning does on this task.

↪ Set `learn_rule` to `PURE_HEBB` and `Apply`.

This changes `lrn.hebb` to 1, and sets `lrn.bias_lrate` to 0.

↪ Do a `Run`.

You will probably notice that the network learns quite rapidly. The network will frequently get perfect performance on the task itself, and on the generalization test. However, every 5 or so runs, the network fails to learn perfectly, and, due to the inability of Hebbian learning to correct such errors, never gets better.

↪ To find such a case more rapidly, you can press `Stop` when the network has already learned perfectly (so you don't have to wait until it finishes the prescribed number of epochs), and then press `Run` again.

Because this task has such obvious correlational structure that is well suited for the Hebbian learning algorithm, it is clear why Hebbian learning helps. However, even here, the network is more reliable if error-driven learning is also used. We will see in the next task that Hebbian learning helps even when the correlational structure is not particularly obvious, but that pure Hebbian learning is completely incapable of learning. These lessons apply across a range of different generalization tests, including ones that rely on more holistic similarity-based generalization, as compared to the compositional (feature-based) domain explored here (O'Reilly, in press, 1996b).

↪ Go to the `PDP++Root` window. To continue on to the next simulation, close this project first by selecting `.projects/Remove/Project_0`. Or, if you wish to stop now, quit by selecting `Object/Quit`.

6.4 Learning to Re-represent in Deep Networks

One of the other critical benefits of combined model and task learning is in the training of deep networks (with many hidden layers). As we explained previously, additional hidden layers enable the re-representation of problems in ways that make them easier to solve. This is clearly true of the cortex, where in the visual system for example the original retinal array is re-represented in a large number of different ways, many of which build upon each other over many "hidden layers" (Desimone & Ungerleider, 1989; Van Essen & Maunsell, 1983; Maunsell & Newsome, 1987). We explore a multi-hidden layer model of visual object recognition in chapter 8.

A classic example of a problem that benefits from multiple hidden layers is the *family trees* problem of Hinton (1986). In this task, the network learns the family relationships for two isomorphic families. This learning is facilitated by re-representing in an intermediate hidden layer the individuals in the family to encode more specifically their functional similarities (i.e., individuals who enter into similar relationships are represented similarly). The importance of this re-representation was emphasized in chapters 3 and 5 as a central property of cognition.

However, the deep network used in this example makes it difficult for a purely error-driven network to learn, with a standard backpropagation network taking thousands of epochs to solve the problem (although carefully chosen parameters can reduce this to around 100 epochs). Furthermore, the poor depth scaling of error-driven learning is even worse in bidirectionally connected networks, where training times are twice as long as in the feedforward case, and seven times longer than when using a combination of Hebbian and error-driven learning (O'Reilly, 1996b).

This example, which we will explore in the subsequent section, is consistent with the general account of the problems with remote error signals in deep networks presented previously (section 6.2.1). We can elaborate this example by considering the analogy of balancing a stack of poles (figure 6.6). It is easier to balance one tall pole than an equivalently tall stack of poles placed one atop the other, because the corrective movements made by moving the base of the pole back and forth have a direct effect on a single pole, while the effects are indirect on poles higher up in a stack. Thus, with a stack of poles, the corrective movements made on the bottom pole have increasingly remote effects on the poles higher up, and the nature of these effects depends on the position of the poles lower down. Similarly, the er-

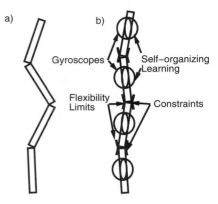

Figure 6.6: Illustration of the analogy between error-driven learning in deep networks and balancing a stack of poles, which is more difficult in **a)** than in **b)**. Hebbian self-organizing model learning is like adding a gyroscope to each pole, as it gives each layer some guidance (stability) on how to learn useful representations. Constraints like inhibitory competition restrict the flexibility of motion of the poles.

ror signals in a deep network have increasingly indirect and remote effects on layers further down (away from the training signal at the output layer) in the network, and the nature of the effects depends on the representations that have developed in the shallower layers (nearer the output signal). With the increased nonlinearity associated with bidirectional networks, this problem only gets worse.

One way to make the pole-balancing problem easier is to give each pole a little internal gyroscope, so that they each have greater self-stability and can at least partially balance themselves. Model learning should provide exactly this kind of self-stabilization, because the learning is local and produces potentially useful representations even in the absence of error signals. At a slightly more abstract level, a combined task and model learning system is generally more constrained than a purely error-driven learning algorithm, and thus has fewer degrees of freedom to adapt through learning. These constraints can be thought of as limiting the range of motion for each pole, which would also make them easier to balance. We will explore these ideas in the following simulation of the family trees problem, and in many of the subsequent chapters.

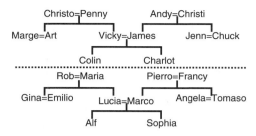

Figure 6.7: The family tree structure learned in the *family trees* task. There are two isomorphic families, one English and one Italian. The = symbol indicates marriage.

6.4.1 Exploration of a Deep Network

Now, let's explore the case of learning in a deep network using the same family trees task as O'Reilly (1996b) and Hinton (1986). The structure of the environment is shown in figure 6.7. The network is trained to produce the correct name in response to questions like "Rob is married to whom?" These questions are presented by activating one of 24 name units in an *agent* input layer (e.g., "Rob"), in conjunction with one of 12 units in a *relation* input layer (e.g., "Married"), and training the network to produce the correct unit activation over the *patient* output layer.

↪ Open project `family_trees.proj.gz` in `chapter_6`.

First, notice that the network (figure 6.8) has `Agent` and `Relation` input layers, and a `Patient` output layer all at the bottom of the network. These layers have *localist* representations of the 24 different people and 12 different relationships, which means that there is no "overt" similarity in these input patterns between any of the people. Thus, the `Agent_Code`, `Relation_Code`, and `Patient_Code` hidden layers provide a means for the network to re-represent these localist representations as richer distributed patterns that should facilitate the learning of the mapping by emphasizing relevant distinctions and deemphasizing irrelevant ones. The central `Hidden` layer is responsible for performing the mapping between these recoded representations to produce the correct answers.

↪ Press `View` and select `EVENTS` on the `family_trees_ctrl` control panel.

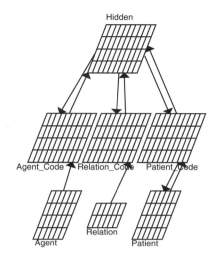

Figure 6.8: The family tree network, with intermediate *Code* hidden layers that re-represent the input/output patterns.

This will bring up a window displaying the first ten training events, which should help you to understand how the task is presented to the network.

↪ Go ahead and scroll down the events list, and see the names of the different events presented to the network (you can click on any that look particularly interesting to see how they are represented).

Now, let's see how this works with the network itself.

↪ Press the `Step` button in the control panel.

The activations in the network display reflect the minus phase state for the first training event (selected at random from the list of all training events).

↪ Press `Step` again to see the plus phase activations.

The default network is using a combination of Hebbian and GeneRec error-driven learning, with the amount of Hebbian learning set to .01 as reflected by the `lrn.hebb` parameter in the control panel. Let's see how long it takes this network to learn the task.

↪ Open up a graph log to monitor training by pressing `View`, `TRAIN_GRAPH_LOG`, turn the `Display` of the network off, and press `Run` to allow the network to train on all the events rapidly.

As the network trains, the graph log displays the error count statistic for training (in red) and the average number of network settling cycles (in orange).

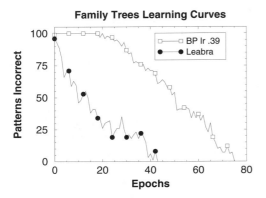

Figure 6.9: Learning curves for family trees task, showing that combination of Hebbian (model) and error-driven (task) learning in Leabra results in faster learning in deep networks compared to pure error-driven learning in a backpropagation network (BP).

Your network should train in around 40 to 50 epochs using the initial default parameters. This may take a while. You can either wait, or you can instead load the results from a fully trained network.

↪   If you decide to wait while your network trains to completion, do `Object/SaveAs` in the network window after training is done, and save it with some descriptive name — we will want to come back to it later.

↪   If you instead opt to load the results from a fully trained network, press `Stop` in the control panel. To load the network's learning curve into the graph log, go to the graph log and select menu `LogFile/Load File`, and choose `family_trees.hebb_err.epc.log`.

The network took 41 epochs to learn, which is indicated in the network file name. Note that the graph log goes from 0 to 40 (41 total).

The 41 epochs it took for the default network to learn the problem is actually relatively rapid learning for a deep network like this one. For example, figure 6.9 shows a comparison of a typical learning curve in Leabra versus the fastest standard feedforward backpropagation network (BP, see box 5.2), which took about 77 epochs to learn and required a very large learning rate of .39 compared to the standard .01 for the Leabra network (O'Reilly, 1996b).

We are not so interested in raw learning speed for its own sake, but more in the facilitation of learning in deep networks from the additional biases or constraints imposed by combining model and task learning. Figure 6.9 shows that these additional constraints facilitate learning in deep networks; the purely task-driven BP network learns relatively slowly, whereas the Leabra network, with both Hebbian learning and inhibitory competition, learns relatively quickly. In this exploration (as in the previous one), we will manipulate the contribution of Hebbian learning. To do this, we can run a network without Hebbian learning and compare the learning times.

↪   If you want to wait while the network trains, set `learn_rule` to `PURE_ERR`, and `Apply`. You will see the `lrn.hebb` change to 0. Then `Run` again.

Again, if you do not want to wait for the network to train, you can just load the results from a fully trained network.

↪   In this case, go to the graph log, and select `LogFile/Load File`, and choose `family_trees.pure_err.epc.log`.

Hebbian learning clearly facilitates learning in deep networks, as demonstrated by the network taking longer to learn without it (81 epochs in this case compared to 41; repeated runs of the networks with different parameters substantiate this effect). Further, kWTA activation constraints play an important facilitatory role in learning as well. The benefits of kWTA activation constraints are somewhat obscured in comparing the purely error-driven Leabra network with the backpropagation (BP) network shown in figure 6.9, because of the very high learning rate used for finding the best performance of the BP network. The benefits of kWTA activation constraints are particularly clear in comparing the purely error-driven Leabra network to a bidirectionally-connected error-driven (GeneRec) network that does not have the kWTA activation constraints, which takes around 300 or more epochs to learn at its fastest (O'Reilly, 1996b).

Now, let's see what pure Hebbian learning can do in this task.

↪   Select `PURE_HEBB` for `learn_rule`, and re-run the network. You can `Stop` it after 10 epochs or so.

This network isn't going to improve at all. You can

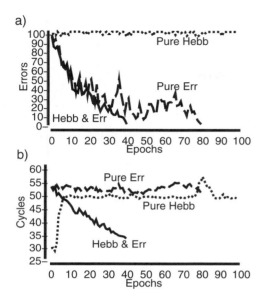

Figure 6.10: Graph log display showing both errors **(a)** And cycles **(b)** Over epochs of training for the three different network learning parameters: pure error driven learning (Pure Err), pure Hebbian learning (Pure Hebb) and combined Hebbian and error-driven learning (Hebb & Err), which performs the best.

see this by loading the graph log for a network trained for 100 epochs.

↪ Select `LogFile/Load File` in the graph log, and choose `family_trees.pure_hebb.epc.log`.

Although Hebbian model learning is useful for helping error-driven learning, the graph shows that it is simply not capable of learning tasks like this on its own.

We next compare all three cases with each other.

↪ Load the `family_trees.all.epc.log` log file.

This log display has the three runs overlaid on each other (figure 6.10). You can identify the lines based on what epoch they end on (40 = HEBB_AND_ERR, 80 = PURE_ERR, and 100 = PURE_HEBB). It is interesting to note that the orange line (average settling cycles) is fairly well correlated with the training error, and only the combined Hebb and error network achieves a significant speedup in cycles. You might also note that the pure Hebb case starts out with very quick settling in the first few epochs, and then *slows down* over training.

Question 6.3 (a) *What do you notice about the general shape of the standard backpropagation (BP) learning curve (SSE over epochs) in figure 6.9 compared to that of the* PURE_ERR *Leabra network you just ran? Pay special attention to the first 30 or so epochs of learning.* **(b)** *Given that one of the primary differences between these two cases is that the* PURE_ERR *network has inhibitory competition via the kWTA function, whereas BP does not, speculate about the possible importance of this competition for learning based on these results (also note that the BP network has a much larger learning rate, .39 vs .01).* **(c)** *Now, compare the* PURE_ERR *case with the original* HEBB_AND_ERR *case (i.e., where do the SSE learning curves (red lines) start to diverge, and how is this different from the BP case)?* **(d)** *What does this suggest about the role of Hebbian learning? (Hint: Error signals get smaller as the network has learned more.)*

To get a sense of how learning has shaped the *transformations* performed by this network to emphasize relevant similarities, we can do a cluster plot of the hidden unit activity patterns over all the inputs. Let's do a comparison between the initial clusters and those after learning for the default network.

↪ First, press `ReInit` on the overall control panel to reinitialize the weights. Then, press `Cluster`.

After a bit (it tests all 100 patterns, so be patient), a cluster plot window will appear. We will compare this cluster plot to one for the trained network.

↪ Go to the network window and select from the menu at the upper left: `Object/Load`, and then select `family_trees.hebb_err.00.041.net.gz` (or the network that you saved). Do `Cluster` again.

Your results should look something like figure 6.11. There are many ways in which people who appear together can be justifiably related, so you may think there is some sensibility to the initial plot. However, the final plot has a much more sensible structure in terms of the overall nationality difference coming out as the two largest clusters, and individuals within a given generation tending to be grouped together within these overall clusters. The network is able to solve the task by transforming the patterns in this way.

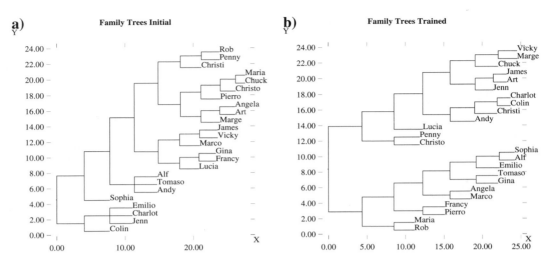

Figure 6.11: Cluster plot of hidden unit representations: **a)** Prior to learning. **b)** After learning to criterion using combined Hebbian and error-driven learning. The trained network has two branches corresponding to the two different families, and clusters within organized generally according to generation.

↪ Go to the `PDP++Root` window. To continue on to the next simulation, close this project first by selecting `.projects/Remove/Project_0`. Or, if you wish to stop now, quit by selecting `Object/Quit`.

6.5   Sequence and Temporally Delayed Learning

[Note: The remaining sections in the chapter are required for only a subset of the models presented in the second part of the book, so it is possible to skip them for the time being, returning later as necessary to understand the specific models that make use of these additional learning mechanisms.]

So far, we have only considered relatively static, discrete kinds of tasks, where a given output pattern (response, expectation, etc.) depends only on the given input pattern. However, many real-world tasks have dependencies that extend over time. An obvious example is language, where the meaning of this sentence, for example, depends on the sequence of words within the sentence. In spoken language, the words themselves are constructed from a temporally extended sequence of distinct sound patterns or *phonemes*. There are many other examples, including most daily tasks (e.g., mak-

ing breakfast, driving to work). Indeed, it would seem that sequential tasks of one sort or another are the norm, not the exception.

We consider three categories of temporal dependency: *sequential*, *temporally delayed*, and *continuous trajectories*. In the **sequential** case, there is a sequence of discrete events, with some structure (*grammar*) to the sequence that can be learned. This case is concerned with just the *order* of events, not their detailed timing.

In the **temporally delayed** case, there is a delay between *antecedent* events and their *outcomes*, and the challenge is to learn causal relationships despite these delays. For example, one often sees lightning several seconds before the corresponding thunder is heard (or smoke before the fire, etc.). The rewards of one's labors, for another example, are often slow in coming (e.g., the benefits of a college degree, or the payoff from a financial investment). One important type of learning that has been applied to temporally delayed problems is called **reinforcement learning**, because it is based on the idea that temporally delayed reinforcement can be propagated backward in time to update the association between earlier antecedent states and their likelihood of causing subsequent reinforcement.

The third case of **continuous trajectories** is one that we will not focus on very much. Here, the relevant information is in the detailed temporal evolution of what might be best described as a continuous system, rather than just in the order of a discrete set of events as characterized by the sequential case. This kind of continuous information is probably quite important for motor control and some perceptual tasks (e.g., perception of motion).

We do not focus on continuous trajectory learning because it is complex and does not fit well within our existing framework. Mechanistically, representing a continuous trajectory depends critically on the detailed temporal response characteristics of neurons. From a biological perspective, many parameters other than weights are likely to be critical, with the self-regulating channels described in chapter 2 providing just one example of the considerable complexities in temporal response that biological neurons can exhibit. Thus, adapting these parameters in a useful way would require very different kinds of mechanisms than we have explored previously. Furthermore, the available computational mechanisms for learning continuous trajectories (e.g., Williams & Zipser, 1989; Pearlmutter, 1989; Williams & Peng, 1990) are far from biologically plausible, and they do not tend to work very well on anything but relatively simple tasks either.

Nevertheless, it may be possible to model some continuous trajectory phenomena by "digitizing" a trajectory into a sequence of events by taking a set of snapshots at regular intervals, and then use the mechanisms developed for sequential tasks. We do not mean to imply that sequential learning is mutually exclusive with temporally delayed learning — indeed, we actually think there may be an intimate relationship between the two, as discussed further in chapters 9 and 11.

Learning in sequential or temporally delayed tasks is generally much more difficult than learning direct input/output mappings. Adding intervening time steps between input-output contingencies can be a lot like adding extra hidden layers to a network. Indeed, there is a way of learning over time with backpropagation where each additional time step is equivalent to adding a new hidden layer between the input and output layers (Rumelhart et al., 1986a). Thus, given the advantages of

the model learning biases (specifically Hebbian learning and inhibitory competition) for learning in deep networks, one might expect that they will also be useful for learning temporally extended tasks. The example we explore below indicates that this is likely the case. We will follow this up with more interesting and complex, cognitively relevant tasks in the second part of the book.

We first explore the use of *context* representations to deal with learning sequential tasks, and then move on to the use of reinforcement learning to handle temporally delayed learning.

6.6 Context Representations and Sequential Learning

The central problem in learning sequential tasks is developing useful **context** representations that capture the information from previous events that is needed to produce an appropriate output (or interpretation) at some later point in time. In the simplest case, called the **Markovian** case, the only prior context necessary to predict the next step in the sequence is contained in the immediately preceding time step. This case is particularly convenient because it avoids the storage problems (and consequent decisions about what information to throw away) that arise when the context must include information from many prior time steps.

In a non-Markovian task, one must expand the context representation (i.e., prior state representation) to contain all the necessary contingencies from prior states. A trivial example of this is one where the context representation literally contains a copy of all prior states. Obviously, such a strategy is impossible with limited capacity memory systems, so some kind of adaptive, strategic memory system must be used to maintain just the right context information. Although the neural network mechanisms we explore here are not particularly powerful in this respect, chapter 9 shows how these mechanisms can be augmented with a more intelligent control mechanism to successfully handle non-Markovian tasks.

Two closely related types of neural network models that incorporate a Markovian-style context representation were developed by Jordan (1986) and Elman (1990), and are often called *Jordan* and *Elman*

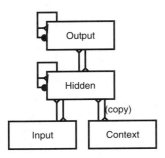

Figure 6.12: Simple recurrent network (SRN), where the context layer is a copy of the hidden layer activations from the previous time step.

networks. The category that includes both models is known as a **simple recurrent network** or **SRN**, which is the terminology that we will use. The context representation in an SRN is contained in a special layer that acts just like another input layer, except that its activity state is set to be a copy of the prior hidden or output unit activity states for the Elman and Jordan nets, respectively (figure 6.12). We prefer the hidden state-based context layer because it gives the network considerable flexibility in choosing the contents of the context representations, by learning representations in the hidden layer. This flexibility can partially overcome the essentially Markovian copying procedure.

We adopt the basic SRN idea as our main way of dealing with sequential tasks. Before exploring the basic SRN, a couple of issues must be addressed. First, the nature of the context layer representations and their updating must be further clarified from a computational perspective. Then we need to examine the biological plausibility of such representations. We then explore a simulation of the basic SRN.

6.6.1 Computational Considerations for Context Representations

In the standard conception of the SRN, the context layer is a literal copy of the hidden layer. Although this is computationally convenient, it is not necessary for the basic function performed by this layer. Instead, the context layer can be any information-preserving transformation of the hidden layer, because there is a set of adapting weights going from the context to the hidden layer that can adapt to a fixed (or slowly updating) transformation of the hidden layer representations by the context layer. This point will be important for the possible biological implementation of context.

Although it is not essential that the context layer be a literal copy of the hidden layer, it is essential that the context layer be updated in a very controlled manner. For example, an alternative idea about how to implement a context layer (one that might seem easier to imagine the biology implementing using the kinds of network dynamics described in chapter 3) would be to just have an additional layer of "free" context units, presumably recurrently connected amongst themselves to enable sustained activation over time, that somehow maintain information about prior states without any special copying operation. These context units would instead just communicate with the hidden layer via standard bidirectional connections. However, there are a couple of problems with this scenario.

First, there is a basic tradeoff for these context units. They must preserve information about the prior hidden state as the hidden units settle into a new state with a new input, but then they must update their representations to encode the new hidden state. Thus, these units need to be alternately both stable and updatable, which is not something that generic activation functions do very well, necessitating a special context layer that is updated in a controlled manner rather than "free" context units. Second, even if free context units could strike a balance between stability and updating through their continuous activation trajectory over settling, the error-driven learning procedure (GeneRec) would be limited because it does not take into account this activation trajectory; instead, learning is based on the final activation states. Controlled updating of the context units allows both preserved and updated representations to govern learning. For these reasons, the free context representation does not work, as simulations easily demonstrate.

For most of our simulations, we use a simple copying operation to update the context representations. The equation for the update of a context unit c_j is:

$$c_j(t) = fm_{hid}h_j(t-1) + fm_{prv}c_j(t-1) \quad (6.2)$$

where the parameter fm_{hid} (meaning "from hidden," a

value between 0 and 1) determines the extent to which the context unit gets updated by new input from the hidden layer, and fm_{prv} ("from previous," also between 0 and 1, and typically set to $1 - k_{hid}$) determines how much it reflects its previous state. The ability of the context units to reflect their prior state (introduced by Jordan, 1986) gives them some limited additional capacity to maintain information beyond the 1 time-step Markovian window. In the basic SRN, fm_{hid} and fm_{prv} are constants (that we typically set to .7 and .3), but we will see in chapter 9 that these parameters can be placed under dynamic control by a specialized *gating mechanism* to control the update of context.

Appendix B contains a detailed description of how to construct an SRN context layer in the simulator.

6.6.2 Possible Biological Bases for Context Representations

Perhaps the most obvious candidate brain area for having something like a context representation is the **frontal cortex**. As discussed in greater detail in chapters 9 and 11, the frontal cortex (especially the prefrontal cortex) seems to be involved in planning and executing temporally extended behaviors. For example, people with frontal lesions are often incapable of executing a sequence of behaviors, even for somewhat routine tasks such as making a cup of coffee, even though they can perform each individual step perfectly well. Thus, they appear to have a specific deficit in *sequencing* these steps.

In addition to sequencing, the frontal cortex appears to be important for maintaining representations over time. Cohen and Servan-Schreiber (1992) argued, and demonstrated with neural network models, that this internal maintenance system is important for what they called *context*. For example, consider ambiguous words such as *pen* that require some kind of context to disambiguate their meaning (e.g., writing implement vs. fenced enclosure). They argued that the frontal cortex is responsible for maintaining the necessary internal context to disambiguate these words, where the context is established by information presented earlier in a text passage. Further, they showed that people with impairments in frontal functioning (schizophrenics) can

use context appearing immediately before an ambiguous word, but not context from a previous sentence.

The intersection of both of these findings, sequencing and internal context maintenance, points directly to something like the SRN context layer, which provides the context necessary for sequential or temporally extended tasks. Further, these data (and many more like them) show that such context representations are used not only to *produce* sequential behavior, but also to *comprehend* sequentially presented information like language (see chapter 10 for a model of this).

In addition to neuropsychological/behavioral data on frontal cortex, there is a lot of evidence that neurons in this brain area exhibit sustained firing over task-relevant delays and sequences (e.g., Goldman-Rakic, 1987; Fuster, 1989; Miller, Erickson, & Desimone, 1996; Barone & Joseph, 1989). Anatomically, the frontal cortex receives from and projects to most other areas of posterior (nonfrontal) cortex, so it has the requisite connectivity to both produce appropriate context representations and have these context representations affect ongoing processing in the posterior system (which is then considered to be like the hidden layer in figure 6.12). As we argued previously, it is not necessary that the frontal context be a literal copy of the posterior cortex.

6.6.3 Exploration: Learning the Reber Grammar

A good example of a task illustrating how the SRN works is the **Reber grammar** task, modeled by Cleeremans, Servan-Schreiber, and McClelland (1989). Reber (1967) was one of the first psychologists to investigate *implicit* learning capabilities, which he explored by having people memorize strings of letters that, unbeknownst to the subject, followed a regular, but probabilistic, grammar. Cleeremans and McClelland (1991) investigated a version of Reber's implicit learning task where participants pushed buttons corresponding to letters that appeared on a computer screen. Subjects ended up pressing the buttons faster and faster for grammatical sequences of letters, but they were not significantly faster for sequences that did not follow the grammar. Thus, they had shown evidence of learning this grammar implicitly, but they explicitly had no knowledge of this grammar.

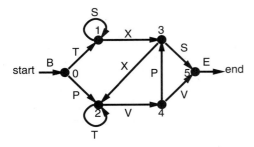

Figure 6.13: The simple finite-state grammar used by Reber (1967). A string from the grammar is produced by starting at the *start*, and generating the letter along the link followed, with links chosen at each node at random with probability .5 for each. The string ends when *end* is reached. An example string would be BTSSSXXTTVVE.

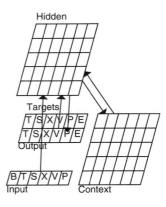

Figure 6.14: The FSA network, with input/output units representing the surface letters, and an SRN-style context layer.

The grammar that Reber (1967) used is shown in figure 6.13. This figure describes a **finite state automaton** (FSA) or **finite state grammar**, which generates a string of letters by emitting the letter corresponding to the link that the automaton takes as it jumps from node to node. Thus, a sequence would be produced as follows: The automaton always starts in the *start* node (0), which generates the letter *B*. Then, with equal (.5) probability, the next node is chosen (either 1 or 2), which generates either the letter *T* or *P*. This process of probabilistically going from node to node and generating the letter along the link continues until the *end* node (and the corresponding letter *E*) have been reached. Thus, the connectivity of the nodes defines the regularities present in the grammar.

Cleeremans et al. (1989) used an SRN to learn the Reber grammar by training the network to predict the next letter in the sequence (as the output of the network) given the prior one as an input. If each link in the FSA had a unique letter, this prediction task would be relatively easy, because the input would uniquely identify the location within the FSA. However, because different links have the same letter, some kind of internal context is necessary to keep track, based on prior history, of where we are within the grammar. This keeping track is what the context layer of the SRN does.

Because the next letter in the FSA sequence is actually chosen at random from among two possible

choices, the best a network can do is either activate both of these choices, or pick one of the two at random. The backpropagation network used by Cleeremans et al. (1989) cannot pick items at random – it always produces a *blend* of the possible outputs. However, as we will see in more detail in chapter 9, a Leabra network can pick one of multiple possible output patterns essentially at random, and we will take advantage of this in this simulation.

↪ **Open project** fsa.proj.gz in chapter_6 **to begin the exploration of FSA learning.**

We begin by exploring the network (figure 6.14).

↪ **Click on** r.wt **and observe the connectivity.**

Note in particular that the context layer units have a single receiving weight from the hidden units. The context units use this connection to determine which hidden unit to update from (but the weight is not used, and just has a random value). Otherwise, the network is standardly fully connected. Notice also that there is a seemingly extraneous Targets layer, which is not connected to anything. This is simply for display purposes — it shows the two possible valid outputs, which can be compared to the actual output.

Let's view the activations, and see a few trials of learning.

↪ **Click on** act **in the network, and make sure the** Display **toggle is on. Then, press** Step **in the control panel.**

This is the minus phase for the beginning of a *sequence* (one pass through the FSA grammar), which always starts with the letter B, and the context units zeroed. The network will produce some random expectation of which letters are coming next. Note that there is some noise in the unit activations — this helps them pick one unit out of the two possible ones at random.

↪ Then, Step again to see the plus phase.

You should see that one of the two possible subsequent letters (T or P) is strongly activated — this unit indicates which letter actually came next in the sequence. Thus, the network only ever learns about one of the two possible subsequent letters on each trial (because they are chosen at random). It has to learn that a given node has two possible outputs by integrating experience over different trials, which is one of the things that makes this a somewhat challenging task to learn.

An interesting aspect of this task is that even when the network has done as well as it possibly could, it should still make roughly 50 percent "errors," because it ends up making a discrete guess as to which output will come next, which can only be right 50 percent of the time. This could cause problems for learning if it introduced a systematic error signal that would constantly increase or decrease the bias weights. This is not a problem because a unit will be correctly active about as often as it will be incorrectly inactive, so the overall net error will be zero. Note that if we allowed both units to become active this would not be the case, because one of the units would always be incorrectly active, and this would introduce a net negative error and large negative bias weights (which would eventually shut down the activation of the output units).

One possible objection to having the network pick one output at random instead of allowing both to be on, is that it somehow means that the network will be "surprised" by the actual response when it differs from the guess (i.e., about 50% of the time). This is actually not the case, because the hidden layer representation remains essentially the same for both outputs (reflecting the node identity, more or less), and thus does not change when the actual output is presented in the plus phase. Thus, the "higher level" internal representation encompasses both possible outputs, while the lower-level output representation randomly chooses one

of them. This situation will be important later as we consider how networks can efficiently represent multiple items (see chapter 7 for further discussion).

To monitor the network's performance over learning, we need an error statistic that converges to zero when the network has learned the task perfectly (which is not the case with the standard SSE, due to the randomness of the task). Thus, we have a new statistic that reports an error (of 1) if the output unit was not one of the two possible outputs (i.e., as shown in the Targets layer). This is labeled as sum_fsa_err in the log displays.

↪ Now, continue to Step into the minus phase of the next event in the sequence.

You should see now that the Context units are updated with a copy of the prior hidden unit activations.

↪ To verify this, click on act_p.

This will show the plus phase activations from the previous event.

↪ Now you can continue to Step through the rest of the sequence. We can open up a training graph log by doing View, TRAIN_GRAPH_LOG, and then we can Run.

As the network runs, a special type of environment (called a ScriptEnv) dynamically creates 25 new sequences of events every other epoch (to speed the computation, because the script is relatively slow). Thus, instead of creating a whole bunch of training examples from the underlying FSA in advance, they are created on-line with a script that implements the Reber grammar FSA.

Because it takes a while to train, you can opt to load a fully trained network and its training log.

↪ To do so, Stop the network at any time. To load the network, do Object/Load in the network window, and select fsa.trained.net.gz. To load the log file, go to the Epoch_0_GraphLog, and do LogFile/Load File and select fsa.epc.log.

The network should take anywhere between 13 and 80 epochs to learn the problem to the point where it gets zero errors in one epoch (this was the range for ten random networks we ran). The pre-trained network took 15 epochs to get to this first zero, but we trained it longer (54 epochs total) to get it to the point where it got 4 zeros in a row. This stamping in of the representations makes them more robust to the noise, but the network still makes occasional errors even with this extra training. The 15 epochs amounts to only 175 different sequences and the 54 epochs amounts to 650 sequences (each set of 25 sequences lasts for 2 epochs).

In either case, the Leabra network is much faster than the backpropagation network used by (Cleeremans et al., 1989), which took 60,000 sequences (i.e., 4,800 epochs under our scheme). However, we were able to train backpropagation networks with larger hidden layers (30 units instead of 3) to learn in between 136 and 406 epochs. Thus, there is some evidence of an advantage for the additional constraints of model learning and inhibitory competition in this task, given that the Leabra networks generally learned much faster (and backpropagation required a much larger learning rate).

Now we can test the trained network to see how it has solved the problem, and also to see how well it distinguishes grammatical from ungrammatical letter strings.

↪ Do View, TEST_GRID_LOG to open a log to display the test results. Then, do Test.

This will test the network with one sequence of letters, with the results shown in the grid log on the right. Note that the network display is being updated every cycle, so you can see the stochastic choosing of one of the two possible outputs. The network should be producing the correct outputs, as indicated both by the fsa_err column and by the fact that the Output pattern matches the Target pattern, though it might make an occasional mistake due to the noise.

To better understand the hidden unit representations, we need a sequence of reasonable length (i.e., more than ten or so events). In these longer sequences, the FSA has revisited various nodes due to selecting the looping path, and this revisiting will tell us about the representation of the individual nodes. Thus, if the total number of events in the sequence was below ten (events are counted in the tick column of the grid log), we need to keep Testing to find a suitable sequence.

↪ To do so, turn the network Display toggle off (to speed things up), and press Test again until you find a sequence with ten or more events. After running the sequence with ten or more events, press the Cluster button on the fsa_ctrl control panel.

This will bring up a cluster plot of the hidden unit states for each event (e.g., figure 6.15). Figure 6.15 provides a decoding of the cluster plot elements.

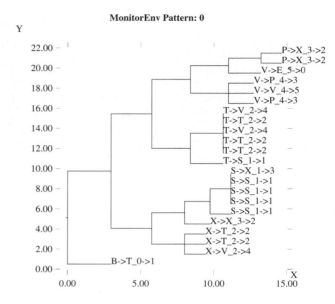

Figure 6.15: Cluster plot of the FSA hidden unit representations for a long sequence. The labels for each node describe the current and next letter and the current and next node (which the network is trying to predict). For example, T→V indicates that T was the letter input when the hidden state was measured for the cluster plot, and the subsequent letter (which does not affect the cluster plot) was V. Similarly, the associated 2→4 indicates that the node was 2 when the hidden state was measured for the cluster plot, and the subsequent node (which does not affect the cluster plot) was 4. The current letter and node are relevant to evaluating the cluster plot, whereas the next letter and node indicate what the network was trained to predict. The letters are ambiguous (appearing in multiple places in the grammar), but the nodes are not.

Question 6.4 *Interpret the cluster plot you obtained (especially the clusters with events at zero distance) in terms of the correspondence between hidden states and the current node versus the current letter. Remember that current node and current letter information is reflected in the letter and number before the arrow.*

↪ Now, switch the test_env from TRAIN_ENV to RANDOM_ENV (Apply). Then Test again.

This produces a random sequence of letters. Obviously, the network is not capable of predicting which letter will come next, and so it makes lots of errors. Thus, one could use this network as a grammaticality detector, to determine if a given string fits the grammar. In this sense, the network has incorporated the FSA structure itself into its own representations.

↪ Go to the PDP++Root window. To continue on to the next simulation, close this project first by selecting .projects/Remove/Project_0. Or, if you wish to stop now, quit by selecting Object/Quit.

6.6.4 Summary

We have seen that the context layer in an SRN can enable a network to learn temporally extended sequential tasks. Later, in chapters 9 and 11, we will also augment the simple and somewhat limited Markovian context of the SRN by introducing two additional mechanisms that introduce greater flexibility in deciding *when* and *what* to represent in the context.

6.7 Reinforcement Learning for Temporally Delayed Outcomes

The context layer in an SRN provides a means of retaining the immediately preceding context information. However, in many cases we need to learn about temporal contingencies that span many time steps. More specifically, we need to be able to solve the **temporal credit assignment** problem. Recall from the discussion of error-driven learning that it solves the credit (blame) assignment problem by figuring out which units are most responsible for the current error signal. The temporal credit assignment problem is similar, but it is about figuring out which *events* in the past are most responsible for a subsequent outcome. We will see that this temporal credit assignment problem can be solved in a very similar way as the earlier *structural* form of credit assignment — by using a time-based form of error-driven learning.

One of the primary means of solving the temporal credit assignment problem is the **temporal differences** (TD) learning algorithm developed by Sutton (1988) based on similar earlier ideas used to model the phenomenon of **reinforcement learning** (Sutton & Barto,

1981). Reinforcement learning (RL) is so named because it is based on the idea that relatively global reinforcement signals (i.e., reward and punishment) can drive learning that seeks to enhance reward and avoid punishment. This is the kind of learning that goes on in *classical* and *operant* **conditioning**. Thus, not only does this form of learning solve the temporal credit assignment problem, it is also closely related to relevant psychological and biological phenomena. In fact, it has recently been shown that the detailed properties of the TD algorithm have a close relationship to properties of various subcortical brain areas (Montague et al., 1996; Schultz, Dayan, & Montague, 1997), as we will review later.

We will start with a discussion of the behavior and biology of reinforcement learning, then review the standard formalization of the TD algorithm, and then show how the notion of activation phases used in the GeneRec algorithm can be used to implement the version of TD that we will use in the Leabra algorithm. This makes the relationship between TD and standard error-driven learning very apparent. We will then go on to explore a simulation of TD learning in action.

Behavior and Biology of Reinforcement Learning

As most students of psychology know, classical conditioning is the form of learning where the conditioned animal learns that stimuli (e.g., a light or a tone) are predictive of rewards or punishments (e.g., delivery of food or water, or of a shock). The stimulus is called the *conditioned stimulus,* or CS, and the reward/punishment is called the *unconditioned stimulus,* or US. In operant conditioning, a behavior performed by the animal serves as the CS. We explore the basic acquisition and *extinction* (unlearning) of conditioned associations in this section.

Some of the brain areas that appear to be specialized for reinforcement learning are the midbrain nuclei (well-defined groups of neurons) such as the ventral tegmental area (VTA) and the substantia nigra (SN), and the cortical and subcortical areas that control the firing of these neurons. Neurons in these midbrain areas project the neurotransmitter **dopamine (DA)** widely to the frontal cortex (VTA) and basal ganglia (SN), and

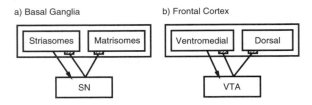

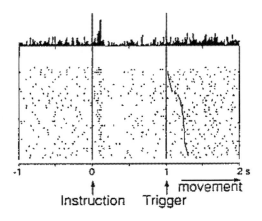

Figure 6.16: Possible arrangement of descending control and ascending distribution of midbrain dopaminergic signals in the basal ganglia and frontal cortex. **a)** Striosomes within the basal ganglia may control the firing of the substantia nigra (SN), which sends dopamine back to the entire basal ganglia. **b)** Ventromedial parts of frontal cortex may control the ventral tegmental area (VTA), which sends dopamine back to the entire frontal cortex.

Figure 6.17: Firing of dopimanergic VTA neurons in anticipation of reward. The top of the plot shows a histogram of spikes, and the bottom shows spikes for individual trials (each trial is a different row). The cue stimulus (instruction) precedes the response trigger by a fixed amount of time, and thus the instruction predicts the reward to be received after the response (movement). VTA fires after the instruction, anticipating the reward. Reproduced from Schultz et al. (1993).

the action of dopamine is likely to *modulate* learning in these areas, among other things. Thus, DA is considered a **neuromodulator**. These midbrain areas provide a relatively global learning signal to the brain areas (frontal cortex and basal ganglia) relevant for planning and motor control. As we will see, the firing properties of these neuromodulatory neurons are consistent with those of the temporal differences learning rule.

Although these midbrain nuclei play the role of broadcasting a global learning signal, other more "advanced" brain areas are required to control the firing of this signal. As we will see, the key idea in reinforcement learning is computing the *anticipation of future reward* — that complex task is likely performed by areas of the frontal cortex and basal ganglia that project to and control the midbrain dopaminergic nuclei. Neural recording studies suggest that the basal ganglia neurons are representing anticipated reward (Schultz, Apicella, Romo, & Scarnati, 1995). Studies of patients with lesions to the ventromedial areas of the frontal cortex (and related structures like the cingulate) suggest that these areas are involved in predicting rewards and punishments (Bechara, Tranel, Damasio, & Damasio, 1996).

Figure 6.16 shows a schematic of a possible relationship between the controlling areas, the midbrain "broadcasters," and the areas that are affected by the dopamine signal. In the case of the basal ganglia system (figure 6.16a), it is fairly well established that the areas (called *striosomes*) that have direct (monosynap-

tic) connections to the substantia nigra constitute a distinct subset of the basal ganglia (Gerfen, 1985; Graybiel, Ragsdale, & Mood Edley, 1979; Wilson, 1990). Thus, although the dopamine signal coming from the SN affects all of the basal ganglia, this signal may be primarily controlled by only a specialized subset of this structure. This notion of a distinct controller system is an essential aspect of the TD learning framework, where it is called the **adaptive critic**. It is also possible that a similar dissociation may exist in the frontal cortex, where certain ventromedial areas play the role of adaptive critic, controlling the dopamine signals for the entire frontal cortex.

The data on the firing properties of the VTA neurons in simple conditioning tasks are particularly compelling (Schultz et al., 1993). Figure 6.17 shows that the VTA neurons learn to fire after the onset of a cue stimulus (instruction) that reliably predicts a subsequent reward (delivered after an arm movement is made in response to a subsequent trigger stimulus). Figure 6.18 shows that this anticipatory firing develops over learning, with firing initially occurring just after the reward is actually

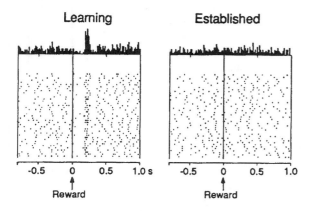

Figure 6.18: Changes in VTA firing with learning (display as in previous figure). During learning, firing occurs only during the delivery of the reward. After acquisition of the task has been established, firing does not occur when the reward is actually delivered, and instead occurs after the instruction stimulus as shown in the previous figure. Schultz et al. (1993).

delivered, but after acquisition of the task has been established, firing occurs for the predictive stimulus, and not to the actual reward.

Thus, VTA neurons seem to fire whenever reward can be reliably anticipated, which early in learning is just when the reward is actually presented, but after learning is when the instruction stimulus comes on (and not to the actual reward itself). This pattern of firing mirrors the essential computation performed by the TD algorithm, as we will see. Note that this anticipatory firing can be continued by performing *second order conditioning*, where another tone predicts the onset of the original tone, which then predicts reward. VTA neurons learn to fire at the onset of this new tone, and not to the subsequent tone or the actual reward.

6.7.1 The Temporal Differences Algorithm

Now, we will see that the properties of the temporal differences algorithm (TD) (Sutton, 1988) provide a strong fit to the biological properties discussed earlier. The basic framework for this algorithm (as for most reinforcement learning algorithms) is that an organism can produce *actions* in an *environment*, and this environment produces *rewards* that are contingent upon

the (often delayed) effects of these actions. The goal of the organism is naturally to produce actions that result in the maximum total amount of reward. Because the organism cares less about rewards that come a long way off in the future, we are typically interested in *discounted* future rewards. This can be expressed mathematically in terms of the following *value function*:

$$V(t) = \langle \gamma^0 r(t) + \gamma^1 r(t+1) + \gamma^2 r(t+2)... \rangle \quad (6.3)$$

where $V(t)$ expresses the *value* of the current state or situation at a given point in time. γ (between 0 and 1) is the *discount factor* that determines how much we ignore future rewards, $r(t)$ is the reward obtained at time t (where time is typically considered relative to some defining event like the beginning of a training trial), and the $\langle ... \rangle$ brackets denote the expectation over repeated trials. Because γ is raised to the power of the future time increments, it gets exponentially smaller for times further in the future (unless $\gamma = 1$).

Equation 6.3 plays a role in TD much like that of the sum-squared error (SSE) or the cross-entropy error (CE) in error-driven learning algorithms — it specifies the *objective* of learning (and is thus called the *objective function* for TD learning). Whereas in error driven learning the goal was to *minimize* the objective function, the goal here is to *maximize* it. However, it should become rapidly apparent that maximizing this function is going to be rather difficult because its value at any given point in time *depends on what happens in the future*. This is just the same issue of temporally delayed outcomes that we have discussed all along, but now we can see it showing up in our objective function.

The approach taken in the TD algorithm to this problem is to divide and conquer. Specifically, TD divides the problem into two basic components, where one component (the **adaptive critic, AC**) learns how to *estimate* the value of equation 6.3 for the current point in time (based on currently available information), while the other component (the **actor**) decides which actions to take. These two components map nicely onto the two components of the basal ganglia shown in figure 6.16a, where the striosomes play the role of the adaptive critic and the matrisomes correspond to the actor. Similarly, the ventromedial frontal cortex might be the adaptive critic and the dorsal frontal cortex the actor.

Of the two TD components, the adaptive critic has the harder job, because the actor can just use the estimated value function for different alternative actions to select which action to perform next (e.g., "if I go right, how much reward will I receive compared to going left.."). Thus, we will focus on the adaptive critic.

The adaptive critic (AC) uses sensory cues to estimate the value of $V(t)$. We will call this estimated value $\hat{V}(t)$ to distinguish it from the actual value $V(t)$. The AC needs to learn which sensory cues are predictive of reward, just as in conditioning. Obviously, the AC only ever knows about a reward when it actually receives it. Thus, the trick is to propagate the reward information backwards in time to the point where it could have been reliably predicted by a sensory cue. This is just what TD does, by using at each point in time the prediction for the *next* point in time (i.e., $\hat{V}(t+1)$) to adjust the prediction for the current point in time.

In other words, the AC "looks ahead" one time step and updates its estimate to predict this look-ahead value. Thus, it will initially learn to predict a reward just immediately (one time step) before the reward happens, and then, the next time around, it will be able to predict this prediction of the reward, and then, predict that prediction, and so on backward in time from the reward.

Note that this propagation takes place *over repeated trials*, and not within one trial (which is thus unlike the error backpropagation procedure, which propagates error all the way through the network at the point that the error was received). Practically, this means that we do not require that the AC magically remember all the information leading up to the point of reward, which would otherwise be required to propagate the reward information back in time all at the point of reward.

To see how the temporal backpropagation happens mathematically, we start by noting that equation 6.3 can be written *recursively* in terms of $V(t+1)$ as follows:

$$V(t) = \langle r(t) + \gamma V(t+1) \rangle \qquad (6.4)$$

Given that this same relationship should hold of our estimates $\hat{V}(t)$, we can now define a *TD error* which will tell us how to update our current estimate in terms of this look-ahead estimate at the next point in time. We do this by just computing the difference (represented as

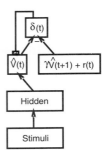

Figure 6.19: The adaptive critic computes estimated total expected future reward ($\hat{V}(t)$) based on the current stimuli, and learns by adjusting the weights to minimize the difference between this estimate and its value based on a one time step look-ahead.

$\delta(t)$) between the value that this estimate should be according to equation 6.4 and our current estimate $\hat{V}(t)$:

$$\delta(t) = \left(r(t) + \gamma \hat{V}(t+1) \right) - \hat{V}(t) \qquad (6.5)$$

Note that we got rid of the expected value notation $\langle ... \rangle$, because we will compute this on each trial and increment the changes slowly over time to compute the expected value (much as we did with our Hebbian learning rule). Note too, that this equation is based on the notion that the predictions of future reward have to be *consistent* over time (i.e., the prediction at time t has to agree with that at time $t+1$), and that the error signal is a measure of the residual inconsistency. Thus, TD learning is able to span temporal delays by building a bridge of consistency in its predictions across time.

The last thing we have to specify for the AC is exactly how $\hat{V}(t)$ is computed directly from external stimuli, and then how this TD error signal can be used to adapt these estimates. As you might expect, we will do this computation using a neural network that computes $\hat{V}(t)$ based on weights from representations of the stimuli (and potentially processed by one or more hidden layers) (figure 6.19). The TD error can then be used to train the weights of the network that computes $\hat{V}(t)$ by treating it the same as the error signal one would get from sum-squared error or cross-entropy error (i.e., like δ_k in equation 5.23 from section 5.6). Thus, to the extent that there is some stimulus in the environment that

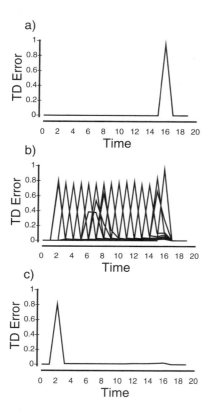

Figure 6.20: Three stages of learning in a simple conditioning experiment, showing TD error ($\delta(t)$) as a function of time. **a)** Shows the initial trial, where the reward is not predicted. **b)** Shows the transition as the estimate of reward gets predicted earlier and earlier. **c)** Shows the final trial, where the tone onset completely predicts the reward.

can be reliably used to produce the correct $\hat{V}(t)$ value, the network will learn this as a function of the TD error. Where no such reliable stimulus predictor exists, the reward will remain unpredictable.

Now, let's see how TD learning works in practice by revisiting the same kind of simple conditioning experiment shown in figure 6.17, where a reward was predicted by a tone which precedes it by some fixed time interval. We can simulate this by having a "tone" stimulus starting at $t = 2$, followed by a reward at $t = 16$. Figure 6.20a shows what happens to the TD error $\delta(t)$ as a function of time on the first trial of learning. There

is a large TD error when the reward occurs at $t = 16$ because it is completely unpredicted. Thus, if you refer to equation 6.5, $\hat{V}(16) = 0$, $\hat{V}(17) = 0$, and $r(16) = 1$. This means that $\delta(16) = 1$ (note we have set $\gamma = 1$ in this case), and thus that the weights that produce $\hat{V}(16)$ will increase so that this value will be larger next time.

This weight increase has two effects. First, it will reduce the value of $\delta(16)$ next time around, because this reward will be better predicted. Second, it will start to propagate the reward backward one time step. Thus, at $t = 15$, $\delta(15)$ will be .2 because the equation at time 15 includes $\hat{V}(16)$. Figure 6.20b shows how this propagation occurs all the way back to $t = 2$. Finally, figure 6.20c shows the "final" state where the network has learned as much as it can. It cannot propagate any further back because there is no predictive stimulus earlier in time. Thus, the network is always "surprised" when this tone occurs, but not surprised when the reward follows it.

The general properties of this TD model of conditioning provide a nice fit to the neural data shown in figure 6.17, suggesting that the VTA is computing something like TD error. One important discrepancy however is that evidence for a continuous transition like that shown in figure 6.20b is lacking. This has some important implications, and can still be explained from within the basic TD framework, as we will discuss further when we explore the simulation that produced these figures later.

We also need to specify something about the other half of TD learning, the *actor*. The TD error signal can easily be used to train an actor network to produce actions that increase the total expected reward. To see this, let's imagine that the actor network has produced a given action a at time t. If this action either leads directly to a reward, or leads to a previously unpredicted increase in estimated future rewards, then $\delta(t)$ will be positive. Thus, if $\delta(t)$ is used to adjust the weights in the actor network in a similar way as in the AC network, then this will increase the likelihood that this action will be produced again under similar circumstances. If there was another possible action at that time step that led to even greater reward, then it would produce larger weight changes, and would thus dominate over the weaker reward.

Intuitively, this thought experiment makes clear that the TD error signal provides a useful means of training both the AC system itself, and also the actor. This dual use of the TD signal is reflected in the biology by the fact that the dopamine signal (which putatively represents the TD error $\delta(t)$) projects to both the areas that control the dopamine signal itself, and the other areas that can be considered the actor network (figure 6.16).

It should also be noted that many different varieties of TD learning exist (and even more so within the broader category of reinforcement learning algorithms), and that extensive mathematical analysis has been performed showing that the algorithm will converge to the correct result (e.g., Dayan, 1992). One particularly important variation has to do with the use of something called an *eligibility trace*, which is basically a time-averaged activation value that is used for learning instead of the instantaneous activation value. The role of this trace is analogous to the *hysteresis* parameter fm_{prv} in the SRN context units (where fm_{hid} is then $1 - fm_{prv}$). The value of the trace parameter is usually represented with the symbol λ, and the form of TD using this parameter as $TD(\lambda)$. The case we have (implicitly) been considering is $TD(0)$, because we have not included any trace activations.

6.7.2 Phase-Based Temporal Differences

Just as we were able to use phase-based activation differences to implement error-driven learning, it is relatively straightforward to do this with TD learning, making it completely transparent to introduce TD learning within the overall Leabra framework. As figure 6.19 makes clear, there are two values whose difference constitutes the TD error δ, $\hat{V}(t)$ and $\gamma\hat{V}(t+1)+r(t)$. Thus, we can implement TD by setting the minus phase activation of the AC unit to $\hat{V}(t)$, and the plus phase to $\gamma\hat{V}(t+1) + r(t)$ (figure 6.21). Thus, to the extent that there is a network of units supporting the ultimate computation of the AC δ value, these weights will be automatically updated to reduce the TD error just by doing the standard GeneRec learning on these two phases of activation. In this section, we address some of the issues the phase-based implementation raises.

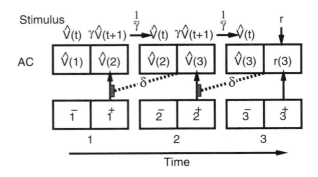

Figure 6.21: Computation of TD using minus-plus phase framework. The minus phase value of the AC unit for each time step is clamped to be the prior estimate of future rewards, $\hat{V}(t)$, and the plus phase is either a computed estimate of discounted future rewards $\gamma\hat{V}(t+1)$, or an actual injected reward $r(t)$ (but not both — requiring an absorbing reward assumption as described in the text).

First, let's consider what happens when the network experiences a reward. In this case, the plus phase activation should be equal to the reward value, plus any additional discounted expected reward beyond this current reward (recall that the plus phase value is $\gamma\hat{V}(t + 1) + r(t)$). It would be much simpler if we could consider this additional $\gamma\hat{V}(t + 1)$ term to be zero, because then we could just clamp the unit with the reward value in the plus phase. In fact, in many applications of reinforcement learning, the entire network is reset after reward is achieved, and a new trial is begun, which is often referred to as an *absorbing reward*. We use this absorbing reward assumption, and just clamp the reward value in the plus phase when an external reward is delivered.

In the absence of an external reward, the plus phase should represent the estimated discounted future rewards, $\gamma\hat{V}(t + 1)$. This estimate is computed by the AC unit in the plus phase by standard activation updating as a function of the weights. Thus, in the absence of external reward, the plus phase for the AC unit is actually an unclamped settling phase (represented by the forward-going arrow in figure 6.21), which is in contrast with the usual error-driven phase schema, but consistent with the needs of the TD algorithm. Essentially, the ultimate plus phase comes later in time when the AC unit is actually clamped by external reward, and intermediate plus phases prior to that in time are all ultimately driven by that later plus phase by the requirement of consistency in reward prediction. Thus, this settling in the plus phase is a kind of "estimated plus phase" in lieu of actually having an external plus phase value.

The minus phase AC unit value is always clamped to the undiscounted value of reward that we estimated on the plus phase of the previous time step. In other words, the minus phase of the next time step is equal to the plus phase of the previous time step. To account for the fact that we assumed that the plus phase computed the *discounted* estimated reward, we have to multiply that plus phase value by $\frac{1}{\gamma}$ to undiscount it when we copy it over to the next time step as our estimate of $\hat{V}(t)$.

In practice, we typically use a γ value of 1, which simplifies the implementational picture somewhat by allowing the next minus phase state to be a direct copy of the prior plus phase state. Thus, one could imagine that this just corresponds to a single maintained activation value across the previous plus phase and the next minus phase. By also using absorbing rewards with $\gamma = 1$, we avoid the problem of accounting for an infinity of future states — our horizon extends only to the point at which we receive our next reward. We will discuss in chapter 11 how the effective choosing of greater delayed rewards over lesser immediate rewards can be achieved by simultaneously performing TD-like learning at multiple time scales (Sutton, 1995).

Figure 6.21 also makes it clear that the weight adjustment computation must use the sending activations at time t but the TD error (plus-minus phase difference) at time $t + 1$. This is because while the AC unit is computing $\hat{V}(t + 1)$ based on stimulus activities at time t, the TD error for updating $\hat{V}(t + 1)$ is not actually computed until the next time step. It is important to note that this skewing of time is not artifactual to the phase-based implementation of TD, but is rather an intrinsic aspect of the algorithm, which requires the use of future states (i.e., $\hat{V}(t + 1)$) to adapt prior estimates. It is this spanning of contingencies across the time step that allows the network to propagate information from the future back in time.

The implementation of TD that we have explained here can be made somewhat more biologically plausible by combining it with the context representations used in the SRN model. As we will explain further in chapters 9 and 11, we can use the TD error signal to control when the context representations get updated, and the use of these context representations simplifies the issues of time skew that we just discussed. Thus, the version of the algorithm that we actually think the brain is implementing is somewhat more biologically plausible than it might otherwise seem.

6.7.3 Exploration of TD: Classical Conditioning

To explore the TD learning rule (using the phase-based implementation just described), we use the simple classical conditioning task discussed above. Thus, the network will learn that a stimulus (tone) reliably predicts the reward (and then that another stimulus reliably predicts that tone). First, we need to justify the use of the TD algorithm in this context, and motivate the nature of the stimulus representations used in the network.

You might recall that we said that the delta rule (aka the Rescorla-Wagner rule) provides a good model of classical conditioning, and thus wonder why TD is needed. It all has to do with the issue of *timing*. If one ignores the timing of the stimulus relative to the response, then in fact the TD rule becomes equivalent to the delta rule when everything happens at one time step (it just trains $\hat{V}(t)$ to match $r(t)$). However, animals are sensitive to the timing relationship, and, more importantly for our purposes, modeling this timing provides a particularly clear and simple demonstration of the basic properties of TD learning.

The only problem is that this simple demonstration involves a somewhat unrealistic representation of timing. Basically, the stimulus representation has a distinct unit for each stimulus for each point in time, so that there is something unique for the AC unit's weights to learn from. This representation is the **complete serial compound** (CSC) proposed by Sutton and Barto (1990), and we will see exactly how it works when we look at the model. As we have noted, we will explore a more plausible alternative in chapter 9 where the TD error signal controls the updating of a context representation that maintains the stimulus over time.

↪ **Open project** `rl_cond.proj.gz` in `chapter_6`.

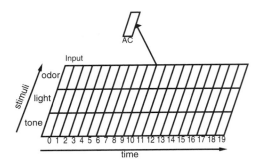

Figure 6.22: The reinforcement learning network with CSC input representation of stimuli by time.

Let's start by examining the network (figure 6.22). The input layer contains three rows of 20 units each. This is the CSC, where the rows each represent a different stimulus, and the columns represent points in time. Then, there is a single AC unit that receives weights from all of these input units.

↪ Click on r.wt and then on the AC unit to see that the weights start out initialized to zero. Then, click back to act.

Let's see how the CSC works in action.

↪ Do Step on the control panel.

Nothing should happen, because no stimulus or reward was present at $t = 0$. However, you can monitor the time steps from the tick: value displayed at the bottom of the network view (a **tick** is one time step in a sequence of events in the simulator).

↪ Continue to Step until you see an activation in the input layer (should be 10 more steps).

This input activation represents the fact that the first stimulus (i.e., the "tone" stimulus in row 1) came on at $t = 10$.

↪ Continue to Step some more.

You will see that this stimulus remains active for 6 more time steps (through $t = 15$). Then, notice that just as the stimulus disappears, the AC unit becomes activated (at $t = 16$). This activation reflects the fact that a reward was received, and the plus-phase activation of this unit was clamped to the reward value (.95 here).

Now, let's see what this reward did to the weights.

↪ Click on r.wt and then on the AC unit.

Notice that the weights have increased for the unit representing the stimulus in its last position just before it went off (at $t = 15$). Thus, the reward caused the AC unit to go from 0 in the minus phase to .95 in the plus phase, and this $\delta(t = 16)$ updated the weights based on the sending activations at the previous time step ($t = 15$), just as discussed in the previous section.

We can monitor the $\delta(t)$ values (i.e., the plus-minus phase difference) for the AC unit as a function of time step using a graph log.

↪ Do View and select GRAPH_LOG. Then, Step once and the graph log should update.

This log clearly shows the blip at $t = 16$, which goes back down to 0 as you continue to Step. This is because we are maintaining the reward active until the end of the entire sequence (at $t = 20$), so there is no change in the AC unit, and therefore $\delta = 0$.

↪ Now, switch back to act and Step again until you get to $t = 15$ again on the second pass through.

Recall that the weight for this unit has been increased — but there is no activation of the AC unit as one might have expected. This is due to the thresholded nature of the units.

↪ To see this, click on net.

You will see that the unit did receive some positive net input.

↪ Continue to Step until you get to trial 3 (also shown at the bottom of the network as trial:3), time step $t = 15$.

Due to accumulating weight changes from the previous 3 trials, the weight into the AC unit is now strong enough to activate over threshold. If you look at the graph log, you will see that there is now a positive $\delta(t)$ at time step 15.

Thus, the network is now *anticipating* the reward one time step earlier. This anticipation has two effects.

↪ First, click on r.wt.

You should notice that the weight from the *previous* time step (now $t = 14$) is increased as a result of this positive $\delta(t = 15)$. These weight changes will eventually lead to the reward being anticipated earlier and earlier.

↪ Now, do one more Step, and observe the graph log.

The second effect is that this anticipation reduced the magnitude of the $\delta(t = 16)$.

↪ Now, click back on r.wt in the network, and let this process play out by doing Continue on the process control panel. Stop the training when the graph log stops changing.

You will see the anticipation creep forward both in the weights and in the graph log, ultimately resulting in activation of the AC unit when the stimulus first comes on at $t = 10$. This is the same process that was shown in figure 6.20, and it represents the heart of the TD algorithm.

At this point, there are many standard phenomena in classical conditioning that can be explored with this model. We will look at two: *extinction* and *second order* conditioning. Extinction occurs when the stimulus is no longer predictive of reward — it then loses its ability to predict this reward (which is appropriate). Second order conditioning, as we discussed earlier, is where a conditioned stimulus can serve as the unconditioned stimulus for another stimulus — in other words, one can extend the prediction of reward backward across two separate stimuli.

We can simulate extinction by simply turning off the reward that appears at $t = 16$. To do this, we need to alter the parameters on the control panel that determine the nature of the stimulus input and reward. First, to familiarize yourself with the controls, look at the stim_1 field — this controls the timing of the first stimulus, with t_on representing the time at which the stimulus comes on, and len being how long it stays on. The two var fields provide for variance around these points, which has been zero (you can explore these on your own later). The timing parameters for reward are in the us (unconditioned stimulus) field. Although these fields determine the timing of the stimulus, another mechanism is used to control their probability of coming on at all. These probabilities are what we want to manipulate. The master control for these probabilities is contained in the probs field, but we will use a shortcut through the StdProbs button.

↪ Press the StdProbs button, and select STIM1_NO_US.

This indicates that stimulus 1 will be presented but no US.

↪ Now, Clear the graph log and Step through a trial.

Question 6.5 (a) *What happened at the point where the reward was supposed to occur?* (b) *Explain why this happened using the TD equations.* (c) *Then,* Continue *the network and describe what occurs next in terms of the TD error signals plotted in the graph log, and explain why TD does this.* (d) *After the network is done learning again, does the stimulus still evoke an expectation of reward?*

One thing you might have noticed is that during this extinction procedure, the weights are not reduced back to zero. Indeed, they are reduced only enough to bring the AC unit below threshold. The effects of this threshold may not be applicable to the real brain because it appears that the AC unit is constantly active at a low level, so either some additional inputs are driving it or the resting potential and threshold are effectively much closer than in this simulation. Thus, we might expect that the weights would have to be reduced much more to bring the AC unit below threshold. However, if the behavior did suggest that extinction was not complete (as it does in at least some situations), then this kind of threshold effect may be at work.

Now, let's explore second order conditioning. We must first retrain the network on the stimulus 1 association.

↪ Press StdProbs and select STIM1_US, and then NewRun (which re-initializes the network) until the onset of the stimulus is clearly driving the expectation of reward.

Now, we will turn on the second stimulus, which starts at $t = 2$ and lasts for 8 time steps (as you can see from the stim_2 field in the control panel).

↪ Do this by selecting StdProbs and STIM1_2_US. Go back to viewing act if you aren't already, and Step through the trial. Then, go back and look at the weights.

Essentially, the first stimulus *acts just like a reward* by triggering a positive $\delta(t)$, and thus allows the second stimulus to learn to predict this first stimulus.

↪ Push Continue, and then Stop when the graph log stops changing.

You will see that the early anticipation of reward gets carried out to the onset of the second stimulus (which comes first in time).

↪ At this point, feel free to explore the many parameters available, and see how the network responds. After you change any of the parameters, be sure to press the `MakeEnv` button to make a new environment based on these new parameters.

Finally, we can present some of the limitations of the CSC representation. One obvious problem is capacity — each stimulus requires a different set of units for all possible time intervals that can be represented. Also, the CSC begs the question of how time is initialized to zero at the right point so every trial is properly synchronized. Finally, the CSC requires that the stimulus stay on (or some trace of it, which you can manipulate using the `tr` parameter) up to the point of reward, which is unrealistic. This last problem points to an important issue with the TD algorithm, which is that although it can learn to bridge temporal gaps, it requires some suitable representation to support this bridging. We will see in chapters 9 and 11 that this and the other problems can be resolved by allowing the TD system to control the updating of context-like representations.

↪ To stop now, quit by selecting `Object/Quit` in the `PDP++Root` window.

6.8   Summary

Combined Model and Task Learning

There are sound functional reasons to believe that both Hebbian model learning and error-driven task learning are taking place in the cortex. As we will see in later chapters, both types of learning are required to account for the full range of cognitive phenomena considered. Computationally, Hebbian learning acts **locally**, and is **autonomous** and **reliable**, but also **myopic** and **greedy**. Error-driven learning is driven by **remote error signals**, and the units **cooperate** to solve tasks. However, it can suffer from **codependency** and **laziness**. The result of combining both types of learning is representations that encode important statistical features of the activity patterns they are exposed to, and also play a role in solving the particular tasks the network must perform. Specific advantages of the combined learning algorithm can be seen in **generalization** tasks, and tasks that use a **deep network** with many hidden layers.

Sequence and Temporally Delayed Learning

Learning to solve tasks having temporally extended **sequential** contingencies requires the proper development, maintenance and updating of **context** representations that specify a location within the sequence. A **simple recurrent network (SRN)** enables sequential learning tasks to be solved by copying the hidden layer activations from the previous time step into a **context layer**. The specialized context maintenance abilities of the **prefrontal cortex** may play the role of the context layer in an SRN. An SRN can learn a **finite state automaton** task by developing an internal representation of the underlying node states.

The mathematical framework of **reinforcement learning** can be used for learning with temporally delayed contingency information. The **temporal differences (TD)** reinforcement learning algorithm provides a good fit to the neural firing properties of neurons in the **VTA**. These neurons secrete the **neuromodulator dopamine** to the frontal cortex, and dopamine has been shown to modulate learning. The TD algorithm is based on minimizing differences in **expectations of future reward** values, and can be implemented using the same phases as in the GeneRec algorithm. Various **conditioning** phenomena can be modeled using the TD algorithm, including acquisition, **extinction**, and **second-order** conditioning.

6.9   Further Reading

The Sutton and Barto (1998) *Reinforcement Learning* book is an excellent reference for reinforcement learning.

Mozer (1993) provides a nice overview of a variety of different approaches toward temporal sequence processing.

The journal *Neural Computation* and the *NIPS* conference proceedings (*Advances in Neural Information Processing*) always have a large number of high-quality articles on computational and biological approaches to learning.

For more detailed coverage of the combination of error-driven and Hebbian learning, see O'Reilly (1998) and O'Reilly (in press).

Part II

Large-Scale Brain Area Organization and Cognitive Phenomena

Chapter 7

Large-Scale Brain Area Functional Organization

Contents

7.1 **Overview** **205**
7.2 **General Computational and Functional Principles 206**
   7.2.1 *Structural Principles* *206*
   7.2.2 *Dynamic Principles* *210*
7.3 **General Functions of the Cortical Lobes and Subcortical Areas** **211**
   7.3.1 *Cortex* *211*
   7.3.2 *Limbic System* *212*
   7.3.3 *The Thalamus* *212*
   7.3.4 *The Basal Ganglia, Cerebellum, and Motor Control* *213*
7.4 **Tripartite Functional Organization** **214**
   7.4.1 *Slow Integrative versus Fast Separating Learning* *214*
   7.4.2 *Active Memory versus Overlapping Distributed Representations* *215*
7.5 **Toward a Cognitive Architecture of the Brain** . . **216**
   7.5.1 *Controlled versus Automatic Processing* . . *217*
   7.5.2 *Declarative/Procedural and Explicit/Implicit Distinctions* *218*
7.6 **General Problems** **219**
   7.6.1 *The Binding Problem for Distributed Representations of Multiple Items* *220*
   7.6.2 *Representing Multiple Instances of the Same Thing* *222*
   7.6.3 *Comparing Representations* *222*
   7.6.4 *Representing Hierarchical Relationships* . . *222*
   7.6.5 *Recursion and Subroutine-like Processing* . *223*
   7.6.6 *Generalization, Generativity, and Abstraction* *224*
   7.6.7 *Summary of General Problems* *224*
7.7 **Summary** **225**

7.1 Overview

We are now in a position to build upon the principles and basic mechanisms developed in the first part of the text to understand a wide range of different cognitive phenomena in the second part. To prepare a suitable foundation for these cognitive models, this chapter provides an overview of the general function and large scale organization of cortical and other brain areas. We focus on the functional and computational bases for the specializations observed in these different brain areas. However, we emphasize how these specializations can be understood against a backdrop of common principles that hold for all areas.

Thus, the goal of this chapter is to provide a useful coherent framework within which the specific models in subsequent chapters can be situated and related. Although this framework is supported by existing data and reflects common threads of thought across a number of researchers over the years, it remains somewhat speculative in certain aspects. Therefore, we suggest that the reader view what follows as a provisional broad-brushstroke framework, and not as established fact.

We begin with a brief summary of some of the general functional and computational principles that underlie all of our cognitive models. Then we provide a brief overview of the different anatomical areas of the cortex and relevant aspects of the subcortical anatomy. We then describe a tripartite functional organization of these areas in terms of the following specialized systems: the **posterior cortex**, the **frontal cortex**, and the **hippocampus and related structures**. This tripartite organization constitutes a kind of **cognitive architecture** — a higher level description of the processes underlying cognitive function, where different cognitive phenomena can be explained in terms of the interactions between these specialized systems (in addition to the common principles and mechanisms applicable to all areas).

A central organizing principle in our framework is the notion of a **tradeoff** between different functional objectives. A tradeoff is where two objectives are mutually incompatible, and thus cannot be simultaneously achieved — achieving one objective trades off against achieving the other. Where such tradeoffs can be identified, and different brain areas associated with different functions, we can provide a principled account for the observed functional specialization — the brain areas are specialized to optimize separately two different functional objectives that would otherwise conflict if a unitary system were to try to achieve both of them. Because these tradeoffs are based on the kinds of mechanisms and principles developed in the first part of this book, they provide a means of leveraging basic properties of neural computation to explain aspects of the large-scale organization of the brain.

The first tradeoff we explore is in the rate of learning and the nature of the resulting representations, with cortex (posterior and frontal) being slow and **integrative** (integrating over instances), and the hippocampus being fast and **separating** (keeping instances separate). The second tradeoff is in the ability to update rapidly and maintain robustly representations in an active state over delays and in the face of interference from ongoing processing (**active maintenance**). The frontal cortex (and particularly the **prefrontal cortex**) appears to be specialized for this kind active maintenance, which plays an important role in both **active memory** and con-

trolled processing (i.e., "executive" control of cognition).

The last part of this chapter addresses a number of general problems that arise in using our framework to model cognitive phenomena. This framework explains a number of aspects of cognition quite naturally, but it is not immediately clear how some other aspects can be explained. We highlight these difficulties as important issues to be addressed by the models presented in subsequent chapters and in future research.

7.2 General Computational and Functional Principles

We can usefully divide our discussion of the general properties of cognition into their **structural** and **dynamic** aspects. The structural aspects describe the ways that information and processing are arranged within the system, determined by the overall patterns of connectivity and relationships between representations at different levels or stages of processing. The dynamic aspects describe the nature of processing over time, determined by how activation flows through the various processing levels and achieves a useful overall outcome.

7.2.1 Structural Principles

Many aspects of processing in the cortex are arranged in a generally **hierarchical** fashion (i.e., having ordered subordinate and superordinate levels), with many different specialized **pathways** of such hierarchies that each operate on and emphasize different aspects of the overall sensory input, motor output, or intermediate processing. However, rich interconnectivity between these different pathways at different levels provides a number of functional benefits, so we do not think of them as completely distinct from one another (i.e., parallel, modular, and strictly hierarchical pathways), but rather as highly interconnected, interdependent, and only approximately hierarchical. It is also clear that processing and memory are **embedded** in the same underlying neural hardware, and **distributed** over a potentially wide range of different processing pathways. These properties have a number of important consequences, as elaborated in subsequent sections.

Hierarchical Structure

We begin by considering the basic building block for our model of the cognitive architecture, the neuron-as-detector presented in chapter 2. Individual neurons are viewed as having relatively stable representations that detect some (difficult to define and complex) set of conditions in their inputs. We saw in chapter 3 that a layer of such detectors can perform a **transformation** of the input patterns that emphasizes some distinctions between patterns and collapses across or deemphasizes others. In chapters 4–6 we saw how these transformations can be shaped by learning so that they both represent important structural or statistical properties of the environment and enable tasks to be solved.

Cognition can be viewed as a hierarchical structure (figure 7.1) of sequences (**layers**) of such transformations operating on sensory inputs and ultimately producing motor outputs (**responses**), or just useful internal states that provide an **interpretation** of the environment, which can be important for subsequent behavior. As discussed in chapter 4, the sensory input contains a large quantity of low quality information, so it must be highly processed before sensible responses or interpretations can be made. For example, the sensory signals from viewing the same object in two different locations can have almost nothing directly in common (i.e., no overlapping activations), but it nevertheless makes sense to interpret these signals as representing the same object. Thus, one wants to transform the inputs to collapse across differences in location, while preserving distinctions between different objects. As we will see in chapter 8, a hierarchical sequence of transformations is necessary to achieve this kind of spatial **invariance**.

This same process of performing transformations that emphasize some dimensions or aspects and collapse across others operates at all levels of processing. For example, the representations that underlie the meanings of words (e.g., dog vs. cat, truth vs. fiction) emphasize those features or properties that define the word, while collapsing across irrelevant ones. An example of a relevant feature for dogs and cats is physical size, but this is irrelevant for truth and fiction, whereas the notion of "reality" is central to truth and fiction, but doesn't affect cats and dogs that much (witness Garfield and Snoopy).

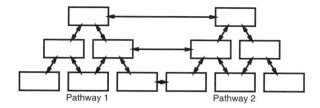

Figure 7.1: Generic hierarchical system, showing two specialized pathways or streams of processing, with inter-pathway connectivity.

Specialized Pathways

An important correlate of a hierarchical structure is the existence of specialized and somewhat distinct **processing pathways** or **streams**, which are necessary because each layer of processing in a hierarchy requires specific types of transformations to be performed in the previous layer(s), to then accomplish their particular job. Thus, subsequent layers build on the transformations performed in previous ones. In addition, there are typically many other potential transformations of the input that are irrelevant for a given transformation. Therefore, it makes sense to group together all the relevant transformations into one coherent stream.

To illustrate the process of building successive levels of transformations upon each other, let's continue with the example of visual object recognition. Consider a layer of processing that transforms visual representations of digits into the appropriate categorical representations (e.g., the digit "8"). If this layer is situated in a specialized pathway after a sequence of transformations that produce a *spatially invariant* visual representation, then it would be relatively simple for one layer of processing to transform the spatially invariant pattern of activity into a categorical representation of a digit (as we saw in chapter 3). In contrast, if this transformation was performed based on the raw sensory input, a huge number of redundant detectors would be required to process images in all the different locations. A visual digit category transformation does not require olfactory, auditory, or somatosensory information, so it makes sense to have specialized visual processing pathways that are distinct from other modalities. In short, it makes sense to collect together all the categorical transformations of visual stimuli into one overall *visual form* or *object* processing stream. Indeed, it appears that this is just what the cortex has done (Ungerleider & Mishkin, 1982).

These same types of specialization pressures operate in many other types of hierarchical structures. For example, the functions of a corporation are typically divided into different specialized divisions (i.e., processing streams), because the details of one division (e.g., manufacturing) typically have little bearing on the details of another (e.g., marketing). However, there is a lot of interdependence *within* a division. For example, all the different manufacturing processes must be tightly coordinated. The same kinds of hierarchical dependencies are also present. For example, a higher-level report on the status of a given division is produced by summarizing, categorizing, and aggregating (i.e., transforming) the lower-level details at various levels of analysis.

Inter-Pathway Interactions

A completely rigid and separate hierarchical structure is not as effective and flexible as one that has many opportunities for communication between the different specialized processing streams at all levels (as many corporations are now discovering). These connections at lower levels can mutually constrain or inform processing across different pathways to better deal with partial, noisy, novel, or particularly complex stimuli. For example, we will explore the idea in chapter 8 that the visual form pathway interacts at many levels with the spatial processing pathway, resulting in the important ability to focus attention at various spatial scales depending on where confusions arise in the visual form pathway. By resolving these confusions at the level at which they occur (instead of waiting for things to go all the way to the top of the hierarchy), the system can deal with them more rapidly and at the appropriate level of detail.

Higher-Level Association Areas

One further deviation from the general hierarchical structure comes when one considers the higher levels of a given processing pathway. These areas will likely receive as much input from different pathways as they

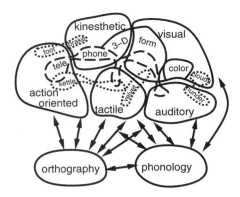

Figure 7.2: Illustration of how semantic information might be distributed across a number of more specific processing pathways, represented here by different sensory modalities. Linguistic representations (orthography, phonology) are associated with corresponding distributed activation patterns across semantics. Figure adapted from Allport, 1985.

will from their own, making the whole hierarchical notion somewhat inapplicable here (figure 7.1). One can better conceive of these **higher-level association** areas as a heterogenous collection of peers, which intercommunicate ("associate") and perform constraint satisfaction processing.

Large-Scale Distributed Representation

The preceding principles converge on the idea that the knowledge associated with a given item is distributed widely across a number of different brain areas, some of which are specialized processing pathways and some of which are higher-level association areas. Figure 7.2 illustrates a version of this general idea proposed by Allport (1985), where the representation of semantic items is distributed across many different specialized systems that together comprise the "semantic memory system." The neuropsychological and neuroimaging evidence generally supports this distributed model (e.g., Saffran & Schwartz, 1994).

This notion of distributed representation across large scale brain areas is similar to the notion of the fine-grained distributed representations across units that we explored in previous models. Both imply that multiple units/areas participate in representing a given thing, and that each unit/area represents multiple things (cf. section 3.3.2). This similarity across the fine-grained properties within an area and the large-scale properties across areas again suggests that the brain has a *fractal* quality, where the small-scale structure is replicated at the larger scale.

This widely distributed view of knowledge conflicts with both popular intuitions and the computer metaphor, which tend to favor the idea that there is a single *canonical representation* of a given knowledge item, with all of the features and attributes stored in one convenient location. This bias toward assuming a canonical representation leads to some of the problems discussed in the last section of this chapter, where we show how a more distributed model avoids these problems.

Dedicated, Content-Specific Processing and Representations

A basic property of neural computation is that knowledge and processing are intimately interrelated. As the preceding discussion makes clear, processing amounts to performing transformations on activity patterns, where these transformations are shaped by accumulated experience (knowledge) through learning. An important consequence of this interrelationship is that processing is relatively *dedicated* and *content specific* for particular types of activation patterns. In other words, unlike a computer, the brain does not have a general purpose CPU.

An advantage of the dedicated, content-specific nature of neural processing is that the selection of transformations to apply in a given situation is determined directly by the specific stimulus (activation pattern) being processed. This makes it easy for the system to treat different stimuli according to their specific properties and consequences. As we saw, this content-specificity becomes even more important as layers are integrated into elaborate hierarchies of processing stages, because subsequent stages can then come to depend on particular types of transformations from their input layers, and can in turn reliably provide specific transformations for subsequent layers. The dedicated, content-specific na-

ture of the transformations also implies a certain amount of stability of over time. This stability enables a rich set of content-specific associations to be built up over time in the connectivity among different representations.

Compare this situation with that of a standard serial computer, where programs (processing) and data (knowledge) are explicitly separated, and processing typically operates *generically* on whatever data it is passed (e.g., as arguments to a function). The advantage of such a system is that it is relatively *concise* and *flexible*, so that a given function need only be written once, and deployed in a wide range of different situations. The ability to do arbitrary *variable binding* (e.g., by passing arguments to a function) is an important contributor to this flexibility. (We will return to this later.) Although there are obvious advantages to flexibility and generality, one disadvantage is that it becomes difficult to treat different stimuli in accordance with their specific properties and consequences — one has to resort to messy sequences of *if-then* constructs and elaborate representational structures that make clear exactly what is different about one stimulus compared to others.

Thus, there is a basic *tradeoff* between specificity and knowledge-dependency on one hand, and generality and flexibility on the other. It appears that the brain has opted to optimize the former at the expense of the latter. This is interesting, given the consensus view that it is precisely the inability to deal with this type of content-specific **real world knowledge** that led to the failure of traditional symbolic (computer metaphor based) models of human cognition (e.g., Lenat, 1995). Thus, it seems that getting all the details right (e.g., knowing the practical differences between tigers and trees) is much more important for surviving in the world than having the kind of flexibility provided by arbitrary variable binding. One compelling demonstration of this point in the domain of language comprehension is made by these two sentences:

Time flies like an arrow.
Fruit flies like a banana.

Clearly, specific, real-world knowledge is necessary to produce the two very different interpretations of the words *flies* and *like* in these sentences. However, we will see that the sacrifice of flexibility in favor of specificity causes a number of other problems, which must be resolved in various different ways as discussed below.

7.2.2 Dynamic Principles

At a dynamic level, we view cognition as the result of activation propagation through the brain's densely interconnected hierarchical structure of bidirectionally connected processing layers as described above. Thus, via the **multiple constraint satisfaction** property of bidirectionally connected networks described in chapter 3, the network will tend to produce an activation state (e.g., a response or interpretation) that satisfies many of the constraints imposed upon it from the environmental inputs and the learned weights. Although many stimuli (e.g., familiar ones) will result in straightforward, rapid settling of the network into a relatively optimal state in response to that stimulus, others may require more extended iterative "searching" for an appropriate activity state.

In either case, the resulting activity state will not typically be the same each time the same stimulus is presented, due to a number of factors (e.g., learning, habituation, and sensitization). Perhaps the most important variable in the response to a stimulus comes from internally maintained activation states carried over from prior processing, which provide additional constraints on the settling process. These internal states (also known as **internal context**) can dynamically alter the interpretation and response to stimuli to provide a more coherent, consistent and/or *strategic* set of responses over time (more on this below). For a simple example of the role of internal context, note that the following two sentences produce very different interpretations of the word "bank":

She swam from the overturned canoe to the bank.
She walked from the post office to the bank.

Thus, the words preceding "bank" establish different internal context representations that then alter its subsequent interpretation (Cohen, Dunbar, & McClelland, 1990).

In addition to multiple constraint satisfaction, all of the *amplification*-like *attractor* dynamics described in

chapter 3 (e.g., pattern completion, bootstrapping, mutual and top-down support, etc.) play an important role in processing. The role of mutual support in providing a form of *active memory* is elaborated further in the following section, because it plays a particularly important cognitive role, despite its relatively simple mechanistic basis. Similarly, the role of inhibition in *attention* is also mechanistically simple and cognitively important, and is covered in the subsequent section.

Mutual Support and Active Memory

Bidirectional excitatory connectivity allows different representations to mutually support (excite) each other. This mutual support is important because it enables representations to remain active even in the absence of externally derived excitation (e.g., from viewing a stimulus), because they can instead rely on *internal* excitation from other mutually supporting representations to remain active over time. This can be viewed as a form of *memory*, because it enables information to persist over time. We will call this **active memory**, which can be contrasted with **weight-based memory** that results from changing weights to store new information (see the following and chapter 9 for more on this distinction).

Active memory is not typically as long-lasting as weight-based memory, because the active neurons either fatigue or are interrupted by ongoing processing. However, active memory has the distinct advantage that it can directly *influence* ongoing processing in other areas (e.g., by providing *internal context* as described above), whereas weight-based memories only directly affect those units whose weights are changed. We will see that there are limits to the capabilities of mutual support for providing active memories, so that other *active maintenance* mechanisms are needed for a more robust and flexible active memory system. However, mutual support provides the basic underlying mechanism, and is the main form of active memory for those brain areas that lack these more sophisticated active maintenance mechanisms.

Inhibition and Attention

Because there is **inhibition** operating at all levels of processing in the cortex as discussed in chapter 3, there is a natural and pervasive limitation on the amount of activation, and thus on the number of things that can be simultaneously represented. This gives rise to the phenomenon of **attention**, where some aspects of the sensory input (or internal context) are ignored in favor of *attention* paid to others (see chapter 8 for more on this). Although cognitive psychologists often view attention as a somewhat discrete and separable mechanism, we view it as an emergent property of constraint satisfaction under the limits of inhibition (for similar ideas, see Desimone & Duncan, 1995; Allport, 1989).

As we have seen, both the external environment and the internal context can determine what is attended to and what is ignored. Further, because all levels of processing are constrained by inhibition, and all levels mutually influence each other to varying degrees via bidirectional connectivity, attentional effects that arise at any level of abstraction can have important consequences for processing at other levels. At a functional level, attention is critical for ensuring some level of **coherence** of processing, so that representations at different levels of processing are all focused on the same underlying thing or set of things. This coherence effect will be important for solving some of the problems discussed later.

7.3 General Functions of the Cortical Lobes and Subcortical Areas

Building on the basic principles and mechanisms summarized above, we now turn to the functional specializations of different brain areas at a relatively large scale of analysis. The emphasis is on the most cognitively relevant brain areas, including the cortex, parts of the limbic system, and other subcortical brain areas.

7.3.1 Cortex

The human cortex is organized into four **lobes** that contain a number of specialized processing pathways and higher-level association areas. The general nature of these specialized functions is described next, illustrated

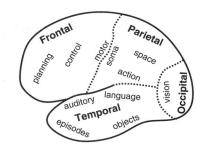

Figure 7.3: Four cortical lobes and associated functions.

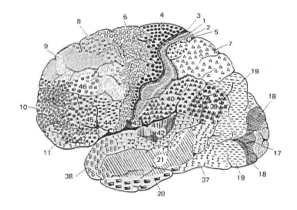

Figure 7.4: Brodmann's areas of the cortex, based on anatomically visible differences in the structure of the cortical layers in different cortical areas. Reproduced from Kandel et al. (1991).

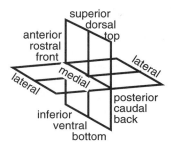

Figure 7.5: Various terms used to refer to locations in the brain.

in figure 7.3, and explored in more detail in subsequent chapters as indicated. Based on anatomical distinctions, primarily in the thicknesses of different cortical layers, the cortical lobes were further subdivided into processing areas by Brodmann, as shown in figure 7.4. We will use the following standard terminology for describing locations (figure 7.5): **superior** or **dorsal** = upper; **inferior** or **ventral** = lower; **posterior** or **caudal** = toward the back; **anterior** or **rostral** = toward the front; **lateral** = toward the sides; **medial** = toward the middle.

Occipital Lobe: Specialized for visual processing, with area V1 (Brodmann area 17) in the central posterior region receiving the main visual inputs from the thalamus, and the other areas (e.g., V2, V4) performing higher levels of transformations (chapter 8).

Temporal Lobe: Specialized for a mix of functions, including primary and higher level auditory perception (superior regions), higher-level visual form and object representations (posterior inferior regions, chapter 8), language processing (superior and medial lateral regions, chapter 10), and longer-term episodic representations (e.g., stories, life events) (anterior inferior regions). Medial regions feed into the *hippocampus* and play an important role in rapid learning of arbitrary information (see following and chapter 9). There is obviously an important relationship between language and audition (i.e., speech perception) that might contribute to their colocalization.

Parietal Lobe: Also specialized for a mix of functions, including spatial processing (e.g., representing where things are located in space, chapter 8), and task specific perceptual processing (e.g., organizing and tuning reaching movements via visual perception). The most anterior and superior regions house the primary and higher-level somatosensory processing areas. Inferior areas near the temporal lobe are important for language (especially in the left hemisphere).

Frontal Lobe: Specialized for maintaining representations in an active state (*active maintenance*), and (consequently) for "executive" control of processing in other areas (more on this below and in chapter 11).

The posterior regions contain the primary and higher-level motor output representations, which is consistent with the executive nature of this lobe in controlling behavior.

7.3.2 Limbic System

The **limbic system** is a group of subcortical brain areas tucked inside the medial surface of the cortex, and consists principally of the **hippocampus**, **cingulate cortex**, and **amygdala**, and also contains the **anterior thalamus**, **hypothalamus**, and the **mammillary bodies**. These areas, which are mutually interconnected, were originally thought to process emotional information. However, it is probably not useful to group them all together as one system, because they are now known to have very different individual roles and can be better understood in terms of their relationship with the cortex.

For example, the hippocampus, which sits just medial to the temporal cortex, is quite important for rapidly learning new information of many different types (not just emotional), is richly interconnected with the medial portions of the temporal cortical association areas, and can be viewed as sitting at the top of the cortical hierarchy by virtue of this connectivity. The cingulate, which is located just inferior to the frontal cortex, appears to be important for tasks that the frontal cortex is also specialized for, including motor control and action selection. Thus, these two areas should probably be thought of more as specialized cortical-like areas, even though they are evolutionarily more ancient *archicortex* (protocortex).

Unlike the hippocampus and cingulate, the amygdala is still thought to be primarily specialized for emotional processing (see Armony, Servan-Schreiber, Cohen, & LeDoux, 1997 for a modeling approach), and the cognitive roles of the other components of the limbic system are not well documented.

7.3.3 The Thalamus

The **thalamus** is a subcortical area with many specialized nuclei (subdivisions) that provides sensory input to the cortex, by relaying information from sensory systems. We will discuss the *lateral geniculate nucleus* of the thalamus and its role in visual processing in chapter 8. Although once thought to be just a relay station, the thalamus is increasingly being appreciated as an active processing system, contributing for example to attentional processing. Several pathways exist within the thalamus that could subserve communication among disparate cortical areas, providing a potential role in coordinating processing in these different areas, for example. However, not much is known at this time about the true extent of thalamic involvement in cortical processing.

7.3.4 The Basal Ganglia, Cerebellum, and Motor Control

For obvious reasons, the brain has devoted a considerable amount of neural resources to motor control. Two brain areas that are known to be very important for motor control are the **basal ganglia** and the **cerebellum**. The basal ganglia starts just below the medial area of the cortex surrounding the third ventricle, and comprises a set of interconnected brain areas including the **caudate** and **putamen** (which are collectively known as the **striatum**), **globus pallidus**, **substantia nigra**, **subthalamic nucleus**, and **nucleus accumbens**. The cerebellum is the large structure that looks like cauliflower at the base of the brain, and is composed of the lateral cerebellar hemispheres and more medial nuclei.

Because of the cognitive focus of this book, we will largely ignore the motor functions of the basal ganglia and cerebellum. However, it has recently become popular to emphasize the cognitive roles of these areas (e.g., Brown & Marsden, 1990; Brown, Schneider, & Lidsky, 1997; Gao, Parsons, & Fox, 1996), and numerous computational models have been developed (e.g., Beiser, Hua, & Houk, 1997; Wickens, 1997). We acknowledge that these areas do probably make an important cognitive contribution, but it is likely to be of a somewhat ancillary or specialized nature that would complement, but not replace, the cortically mediated processing that is the focus of this book.

In keeping with the emphasis in this chapter on functional tradeoffs for understanding brain area specializations, we offer the following idea as to what the cognitive role of the basal ganglia might be, and how this complements the frontal cortex, which is also a motor control structure. In short, there is a tradeoff between the kind of continuous, constraint-satisfaction processing that is thought to occur in the cortex, and the need for a more discrete, high-threshold system for deciding when the accumulated evidence warrants some kind of action. Thus, the basal ganglia might be specialized for performing this high-threshold decision-making process. So, whereas cortical neurons are constantly firing and shaping the flow and integration of information, the basal ganglia neurons are quietly waiting until they receive just the right pattern of input activation from the cortex to trigger an action.

The continuous versus discrete tradeoff idea is consistent with the oft-discussed notion that the basal ganglia are important for *action selection* — choosing an appropriate action given the current sensory-motor context. Furthermore, neural recordings of neurons in the striatum, which is the principal area where action selection is thought to occur, show that the neurons there are mostly completely silent, which is consistent with the high-threshold notion. This idea is also consistent with one of the main effects of Parkinson's disease, which affects the basal ganglia, where patients are unable to initiate movements — this is just what one would expect if the system that is responsible for detecting when to make an action is impaired. Interestingly, these patients are otherwise capable of making relatively normal movements once they have been induced, which would suggest that the basal ganglia are really just specialized for the *initiation* of action, but not its execution. Probably the execution depends more on the frontal cortical areas, which are bidirectionally connected with the basal ganglia.

It should be clear that a high-threshold detection system is appropriate for initiating motor outputs — moving muscles uses a lot of energy, and should not be done needlessly. By the same token, it should also be clear that such a high-threshold system would be useful for controlling the initiation of purely cognitive "actions." In chapters 9 and 11, we consider the possibility that the symbiotic relationship between the frontal cortex and basal ganglia that likely has evolved for motor control could have been coopted for controlling the updating and storage of activation-based memories in the frontal cortex. However, we stop short of actually including simulations of this idea, opting instead to focus on another, simpler control mechanism based on the brain area that provides the neuromodulator *dopamine* to the cortex. These two mechanisms may work in tandem, or there may be some finer division of labor between them that we have yet to identify.

Interestingly, the dopaminergic brain area innervating the frontal cortex, the *ventral tegmental area* (VTA) is adjacent to the substantia nigra, which is part of the basal ganglia. Thus, the VTA constitutes another important subcortical area, one that we actually do include in some of our models. As we discussed in chapter 6, the VTA and substantia nigra likely play a role in controlling learning as well, and there may be some homologies between this kind of learning in the basal ganglia and frontal cortex. Thus, much like the hippocampus and cingulate cortex, the basal ganglia are richly intertwined with cortical processing and learning, and future modeling work will better illuminate the precise nature of this relationship.

Even less is known about the cognitive role of the cerebellum than that of the basal ganglia. One speculation is that the cerebellum may be specialized for timing intervals between events. This would explain its important role in fine motor control, where the timing of muscle firing is critical. Clearly, such timing information could also have a cognitive role. Several detailed models of cerebellar involvement in motor control exist (e.g., Schweighofer, Arbib, & Kawato, 1998a, 1998b; Contreras-Vidal, Grossberg, & Bullock, 1997).

7.4 Tripartite Functional Organization

We now attempt to provide a more principled framework for understanding the different characteristics of some of the brain areas described above, based on two functional tradeoffs that are optimized by three broadly characterized systems of brain areas. One tradeoff is in the rate of learning and the way this interacts with knowledge representations. The other is in the ability to update rapidly and maintain actively information over delays and in the face of interfering stimuli, and how this interacts with the ability to use graded, distributed representations with dense interconnectivity.

Interestingly, both of these tradeoffs arise in the context of memory, suggesting that the functional demands of memory play a central role in shaping the overall cognitive architecture. As such, a more detailed account of these tradeoffs is provided in chapter 9.

The three brain systems are as follows:

Posterior cortex: consisting of the occipital, temporal, and parietal areas of the cortex. These areas are either directly responsible for analyzing sensory inputs and producing motor outputs, or are higher level association areas that serve to coordinate and integrate these activities. We characterize this system as having rich *overlapping distributed* representations built up *slowly* through learning to capture the stable, salient aspects of the environment and to solve the kinds of tasks the organism is typically faced with.

Frontal cortex: consisting of the frontal lobe, which is nearly as large as the posterior cortex in humans (but considerably smaller in "lower" animals). Our characterization of the frontal cortex is based primarily on studies of the *prefrontal cortex*, which are the frontal areas anterior of the motor areas (it is not clear if the motor cortex should be considered on functional grounds to be part of the frontal or posterior cortex, see chapter 11 for more discussion). The frontal cortex appears to be specialized for the *active maintenance* of information over time, which is particularly useful for *controlled processing*, where responses are *mediated* by various task-specific constraints, and not simply *automatic* responses to incoming stimuli (as is more characteristic of the posterior cortex).

Hippocampus and related structures: consisting of the the hippocampus proper and other areas which feed into it including the entorhinal cortex and the subiculum. The hippocampus appears to play a critical role in the *rapid acquisition of novel information*, in contrast to the slow learning in both the posterior and frontal cortex.

7.4.1 Slow Integrative versus Fast Separating Learning

Our functional analysis begins by assuming that the cortical systems (posterior and frontal) use the learn-

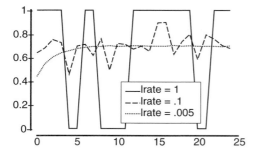

Figure 7.6: Effect of learning rate *lrate* on the ability of a weight to represent underlying conditional probability of the input unit activity given the output unit activity (i.e., the CPCA Hebbian learning objective). This conditional probability was .7, as is reflected by the .005 lrate case. With lrates of .1 or 1, the weight bounces around too much with each training example (which is binary), making it impossible to represent the overall probability that is only apparent across a number of individual examples.

ing mechanisms described in chapters 4–6 to develop representations of the important underlying structural and statistical characteristics of the world, to process perceptual inputs effectively, and to produce systematic and useful motor outputs. Given this, learning in the cortex must necessarily be *slow* to *integrate* over many individual experiences and extract the general underlying regularities of the environment (McClelland, Mc-Naughton, & O'Reilly, 1995; White, 1989b).

Figure 7.6 shows a simple example of this point, taken from the exploration described in section 4.6, demonstrating that a slow learning rate enables the weight to converge on the actual underlying conditional probability of an event occurring in the environment. If somehow the world were to provide underlying statistical regularities *all in one experience*, then you might be able to get away with a faster learning rate. However, because each experience is typically just a small and probably noisy fragment of the overall picture, slow learning must be used to blend this fragment smoothly together with all the others. Note that by virtue of integrating each episode together with previous ones, the unique details specific to these episodes are lost, with only some faint residue remaining.

However, survival in the world demands that rapid learning also occur, because specific, arbitrary information is also very important (e.g., remembering where you parked your car today, or remembering which cave you hid your food in and distinguishing that from the cave you saw the bear family enter last night). Notice also that in this rapid form of learning, the memories of individual episodes should be kept *separate* instead of integrating across them (e.g., today's parking spot should not be confused with yesterday's, nor should one cave be confused with the other). Because learning cannot be both fast and slow (or both integrating and separating), there is a basic *tradeoff* between the demands of slow integration and rapid separating.

It seems that the brain has resolved this tradeoff by allowing the cortex to learn slowly and integrate over experiences, while the hippocampus provides a complementary rapid, separating learning system. This idea is consistent with a large amount of data on people and animals with hippocampal lesions (see McClelland et al., 1995, for a review). For example, a famous patient, known by his initials "HM," had large chunks of his medial temporal cortex (including the hippocampus) removed bilaterally to prevent epilepsy that was originating there. HM was subsequently unable to learn much of any new information about the people he met, the events that occurred, and the like. However, he was able to learn a number of relatively complex perceptual-motor tasks, and showed other forms of intact learning that is characteristic of posterior-cortical learning. Perhaps the clearest distinction between the role of the hippocampus and that of the cortex comes from a group of people who had relatively pure hippocampal lesions early in life, and yet have acquired normal levels of long-term knowledge about the world and tasks like reading (Vargha-Khadem, Gadian, Watkins, Connelly, Van Paesschen, & Mishkin, 1997). Their primary deficit is on tasks that require rapid learning of arbitrary information. Chapter 9 explores these ideas further.

7.4.2 Active Memory versus Overlapping Distributed Representations

A different type of tradeoff can be used to understand the difference between the posterior and frontal cortex, this time involving the *active memory* (maintenance) of information instead of learning rate. As described earlier, active memories can be supported by bidirectional connectivity, and they are important for both memory and influencing processing in other brain areas. However, a couple of specializations are necessary to support a robust form of active maintenance that can also be rapidly updated (Cohen, Braver, & O'Reilly, 1996; O'Reilly, Braver, & Cohen, 1999a).

For example, if active memories are used in conjunction with highly overlapping distributed representations, information tends to spread to the overlapping representations when it is supposed to be maintained. Although this spreading activation can be useful for performing *inference* (e.g., when you see smoke, spreading activation can activate "fire"), it is not useful for accurately maintaining information over time. Furthermore, active maintenance needs to be considerably more robust than the more transient activation signals used in performing sensory motor mappings, because the effects of noise and interference from other activity in the network tend to accumulate over time.

As we will see in chapter 9, one way to produce a more robust active maintenance system is to *isolate* the representations more. This prevents spread, but also eliminates all of the potential benefits of spreading activation. This tradeoff can be resolved by having a specialized system for active maintenance, that uses more isolated representations (i.e.., the frontal cortex), in conjunction with a posterior cortical system that has overlapping distributed representations and can therefore perform inference and generalization.

Another specialization that the active maintenance system requires is a mechanism that allows for both rapid updating when new information is to be maintained and robust maintenance in the face of noise and activation elsewhere in the system. These are contradictory, but both can be achieved by using a neuromodulatory mechanism that dynamically regulates ("gates") the strengths of the inputs to the active maintenance system (Cohen et al., 1996; Hochreiter & Schmidhuber, 1995). Because this specialization would presumably be unnecessary for a nonactive maintenance system, it provides further motivation for having a specialized active maintenance system.

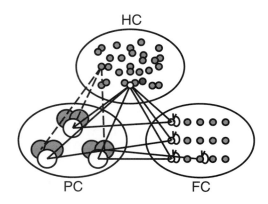

Figure 7.7: Diagram of key properties of the three principal brain areas. Active representations are shown in white; highly overlapping circles are distributed representations; non-overlapping are isolated; in between are separated. Weights between active units are shown in solid lines; those of nonactive units in dashed. Three active representations are shown, which can be thought of as feature values along three separate "dimensions" (e.g., modalities). **PC** posterior cortex representations are distributed and embedded in specialized (e.g., modality specific) processing areas. **FC** frontal cortex representations are isolated from each other, and combinatorial, with separate active units representing each feature value. Unlike other areas, frontal cortex units are capable of robust self-maintenance, as indicated by the recurrent connections. **HC** hippocampal representations are sparse, separated (but still distributed), and conjunctive, so that only a single representation is active at a time, corresponding to the conjunction of all active features.

7.5   Toward a Cognitive Architecture of the Brain

The central characteristics of the three different brain systems described previously are illustrated in figure 7.7. The basic picture is that the posterior cortex learns slowly to form integrative, distributed, overlapping representations with dense interconnectivity. It can exhibit short term active memory, but this is relatively easily interrupted by new incoming stimuli. The frontal cortex also learns slowly, but has more isolated representations and dynamic regulation mechanisms that enable it to maintain active memories over longer delays and in the face of new incoming stimuli. Finally, the hippocampus learns rapidly to form separated representations that minimize the interference between even similar memories. Taken together, these interacting systems, together with the basic principles outlined earlier, constitute a description of the *cognitive architecture* of the brain. Although aspects of this architecture are speculative, much of its general character is well supported by available data.

This cognitive architecture provides a framework for explaining the cognitive phenomena explored in detail in the subsequent chapters. In chapter 8, we will explore models of sensory processing in the posterior cortex, that exploit overlapping distributed representations and slow, integrative learning to shape these representations according to the structure of the sensory environment. Chapter 10 also mostly explores models of the posterior cortex, but in the context of language processing and mappings between different kinds of representations (principally orthographic, phonological and semantic). Chapter 9 focuses on memory, and explores the main tradeoffs and specializations that underlie the major components of the cognitive architecture. Finally, chapter 11 explores models that incorporate interacting posterior and frontal components of this cognitive architecture in the service of understanding how complex, temporally extended cognitive processing can emerge therefrom.

In the sections that follow, we elaborate some of the properties of this cognitive architecture by comparing it with more traditional cognitive architectures, and by mapping some of the main architectural distinctions in the literature onto this architecture.

7.5.1 *Controlled versus Automatic Processing*

Some of the main differences between more traditional cognitive models and the cognitive architecture sketched above can be highlighted by considering the distinction between *controlled* versus *automatic* processing. Generally speaking, controlled processing has to do with the ability to flexibly adapt behavior to different task demands, and generally act like an "intelligent" agent in the world. This kind of processing has classically been described in contrast with automatic processing (Schneider & Shiffrin, 1977; Shiffrin & Schneider,

1977), which is characterized as a simpler, more direct association of a stimulus input with a response. Another way of stating this distinction is that controlled processing is "higher level" cognition, whereas automatic processing is "lower level."

As a general characterization, the more traditional cognitive models based on production systems and the computer metaphor (e.g., Anderson, 1983; Newell, 1990) have been concerned with controlled processing (e.g., problem solving, mathematical theorem proving, logical reasoning), whereas neural network models have been concerned with automatic processing (e.g., perception, input-output mappings). Thus, it is important to see how our neural network-based cognitive architecture gives rise to controlled processing, and compare this with more traditional models. Although this is the primary topic of chapter 11, we will briefly sketch some of the main ideas here, because they are important for framing the entire endeavor.

Perhaps the best way to contrast the traditional approach to controlled processing from our own is in terms of centralized versus distributed processing. In many traditional models there is a centralized, controlling agent of some sort, one that is surrounded by a number of more automatic processing systems. Thus, we see a kind of Cartesian dualism here between the controller and the controlled, that probably reflects the compelling and widely shared intuition that a central soullike entity operates the levers of the complex biological apparatus of our brains. Needless to say, this approach begs the question as to how this internal *homunculus* ("little man") got to be so smart.

This centralized model is very clear in Baddeley's (1986) framework, where there is a "central executive" responsible for all the intelligent controlled processing, while a number of relatively "dumb" slave systems carry out more basic automatic processes. In Fodor's (1983) model, the mind is construed as having a central realm of intelligent, controlled processing, surrounded by a large number of highly encapsulated modules that automatically carry out sensory and motor processing. Perhaps the best example of this kind of architecture is the source metaphor itself — the standard serial computer. A computer has a centralized processing unit (CPU) that is surrounded by a number of "dumb" peripherals that service various needs (e.g., the hard disk is a memory module, the terminal is a response module, and the keyboard is a perceptual module).

In contrast, the neural network principles summarized in this chapter are fundamentally based on distributed knowledge and processing. Thus, our basic assumption is that controlled processing is an emergent property of the huge neural network that is the brain, and is not a reflection of some kind of dualistic distinction between central and peripheral systems. Nonetheless, the different components of our tripartite cognitive architecture are probably differentially involved in controlled versus automatic processing. Thus, we are led to an explanation of this distinction that is based on emergent properties of the entire network, but that also incorporates the unique contributions that specialized brain areas may make.

As we will see in chapter 11, the specializations of the frontal cortex (specifically the prefrontal areas) for rapidly updatable, robust active maintenance enable this area to provide a sustained, top-down biasing influence over processing elsewhere in the system. These actively maintained frontal cortex representations can guide behavior according to goals or any other types of internal constraints. Thus, the frontal cortex likely plays a more central role in cognitive control than other areas. However, it is through global constraint satisfaction processing across all three areas (posterior and frontal cortex and hippocampus) that representations are activated in the frontal cortex in the first place, so controlled processing remains essentially distributed and emergent. Furthermore, we emphasize the importance of using powerful learning mechanisms to explain how controlled behavior can be "smart," thereby avoiding the need for a homunculus.

7.5.2 Declarative/Procedural and Explicit/Implicit Distinctions

Another set of terms are used to denote distinctions similar to controlled versus automatic processing, but not completely synonymous. One such distinction is *implicit* versus *explicit* knowledge and processing. A related distinction is *procedural* versus *declarative* knowledge. Both explicit and declarative connote much

the same thing as controlled processing, implying deliberate, conscious, intentional processing, whereas implicit and procedural imply the lack of these attributes. However, declarative also appears to imply the use of linguistic representations, in that the information can be "declared." Explicit is not as tied to language, but does seem to imply conscious access to information. Meanwhile, procedural seems to imply action-oriented behaviors, whereas implicit implies the lack of conscious access.

Thus, understanding the meaning of these terms within our cognitive architecture requires us to deal with the issues of conscious awareness and the role of language. Although a comprehensive discussion of these issues is beyond our present scope, we can summarize a few relevant points.

First, regarding conscious awareness, a group of related ideas in the literature focuses on the importance of the duration, persistence, stability, and level of influence of representations (e.g., Kinsbourne, 1997; Mathis & Mozer, 1995). Under this general view, one can have conscious awareness of something to the extent that its representation has some or all of these characteristics. Within a neural network perspective, this amounts to saying that conscious awareness requires an activation pattern that is sufficiently strong to drive activations elsewhere in the network. In other words, we are aware of those things that are playing a prominent role in constraining the global constraint satisfaction settling process within the brain.

As a result, one should generally have greater conscious awareness of things that are active in the frontal cortex and hippocampus, as compared to the posterior cortex. The frontal cortex and hippocampus sit in a relatively powerful position at the top of the cortical hierarchy, and the frontal cortex in particular is specialized for constraining (biasing) processing in task or goal appropriate ways. This is consistent with the idea that these two areas also play a particularly important role in controlled processing, as discussed in chapter 11.

Thus, we think there is a coherent story here that ties together consciousness and the roles of the controlled-processing areas of the frontal cortex and hippocampus. Interestingly, this story does not need to make reference to language, allowing that non-human animals can be conscious and can have both "explicit" and "implicit" representations.

However, there is reason to believe that the intuitive notion captured by the term "declarative," that consciousness is strongly associated with language, also has some validity. Specifically, language input/output pathways become strongly associated with so many other internal representations that they can exert considerable influence over the general state of the system, making them likely to be within conscious awareness according to our working definition (e.g., when someone says something to you, the words are likely to strongly influence your conscious state).

7.6 General Problems

We next address a number of general problems that arise from the general functional principles described above. All too often, people tend to leap to the conclusion that because neural networks exhibit some kind of problem, they are somehow bad models of cognition. A classic example of this can be found in the case of *catastrophic interference*, where McCloskey and Cohen (1989) found that generic neural networks suffered much more interference from simple sequential list learning than humans did. This led them to conclude that neural networks were not good models of cognition. However, McClelland et al. (1995) showed that this failure actually tells us something very important about the way the brain works and helps to make sense of why there are two fundamentally different kinds of memory systems (the cortex and the hippocampus, as described previously and in chapter 9).

It is also important to emphasize that in many cases these problems actually reflect documented limitations of human cognition. Thus, instead of taking some kind of "optimality" or "rational analysis" approach that would argue that human cognition is perfect, we suggest that instead cognition reflects a number of tradeoffs and compromises. The fact that neural network models seem to provide useful insight into the nature of these human cognitive limitations is a real strength of the approach.

Many of the following problems have to do with the lack of flexibility resulting from the use of dedicated, content-specific representations. As we indicated earlier, there is a tradeoff along this flexibility–specialization dimension, and it appears that the brain has generally opted for the knowledge-dependency benefits of content-specific representations. Thus, the challenge posed by these problems is to understand how some measure of flexibility can emerge from within the context of a system with these knowledge-dependent representations.

One general category of approaches to the following problems has been to try to implement structured, symbolic-style representations in neural-like hardware (e.g., Touretzky, 1986; Hummel & Biederman, 1992; Hummel & Holyoak, 1997; Smolensky, 1990; Shastri & Ajjanagadde, 1993). Most of these models adopt a dynamic temporal binding mechanism and therefore use mechanisms that go beyond the standard integration of weighted activation signals that we use in the models in this book. The appeal of such models is that their representations transparently exhibit the kinds of flexibility and structure that are characteristic of symbolic models (e.g., binding is explicitly achieved by a binding mechanism, and hierarchical representations are literally hierarchical). The limitations of such models are also similar to the limitations of symbolic models — learning mechanisms for establishing the necessary structured representations and the systems that process them are limited at best, and it is unclear how the needed mechanisms relate to known biological properties.

We do not think that the advantages of the structured models outweigh their disadvantages — there are reasonable solutions to the following problems that are more consistent with the basic set of principles developed in this text. Whereas the structured model solutions to these problems provide formal and transparent solutions, the solution we generally advocate relies on the emergent powers of complex distributed representations across many different brain areas. As we mentioned previously, the following problems often arise because of the pervasive assumption that a single canonical representation must satisfy all possible demands — if one instead considers that a distributed collection of different kinds of representations can work together to satisfy different demands, the problem disappears.

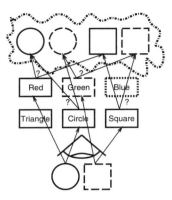

Figure 7.8: Illustration of the binding problem, where encoding in terms of separate features leads to confusion when multiple items are present in the input. Here, a red circle and green square are present in the input, but the same representation would be activated by a green circle and a red square, so the system does not really know which was present (as illustrated by the "imagination bubble" above the representation).

We will discuss in more detail examples of structured approaches in the context of object recognition (i.e., having a full 3-D structured representation akin to one you might find in a computer-aided design program) and sentence-level processing (i.e., representing the full parse-tree grammatical structure of a sentence) in chapters 8 and 10, respectively. We will find that the alternative distributed approach adopted in the models we explore offers a number of advantages in these contexts. Finally, note that although we focus on examples from visual perception in the following discussion, the issues generalize to many other aspects of cognition.

7.6.1   The Binding Problem for Distributed Representations of Multiple Items

One of the most commonly raised problems with neural networks is known as the **binding problem**, which arises whenever different features of a given stimulus are represented completely separately by different underlying representations, and multiple items need to be represented. Let's imagine we have a set of units that encode color information (e.g., red, green, and blue), and another set that encode shape information (e.g., cir-

cle, square, triangle). The binding problem arises when you present both a red circle and a green square to such a system — how does it know that it is the circle that is red and the square that is green, and not the other way around (see figure 7.8 for an illustration)? In other words, how does the system *bind* these separate features together as applying to the same object?

This is a good example of a problem that arises from a simplified, transparent, symbol-like set of representational assumptions, which can be resolved by adopting a more complex and less transparent distributed framework. The simplification in question is that stimulus information (e.g., shape and color) is represented completely separately — if instead representations incorporate aspects of both shape and color, then the *conjunctions* between these stimulus dimensions (e.g., red-and-circle, vs. green-and-circle) can be represented.

The standard objection to this conjunctive solution is that it is impossible to represent all possible such combinations in the world — way too many units would be required for realistic numbers of features. However, the alternative implicit in this objection is also overly simplistic — instead, individual units can represent *multiple combinations* of conjunctions, thereby covering the space much more efficiently (Wickelgren, 1969; Mel & Fiser, 2000). We can analyze this solution by considering combinations of conjunctions used together with the separate feature representations. The critical test is whether the overall distributed pattern of activity across all the units uniquely identifies the combination and binding of features present in the input.

Table 7.1 shows how the combination-of-conjunctions scheme works, with only a single additional unit required. This additional unit responds to a red circle *or* a green square *or* a blue triangle, and is enough to disambiguate the cases where the network would otherwise be confused on the basis of the separate features alone (e.g., confusing a red square and a green circle for a green square and a red circle). Thus, the total number of units required is 7 (6 separate features and 1 conjunction unit), which is only 2 less than the 9 units that would be needed to encode all possible conjunctions. However, when you scale the problem up, the advantages become more apparent. For example, if you have 4 colors and 4 shapes, then 16 conjunctive

obj1	obj2	R	G	B	S	C	T	RC GS BT
RS	GC	1	1	0	1	1	0	0
RC	GS	1	1	0	1	1	0	1
RS	GT	1	1	0	1	0	1	0
RT	GS	1	1	0	1	0	1	1
RS	BC	1	0	1	1	1	0	0
RC	BS	1	0	1	1	1	0	1
RS	BT	1	0	1	1	0	1	1
RT	BS	1	0	1	1	0	1	0
RC	GT	1	1	0	0	1	1	1
RT	GC	1	1	0	0	1	1	0
RC	BT	1	0	1	0	1	1	1
RT	BC	1	0	1	0	1	1	0
GS	BC	0	1	1	1	1	0	1
GC	BS	0	1	1	1	1	0	0
GS	BT	0	1	1	1	0	1	1
GT	BS	0	1	1	1	0	1	0
GC	BT	0	1	1	0	1	1	1
GT	BC	0	1	1	0	1	1	0

Table 7.1: Solution to the binding problem by using representations that encode combinations of input features (i.e., color and shape), but achieve greater efficiency by representing multiple such combinations. Obj1 and obj2 show the features of the two objects. The first six columns show the responses of a set of representations that encode the separate color and shape features: R = Red, G = Green, B = Blue, S = Square, C = Circle, T = Triangle. Using only these separate features causes the binding problem: observe that the two configurations in each pair are equivalent according to the separate feature representation. The final unit encodes a combination of the three different conjunctions shown at the top of the column, and this is enough to disambiguate the otherwise equivalent representations.

units would be required, but only 11 are needed with the features plus combinations-of-conjunctions scheme described here (8 feature units and 3 conjunctive units). We will explore more complex conjunctive binding representations that develop naturally from learning in chapter 8.

Another proposed solution to the binding problem, mentioned previously, uses processing dynamics to establish bindings between different feature elements on the fly (i.e., without using dedicated, content-specific

representations that encode conjunctive information). The most prominent idea of this type is that the synchronous oscillation of features belonging to the same object could encode binding information (e.g., Gray, Engel, Konig, & Singer, 1992; Engel, Konig, Kreiter, Schillen, & Singer, 1992; Zemel, Williams, & Mozer, 1995; Hummel & Biederman, 1992). However, the available evidence does not establish that the observed synchrony of firing is actually used for binding, instead of being an epiphenomenon. This is important, because such synchrony (which has been observed) is very likely to be a natural consequence of simple activation propagation in the spiking neurons of the brain (i.e., neurons that are communicating with each other will tend to drive each other to spike at roughly the same time).

Another problem with the synchrony-based binding idea is that it requires entirely new mechanisms for processing the bound information. Because feature bindings are transient and dynamic in these systems, any further processing of the bound representations would also have to rely on dynamic mechanisms — standard weight-based detectors and transformations would not work. For example, if there is some unique consequence or set of associations for red circles that does not apply to green or blue circles, how can this information become associated with a representation that only exists as a relatively fleeting temporal synchronization? This problem does not arise when a unique pattern of activity across a set of dedicated representational units is used (as with the combination of conjunctive representations scheme described earlier).

Finally, it is essential to realize that in many cases, people *fail* to solve the binding problem successfully, and such failures can provide important clues as to the underlying representations involved. For example, it is well known that searching for some combinations of visual features requires slow, serial-like processing, while other combinations can be found with fast, parallel-like speed (Treisman & Gelade, 1980). The simple interpretation of this phenomenon is that people sequentially restrict their object processing to one object at a time using spatial attention, so that there is no possibility of a binding problem between the features of multiple objects. The details of the visual search process are more complicated than this simple story, but the basic idea still holds. We will explore this kind of attentional interaction between spatial and object processing in chapter 8.

7.6.2 Representing Multiple Instances of the Same Thing

An extreme case of the binding problem occurs with multiple instances of the *same item*. Clearly, it is not possible to to distinguish these instances on the basis of object-centered features like color and shape. However, there are at least two other ways that the actual number of items can be accurately represented. First, the sequential application of an attentional mechanism directed at each of the items in turn, when combined with some kind of counting mechanism, could result in an appropriate representation.

Alternatively, unless the items are presented in the same location, spatial location representations can be used to disambiguate the case where only one item is present from the case with multiple instances of the same item. Thus, it is important to take into account the full range of possible representations, not just a single canonical object-based representation, when considering whether there really is a problem.

7.6.3 Comparing Representations

Another problem (related to the representation of multiple items) arises whenever you have to compare two different representations. Although one can use attention to time-share the same representational space across two different items, this does not work when you need to actually compare the two items, because you must have both of them represented at the same time. We suggest two solutions that use a single representational space without requiring that both representations be distinctly active in that space, and another that uses two distinct sets of representations with a comparison between them.

One potential solution using a common representational space would be that the natural network dynamics of inhibition and pattern overlap will result in a representation of what the two items have in common, which can be used as a basis for the comparison judgment (re-

call the exploration of presenting multiple digits to the same network in chapter 3).

Relatedly, it is possible to compare a visible stimulus with a stored representation of another stimulus by just assessing how well the visible stimulus activity pattern fits with the pattern of weight values that encode the stored stimulus. The speed with which the network settles, or the *goodness* (see chapter 3) of the resulting activation state are measures that can be used to assess the general fit of that stimulus with a stored one. Assuming that there is one stored pattern that is obviously closest to the visible one, then this measure will tell you how close these two are.

Although it may initially seem unnecessarily redundant, it is actually quite likely that the brain has multiple representations that could be used for comparison purposes. For example, we think that the frontal cortex has somewhat redundant representations of much of the content of posterior cortex, because this information must be represented in the specialized frontal cortex for active maintenance purposes. Thus, frontal cortex could hold the representation of one of the items, and the other could be represented in the posterior system (e.g., by viewing the item). The comparison would then be based on overlap or some kind of goodness measure that indicates how consistent these two representations are. The idea that the frontal cortex is somehow involved in comparisons is intriguingly consistent with the existence of the same capacity limitations for both relative judgments (comparisons) and active memory (Miller, 1956). It is also possible that multiple, somewhat redundant representations within the posterior cortex, each with a different emphasis but probably some overlap, could be used in a similar fashion.

Thus, there are a number of possible solutions to this problem, but we are not aware of implemented models that demonstrate the actual viability of these ideas.

7.6.4 Representing Hierarchical Relationships

Although we have emphasized the notion of a structural hierarchy of representations at increasing levels of abstraction, there are many other forms of hierarchical structure in the world that need to be represented in some systematic fashion. One problem is that most things have both subordinate components and are themselves a component of a superordinate entity. For example, a person's face is composed of components such as eyes, a nose, and a mouth, and at the same time is a component of the body. We think that there are spatially invariant representations of the visual aspects of such objects (e.g., an invariant representation of a nose, mouth, face, etc.).

The question is therefore how the structural relationship information of the parts as components (e.g., the relative position of the nose within the face) can be reconciled with the invariant representations of the parts as objects unto themselves (e.g., Hinton et al., 1986). Are there separate "relationship" representations that somehow bind together the invariant nose representation with the containing face representation? As you can tell, these kinds of questions presume canonical representations of the object parts, and the structuralist, symbolic solution is somehow to connect up these canonical face-part representations within a larger structure for the entire face, with relationship-binding associations that convey the relationship information.

In contrast, the multiple, distributed representations solution to this problem is to allow that there can be many invariant representations active at some higher level in the system, instead of just one canonical representation. These higher-level representations can all feed off of lower-level visual feature representations that encode structural information via the same kind of limited conjunctive-style representations as were suggested as a solution to the binding problem (we will explore the role of these kinds of representations in object recognition in chapter 8). Thus, there can be a shared representation of the nose in a face and the invariant nose to the extent that they both build off of the same lower-level features. The higher-level face representation can retain the conjunctive information that encodes the relationship between the nose and the rest of the face, while the invariant nose representation abstracts away from this context.

It is also likely that sequential attentional mechanisms can be used to focus on different aspects of hierarchically structured objects. Thus, the state of the visual system when one is focusing on the face as a whole will be different than when one is focusing just on the nose — higher levels of the system can maintain the invariant representations (and integrate over the sequential attentional shifts), while the lower levels are modulated by attention in a way that emphasizes the information necessary to process the object in the current focus of attention. Thus, when you focus on the nose, this deemphasizes those lower-level features that encode the face, while emphasizing those that encode the nose. This would make the job of abstracting away from the facial context easier.

As it happens, the example of face recognition is a particularly interesting one for these issues, because it appears that the representation of the face is much more than the sum of the representations of the individual parts — faces appear to be encoded more "holistically" (conjunctively) than other objects like houses (e.g., Farah, 1992). Thus, the representation of a nose in a face is not likely to have much in common with the representation of the nose alone.

7.6.5 Recursion and Subroutine-like Processing

Another challenge for dedicated, content-specific representations is the problem of **recursion** or executing **subroutines**, where either the same type of processing (recursion) or a different type of processing (subroutine) needs to be performed in the middle of a given processing step to obtain a result that is needed before processing can proceed. In a serial computer, the current set of state variables is simply pushed onto the stack (i.e., stored in a temporary memory buffer), and the subroutine (possibly the same one) is called with appropriate arguments.

This recursion is not easy when data and processing are not separable, particularly in the case of recursion where the same type of processing has to be performed on different data, without forgetting the previous data! This issue arises in the processing of sentences with embedded clauses (e.g., "The mouse the cat the dog bit chased squeaked."), where one might imagine that the overall processing of the sentence is composed of a number of "subroutine calls" to process each clause. However, as you can probably tell, people cannot easily parse such sentences, indicating a limitation in exactly this type of processing.

It is likely that the limited recursion or subroutining that does appear to exist in human cognition uses specialized memory systems to keep track of prior state information. For example, rapid hippocampal learning could be very useful in this regard, as could the frontal active memory system. Indeed, there is some recent evidence that the frontal pole may be specifically important for subroutine-like processing (Koechlin, Basso, & Grafman, 1999). In addition, the same kinds of combinations-of-conjunctive binding representations as discussed above could be useful, because they can produce different representations for the same items at different places within a sequence, for example.

7.6.6 Generalization, Generativity, and Abstraction

How do you get dedicated, content-specific representations to appropriately recognize novel inputs (generalization) and produce novel outputs (generativity)? This problem has often been raised as a major limitation of neural network models of cognition. One important point to keep in mind is that people are actually not particularly good at transferring knowledge learned in one context to a novel context (Singley & Anderson, 1989). Nevertheless, we are clearly capable of a significant amount of generalization and generativity.

One of the most important means of achieving generalization and generativity is by learning associations at the appropriate level of *abstraction*. For example, let's imagine that one learns about the consequences of the visual image corresponding to a tiger (e.g., "run away"). Because the actual visual image in this instance could have been anywhere on the retina, it is clear that if this learning took place on a lower-level retinally-based representation, it would not generalize very well to subsequent situations where the image could appear in a novel retinal location. However, if the learning took place on a more abstract, *spatially invariant* representation, then images of tigers in any location on the retina would trigger the appropriate response. This same argument applies at all different levels of representation in the system — if you learn something such that the same (or very similar) representation will be reactivated by the class of instances it is appropriate to generalize over, then generalization ceases to be a problem.

Given that we think the cortex is organized according to rough hierarchies of increasingly abstract representations, the abstraction solution to generalization is quite plausible. Further, it is likely that learning will automatically tend to form associations at the right level of abstraction — in the example above, the invariant representation will always be predictive of (correlated with) things associated with tigers, whereas the lower-level representations will be less so. Learning (of both the task and model variety) is very sensitive to predictability, and will automatically use the most predictable associations.

In addition to abstraction, distributed representations are important for generalization because they can capture the similarity structure of a novel item with previously learned items. Here, a novel item is represented in terms of a combination of "known" distributed features, such that the previously-learned associations to these features provide a basis for correct responding to the novel item. Neurons will naturally perform a weighted average of the feature associations to produce a response that reflects an appropriate balance of influences from each of the individual features. We will see many examples of this in the chapters that follow.

Although generativity has been somewhat less well explored, it also depends on the recombination of existing outputs. For example, novel sentences are generated by recombining familiar words. However, exactly what drives this novel recombination process (i.e., "creativity") has yet to be identified.

7.6.7 Summary of General Problems

It should be clear that most of the preceding problems are caused by a somewhat impoverished set of assumptions regarding the nature of the representations involved. For example, the binding problem is not as much of a problem if there is some element of conjunctivity in the representations, and generalization is fine as long as knowledge is encoded at the proper level of abstract representations. Thus, a general lesson from these problems is that it is important to question the representational assumptions that give rise to the problem in the first place.

We should also emphasize that we have no guarantee that the cognitive architecture we have sketched will result in something as powerful as human cognition. At this stage, we can say only that these properties are sufficient to simulate a wide range of cognitive phenomena, but that many challenging issues remain to be solved before the full scope of human cognition can be understood at a mechanistic, and ultimately biological level. See chapter 12 for more discussion of the limitations of the current framework and directions for future research.

7.7 Summary

In this chapter we have sketched an overall framework for modeling cognitive phenomena based on neural network principles. We were able to leverage these basic principles to understand the large-scale specializations of different brain areas. The interactions between these specialized brain areas constitute a kind of cognitive architecture. Now we are ready to explore a wide range of cognitive phenomena in the subsequent chapters.

Chapter 8

Perception and Attention

Contents

8.1   **Overview** **227**
8.2   **Biology of the Visual System** **228**
     8.2.1   The Retina *228*
     8.2.2   The LGN of the Thalamus *230*
     8.2.3   Primary Visual Cortex: V1 . . . . *230*
     8.2.4   Two Visual Processing Streams *232*
     8.2.5   The Ventral Visual Form Pathway: V2, V4,
           and IT *233*
     8.2.6   The Dorsal Where/Action Pathway *233*
8.3   **Primary Visual Representations** **234**
     8.3.1   Basic Properties of the Model *235*
     8.3.2   Exploring the Model *237*
     8.3.3   Summary and Discussion *240*
8.4   **Object Recognition and the Visual Form Pathway** **241**
     8.4.1   Basic Properties of the Model *243*
     8.4.2   Exploring the Model *246*
     8.4.3   Summary and Discussion *255*
8.5   **Spatial Attention: A Simple Model** **257**
     8.5.1   Basic Properties of the Model *258*
     8.5.2   Exploring the Simple Attentional Model . . *261*
     8.5.3   Summary and Discussion *268*
8.6   **Spatial Attention: A More Complex Model** **269**
     8.6.1   Exploring the Complex Attentional Model . *269*
     8.6.2   Summary and Discussion *272*
8.7   **Summary** **272**
8.8   **Further Reading** **273**

8.1   Overview

In this chapter we explore models of visual perception from the lowest level cortical representations to the more abstract high-level, spatially invariant object representations. We demonstrate how attentional effects emerge at multiple levels of representation and in the interactions between different specialized processing streams. We focus on vision because it is the most studied and relied-upon of our senses, and similar principles are likely to apply to other senses.

As we observed in chapter 7, perceptual processing is conceived of as a sequence of *transformations* that emphasize some aspects of the perceptual input while collapsing across others. Our somewhat unitary and transparent subjective visual experience is constructed from a wide array of processing areas, each specialized to some extent for a particular aspect of the visual world (e.g., shape, color, texture, motion, depth, location, and so on). Thus, the general structural principles of specialized, hierarchical processing streams discussed in chapter 7 are quite relevant here.

We focus primarily on two pathways, one that emphasizes *object identity* information and collapses across other aspects of the input such as spatial location (the "what" pathway), and one that emphasizes spatial location information while collapsing across object identity information (the "where" pathway). These two pathways interact with each other, and produce a complex pattern of spatial and object-based *attention*. The principles derived from exploring this subset of phe-

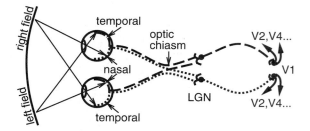

Figure 8.1: Pathway of visual information from retina to cortex. Light is reflected off of surfaces, transduced in the retina, and routed according to left and right visual fields (with the projections from the nasal retina crossing at the optic chiasm), to the LGN of the thalamus, which then projects up to the primary visual cortex, V1, and from there to specialized cortical processing areas (V2, V4, and beyond).

nomena should apply more generally to other aspects of visual processing, and to cortical processing in general. For example, the object recognition model provides an excellent demonstration of the power of rich, overlapping distributed representations developed over many specific training experiences to solve difficult problems.

8.2 Biology of the Visual System

The biology of the visual system begins with the eyes, but it is not completely clear where it ends, as increasingly abstract levels of visual processing merge gradually into multimodal or amodal "cognitive" processing. Indeed, there is considerable evidence that putatively visual brain areas are activated when a person is thinking about the semantic properties of an object (see chapter 10). In this section, we cover the brain areas widely regarded as visual processing areas, starting with the *retina*, going next to the *lateral geniculate nucleus* (LGN) of the *thalamus*, then into the primary and higher visual cortex in the *occipital lobe* (V1, V2, etc.), and continuing up into the *parietal* and *temporal* lobes (figure 8.1).

Although a vast amount is known about the visual system, particularly the early stages of processing, we provide only a sketch of the main findings here. Our objective is to provide sufficient orientation and empir-

ical grounding for the models described in this chapter. Thus, we have focused our presentation on those aspects of visual processing that are particularly important for object recognition, to the exclusion of many other aspects that are important for processing motion, color, surface, depth, and so on. Although these other visual properties play a role in object recognition (and attention), people are remarkably good at recognizing objects from simple line drawings, which indicates that basic shape or form information is at least sufficient for object recognition.

One of the key properties necessary for object recognition, in addition to representing basic *form* information (e.g., outline or general shape) is **spatial invariance**, where a given object can be recognized in a relatively wide range of spatial locations, sizes, rotations, and the like. In our models, we explore location and size invariance, which are the best documented aspects of spatial invariance in terms of the underlying neural representations. We will see that the visual system seems to gradually build up this invariance over subsequent stages of processing.

8.2.1 The Retina

The retina is much more than a passive light transduction device — it provides a relatively highly processed signal to the cortical visual areas (via the thalamus). It is important to understand the nature of this processing because it is incorporated into our models, in some cases by performing some appropriate form of preprocessing on actual images, and in others by directly providing input representations that roughly capture the effects of retinal processing.

Retinal processing performs **contrast enhancement** that emphasizes visual signal *changes* over space (and time). This processing tends to enhance the *edges* of objects, at the expense of coding the absolute values of regions with relatively constant illumination (i.e., surfaces). One benefit of this processing is that it greatly *compresses* the representation of a visual scene — instead of conveying every "pixel" of illumination, fewer and more informative edges are represented.

A complex three-layered circuit is responsible for the retinal processing. Everything starts with the light-

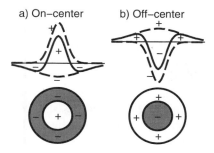

a) On–center   b) Off–center

Figure 8.2: On- and off-center receptive fields computed by the retina. The bottom shows a two-dimensional picture of the receptive field, with central and surround regions. The upper profiles show a slice through the center of the two-dimensional receptive fields, showing how a broad surround field and a narrow central field (in dashed lines) can be combined to form the overall receptive field (in solid line) as the difference of the two fields modeled as Gaussians.

sensitive **photoreceptor** cells that turn photons into electrical signals. There are two types of photoreceptors, *rods* and *cones*. Rods are primarily responsible for vision under low light levels (*scotopic* vision). Cones have three different wavelength sensitivities, and are primarily responsible for vision with high levels of light (*photopic* vision). Cones are primarily found in the **fovea**, the central part of the retina, which processes the portion of the image one is directly looking at.

Subsequent stages of retinal processing combine these electrical signals across local regions of photoreceptors, and then perform various types of *subtractions* of different regions using specialized, retina-specific mechanisms. These subtractions provide the crucial contrast enhancement effect, and are also responsible for enhancing the wavelength-selective properties of the photoreceptors to enable the perception of color. Finally, the **ganglion** neurons provide the output signals from the retina to the thalamus, described in the next section. The retina represents the central region of visual space, called the **fovea**, with the highest level of resolution for a highly detailed picture of things in the focus of one's gaze.

Most of the subtractions computed by the retina involve a **center-surround** receptive field. The **receptive field** (RF) of a neuron generally refers to the spatial dis-

tribution (in the retina) of inputs (light) that affect the firing of that neuron (more generally, this term refers to the set of inputs that activate a given neuron). You can picture the center-surround RF as a target, with a central region and a surrounding ring. Figure 8.2 shows the two main categories of center-surround receptive fields: an **on-center** RF, where the neuron is more active when the central portion of its receptive field is brighter than the surrounding portion, and an **off-center** RF, where the neuron is more active when the center is darker than the surround.

As illustrated in the figure, the on-center RF is constructed by subtracting a broadly-tuned but somewhat shallow surround region from a more sharply tuned and more peaked center region, and vice-versa for the off-center RF. Because each of the individual tuning functions can be modeled by a Gaussian (normal, bell-shaped) distribution function, the resulting center-surround field has been called a **difference of Gaussians** (DOG).

Consider what would happen if a uniform region of light covered the entire receptive field of either an on- or off-center neuron — the excitation would cancel out with the inhibition, leaving no net effect. However, if light were to fall more in the excitatory center of an on-center neuron than in its inhibitory surround, there would be net excitation. Conversely, if there was *less* light on the inhibitory center of an off-center neuron compared to its excitatory surround, it would become excited. These receptive field properties lead to the compression effect mentioned above, because the retinal output neurons (ganglion cells) fire maximally when there is a change in illumination level over their receptive fields, not when there is constant illumination. Although we have focused only on intensity (brightness) coding, retinal neurons also have on- and off-center coding of different wavelength tunings based on inputs from the different cone types (i.e., for color perception).

We will see in subsequent sections how these basic retinal receptive field properties provide useful building blocks for subsequent processing areas.

8.2.2 The LGN of the Thalamus

The thalamus is generally regarded as the "relay station" of the brain, because its many different nuclei relay sensory signals up to the cortex (and other places). The visual nucleus of the thalamus is called the **lateral geniculate nucleus** or **LGN**, and it relays information from the retina to the visual cortex. The LGN also organizes the retinal signals somewhat, using a six-layered structure (though there is recent evidence for six more layers). This organization is based in part on the eye of origin, with 3 layers for one eye and 3 for the other, and the spatial layout of the visual inputs that retains the topography of the retina (i.e., it is a **retinotopic** mapping, preserved in many cortical areas as well). The on- and off-center cells may also be organized into different thalamic layers.

Another aspect of LGN organization involves two different categories of neurons, called *magnocellular* (M, magno meaning big) and *parvocellular* (P, parvo meaning small). Generally speaking, the M cells have broader receptive fields (i.e., poorer acuity), poor wavelength selectivity, better motion selectivity, and better contrast sensitivity (i.e., low light or small brightness differences) compared to the P cells, which are high resolution (small receptive fields), and have better wavelength sensitivity. Thus, it is tempting to think of P cells as uniquely contributing to form processing, and M cells to motion processing. This is not correct, however, as both types participate in form processing, although to varying degrees.

Increasingly, people are finding that the thalamus is responsible for a number of important forms of processing beyond simply organizing and relaying information from the retina. However, the fact remains that the basic on- and off-center coding of information from the retina is passed on relatively intact to the visual cortex. Thus, instead of elaborating the complexity of the *structural* information being conveyed by the visual signal (i.e., what it reflects about the structure of the visual scene), the thalamus appears to contribute more to the *dynamic* aspects of this information. For example, aspects of the temporal dynamics of the magnocellular cells, that are important for motion processing, appear to be computed in the LGN itself.

Another dynamic aspect of thalamic processing has to do with *attention*. Indeed, one of the biggest clues about thalamic function comes from the large number of *backprojections* from the visual cortex back into the thalamus. According to some estimates, these backprojections outnumber the forward-going projections by an order of magnitude (Sherman & Koch, 1986)! These backprojections are generally thought to play a role in controlling the attentional processing performed by the thalamus, where some aspects or regions of the visual scene are dynamically focused on to the exclusion of others (e.g., LaBerge, 1990; Crick, 1984). Because the thalamus has all of the visual input concentrated in a relatively compact structure, it may be uniquely suited for implementing the kind of competitive activation dynamics across the entire visual scene that result in attentional effects. A similar argument can be made regarding attentional competition across modalities, because all sensory modalities except olfaction go through the thalamus, and could potentially compete with each other there. Further, the thalamus is thought to be important for modulating levels of arousal (e.g., sleep versus waking) by controlling cortical sensory input.

Although we will explore models of visual attention in this chapter, these models are based on cortically-mediated attentional processing, not thalamic attention. However, similar principles are likely to apply. Given that we also are not focusing on motion processing, this means that our models do not really capture the contributions of the LGN. We will however, take advantage of the laminar (layered) organization of the LGN to organize the on- and off-center inputs to our models.

8.2.3 Primary Visual Cortex: V1

The next major processing area in the visual stream is the **primary visual cortex**, also known as area **V1**, which is at the very back of the occipital lobe in primates.[1] Area V1 builds on the thalamic input by producing a richer set of representations that provide the basis for subsequent cortical processing. We will focus on those representations that capture more complex and useful aspects of visual form.

---

[1] Visual information is also subsequently processed in various subcortical brain areas as well.

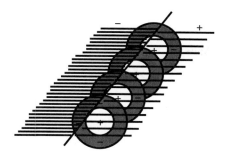

Figure 8.3: A string of on-center receptive fields can represent an edge of a surface, where the illumination goes from darker (on the left) to lighter (on the right). The on-center part of the receptive field is excited more than the off-surround due to the placement of the edge, resulting in net excitation.

Considering the on- and off-center coding scheme provided by the retina (and LGN) in isolation, one might expect that the world consisted of little points of light surrounded by darkness (like the night sky), or the opposite (points of darkness surrounded by light). However, one can combine these basic receptive field elements together to represent what are arguably the basic building blocks of visual form, **edges** (figure 8.3). An edge is simply a roughly linear separation between a region of relative light and dark. Hubel and Wiesel (1962) showed that some neurons in V1 called **simple cells** encode *oriented* edges or bars of light. They proposed something very much like figure 8.3 to explain how these **edge detectors** could be constructed from a set of LGN center-surround neurons. Although this proposal is still controversial, it is consistent with some recent evidence (Reid & Alonso, 1995).

Edge detectors make sense functionally, because edges provide a relatively compact way of representing the form of an object — with the assumption that the region between edges is relatively homogeneous, the visual system can capture most of the form information with just the outline. However, this is not to suggest that the visual system only encodes the outline — other types of neurons encode things like the color and texture of surfaces. These surface coding neurons can also be more efficient by summarizing the surface properties over larger regions of space. Again, we will focus primarily on the visual form information encoded by the

edge detector neurons.

As one might imagine, there are many different kinds of edges in the visual world. Edges differ in their orientation, size (i.e., spatial frequency, where low frequency means large, and high frequency means small), position, and *polarity* (i.e., going from light-to-dark or dark-to-light, or dark-light-dark and light-dark-light). The V1 edge detectors exhibit sensitivity (*tuning*) for different values of all of these different properties. Thus, a given edge detector will respond maximally to an edge of a particular orientation, size, position, and polarity, with diminished responses as these properties diverge from its optimal tuning. This is an example of the **coarse coding** of these visual properties. A particularly useful way of summarizing the tuning properties of simple cells is in terms of a *Gabor* wavelet function, which is the product of an oriented sine wave (capturing the orientation, polarity and size properties) and a Gaussian (which restricts the spatial extent of the sine wave). We will see what these look like in a subsequent exploration.

The different types of edge detectors (together with the surface coding neurons) are packed into the two-dimensional sheet of the visual cortex according to a **topographic** organization. This topography is probably a result of both innate biases in initial connectivity patterns, and learning influenced by factors such as the lateral connectivity among neurons within V1. At the broadest level of organization, all the neurons are roughly arranged according to the retinal position that they encode (i.e., a retinotopic organization, like the LGN). Thus, V1 can be thought of as a two-dimensional *map* organized according to retinal space. This map is distorted, in that there is a disproportionate number of neurons encoding positions within the fovea in the center of the visual field, because this is the most sensitive, high-resolution area.

Within the large-scale positional map, neurons are generally organized topographically according to their different tuning properties. One account of this organization (Livingstone & Hubel, 1988) is that the surface coding neurons and the oriented edge detectors are separated, with the surface neurons grouped together in a structure called a **blob**, which is surrounded by the **interblob** region where the edge detectors are found.

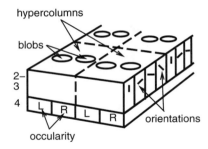

Figure 8.4: Structure of a cortical hypercolumn, that represents a full range of orientations (in layers 2–3), ocular dominance columns (in layer 4, one for each eye), and surface features (in the blobs). Each such hypercolumn is focused within one region of retinal space, and neighboring hypercolumns represent neighboring regions.

Within the interblob region, the edge detectors appear to be organized according to orientation, such that neighboring neurons encode similar orientations, with a relatively smooth progression of orientation found by moving along a given direction. The **ocular dominance columns**, in which V1 neurons respond preferentially to input from one eye or the other, but not both, are organized orthogonally to the orientation dimension. These ocular dominance columns might be important for stereo depth coding, although they are not present in all mammals.

This topographic arrangement can be summarized with the notion of a **hypercolumn**, that contains a full range of orientation codings and ocular dominance columns (i.e., one for each eye), in addition to two blobs (figure 8.4). All the neurons within a given hypercolumn process roughly the same region of retinal space, and neighboring hypercolumns process neighboring regions of space. Inevitably, one must view this hypercolumn topology as more of a continuum than as the discrete structure described here. One way of viewing such a continuum is that the blob regions contain the neurons tuned to a low spatial frequency (i.e., broad areas), while the interblob regions contain higher spatial frequency cells. Nevertheless, we will see that this notion of a hypercolumn is a useful abstraction for organizing models.

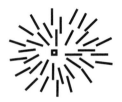

Figure 8.5: A pinwheel structure, where orientation coding of V1 neurons (indicated by the orientation of the lines) moves around in a circle of neurons, with a singularity in the middle where orientation is not clearly coded (indicated by the small square).

Another interesting topographic feature of V1 is the *pinwheel* (e.g., Blasdel & Salama, 1986), where all orientations are represented around a circle of neurons, with a *singularity* in the middle of the circle where orientation is not clearly coded (figure 8.5). We will see in the first simulation below that this pinwheel structure, along with many of the other key properties of V1 edge detector neurons and their topographic organization, can emerge from CPCA Hebbian learning with the kWTA activation function, together with neighborhood interactions between neurons.

8.2.4 Two Visual Processing Streams

Beyond V1, visual processing appears to separate into two major streams (figure 8.6). Initially, this split was described in terms of a *ventral* "what" pathway for processing object identity information, and a *dorsal* "where" pathway for processing spatial location and motion information (Ungerleider & Mishkin, 1982). The ventral stream goes along the lower part of the cortex from the occipital lobe to the inferior temporal cortex (IT). The dorsal stream goes along the upper part of the cortex from the occipital lobe to the parietal lobe. The reality of what these brain areas do is probably a bit more complex than this simple story. For example, it is likely that the dorsal pathway plays a role in using visual information to guide motor actions, which certainly involves spatial location information, but also certain kinds of visual form information (Goodale & Milner, 1992). There is clearly intercommunication between these pathways, so they cannot be considered

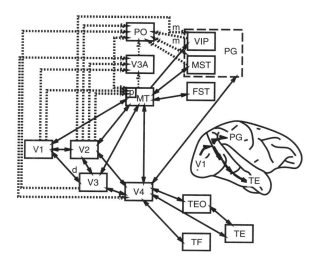

Figure 8.6: Diagram of the monkey visual system, showing the dorsal "where" pathway (to PG) and the ventral "what" pathway to TE. Solid lines indicate full visual field projections, whereas dotted lines are only the peripheral visual field. Adapted from Desimone & Ungerleider (1989), which contains further details.

to be functionally isolated processing "modules." We will explore one idea about what these interconnections might be doing in the models described later in this chapter.

8.2.5 The Ventral Visual Form Pathway: V2, V4, and IT

The ventral pathway for representing visual form information (i.e., object recognition) can be thought of as successive stages that lead to increasingly spatially invariant representations. In addition, the complexity of the form information encoded by these representations increases in successive stages, and the receptive fields get larger.

The next area after V1, called **V2**, appears to contain a number of interdigitated regions (called *stripes*) of specialized neurons that emphasize different aspects of visual information (e.g., form (edges), surface properties (color, texture), and motion). As emphasized by Desimone and Ungerleider (1989), one critical difference between V2 and V1 representations is that some

V2 neurons exhibit their feature selectivity *across a range of different positions*. Thus, these neurons can be seen as the initial steps toward spatially invariant object representations. We will see in section 8.4 how these kinds of partially invariant V2 receptive fields might develop, and how the weights need to be configured to achieve this property.

The next major area after V2 is **V4**, which receives inputs from V2, and is the first visual area that appears to be primarily focused on visual form processing and object recognition. Here, neurons continue the process of spatial invariance coding begun in V2, and also exhibit more complex feature detection.

In the inferior temporal cortex (**IT**), neurons achieve a high level of both size and location invariance, and some measure of rotational invariance. Further, the neurons encode complex (and often very difficult to characterize) properties of shapes. Thus, it seems likely that IT neurons provide a distributed basis for invariant object recognition. Lesions in this area can produce *visual agnosias*, or the inability to recognize objects visually (Farah, 1990). One particularly interesting form of agnosia is *prosopagnosia*, where a lesion results in the inability to recognize faces (see Farah et al., 1993 for a neural network model). For more details on some of the specific properties of this neural code, see Tanaka (1996) and Desimone and Ungerleider (1989).

8.2.6 The Dorsal Where/Action Pathway

The dorsal pathway represents spatial information and other information relevant for action. Neurons in this pathway have large receptive fields, often have preferred directions of motion, and incorporate information about the position of an animal's head and eyes. All of these properties support the processing of information about the location of objects in this pathway.

The dorsal pathway areas proceed up to the parietal lobe, and they include areas such as **MT** and **MST** (important for motion processing) and posterior parietal areas such as **VIP** and **LIP**. There is considerable evidence that these areas process spatial information (e.g., Andersen, Essick, & Siegel, 1985; Ungerleider & Mishkin, 1982). Perhaps the most dramatic evidence comes from patients with **hemispatial neglect**. These patients, who typically have damage to the right parietal lobe, exhibit deficits in processing information that appears in the left-hand side of space. For example, they are impaired at detecting stimuli that appear in the left, and they fail to reproduce the left-hand side of scenes that they are asked to draw. They also have problems that appear to be specific to the left-hand sides of objects (Tipper & Behrmann, 1996), suggesting that parietal spatial representations have multiple reference frames (see also Snyder, Grieve, & Andersen, 1998).

Neural recordings from posterior parietal areas in monkeys clearly show that these areas encode combinations of both visual location and eye position (Zipser & Andersen, 1988). Furthermore, Colby et al. (1996) have shown that neurons in LIP that encode spatial location information are dynamically updated to anticipate the effects of eye movements.

The dorsal pathway may provide a spatially organized form of attention. We explore a model of this kind of attention in section 8.5, where we see that neglect can be simulated by damaging a pathway that has spatially mapped representations. The attentional effect produced by the spatial pathway in this model interacts in important ways with the object-processing pathway, enabling multiple objects to be processed without confusion. Thus, although it is important to understand how different aspects of visual information are processed in different pathways, it is also important to understand how these pathways interact with each other.

8.3 Primary Visual Representations

The first model we explore deals with the lowest level representations in the visual cortex (i.e., in area **V1**), that provide the basis upon which most subsequent visual cortical processing builds. This model demonstrates why the known properties of these representations are computationally useful given the nature of the visual world. This demonstration emphasizes one of the main benefits of computational models in cognitive neuroscience — they can explain *why* the brain and/or cognition has certain properties, which provides a much deeper level of understanding than merely documenting these properties.

The **correlational structure** of the visual environment provides a computationally oriented way of thinking about why edges are represented in V1. As we discussed in chapter 4, there are reliable correlations among the pixels that lie along an edge of an object, and because objects reliably tend to have such edges, they provide the basis for a particularly useful and compact representation of the environment. Once these basic pixelwise correlations are represented as edges, then subsequent levels of processing can represent the higher level correlations that arise from regularities in the arrangement of edges (e.g., different kinds of edge intersections or junctions, basic shape features, etc.), and so on up to higher and higher levels of visual structure (as we will see in the next model).

The objective of the first model is to show how a V1-like network can learn to represent the correlational structure of edges present in visual inputs received via a simulated thalamus. Olshausen and Field (1996) showed that a network that was presented with natural visual scenes (preprocessed in a manner generally consistent with the contrast-enhancement properties of the retina) could develop a realistic set of oriented edge-detector representations. However, this network was not based on known biological principles and was mainly intended as a demonstration of the idea that *sparse* representations provide a useful basis for encoding real-world (visual) environments. Many other computational models of these early visual representations have been developed, often emphasizing one or a few aspects of the many detailed properties of V1 representations (for recent reviews, see Swindale, 1996; Erwin, Obermayer, & Schulten, 1995). These models have been very useful in illuminating the potential relationships between various biological and computational properties and the resulting V1 representations.

The model we present incorporates several of the properties that have been identified in other models as important, while using the principled, biologically based mechanisms developed in the first part of this text. This relatively simple model — a standard Leabra model with one hidden layer — produces fairly realistic V1 representations based on natural visual inputs. The model uses the CPCA Hebbian learning algorithm on the same preprocessed visual scenes used by Olshausen and Field (1996). Recall from chapter 4 that the sequential PCA algorithm (SPCA) does not produce the appropriate edge detector representations, giving instead the "blob" representation and its orthogonal subcomponents as shown in figure 4.8. However, the conditional PCA (CPCA) Hebbian algorithm should *self-organize* representations of the appropriate conditional correlational structure present in image edges.

Because we use only Hebbian model learning in this case, we are effectively treating the very earliest levels of perceptual processing as sufficiently removed from any particular task that error-driven learning does not play a major role. Put another way, we assume that the statistical structure of the input (visual images) is sufficiently strong to constrain the nature of the representations developed by a purely model learning system, without the need for extra task-based constraints. The success of the model in producing realistic-looking receptive fields justifies this assumption to some extent. We will see in the next model that even the next layer up in the network benefits from a combination of model and task learning.

The model focuses on several important properties of V1 representations — orientation, position, size, and polarity — that have been emphasized to varying extents in existing models. For each of these properties or *dimensions*, the model develops *coarse coding* representations that cover the space of possible values along each dimension, as with actual V1 neurons. For example, in the case of orientation, the units have a preferred orientation where they respond maximally, and progressively weaker responses for increasingly different orientations. Further, individual units have a particular tuning value along each of these dimensions (e.g., coding for a low spatial frequency (large) edge with dark-light polarity at 45 degrees in a given location). Finally, we explore the topographic arrangement of these dimensions (with neighboring units representing similar values) that is produced by having excitatory lateral connectivity within V1.

8.3.1 Basic Properties of the Model

The inputs to the model are based on the on- and off-center neurons of the LGN that project to V1. For con-

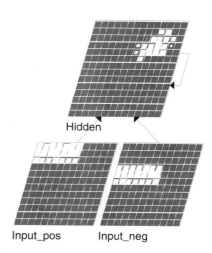

Figure 8.7: V1 receptive field network, showing both on- and off-center LGN inputs and the single V1 hidden layer with lateral excitatory connectivity.

venience, we have organized these two different types of inputs into two separate layers (figure 8.7), which may actually be a characteristic of LGN inputs. V1 itself is modeled as a single layer, which actually corresponds to the hidden layer of this area (cortical layers 2, 3), because many of the input layer neurons (cortical layer 4) have basically the same unoriented on- and off-center receptive fields as the LGN (and retina). Thus, the inputs in our model could probably be viewed as either the cortical input layer or the LGN, but we refer to them as LGN inputs.

The network was presented with images of natural scenes (mountains, plants, etc.) that had been preprocessed by Olshausen and Field (1996) to mimic the effects of contrast enhancement in the retina (using a spatial filtering that approximates the effects of the center-surround processing). Because the units in the Olshausen and Field (1996) network had both positive and negative weights and activations (which is biologically implausible), they did not separate on- and off-center components. However, we must separate these components because our activations and weights obey the biological constraints. We do this separation by presenting the positive-valued processed image pixels in the "on-center" input layer, and the absolute values of the negative-valued ones in the "off-center" input layer. The absolute values capture the fact that off-center neurons get more excited (positively) when the input is darker (more negative in the filtered images) in their center than in their surround.

One critical aspect of any model is its scale relative to the actual brain. This model is intended to simulate roughly one cortical hypercolumn, a relatively small structural unit in the cortex. As we discussed previously, a hypercolumn in V1 is generally thought to contain one full set of feature dimensions, e.g., orientations, sizes, etc., for a given area of the retina. However, a hypercolumn has many thousands of neurons, so our model of one hypercolumn is considerably reduced. The main factor in determining the scale of the model is not its raw number of units, but rather its patterns of connectivity (and inhibition), because these determine how units interact and whether they process the same or different input information.

The present model's connectivity reflects the following aspects of a hypercolumn: (1) All of the units receive from the same set of LGN inputs (actual V1 neurons within a hypercolumn probably have different individual connectivity patterns, but they receive from roughly the same part of the LGN); (2) The lateral connectivity extends to a relatively large portion of the neighboring units; (3) All of the units compete within a common inhibitory system (i.e., one kWTA layer). The kWTA average-based inhibitory function ensures that no more than about 10 percent of the units can be active at any given time, which is critical for specialization of the units, as discussed in chapter 4.

One consequence of the model's scale is that only a small patch of an overall image is presented to the inputs of the network, because a hypercolumn similarly processes only one small patch of the overall retinal input. In contrast with many other models of V1 that require initial spatially topographic connectivity patterns to obtain specialization in the V1 units (e.g., the *arbor function* in the Miller et al., 1989 and subsequent models), the V1 units in our model are also fully connected with the input layers. If we were simulating a larger patch of visual cortex in the model, we would probably need to include spatially restricted topographic connectivity patterns, and we would expect that this rough initial topography would be refined over learning into more well-defined hypercolumn structures.

The mechanism for inducing topographic representations in the model relies on excitatory interactions between neighboring units. These interactions were implemented by having a circle of connections surrounding each unit, with the strength of the connections falling off as a Gaussian function of distance. Thus, if a given unit becomes active, it will tend to activate its (closest) neighbors via the lateral excitation. Over learning, this will cause neighboring units to become active together, and therefore develop similar representations as they will have similar conditionalized responses to subsets of input images.

As discussed in chapter 4, this neighborhood excitation is the key idea behind Kohonen networks (Kohonen, 1984; von der Malsburg, 1973), which explicitly clamp a specific activation profile onto units surrounding the single most active unit in the layer. The main advantage of the current approach is that it has considerably more flexibility for representing complex images with multiple features present. This flexibility is due to the use of the kWTA inhibitory function, which just selects the best fitting (most excited) units to be active regardless of where they are located (though this is obviously influenced by the excitatory neighborhood connectivity). In contrast, the Kohonen function essentially restricts the network to representing only one feature (and its neighbors) at a time. Furthermore, the current model is closer to the actual biology, where a balance between lateral excitation and inhibition must be used to achieve topographic representations.

In our model, the lateral excitatory connectivity *wraps around* at the edges, so that a unit on the right side of the hidden layer is actually the neighbor of a unit on the left side (and the same for top and bottom). This imposes a toroidal or doughnut-shaped functional geometry onto the hidden layer. This wrap-around is important because otherwise units at the edges would not have as many neighbors as those in the middle, and would thus not get activated as much. This is not a problem in the cortex, where the network is huge and edge units constitute a relatively small percentage of the population.

Noise is added to the membrane potentials of the V1 units during settling, which is important for facilitating the constraint-satisfaction settling process that must balance the effects of the lateral topography inducing connections with the feedforward connections from the input patterns. Noise is useful here for the same reasons it was useful in the Necker cube example in chapter 3 — it facilitates rapid settling when there are many relatively equally good states of the network, which is the case with the lateral connectivity because each unit has the same lateral weights, and so every point in the hidden unit space is trying to create a little bump of activity there. Noise is needed to break all these ties and enable the "best" bump (or bumps) of activity to persist.

Finally, because the V1 receptive fields need to represent graded, coarse-coded tuning functions, it is not appropriate to use the default weight contrast settings that are useful for more binary kinds of representations (e.g., where the input/output patterns are all binary-valued). Thus, the results shown below are for a weight gain parameter of 1 (i.e., no weight contrast) instead of the default of 6. Because weight gain and the weight offset interact, with a higher offset needed with less gain, the offset is set to 2 from the default of 1.25, to encourage units to represent only the strongest correlations present in the input (see section 4.7 in chapter 4 for details).

8.3.2 Exploring the Model

[Note: this simulation requires a minimum of 64Mb of RAM to run.]

↪ Open the project `v1rf.proj.gz` in `chapter_8` to begin.

You will notice that the network (figure 8.7) has the two input layers, each $12x12$ in size, one representing a small patch of on-center LGN neurons (`Input_pos`), and the other representing a similar patch of off-center LGN neurons (`Input_neg`). Specific input patterns are produced by randomly sampling a $12x12$ patch from a set of ten larger ($512x512$ pixels) images of natural scenes. The single hidden layer is $14x14$ in size.

↪ Let's examine the weights of the network by clicking on `r.wt` and then on a hidden unit.

You should observe that the unit is fully, randomly connected with the input layers, and that it has the circular *neighborhood* of lateral excitatory connectivity needed for inducing topographic representations.

↪ Select `act` again in the network window. Locate the `v1rf_ctrl` control panel, and press the `LoadEnv` button.

This loads a single preprocessed $512x512$ image (ten such images were loaded in training the network, but we load only one in the interest of saving memory and time).

↪ Now, do `StepTrain` in the control panel, and observe the activations as the network settles in response to a sampled input pattern.

The hidden units will initially have a somewhat random and sparse pattern of activity in response to the input images.

You should observe that the on- and off-center input patterns have complementary activity patterns. That is, where there is activity in one, there is no activity in the other, and vice versa. This complementarity reflects the fact that an on-center cell will be excited when the image is brighter in the middle than the edges of its receptive field, and an off-center cell will be excited when the image is brighter in the edges than in the middle. Both cannot be true, so only one is active per image location. Keep in mind that the off-center units are active (i.e., with positive activations) to the extent that the image contains a relatively dark region in the location coded by that unit. Thus, they do not actually have negative activations to encode darkness.

↪ Continue to do `StepTrain` for several more input patterns.

Question 8.1 (a) *What would you expect to see if the lateral, topography-inducing weights were playing a dominant role in determining the activities of the hidden units?* **(b)** *Are the effects of these lateral weights particularly evident in the hidden unit activity patterns? Now, increase the control panel parameter* `lat_wt_scale` *to .2 from the default of .04 and continue to* `StepTrain`*. This will increase the effective strength of the lateral (recurrent) weights within the hidden layer.* **(c)** *How does this change the hidden unit activation patterns? Why?*

↪ Set `lat_wt_scale` back to .04.

We use this relatively subtle strength level for the lateral weights so the network can have multiple bumps of activity, not just one dominant one. This is important if there are multiple different edges with different orientations present in a given image, which is sometimes (but not always) the case.

If we let this network run for many, many more image presentations, it will develop a set of representations in V1 that reflect the correlational structure of edges that are present in the input. Because this can take several hours, we will just load a pre-trained network at this point.

↪ Press LoadNet on the control panel.

This loads a network that has been trained for 10,000 epochs of 10 image presentations, or 100,000 total image presentations.

↪ Select r.wt, and then click on the upper left-most hidden unit.

You should see in the weights projected onto the input layers some faint indication of a vertical orientation coding (i.e., a vertical bar of stronger weight values), with the on-center (Input_pos) bar in the middle of the input patch, and the off-center (Input_neg) bar just adjacent to it on the left. Note that the network always has these on- and off-center bars in adjacent locations, never in the same location, because they are complementary (both are never active in the same place). Also, these on- and off-center bars will always be parallel to each other and perpendicular to the direction of light change, because they encode edges, where the change in illumination is perpendicular to the orientation of the edge (as depicted in figure 8.3).

↪ To see these more clearly (because the weights have a somewhat small magnitude), click on the down arrow on top of the color scale bar on the right of the network window until there is good visual contrast in the weight display.

This shrinks the overall range of values represented, providing better contrast for the smaller weight values.

↪ Then click on the next unit to the right, and then the next one over, and click back and forth between these 3 units.

You should observe that the on-center bar remains in roughly the same position, but the off-center weights for the second unit switch from being just on the left

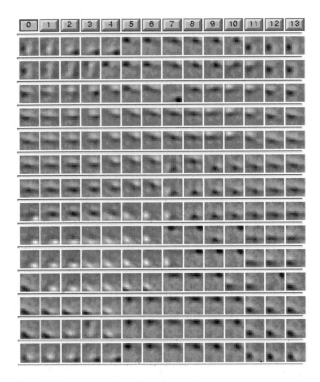

Figure 8.8: The receptive fields of model V1 neurons. Lighter shades indicate areas of on-center response, and darker shades indicate areas of off-center response.

to surrounding the central on-center bar. This reflects a transition in the *polarity* of the receptive field, with the left-most unit having a *bipolar* organization with one on-center and one off-center region, while the next unit over has a *tripolar* organization with one on-center region and two off-center ones. The third unit from the left goes back to a bipolar field, but with the off-center bar on the right. Further, it has an off-vertical orientation going up-right, representing a transition to a different but related orientation coding compared to the vertical of the previous two units. It also looks somewhat smaller in size.

Although this examination of the individual unit's weight values reveals both some aspects of the dimensions coded by the units and their topographic organization, it is difficult to get an overall sense of the unit's representations by looking at them one at a time. Instead, we will use a single display of all of the receptive fields at one time.

↪ To view this display, press `View`, `RFIELDS` in the control panel, and select `v1rf.rfs.log` in response to the file dialog that appears (you should be able to just press `Open`).

You will now see a grid log that presents the pattern of receiving weights for each hidden unit, which should look just like figure 8.8 (note that this is the same as figure 4.9). To make it easier to view, this display shows the off-center weights subtracted from the on-center ones, yielding a single plot of the receptive field for each hidden unit. Positive values (in red tones going to a maximum of yellow) indicate more on-center than off-center excitation, and vice versa for negative values (in blue tones going to a maximum negative magnitude of purple). The receptive fields for each hidden unit are arranged to correspond with the layout of the hidden units in the network. To verify this, look at the same 3 units that we examined individually, which are along the upper left of the grid log. You should see the same features we described above, keeping in mind that this grid log represents the *difference* between the on-center and off-center values. You should clearly see the topographic nature of the receptive fields, and also the full range of variation among the different receptive field properties.

Question 8.2 *Which different properties of edges are encoded differently by different hidden units? In other words, over what types of properties or dimensions do the hidden unit receptive fields vary? There are four main ones, with one very obvious one being orientation — different hidden units encode edges of different orientations (e.g., horizontal, vertical, diagonal). Describe three more such properties or dimensions.*

You should observe that the topographic organization of the different features, where neighboring units usually share a value along at least one dimension (or are similar on at least one dimension). Keep in mind that the topography wraps around, so that units on the far right should be similar to those on the far left, and so forth. You should also observe that a range of different values are represented for each dimension, so that the

space of possible values (and combinations of values) is reasonably well covered.

One of the most interesting aspects of the topography of these representations (in the network as well as in V1 neurons) are *pinwheels*, where the orientation of the receptive fields varies systematically around 360 degrees in the topographic space of the units.

Start at the hidden unit located 3 rows from the top in column number 7, and note the orientation of the units as you progress around a circle several units wide in the surrounding units — they progress around the circle of orientations. This structure can be seen as a consequence of having smoothly varying neighborhood relationships — if each unit has an orientation coding similar but distinct from its neighbor, then one would expect that they might proceed around the circle as one goes further away.

The unit at the middle of the pinwheel represents a *singularity*, which does not smoothly relate to neighboring unit values. Singularities also occur where there are relatively abrupt changes in orientation mapping across a short distance in the hidden unit topographic space. Both of these phenomena are found in the topographic representations of real V1 neurons, and provide an important source of data that models must account for to fully simulate the real system (Swindale, 1996; Erwin et al., 1995).

We can directly examine the weights of the simulated neurons in our model, but not in the biological system. Thus, more indirect measures must be taken to map the receptive field properties of V1 neurons. One commonly used methodology is to measure the activation of neurons in response to simple visual stimuli that vary in the critical dimensions (e.g., oriented bars of light). Using this technique, experimenters have documented all of the main properties we observe in our simulated V1 neurons — orientation, polarity, size, and location tuning, and topography. We will simulate this kind of experiment now.

↪ First, do `View`, `PROBE_ENV` in the control panel to bring up the probe stimuli.

This will bring up an environment containing 4 events, each of which represents an edge at a different orientation and position.

Question 8.3 *Explain the sense in which these probe stimuli represent edges, making reference to the relationship between the* Input_pos *and* Input_neg *patterns.*

Now, let's present these patterns to the network.

↪   Select act in the network window, and then do StepProbe in the control panel. Continue to StepProbe through the next 3 events, and note the relationship in each case to the weight-based receptive fields shown in the grid log.

You should observe that the units that coded for the orientation and directionality of the probe were activated.

If you are interested, you can draw new patterns into the probe events, and present them by the same procedure just described. In particular, it is interesting to see how the network responds to multiple edges present in a single input event.

Finally, to see that the lateral connectivity is responsible for developing topographic representations, you can load a set of receptive fields generated from a network trained with lat_wt_scale set to .01.

↪   Do View,   RFIELDS, and select v1rf_lat01.rfs.log.

You should see little evidence of a topographic organization in the resulting receptive field grid log, indicating that this strength of lateral connectivity provided insufficient neighborhood constraints. Indeed, we have found that these patterns look similar to those with networks trained without any lateral connectivity at all.

There appears to be an interaction between the topographic aspect of the representations and the nature of the individual receptive fields themselves, which look somewhat different in this weaker lateral connectivity case compared to the original network. These kinds of interactions have been documented in the brain (e.g., Das & Gilbert, 1995; Weliky, Kandler, & Katz, 1995), and make sense computationally given that the lateral connectivity has an important effect on the response properties of the neurons, which is responsible for tuning up their receptive fields in the first place.

↪ Go to the PDP++Root window. To continue on to the next simulation, close this project first by selecting

.projects/Remove/Project_0. Or, if you wish to stop now, quit by selecting Object/Quit.

8.3.3   Summary and Discussion

This model showed how Hebbian learning can develop representations that capture important statistical correlations present in natural images. These correlations reflect the reliable presence of edges in these images, with the edges varying in size, position, orientation, and polarity. Because the resulting representations capture many of the important properties of actual V1 receptive fields, this model can provide a computational explanation of why these properties arise in the brain. This is an important advantage of computational models — experimentalists can record and document the properties of visual representations, and a computational model can show how these properties result from the interaction between general learning and architectural principles and the structure of the natural environment.

Another advantage of understanding the principled basis for these visual representations is that we can potentially understand the commonalities between these representations and those in other sensory modalities. For example, the phenomenon of topography is widely observed throughout all primary sensory representations (e.g., somatosensory representations are arranged like a miniature human or *homunculus* in the brain). We can expect that other sensory modalities will tend to represent the strong correlational features present in the input.

One interesting indication that general principles are at work in shaping perceptual representations comes from an experiment by Sur, Garraghty, and Roe (1988). They rerouted visual projections from the thalamus into the auditory cortex of ferrets and found that neurons in the auditory cortex developed several response properties typical of visual neurons. Although this and other similar experiments are far from conclusive, they do provide suggestive evidence that the different areas of cortex use the same basic kinds of learning principles.

Finally, we should note that the early visual system has been the subject of a large number of computational models, exploiting a range of different principles (for recent reviews, see Swindale, 1996; Erwin et al.,

1995). The model presented here is comparatively simple, and has not been analyzed as extensively as some of the other models in the literature. Nevertheless, the current model may be unique in the number of known properties of V1 representations that it captures based on processing natural images. Although the Olshausen and Field (1996) model used natural images, it did not capture the topographic aspects of V1 representations. Most other models use artificial input stimuli that may not provide an accurate rendition of the statistics of natural images.

In the next section, we will see how these V1 representations can provide the building blocks for more elaborate representations in subsequent areas of the visual system.

8.4 Object Recognition and the Visual Form Pathway

The next model simulates the object recognition pathway that processes the visual form of objects (i.e., the ventral "what" pathway). This model uses V1-like edge detector representations at the lowest level and builds all the way up to **spatially invariant** representations that enable recognition of objects regardless of where they appear in the visual input space, and over a range of different sizes. Because we focus on shape over other visual properties of objects (e.g., color, motion), it might be more appropriate to consider the model one of *shape recognition*, but the same basic principles should generalize to these other object properties.

We take the development of spatially invariant representations to be the defining characteristic of processing in the ventral pathway: transformations collapse across different spatial locations and sizes while preserving distinctions among different objects. Although only two forms of invariance (location and size) are simulated here, the same mechanisms should lead to at least some degree of rotation invariance as well (note that it appears that the brain does not exhibit a very high degree of rotational invariance in its representations; Tanaka, 1996).

The traditional approach to spatially invariant object recognition (e.g., Marr, 1982) involves creating an internal 3-D model of the structure of the object based on

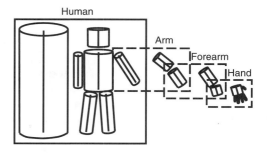

Figure 8.9: Schematic of Marr's view of object recognition based on a creating an internal 3-D model of the object, here using a hierarchical system of cylinders.

the visual properties of the object's surfaces (figure 8.9). Object recognition then amounts to matching the model constructed from the perceptual input to the closest fitting 3-D structure associated with known objects. The advantage of this approach is that the 3-D structural representation is completely invariant with respect to particular 2-D views, so that one only needs to store a single canonical representation of an object, and it can then be recognized from any viewpoint.

Hinton (1981) proposed a neural-network approach to invariant object recognition that bears some resemblance to the Marr approach (see also Zemel, Mozer, & Hinton, 1989). In Hinton's model, a combined constraint-satisfaction search is performed simultaneously at two levels: (1) the parameters of a set of transformation functions that operate on the input image (e.g., rotation, translation, dilation, etc.), which are used to transform the image into a canonical form; (2) the match between the transformed image and a stored canonical view. Again, the objective is to dynamically construct a canonicalized representation that can be easily matched with stored, canonical object representations.

Both Marr's approach of producing a full 3-D structural model based on a given 2-D view, and Hinton's approach of finding an appropriate set of canonicalizing transformations, are exceedingly difficult search problems. Essentially, there are many 2-D projections that map onto many 3-D structures (or many transformations that map onto many canonical representations), resulting in an underdetermined combinatorial many-to-many search problem. A successful implementation of this type of approach has yet to be demonstrated. Furthermore, the evidence from neural recording in monkeys suggests that visual object representations are somewhat more view-specific (e.g., Tanaka, 1996), and not fully 3-D invariant or canonical. For example, although IT neurons appear to be relatively location and size invariant, they are not fully invariant with respect to rotations either in the plane or in depth. Behavioral studies in humans appear to provide some support for view-specific object representations, but this issue is still strongly debated (e.g. Tarr & Bülthoff, 1995; Biederman & Gerhardstein, 1995; Biederman & Cooper, 1992; Burgund & Marsolek, in press).

For these reasons, we and others have taken a different approach to object recognition based on the gradual, hierarchical, parallel transformations that the brain is so well suited for performing. Instead of casting object recognition as a massive dynamic search problem, we can think of it in terms of a gradual sequence of transformations (operating in parallel) that emphasize certain distinctions and collapse across others. If the end result of this sequence of transformations retains sufficient distinctions to disambiguate different objects, but collapses across irrelevant differences produced by different viewing perspectives, then invariant object recognition has been achieved. This approach is considerably simpler because it does not try to recover the complete 3-D structural information or form complex internal models. It simply strives to preserve sufficient distinctions to disambiguate different objects, while allowing lots of other information to be discarded. Note that we are not denying that people perceive 3-D information, just that object recognition is not based on canonical, structural representations of this information.

One of the most important challenges for the gradual transformation approach to spatially invariant object recognition is the *binding problem* discussed in chapter 7. In recognizing an object, one must both encode the spatial relationship between different features of the object (e.g., it matters if a particular edge is on the right or left hand side of the object), while at the same time collapsing across the overall spatial location of the object as it appears on the retina. If you simply encoded

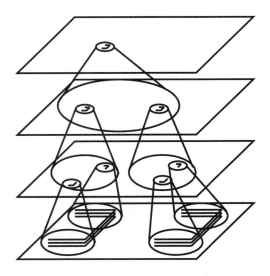

Figure 8.10: Hierarchical sequence of transformations that produce spatially invariant representations. The first level encodes simple feature conjunctions across a relatively small range of locations. The next level encodes more complex feature conjunctions in a wider range of locations. Finally, in this simple case, the third level can integrate across all locations of the same object, producing a fully invariant representation.

each feature completely separately in a spatially invariant fashion, and then tried to recognize objects on the basis of the resulting collection of features, you would lose track of the spatial arrangement (binding) of these features relative to each other, and would thus confuse objects that have the same features but in different arrangements. For example the capital letters "T" and "L" are both composed of a horizontal and a vertical line, so one needs to represent the way these lines intersect to disambiguate the letters.

As perhaps most clearly enunciated by Mozer (1987) (see also Mozer, 1991; Fukushima, 1988; LeCun, Boser, Denker, Henderson, Howard, Hubbard, & Jackel, 1989), the binding problem for shape recognition can be managed by encoding limited combinations of features in a way that reflects their spatial arrangement, while at the same time recognizing these feature combinations in a range of different spatial locations. By repeatedly performing this type of transformation over many levels of processing, one ends up with spatially invariant representations that nevertheless encode the spatial arrangements between features (figure 8.10).

Thus, our model depends critically on learning a hierarchical series of transformations that produce increasingly more complex (in terms of object features) and spatially invariant representations. Hierarchical representations are likely to be important for many aspects of cortical processing (see chapter 10 for more examples). Our model's ability to learn such representations using both task and model learning provides a key demonstration of this general principle.

Many researchers have suggested that object recognition operates in roughly a hierarchical fashion, and several existing models implement specific versions of this idea (Fukushima, 1988; Mozer, 1987; LeCun et al., 1989). These models separate the process of creating increasingly complex featural representations and that of creating increasingly invariant representations into two different interleaved stages of processing. One stage collapses over locations, and the other builds more complex feature representations. This makes the training easier, because the model can be specifically constrained to produce the appropriate types of representations at each layer.

In contrast, the present model is not constrained in this stagelike way and develops both aspects of the representation simultaneously and in the same units. This accords well with the properties of the visual system, which appears to achieve both increased featural complexity and spatial invariance in the same stages of processing.

Our model also demonstrates how a hierarchical sequence of transformations can work effectively on novel inputs (i.e., generalization). Thus, we will see that a new object can be learned (relatively rapidly) in a small set of retinal positions and sizes, and then recognized fairly reliably without further learning in the other (untrained) positions and sizes. It is important to demonstrate generalization because it is unreasonable to expect that one must have already seen an object from all possible viewpoints before being able to reliably recognize it. Generalization also falls naturally out of the traditional approaches, but the gradual transformation approach has not previously been shown to be capable of generalizing the invariance transformation (but

other kinds of generalization have been explored; Le-Cun et al., 1989). Furthermore, the behavioral literature shows that people can generalize their object recognition across locations, although with some level of degradation (Peterson & Zemel, 1998; Zemel, Behrmann, Mozer, & Bavelier, submitted).

Our model accomplishes generalization of the invariance transformation by extracting and transforming complex structural features shared by all objects. The higher levels of the network contain spatially invariant representations of these complex object features, the combinations of which uniquely identify particular objects. This assumes that there is a roughly fixed set or vocabulary of underlying structural regularities shared by all objects, that are also distinctive enough so that the combination of such features disambiguates the objects. We ensure this in the model by constructing objects from a fixed set of line features, but it is also likely to be true of objects in the real world, which can all be seen as composed from a pallet of different surfaces, textures, colors, component shapes, etc. Although one particular suggestion exists as to what these component shapes might be (Biederman, 1987), we do not have to commit to such specifics because learning will automatically find them (as it does in the model).

Finally, one important limitation of the current model is that it processes only a single object at a time. However, we will see in a later section how spatial and object-based representations interact to enable the perception of complex and potentially confusing visual displays containing multiple objects.

8.4.1 Basic Properties of the Model

The basic structure of the model (figure 8.11) is much like that of figure 8.10. Whereas the previous model represented roughly a single cortical hypercolumn, this model simulates a relatively wide cortical area spanning many hypercolumns (the individual hypercolumns are shown as smaller boxes within the layers in figure 8.11). Even more so than in the previous case, this means that the model is very scaled down in terms of the number of neurons per hypercolumn. As before, the connectivity patterns determine the effective scale of the model, as indicated below.

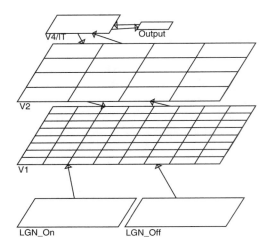

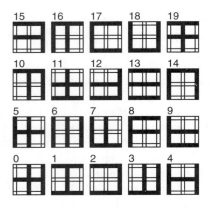

Figure 8.12: Objects used in the object recognition model.

Figure 8.11: Structure of the object recognition model, having on- and off-center LGN inputs, a V1-like oriented edge detector layer, followed by V2 and V4/IT that produce increasingly invariant and featurally complex representations (V4 and IT are collapsed together due to the simplicity of the objects and scale of the model). The output represents some further use of object representations by other parts of the brain. Hypercolumns are indicated by smaller boxes within layers.

The need to represent a large cortical scale requires the introduction of some additional structure, particularly with respect to the way that inhibition is computed. The idea behind this structure is that inhibition acts at multiple scales, with stronger inhibition among neurons relatively close together (i.e., within a single cortical hypercolumn), but also significant inhibition communicated across larger distances via longer range excitatory cortical connectivity that projects onto local inhibitory interneurons.

These multiscale inhibitory dynamics are implemented in the model with two nested levels of kWTA inhibition. Units within a single hypercolumn compete amongst themselves for a given kWTA activity level, while at the same time all the units across hypercolumns within the layer compete for a larger kWTA activity level reflecting the longer-range inhibition. The net inhibition for each unit is then the maximum of that computed by each of these kWTA computations.

The connectivity patterns also reflect the relatively large scale of this model. As in the previous model, we assume that all of the units within a given hypercolumn are connected to the same inputs. We further assume that neighboring hypercolumns connect with partially overlapping, but correspondingly offset, inputs. Thus, there is some redundancy (due to the overlap) in the coding of a given input area across multiple hypercolumns, but basically different hypercolumns process different information.

Although each hypercolumn of units processes different parts of the input, the hypercolumns are basically doing the same thing — extracting features over multiple locations and sizes. Furthermore, no part of the input is any different than any other — objects can appear anywhere. Thus, each hypercolumn of units can share the same set of weights, which saves significantly on the amount of memory required to implement the network. We use this *weight linking* or *weight sharing* (LeCun et al., 1989) in all the multihypercolumn layers in this model. Weight sharing allows each hypercolumn to benefit from the experiences in all the other hypercolumns, speeding up learning time (see following details section for more information).

The environment experienced by the model contains 20 objects composed of combinations of 3 out of 6 horizontal and vertical lines (figure 8.12). The regularity to these objects in their basic features is critical for enabling the network to generalize to novel objects, as described above. The network is trained on only the first 18 objects in a range of positions and sizes. The last two objects are used later for testing generalization.

This model can be seen as an extension of the previous one, in that the input is LGN-like, with separate on- and off-center layers. Objects are represented using bars of light (activity in the on-center LGN input) one pixel wide. The off-center input had activity at the ends of each bar, representing the transition from light to dark there. This *end stopping* information is widely thought to be encoded by neurons in the early visual cortex to represent lines of a particular length, for example.

The LGN is 16x16 units and wraps around like the previous simulation (i.e., the right-most unit is a neighbor of the left-most one and same for top-bottom). Objects are one of four sizes, corresponding to 5, 7, 9, and 11 pixel-length bars. The lower left hand side of the objects can be located anywhere within the 16x16 grid, for a total of 256 different unique locations. Thus, all combined, there were 1024 different unique "images" of a given object.

As in the previous model, a V1-like area processes the LGN input using simple oriented edge-detector representations. We fixed these representations from the outset to encode horizontal and vertical lines in all possible locations within the receptive field so that we could use the smallest number of V1 units possible. Instead of trying to make combinations of different polarities between the on- and off-center inputs, we just had one set of units encode bars in the on-center field, and another encode bars in the off-center field. Given that the receptive field size is 4x4 from each LGN input, there are 8 horizontal and vertical bars for the on-center and eight for the off-center, for a total of 16 units (4x4) in each V1 hypercolumn. Thus, we have considerably simplified the V1 representations to make the model simpler and more compact, but the essential property of orientation tuning is retained.

The next layers in the pathway represent the subsequent areas in the cortical object recognition pathway, V2 and V4. These areas have successively larger, more complex, and more spatially invariant receptive field properties. Due to the limited size of this model, V4 representations encompass all of the visual input

space, and thus can produce fully invariant representations over this entire space. The relative simplicity of the objects in our simulated environment also enables the V4 representations to have sufficient complexity in terms of feature combinations to distinguish among the different objects. In a larger, more realistic model of the cortex, full invariance and object-level complexity would not be possible until the next layer of processing in the inferior temporal cortex (IT). Thus, we have effectively just collapsed the V4 and IT layers into one layer.

The last layer in the network is the "output" layer, which enables us to use task-based, error-driven learning (in addition to model-based Hebbian learning) to train the network. It can be viewed as corresponding to any of a number of possible task-like outputs. For example, the different objects could have different sounds, textures, or smells, and the network could be predicting the corresponding representation in one of these other modalities, with the feedback being used to improve the ability of the visual system to identify the different objects to accurately predict these other correlates. Similarly, the objects may have different physical consequences (e.g., some can stand by themselves, others can roll, etc.), or they may serve as symbols like digits or letters. In any case, we simply have a distinct output unit for each object, and the network is trained to produce the correct output unit given the image of the object presented in the input. This task-based training is important for successful learning in the network.

Additional Model Details

This section contains additional details and substantiation of the basic features just described.

To verify that the weight linking shortcut does not play a substantial role in the resulting performance of the network, a control network was run without weight sharing. This network took much more memory and training time, as expected, but the resulting representations and overall performance were quite similar to the network using weight sharing that we explore here. This result makes sense because each hypercolumn should experience the same input patterns over time, and thus should develop roughly the same kinds of weight patterns. The use of Hebbian learning is undoubtedly important for the similarity between the weight shared and separate weight networks, because this form of learning tends to reliably produce the same weight patterns. A purely error driven backpropagation network run for comparison did not perform similarly in these two cases; each hypercolumn in the separate weight backpropagation network ended up doing very different things, leading to worse performance in terms of the spatial invariance properties of the resulting network. This is consistent with the general finding that backpropagation networks tend to have a high level of variance in their learned solutions.

One further architectural feature of the model is that we did not include the excitatory lateral interconnections among units within the same layer that were important for developing topography in the previous model. This was done because including such connections makes the model that much slower, and they do not appear to be essential given the model's good performance. However, were they included, they could presumably impose various kinds of topographic orderings of the object-based representations (see Tanaka, 1996, for neurophysiological evidence of this), and would likely be important for filling-in obscured parts of images and other similar kinds of pattern-completion phenomena (as explored in chapter 3).

We did not include off-center activity along the length of each bar because this would have been redundant with the on-center representation for the barlike stimuli we used. If our stimuli had surfacelike properties (as in the previous simulation), then this additional off-center information would not have been redundant, as it could indicate the relative brightness of different surfaces.

If we let the V1 receptive fields develop through learning instead of fixing them to be the minimal set required by the task, extra units would be required as we discussed in chapter 4. We have already demonstrated that these kinds of representations will develop in response to natural images, and we also ran a larger model and verified that these representations do develop here.

The parameters for the network are all standard, with the amount of Hebbian learning set to .005 except for the connections between V1 and V2, which are at .001. This lower amount of Hebbian learning here is necessary due to the weight sharing, because the same weights are being updated many times for each input, causing the Hebbian learning to be even more dominant. The learning rate was also dropped to .001 from .01 after 150 epochs, which helped to reduce the interference effects of weight changes from one pattern on other patterns. The slower learning rate could have been used from the start, but this significantly slows overall learning.

8.4.2 Exploring the Model

[*Note: this simulation requires a minimum of 128Mb of RAM to run.*]

↪ **Open the project** `objrec.proj.gz` **in** `chapter_8` to begin.

You will see that the network looks like a skeleton, because it is too big to save all the units and connections in the project file. We will build and connect the network in a moment, but first, the skeleton reveals some important aspects of the network structure. You can see the LGN input layers, which are $16x16$ units in size. Above that, you can see the V1 layer, which has an $8x8$ grid structure, where each of these 64 grid elements represents one hypercolumn of units. Each hypercolumn will contain a group of 16 ($4x4$) units when the network is built, and these units will all be connected to the same small ($4x4$) region of both LGN inputs. As discussed earlier, neighboring groups will be connected to half-overlapping regions of LGN, as we will see more clearly when the network is connected. In addition to connectivity, these groups organize the inhibition within the layer, as described above. The kWTA level is set to 6 out of 16 units within a hypercolumn, and 60 across the entire layer (i.e., ten hypercolumns out of 64 could have their maximal activity of 6, though activity need not be distributed in this manner).

The V2 layer is also organized into a grid of hypercolumns, this time $4x4$ in size, with each hypercolumn having 64 units ($8x8$). Again, inhibition operates at both the hypercolumn and entire layer scales here, with 8 units active per hypercolumn and 48 over the entire layer. Each hypercolumn of V2 units receives from a quarter of the V1 layer, with neighboring columns again having half-overlapping receptive fields. Next, the V4/IT layer represents just a single hypercolumn of units ($10x10$ or 100 units) within a single inhibitory group, and receives from the entire V2 layer. Finally, the output layer has 20 units, one for each of the different objects.

Now, let's build and connect the network.

↪ Press `BuildNet` on the `objrec_ctrl` overall control panel.

You will see the network fill in with units, and it will also be connected.

↪ Now, switch to `r.wt`, and click on units in the V1 layer.

You should see that each V1 unit receives from a set of 4 input units, arranged either horizontally or vertically. You may also be able to see that each hypercolumn of V1 units has a potential receptive field of a $4x4$ patch of the input layers (as indicated by the slightly darker gray color of those units), and neighboring hypercolumns receive from half-overlapping such patches.

↪ Now click on V2 units.

You should see that their connectivity patterns are similar in form, but larger in size.

Now, let's see how the network is trained.

↪ First, go back to viewing `act` in the networks display. Then, do `StepTrain` in the control panel.

You will see the negative phase of settling for the input image, which is one of the shapes shown in figure 8.12 at a random location and size.

↪ Press `StepTrain` again to see the plus phase. You can then continue to `StepTrain` through a series of inputs to get a feel for what some of the different input patterns look like.

Because it takes more than 24 hours for this network to be trained, we will just load the weights from a trained network. The network was trained for 460 epochs of 150 object inputs per epoch, or 69,000 object presentations. However, it took only roughly 200 epochs (30,000 object presentations) for performance to approach asymptote. This corresponds to the network having seen each object in each location and size (i.e., 1024 locations and sizes per object for 18 objects) only twice (assuming a perfect uniform distribution, which was not the case). Thus, it is clear that there is a consid-

erable amount of generalization during training, some of which is due to the weight sharing, but probably not all of it (weight sharing doesn't help with size invariance, for example).

Because this network is relatively large, only the actual weight values themselves have been saved in a file.

↪ Load the weights using `LoadNet` on the control panel. Then, `StepTrain` a couple of times to see the minus and plus phases of the trained network as it performs the object recognition task. To enhance the excitement of seeing the network perform this difficult task, you can set the `net_updt` to `CYCLE_UPDT` and see the activation patterns evolve as the network settles over cycles of processing.

You should see that the plus and minus phase output states are the same, meaning that the network is correctly recognizing most of the objects being presented. To view a record of this performance, we can open a training log.

↪ Do `View`, `TRAIN_LOG`, and press the rewind VCR button in the log to see prior results.

The `sum_se` column of this log shows the error for each pattern. Although you may see an occasional error, this column should be mostly zeroes (the errors are usually associated with the smallest sizes, which are just at the low end of the resolution capabilities of the network given its feature detectors). Thus, the network shows quite good performance at this challenging task of recognizing objects in a location-invariant and size-invariant manner.

Activation-Based Receptive Field Analysis

Unfortunately, it is not particularly informative to watch the patterns of activity in the various layers of the network in response to the different inputs. Further, because most of the units are not directly connected to the input, we can't just view their weights to easily see what they are representing. We can instead generate an *activation based receptive field* for the hidden units in the network.

The activation based receptive field shows how a unit's activity is correlated with another layer's activity patterns, as measured over a large sample of patterns. For example, we might want to know how a V2 unit's activity correlates with LGN patterns of activity. If the V2 unit reliably responds to only one input pattern, the resulting activation based receptive field will just be that input pattern. If the V2 unit responds equally to a set of ten input patterns, the result will be the average of these ten patterns. The corresponding mathematical expression for a given receptive field element r_i (corresponding to an LGN unit i, in the example above) is:

$$r_i = \frac{\sum_t y_j(t) x_i(t)}{\sum_t y_j(t)} \qquad (8.1)$$

where $y_j(t)$ is the activation of the unit whose receptive field we are computing (the V2 unit in the example above), $x_i(t)$ is the activation of the unit in the layer on which we are computing the receptive field (LGN in the example above), and t is an index over input patterns, as usual. Note that this is very similar to what the CPCA Hebbian learning rule computes, as we saw in the previous simulation. However, as in the V2-LGN example above, we can use the activation based receptive field procedure to compute "weights" (receptive field values) for layers that a given unit is not directly connected to. For example, it can also be useful to look at a unit's activation based receptive field by averaging over the output images, to see what object the unit participates in representing.

Now, let's take a look at the activation based receptive fields for the different layers of the network.

↪ Press View on the overall control panel, and select ACT_RF. Press Open in the file selection window to pull up the input receptive field for the V2 units from the on-center LGN layer (figure 8.13). Another file selection window will also appear; you can move that aside while you examine the current display.

Because we are doing weight sharing, we need only look at one hypercolumn's worth of V2 units, which are displayed in the large-scale 8x8 grid in this window. Within each of these grid elements is another grid representing the activation-weighted average over the input patterns, which is the activation based receptive field for this unit. Note that these units are in the first (lower left hand) hypercolumn of the V2 layer, so they receive from the corresponding lower left hand region of the input, which is why the receptive fields emphasize this region.

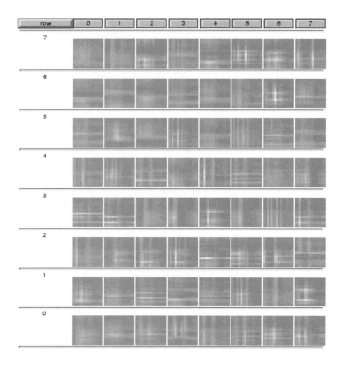

Figure 8.13: V2 activation-based receptive fields from on-center LGN inputs. The large-scale 8x8 grid represents one hypercolumn's worth of units, with each large grid containing a grid representing the on-center LGN input. The colors represent the values of the activation-weighted averages over input patterns. The neurons appear to represent low-order conjunctions of features over a (small) range of locations.

Notice that some units have brighter looking (more toward the yellow end of the scale) receptive fields and appear to represent only a few positions/orientations, while others are more broadly tuned and have dimmer (more toward the dark red end of the scale) receptive fields. The brightness level of the receptive field is directly related to how *selective* the unit is for particular input patterns. In the most selective extreme where the unit was activated by a single input pattern, the receptive field would have just maximum bright $r_i = 1$ values for that single pattern. As the unit becomes less selective, the averaging procedure dilutes the receptive field values across all the patterns that the unit represents, resulting in dimmer values. We can use this brightness/dimness feature to evaluate to what extent these V2 units encode conjunctions of features (responding only when the features are present together), and to what extent they exhibit spatial invariance (responding to a feature or features in a range of different locations).

We first consider conjunctions of features. If a unit responds only when two features are present together, thus representing the conjunction of these features, the unit will have a bright encoding of those features. For example, the unit in column 5, row 7, has two bright vertical lines, and the unit at 1, 3 has two bright horizontal lines, suggesting that each of these units represents the conjunction of their respective features. In contrast, if a unit had responded to one feature in one input and the other feature in another input (thus not representing the conjunction of those features), then the lines would be dimmer, due to the diluting of the activation based receptive field. Thus, we see some evidence for conjunctive representations in the V2 units in the multiple bright features encoded by some of the units.

We next consider spatial invariance. If a unit responds to the same feature in a number of different locations (across inputs), thus representing that feature in a spatially invariant manner, the unit will have a dim encoding of the feature in each of those locations. The dim receptive fields are produced by the process of averaging across different inputs, with activation based receptive fields becoming more diluted the more a unit responds to different inputs (the less selective the unit is). For example, the unit at 5, 5 has several dim vertical lines, suggesting that the unit represents this feature across those different locations. Thus, we see some evidence of spatially invariant encoding in the V2 units in these dimmer receptive fields for the same feature in different locations.

Question 8.4 *Explain the significance of the level of conjunctive representations and spatial invariance observed in the V2 receptive fields, in terms of the overall computation performed by the network.*

↪ Press `Open` in the file selection window to bring up the next receptive field display, which shows the input receptive fields from the off-center LGN input layer (figure 8.14). Again put aside the next dialog for a moment.

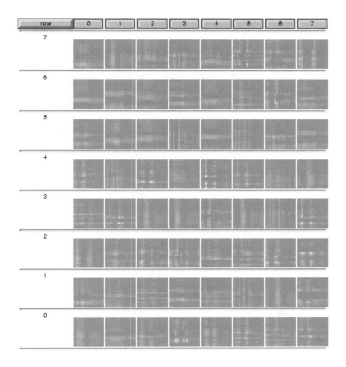

Figure 8.14: V2 activation-based receptive fields from off-center LGN inputs. Layout is the same as the previous figure.

You should observe a clear correspondence between the receptive field patterns for the on- and off-center inputs, indicating that the V2 neurons have encoded the linear elements represented in the on-center fields, and also where these lines should end as represented in the off-center fields.

↪ Now press `Open` in the next file selection window to view the *output* layer receptive fields for these same V2 units (figure 8.15).

This enables you to see which objects the units participate in representing. You may notice there does not appear to be a correlation between input and output selectivity — units with highly selective input coding participated in the representation of many objects, and vice versa. You might have expected that highly selective input tuning would make units highly selective for what objects they represent, but in fact they are representing shared features of objects and so can participate in the representation of multiple objects.

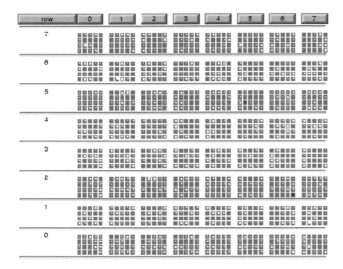

Figure 8.15: V2 activation-based projection fields to the output units, showing that each unit participates in representing multiple objects.

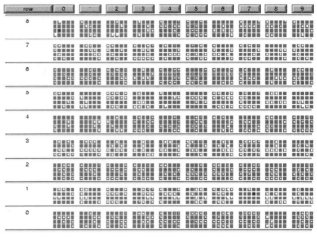

Figure 8.16: V4 activation-based projection fields to the output units.

Question 8.5 *Using the images of the objects shown in figure 8.12 (which are in the same configuration as the output units), explain one unit's participation in a particular output representation based on the features shown in its input receptive fields. (Hint: Pick a unit that is particularly selective for specific input patterns and specific output units, because this makes things easier to see.)*

↪ Press Open in the next file selection window to view the input receptive fields for all of the V4 units.

Be sure to notice the scale shown at the bottom of the window, that tells you how large the maximum values are in this window. This scale shows that even though the receptive fields appear yellow, the maximum value represented by yellow is very small on the 0–1 scale (around .1). Thus, each of these units is active across a wide range of different input patterns. Furthermore, these patterns appear to be uniformly distributed across the input space, suggesting that in fact these units are fully spatially invariant.

↪ Finally, press Open once more to view the output receptive fields for the V4 units (figure 8.16).

Again, be sure to notice the scale shown at the bottom of the window. You may want to manipulate the scale (by typing in new numbers or pressing the control buttons in the bottom right) to match the scale in the grid log for the V2 receptive fields when making comparisons.

Question 8.6 (a) *Based on this latest display, do V4 units appear to code for entire objects, or just parts of different objects? Explain.*

One can also compare the relative selectivity of these V4 units for particular output units (objects) as compared to the V2 units. By focusing specifically on the number of objects a given unit clearly *doesn't* participate in, it should be clear that the V4 units are more selective than the V2 units, which substantiates the idea that the V4 units are encoding more complex combinations of features that are shared by fewer objects (thus making them more selective to particular subsets of objects). Thus, we see evidence here of the hierarchical increase in featural complexity required to encode featural relationships while also producing spatial invariance.

↪ Iconify all the receptive field windows.

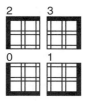

Figure 8.17: Probe stimuli used to test the response properties of V2 and V4 units in the model.

Probe Stimulus-Based Receptive Field Analysis

For another perspective on how the V2 and V4 units are encoding the visual inputs, we can use the probe stimulus technique and observe the unit's responses, just like we did in the previous simulation. In the present case, we present the 4 different probe stimuli shown in figure 8.17, and record the V2 and V4 unit's responses, which can be displayed in a grid log much like the activation-based receptive fields we just examined.

↪ Select View, PROBE_RF in the control panel. Press Open in the file selection window that appears as before, and a grid log window will appear (figure 8.18). Another file selection window will also appear, and you can again move that aside while you examine the current display.

This log displays the responses of a hypercolumn of V2 units to the probe stimuli. To view the responses to all 4 probes in one display, we presented the probes in only one quarter of the possible locations (the lower left set of 8x8 LGN locations), and then plotted the units' responses for each probe as one quarter of the 16x16 grid shown in the display, with the position of the probe corresponding to those shown in figure 8.17. Figure 8.19 illustrates this arrangement. Thus, the responses over the 8x8 locations for the lower left hand probe in the figure (probe 0) are shown in the lower left 8x8 cells of the overall grid, and those for the upper right probe in the figure (probe 3) are in the upper right 8x8 cells of the overall grid. Thus, a unit that responded selectively to only one probe, but did so in all of its locations (i.e., had a highly spatially invariant representation), would show up in the display as having a solid yellow (active) color in the corresponding quarter of its grid.

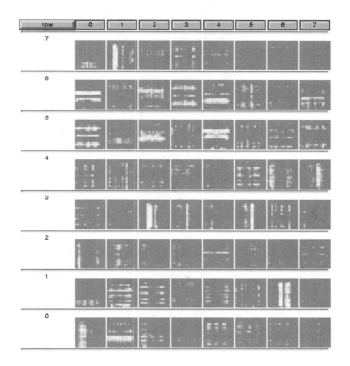

Figure 8.18: V2 probe response fields. The large 8x8 grid represents one hypercolumn's worth of units, with each cell containing the probe receptive field for that unit as described in the previous figure.

Question 8.7 **(a)** *Based on the number of units that responded to this small subset of features compared to those that did not significantly respond (i.e, did not have at least one yellowish dot of activity), what can you conclude about the selectivity of the V2 units for responding to particular features?* **(b)** *For those units that were significantly active, based on the number of different locations for which the unit was active (i.e., the area of colored pixels in the display), would you say that these units exhibited at least some degree of spatial invariance? Explain.* **(c)** *How do these results correspond with the conclusions based on the activation based receptive fields examined previously?*

↪ Press Open to the next file selection window, which will bring up the probe receptive fields for the V4 units.

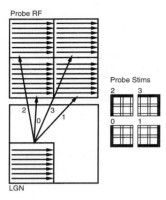

Figure 8.19: Organization of the probe receptive fields for all 4 probe stimuli as displayed in one plot. The 4 probes (0–3) were each swept across the lower-left quadrant of the LGN input, and the activations of V2 and V4 units recorded. For each V2/V4 unit, its response when the probe was in a given location (indexed by the lower left-hand corner of the probe) is plotted in the probe RF, with the quadrants of the probe RF arranged in the same way the probes themselves are.

You should observe much greater levels of spatial invariance in the V4 units (figure 8.20) compared to the V2 units, as we would expect from previous analyses. Several of these V4 units responded to a single feature across most of the locations it was presented, which corresponds to a single yellow quadrant of nearly-solid activity in the probe display. Other units responded to two different features in this invariant fashion, corresponding to two quadrants of activity. Some of the units even appear to respond to all probes across all locations. Given that the probes all involved a simple combination of a vertical and horizontal line, these units that did not discriminate the different probes are likely encoding less specific aspects about the vertical-horizontal line junction (and even just the very fact of such a junction in the least specific case).

Sweep Analysis

A similar way of testing the representations in the network is to sweep all of the actual object stimuli systematically across all of the positions in the input, at all the different sizes, and record some statistics on the result-

Item Summary					
itm	err	%tot	%itm	correl	uniq
0	19	0.64	1.85	97.76	4.22
1	65	2.22	6.34	91.85	7.74
2	71	2.42	6.93	92.70	8.37
3	35	1.19	3.41	96.44	5.52
4	42	1.43	4.10	95.66	5.27
5	42	1.43	4.10	95.78	5.53
6	23	0.78	2.24	97.80	4.65
7	42	1.43	4.10	95.96	4.63
8	70	2.39	6.83	92.90	8.70
9	70	2.39	6.83	93.38	6.08
10	35	1.19	3.41	96.47	5.56
11	43	1.46	4.19	96.09	4.96
12	61	2.08	5.95	94.25	7.97
13	28	0.95	2.73	96.98	4.59
14	41	1.40	4.00	95.37	5.31
15	62	2.11	6.05	94.06	6.21
16	57	1.94	5.56	94.49	7.47
17	72	2.46	7.03	92.03	6.37
18	1024	34.99	100	73.29	9.43
19	1024	34.99	100	55.47	8.19
size	Size Summary				
0	1012	34.58	19.76	88.77	6.33
1	614	20.98	11.99	90.03	6.34
2	612	20.91	11.95	95.34	6.34
3	688	23.51	13.43	93.62	6.35

Table 8.1: Summary of sweep testing results prior to generalization training on novel items (18 and 19). *itm* gives the object by number, *err* is the total number of errors across all positions and sizes for that object, *%tot* is the percentage of errors for that item out of total errors, *%itm* is the percentage of errors out of total presentations of the item, *correl* is the average correlation between subsequent V4 representations for the item, and *uniq* is the average number of unique V4 representations across all 256 different locations. The last four rows show the same kinds of statistics tabulated instead for the four different sizes — more errors are made on the smallest size. The *uniq* value for the novel items (18 and 19) indicate relatively invariant representations without any specific training on these items.

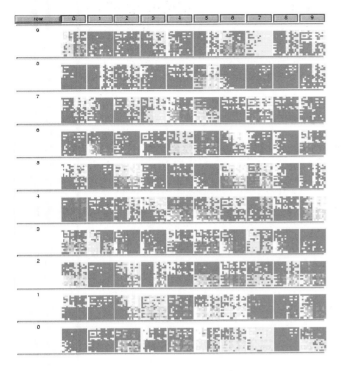

Figure 8.20: V4 probe response fields. See figure 8.18 for explanation.

ing activity patterns (table 8.2). One important statistic is the number of different unique patterns (after binarizing to 0–1 values based on a threshold of .5) that occur on the V4 layers across all the 256 different positions of a given object (recall that position is indexed by where the lower left-hand corner of the object appeared) and four different sizes. When we do this, there are on average around ten or so different V4 patterns, compared to 1024 different object images. Thus, we might conclude that most of the time the V4 representation is fully invariant for a given object. Interestingly, this is true even for the two novel objects that the network has never seen before. This will prove critical for the generalization test described below. A detailed report of the sweep analysis can be found in the `objrec.swp_pre.err` file in `chapter_8`, which summarizes the results by object (Item), size, object by size, and X, Y and XY spatial coordinates, reporting errors, pairwise correla-

tions between subsequent V4 representations, and the number of unique activation patterns.

Summary and Discussion of Receptive Field Analyses

Using these techniques, we have obtained some insight into the way this network performs spatially invariant object recognition, gradually over multiple levels of processing. Similarly, the complexity of the featural representations increases with increasing levels in the hierarchy. By doing both of these simultaneously and in stages over multiple levels, the network is able to recognize objects in an environment that depends critically on the detailed spatial arrangement of the constituent features, thereby apparently avoiding the binding problem described previously.

You may be wondering why the V2 and V4 representations have their respective properties — why did the network develop in this way? In terms of the degree of spatial invariance, it should be clear that the patterns of connectivity restrict the degree of invariance possible in V2, whereas the V4 neurons receive from the entire visual field (in this small-scale model), and so are in a position to have fully invariant representations. Also, the V4 representations can be more invariant, and more complex because they build off of limited invariance and featural complexity in the V2 layer. This ability for subsequent layers to build off of the transformations performed in earlier layers is a central general principle of cognition (see chapter 7).

The representational properties you observed here can have important functional implications. For example, in the next section, we will see that the nature of the V4 representations can play an important role in enabling the network to generalize effectively. To the extent that V4 representations encode complex object features, and not objects themselves, these representations can be reused for novel objects. Because the network can already form relatively invariant versions of these V4 representations, their reuse for novel objects will mean that the invariance transformation itself will generalize to novel objects.

Generalization Test

In addition to all of the above receptive field measures of the network's performance, we can perform a behavioral test of its ability to generalize in a spatially invariant manner, using the two objects (numbers 18 and 19 in figure 8.12) that were not presented to the network during training. We can now train on these two objects in a restricted set of spatial locations and sizes, and assess the network's ability to respond to these items in novel locations and sizes. The sweep test above indicates that the network should generalize, because it produced spatially invariant responses in layer V4 for these novel stimuli. Thus, presumably the bulk of what the network needs to do is learn an association between these V4 representations and the appropriate output units, and good generalization should result to all other spatial locations.

In addition to presenting the novel objects during training, we also need to present familiar objects; otherwise the network will suffer from *catastrophic interference* (see chapters 7 and 9 for more discussion of this issue). The following procedure was used. On each trial, there was a 1 in 4 chance that a novel object would be presented, and 3 in 4 chance that a familiar one was presented. If a novel object was presented, its location was chosen at random from a 6x6 grid at the center of the visual field (i.e., 36 possible locations, out of a total of 256, or roughly 14% of the locations), and its size was chosen at random to be either 5 or 9 pixels (i.e., 2 out of the 4 possible sizes, or 50% of the sizes). If a familiar object was presented, then its size and position was chosen completely at random from all the possibilities. This procedure was repeated for 60 epochs of 150 objects per epoch, with a learning rate of .001. Although the network started getting the novel objects correct after only 3 epochs, the longer training ensured that the new knowledge was well consolidated before testing.

Testing entailed another sweep analysis after training on the new objects (table 8.2). The detailed results are contained in the file `objrec.swp.err`. In particular, pay attention to the *%itm* column, which shows the errors as a function of total presentations of that item (object). The overall results were that object 18 had roughly 15 percent errors (85% correct) during testing

		Item Summary			
itm	err	%tot	%itm	correl	uniq
0	38	1.71	3.71	96.02	5.93
1	110	4.96	10.74	88.53	9.53
2	22	0.99	2.14	97.54	3.97
3	142	6.40	13.86	90.04	5.76
4	66	2.97	6.44	92.70	7.57
5	39	1.75	3.80	96.19	7.18
6	42	1.89	4.10	96.03	5.71
7	176	7.94	17.18	87.56	7.74
8	57	2.57	5.56	94.41	5.99
9	150	6.76	14.64	86.93	8.54
10	99	4.46	9.66	90.65	6.95
11	106	4.78	10.35	91.99	4.96
12	159	7.17	15.52	87.13	8.26
13	64	2.88	6.25	94.30	6.23
14	55	2.48	5.37	93.80	5.93
15	229	10.33	22.36	83.39	6.26
16	82	3.70	8.00	92.28	9.25
17	65	2.93	6.34	92.94	8.27
18	162	7.31	15.82	85.10	10.74
19	353	15.92	34.47	73.74	9.16
size		Size Summary			
0	921	41.56	17.98	86.35	7.19
1	353	15.92	6.89	89.03	7.19
2	290	13.08	5.66	94.75	7.20
3	652	29.42	12.73	92.12	7.21
itm,size		Item by Size Summary			
18,0	27	1.21	10.54	84.98	10.72
18,1	70	3.15	27.34	82.99	10.73
18,2	31	1.39	12.10	84.67	10.74
18,3	34	1.53	13.28	87.76	10.75
19,0	122	5.50	47.65	66.16	9.14
19,1	102	4.60	39.84	70.40	9.16
19,2	33	1.48	12.89	79.15	9.16
19,3	96	4.33	37.5	79.24	9.18

Table 8.2: Summary of sweep testing results after generalization training on the novel items (18 and 19) in a limited number of positions and sizes. Columns are as in previous table, with additional data for novel items in different sizes shown. The *%itm* column for the novel items (15.82 and 34.47) gives the generalization error, which is not bad considering the limited range of training locations and sizes (covering only 7% of the total possible). The Item by Size data shows that size generalization to the untrained sizes (1 and 3) is also fairly good (27.34 and 13.28 for object 18, 39.84 and 37.5 for 19). More errors are also generally made in the smaller sizes. Finally, there is some evidence of interference from the generalization training in comparison with table 8.1.

across all possible locations and sizes, and object 19 had 34 percent errors (66% correct). Considering that the network had been trained on only 72 out of 1024 possible input images (7%), that is quite a good generalization result. The network performed correctly on roughly twelve times as many images as it was trained on for object 18, and 9.4 times for object 19. We also note that there was some evidence of interference from the training on some of the other objects, which can be observed in detail by comparing this file with `objrec.swp_pre.err` (table 8.1).

Looking specifically at the size generalization performance, the network generalized to object 18 in the novel sizes (which show up as sizes 1 and 3 in the table) at a level of 27d percent and 13 percent errors, which is not wildly different from the trained sizes (10% and 12%). Similar results held for object 19, which had 40 percent and 37 percent errors in the novel sizes, compared to 48 percent and 13 percent for the trained ones. Thus, there is good evidence that the network was able to generalize its learning on one set of sizes to recognizing objects at different sizes that it had never seen before. Note also that the smaller sizes produced many more errors, because they are near the level of acuity of the model (i.e., object features are basically the same size as the individual oriented line detectors in V1). Thus, we would expect better performance overall from a larger network.

To determine where the learning primarily occurred, we can examine the difference between the pregeneralization and postgeneralization training weights (i.e., for each weight, we subtracted its value before generalization training from its value after training, and then saved that value as the weight value for the connection in question). We can load these weight differences into the network where they will appear instead of the normal weight values, and can thus be viewed using our standard weight viewing technique.

↳ Do `Actions/Read Weights` in the NetView window, and select `objrec.diff.wts.gz` (this is what the `LoadNet` button does, but it loads the trained weights). Click on `r.wt`, and then click on objects 18 and 19 in the output layer.

You should see that the magnitude of the weight changes from V4 to these units was about .25 or so. Now, if you compare that with other output units and

other layers lower in the network, it is clear that this is where the primary learning occurred. Nevertheless, there is evidence of some weight change in the other units, which probably accounts for the observed interference. This kind of interference is probably inevitable because learning will constantly be jostling the weights.

To summarize, these generalization results demonstrate that the hierarchical series of representations can operate effectively on novel stimuli, as long as these stimuli possess structural features in common with other familiar objects. The network has learned to represent combinations of these features in terms of increasingly complex combinations that are also increasingly spatially invariant. In the present case, we have facilitated generalization by ensuring that the novel objects are built out of the same line features as the other objects. Although we expect that natural objects also share a vocabulary of complex features, and that learning would discover and exploit them to achieve a similarly generalizable invariance mapping, this remains to be demonstrated for more realistic kinds of objects. One prediction that this model makes is that the generalization of the invariance mapping will likely be a function of featural similarity with known objects, so one might expect a continuum of generalization performance in people (and in a more elaborate model).

↳ Go to the `PDP++Root` window. To continue on to the next simulation, close this project first by selecting `.projects/Remove/Project_0`. Or, if you wish to stop now, quit by selecting `Object/Quit`.

8.4.3 Summary and Discussion

This model achieves two important objectives for a biologically realistic model of object recognition. First, the response properties of the units in the different layers of the model provide a good qualitative fit to those of corresponding areas in the ventral visual pathway. Second, the model does a good job of discriminating between different objects regardless of what position or size they appeared in. Furthermore, this ability to perform spatially invariant object recognition generalized well to novel objects. All of this was achieved with relatively minimal built-in constraints through the use of the generic learning principles of the Leabra algorithm.

One of the most important contributions of this model is the ability to understand the functional implications of the observed neural response properties, and how these contribute to a sensible computational algorithm for doing object recognition. Thus, we can see how the binding problem in object recognition can be averted by developing representations with increasingly complex featural encodings and increasing levels of spatial invariance. Further, we can see that by developing complex but still distributed (i.e., subobject level) featural encodings of objects, the system can generalize the invariance transformation to novel objects.

One major unresolved issue has to do with the nature of the complex representations that enable generalization in the model. What should these representations look like for actual objects, and can computational models such as this one provide some insight into this issue? Obviously, the objects used in the current model are too simple to tell us much about real objects. To address this issue, the model would have to be made significantly more complex, with a better approximation to actual visual feature encoding (e.g., more like the V1 receptive field model), and it should be trained on a large range of actual objects. This would require considerably faster computational machinery and a large amount of memory to implement, and is thus unlikely to happen in the near future.

As we mentioned earlier, Biederman (1987) has made a proposal about a set of object components (called *geons*) that could in theory correspond to the kinds of distributed featural representations that our model developed in its V4 layer. Geons are relatively simple geometrical shapes based on particularly informative features of objects that are likely to provide useful disambiguating information over a wide range of different viewpoints (so-called *non-accidental* properties; Lowe, 1987). Although we obviously find the general idea of object features important, we are not convinced that the brain uses geons. We are not aware of any neural recording data that supports the geon model. Furthermore, the available behavioral support mostly just suggests that features like corners are more informative than the middle portions of contours (Biederman & Cooper, 1991). This does not specifically support the geon model, as corners (and junctions more

generally) are likely to be important for just about any model of object recognition. We also suspect that the representations developed by neural learning mechanisms would be considerably more complex and difficult to describe than geons, given the complex, high-dimensional space of object features. Nevertheless, we are optimistic that future models will be able to speak to these issues more directly.

One objection that might be raised against our model is that it builds the location invariance solution into the network architecture by virtue of the spatially localized receptive fields. The concern might be that this architectural solution would not generalize to other forms of invariance (e.g., size or rotation). However, by demonstrating the ability of the model to do size invariant object recognition, we have shown that the architecture is not doing all the work. Although the scale and featural simplicity of this model precludes the exploration of rotational invariance (i.e., only 90-degree rotations are possible, with the horizontal and vertical input features, such rotations turn one object into another), we do think that the same basic principles could produce at least the somewhat limited amounts of rotational invariance observed in neural recording studies. As we have stated, the network achieves invariance by representing conjunctions of features over limited ranges of transformation. Thus, V2 neurons could also encode conjunctions of features over small angles of rotation, and V4 neurons could build on this to produce more complex representations that are invariant over larger angles of rotation, and so on.

Finally, it is important to emphasize the importance of using both error-driven and Hebbian learning in this model. Neither purely error-driven nor purely Hebbian versions of this network were capable of learning successfully (the purely error-driven did somewhat better than the purely Hebbian, which essentially did not learn at all). This further validates the analyses from chapter 6 regarding the importance of Hebbian learning in deep, multilayered networks such as this one. Error-driven learning is essential for the network to form representations that discriminate the different objects; otherwise it gets confused by the extreme amount of featural overlap among the objects. Although it is possible that in the much higher dimensional space of real object recognition this problem would be so reduced to enable Hebbian learning to be successful on its own, we suspect that error-driven learning will still play an important role.

8.5 Spatial Attention: A Simple Model

The models we develop next build on the previous model by showing how attention to specific spatial locations, mediated by the dorsal "where" visual pathway, can enable objects to be recognized in a crowded scene that would otherwise overwhelm the ventral object recognition pathway. Objects tend to be spatially contiguous, so object recognition benefits from grouping together and focusing processing on visual features located within a contiguous spatial region.

As described in chapter 7, attention plays an important role in solving the binding problem by restricting the focus of processing to one related set of features (e.g., one object). This focus enables the resulting pattern of distributed representations to be interpretable, because they will apply to features that should actually be related to each other, as opposed to random combinations of features from different objects (or other aspects of the environment). We avoided this problem in the previous model by presenting the simulation with only one object at a time.

This multiple-object binding problem is somewhat different than the multiple-feature binding problem confronted in the previous model. With multiple objects, we do not necessarily want to form conjunctive representations that encode multiple objects simultaneously, especially if these objects are completely unrelated. However, for objects commonly seen together (e.g., eyes within a face), the network could use the same kind of hierarchical feature-conjunctions and spatial invariance solution to the multiple object binding problem as it did with the multiple-feature one.

In this section and the next we develop two closely related models of attention, with the second model (which is an extension of the above object recognition model) perceiving multiple objects in the environment by sequentially focusing attention on each in turn. Although we focus on this case of attentional effects in object recognition (specifically the role of spatial representa-

tions in controlling attention), the principles apply quite generally across many other domains and processing pathways.

Before we turn to the models, we need to reemphasize the point made in chapter 7 that attention is not a separate mechanism in our framework, but rather an emergent property of the activation dynamics and representational structure of the network. This contrasts with the traditional view, where attention is seen as a distinct mechanism. In the context of visual processing, attention has specifically been associated with the types of spatially mediated effects that we model here. Attention has also been used to refer to the role of the prefrontal cortex in focusing processing in a task-relevant manner (see chapters 7 and 11).

In our models, attention emerges from inhibitory competition (which is responsible for imposing a limitation on the total amount of activity within a given set of representations), and constraint satisfaction operating throughout the network (which determines the representations that will become active in a given context). Similar views of attention as a ubiquitous property of the cortex have been articulated by Desimone and Duncan (1995) and Allport (1989). Even though we consider attention to be an emergent property, we often refer to it as though it were a single mechanism for convenience.

Because the mechanisms that underlie attention are ubiquitous throughout the cortex, one would expect to find attentional effects associated with all different sorts of processing. Furthermore, the same kinds of processing capacity limitations and binding problems discussed here in the context of object recognition apply generally as well. Thus, the models here provide a good demonstration of a very general cortical function. Also, you will see that although spatial representations provide a useful organizing substrate for visual attention, other kinds of representations (e.g., in the object processing pathway) can also make contributions to visual attention.

In the models that follow, we will also see that the structural principles developed in chapter 7 (hierarchies of specialized processing pathways with lateral interactions) are critical for determining the ways in which these functional considerations are resolved in the spe-

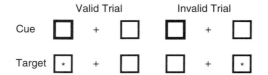

Figure 8.21: The Posner spatial attention task. The cue is a brightening or highlighting of one of the boxes that focuses attention to that region of space. Reaction times to detect the target are faster when this cue is valid (the target appears in that same region) than when it is invalid.

cific case of the interactions between spatial and object representations. Specifically, more parallel processing takes place at lower levels within the system, and higher levels enforce greater focus on single objects or locations in space.

8.5.1 Basic Properties of the Model

In the first attentional model, we begin to explore the ways that spatial representations can interact with the kinds of object-based processing developed in the previous model. Thus, we are simulating some of the ways in which the dorsal "where" processing stream can interact with the ventral "what" processing stream. As discussed previously, parietal cortex contains many different types of spatial representations, and lesions in this lobe cause deficits in spatial processing. Although there are probably many different types of spatial representations in the parietal cortex (e.g., having different reference frames), we will not make many assumptions about the nature and other functions of these parietal representations — we will just use a simple maplike spatial representation.

One of the simplest and most influential paradigms for studying spatial attention is the Posner task (Posner et al., 1984), illustrated in figure 8.21. When attention is drawn or *cued* to one region of space (e.g., by highlighting a box on one side of the display), this affects the speed of target detection in different locations. When attention is drawn to the same region where the target subsequently appears (i.e., a validly cued trial), subjects are faster to detect the target than when attention is drawn to the opposite region (an invalidly cued

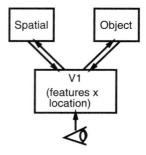

Figure 8.22: Representations of space and object could both interact via a low-level spatially mapped feature array like V1. Spatial attention would result from top-down activation by the spatial pathway of corresponding regions in V1, which would then be the focus of processing by the object pathway.

trial). Although the target is typically a rather simple shape, we will assume that its detection occurs via the object processing pathway, or at least the relatively early stages thereof.

The Posner task provides a simple way of exploring the interactions between the spatial and object processing pathways. Specifically, activation in a specific location in the spatial processing pathway should facilitate the processing of objects (targets) that appear within that part of space, and impede processing of objects in other parts of space. In addition to this basic attentional modulation effect, the model must also be capable of shifting attention to new locations in space as new cues or objects come into view. For example, in the Posner task, one must be able to switch attention to the location where the target appears, even though doing so may take longer on invalidly cued trials. In general, there is a tradeoff between focusing attention in one location and switching it to a new one — by focusing attention on one location and impeding processing elsewhere, this makes it less likely that the system will process and shift attention to other locations. However, attention must be dynamic and movable if it is to be useful, so a reasonable balance must be achieved.

The model could be constructed such that both spatial and object representations interact via top-down effects on a V1-like spatial feature map, that provides the inputs for both subsequent levels of processing (figure 8.22). In such a model, the activation of a region in

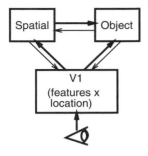

Figure 8.23: Spatial representations can have an attentional effect via direct connections to the object processing system (which is spatially organized at its lower levels). The spatial pathway can have a strong impact (thicker arrow) on object processing, while remaining sensitive to bottom up inputs (thicker bottom-up arrows than top-down ones).

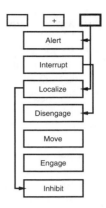

Figure 8.24: Attentional selection theory proposed by Posner et al. (1984). The parietal cortex is thought to be responsible for the disengage process.

the spatial pathway would provide top-down support for this region in V1, meaning that the features in this region will be preferentially processed by the object pathway. With the presence of lateral inhibition, the regions not supported by the top-down spatial input will be at a competitive disadvantage, and therefore less likely to be active.

Although this model is simple and elegant, it has an important limitation — it exacerbates the tradeoff between the ability to focus attention at a given location, and the ability to respond to new inputs in novel locations. The attentional effects are mediated by what is effectively the input layer of the network (V1). Thus, the top-down spatial activation focused on a specific location inhibits the ability of other locations in the input layer to become active. However, these other locations need to become active before attention can be switched to them, creating a catch-22 situation — you have to allow other locations to be active for attention to switch, but these other locations have to be suppressed to implement attention in the first place. Thus, for this kind of system to be able to switch attention to a new location, the top-down projections from the spatial system to V1 must be made relatively weak — so weak that the resulting level of spatial attention is often incapable of sufficiently focusing the object processing pathway on one object over another.

The alternative model that we explore here is shown in figure 8.23. The key difference is that this model includes lateral interconnectivity between the spatial pathway and the object processing pathway, that enables spatial attention to affect object processing directly without having to go through the V1 input layer first. This configuration avoids the catch-22 situation by enabling strong attentional effects on object recognition without requiring the model to ignore novel inputs via strong top-down attentional modulation. Thus, the efficacy of the spatial modulation of object processing is not limited by the need to keep the spatial system sensitive to bottom-up input. The strong influence of spatial processing on the object pathway is emphasized in the figure by the thicker arrow. Similarly, the ability of the model to be sensitive to bottom-up input is emphasized by thicker bottom-up arrows than top-down ones. For this model to work, the spatial pathway must interact with the lower, spatially organized levels of the object processing pathway (e.g., areas V2 and V4 in the object recognition model described in the previous section). Our model also includes multiple spatial scales of processing both in the object pathway (as in the previous model), and correspondingly in the spatial pathway.

Effects of Spatial Pathway Lesions

The effects of lesions in the parietal cortex on performance in the Posner spatial cuing task provide an important source of constraint on the model. As discussed previously, unilateral lesions (i.e., to only one hemisphere) of the parietal cortex generally lead to the phenomenon of hemispatial neglect — the inability to focus attention to the corresponding half of visual space (i.e., the left half of visual space for a right hemisphere lesion). Unilateral parietal damage can result in varying degrees of behavioral deficit. Patients with relatively mild impairments exhibit disproportionately slower attention switching on invalidly cued trials when the target appeared in the damaged half of space. More severely impaired neglect patients can be completely unable to switch attention into the damaged half of space. Although this pattern of data is generally consistent with the idea that parietal damage results in difficulty focusing attention on the damaged side, Posner et al. (1984) have argued based on a box-and-arrow model that the parietal cortex implements a *disengage* mechanism (figure 8.24). They conclude that the observed behavior comes from the inability to disengage attention from the good side of space.

Using a model of spatial attention based on the architecture shown in figure 8.22, Cohen et al. (1994) were able to account for the observed parietal lesion data on the Posner spatial cuing task. This model has no specific "disengage" mechanism. Instead, the process of disengaging attention from one location occurs as a natural consequence of engaging attention elsewhere. Thus, in these terms, the parietal lesion data can be explained as the inability of the damaged spatial representations to provide sufficient top-down support to the corresponding half of visual space. Thus, when the target appears in the damaged half of space, patients are impaired in engaging attention there. This explanation is also generally consistent with the hemispatial neglect syndrome in patients with more severe damage, where patients have difficulty focusing attention in the damaged half of visual space.

An interesting source of empirical support for the Cohen et al. (1994) model over the Posner et al. (1984) disengage model comes from the effects of bilateral

parietal lesions, which are associated with **Bálint's syndrome** (Husain & Stein, 1988). Under the disengage model, one would expect that bilateral parietal damage would produce bilateral deficits in disengaging, and greater amounts of slowing in the invalidly cued trials in both directions. However, Bálint's syndrome patients instead exhibit smaller amounts of slowing on invalidly cued trials, and in general show deficits in deploying attention. This is consistent with what happens in the Cohen et al. (1994) model, namely that there is a bilateral reduction in top-down spatial activation, and thus an overall reduction in the size of attentional effects.

Our model provides a more robust (and somewhat richer) instantiation of the basic points made by Cohen et al. (1994), in part because our model is based on the architecture shown in figure 8.23, which has lateral interactions between the spatial and object processing pathways as discussed previously. Thus, whereas Cohen et al. (1994) had to use very carefully chosen parameter values to achieve reasonable performance, our model behaves reasonably over a wider parameter range. Overall, this modeling exercise provides an excellent example of how the use of biologically based principles for understanding cognition can give rise to very different functional descriptions of cognitive phenomena than traditional box-and-arrow models.

Object-Based Attention

Our model includes top-down projections from the object pathway to V1, and lateral projections to the spatial system from the object pathway, both of which allow for the possibility of object-based attentional effects. There is considerable debate in the literature regarding the exact nature of object-based attention — is it essentially just attention to the spatial region (and features) where the object is located (e.g., Mozer, Zemel, Behrmann, & Williams, 1992; Vecera & Farah, 1994), or is it specifically attention in the object pathway (e.g., Duncan, 1984)? Our model allows for both, with potentially complex interactions between the two processing pathways that could give rise to all sorts of interesting effects, some of which are explored later.

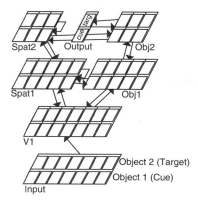

Figure 8.25: The simple spatial attention model.

8.5.2 Exploring the Simple Attentional Model

↪ Open the project `attn_simple.proj.gz` in `chapter_8` to begin.

Let's step through the network structure and connectivity, which was completely pre-specified (i.e., the network was not trained, and no learning takes place, because it was easier to hand-construct this simple architecture). As you can see, the network basically resembles figure 8.23, with mutually interconnected `Spatial` and `Object` pathways feeding off of a V1-like layer that contains a spatially mapped feature array (figure 8.25). In this simple case, we're assuming that each "object" is represented by a single distinct feature in this array, and also that space is organized along a single dimension. Thus, the first row of units represents the first object's feature (which serves as the cue stimulus) in each of 7 locations, and the second row represents the second object's feature (which serves as the target) in these same 7 locations.

↪ Now select `r.wt` in the network window and click on the object and spatial units to see how they function via their connectivity patterns.

The object processing pathway has a sequence of 3 increasingly spatially invariant layers of representations, with each unit collapsing over 3 adjacent spatial locations of the object-defining feature in the layer below. Note that the highest, fully spatially invariant level of the object pathway plays the role of the output layer, and is used for measuring the reaction time to detect ob-

jects. This happens by stopping settling whenever the *target* output (object 2) gets above an activity of .6 (if this doesn't happen, settling stops after 200 cycles).

The spatial processing pathway has a sequence of two layers of spatial representations, differing in the level of spatial resolution. As in the object pathway, each unit in the spatial pathway represents 3 adjacent spatial locations, but unlike the object pathway, these units are not sensitive to particular features. Two units per location provide distributed representations in both layers of the spatial pathway. This redundancy will be useful for demonstrating the effects of partial damage to this pathway.

↪ Locate the `attn_ctrl` overall control panel.

This control panel contains a number of important parameters, most of which are `wt_scale` values that determine the relative strength of various pathways within the network (and all other pathways have a default strength of 1). As discussed in chapter 2, the connection strengths can be uniformly scaled by a normalized multiplicative factor, called `wt_scale` in the simulator. We set these weight scale parameters to determine the relative influence of one pathway on the other, and the balance of bottom-up (stimulus driven) versus top-down (attentional) processing.

As emphasized in figure 8.23, the spatial pathway influences the object pathway relatively strongly (as determined by the `spat_obj` parameter with a value of 2), whereas the object pathway influences the spatial pathway with a strength of .5. Also, the spatial system will be responsive to bottom-up inputs from V1 because the `v1_spat` parameter, with a value of 2, makes the V1 to `Spat1` connections relatively strong. This strength allows for effective shifting of attention (as also emphasized in figure 8.23). Finally, the other two parameters in the control panel show that we are using relatively slow settling, and adding some noise into the processing to simulate subject performance.

Perceiving Multiple Objects

Although much of the detailed behavioral data we will explore with the model concerns the Posner spatial cueing task, we think the more basic functional motivation for visual attention is to facilitate object recog-

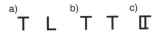

Figure 8.26: The three different MULTI_OBJS conditions illustrated with letters. **a)** has two different objects in different locations. **b)** has the same object in different locations. **c)** has two different objects in the same location. This last condition is clearly the most difficult for object identification.

nition when multiple objects are presented simultaneously. Therefore, we will start with a quick exploration of the network's object recognition capacities as a function of the spatial distribution of two objects. This will provide an introduction to the kinds of interactions between spatial and object processing that can happen using this relatively simple model. Let's begin by viewing the events that we will present to the network.

↪ **Press** View, EVENTS **in the control panel.**

The environment window shows 3 events (figure 8.26). The first event has two different objects (features) present in different spatial locations. Note that the target object has slightly higher activation (i.e., it is more salient), which will result in the reliable selection of this object over the other. The next event has two of the same objects (targets) presented in different locations. Finally, the last event has the two different objects in the same spatial location. As the figure makes clear, recognizing objects when they overlap in the same location is considerably more difficult than when they appear in different locations. Although it is clearly easier to recognize objects if only copies of the same object are present as opposed to different objects, this difference is not likely to be significant for small numbers of presented objects.

Now, let's test these predictions in the model.

↪ **Switch back to viewing** act **in the network window. Do a** Step **in the control panel.**

This will present the first event to the network, which will stop settling (i.e., updating the network's activations a cycle at a time) when the target unit's activation exceeds the threshold of .6 in the Output layer.

↪ **Then** Step **through the remaining events.**

You should have seen that the network settled relatively quickly for the first two events, but was slowed

on the third event where the objects overlap in the same region of space. To see this pattern more precisely, we can open a graph log of the settling times.

↪ **Do** View, GRAPH_LOG **to open the log. Then do** Run **on the control panel to re-run the 3 events.**

This graph log shows the settling times (number of cycles to reach threshold) for each event. You should see that the network did indeed have more difficulty with the objects appearing in the same spatial location (although sometimes it doesn't take as long — there is some noise added to the processing and this can activate the target unit relatively quickly in a minority of cases). To get a better sense of the overall reaction times in this simulation, we can run multiple runs and record the results in text logs.

↪ **Do** View, TEXT_LOG **and** View, BATCH_TEXT_LOG **to open the logs. Then run a batch of 10 runs by pressing** Batch. **Note that the log column labels (Neutral, Valid, Invalid) relate to the Posner spatial cuing task, but they correspond to the three events in this case.**

Question 8.8 (a) *Describe the network's reaction to each event and explain it in terms of the interactions between the excitation and inhibition as it flows through the spatial and object pathways in the network.* **(b)** *Report the resulting average settling times in the batch text log (*Batch_0_TextLog*). Were your original results representative?*

You should have observed that spatial representations can facilitate the processing of objects by allocating attention to one object over another. The key contrast condition is when both objects lie in the same location, so that spatial attention can no longer separate them out, leaving the object pathway to try to process both objects simultaneously.

The Posner Spatial Cuing Task

Now, let's see how this model does on the Posner spatial cuing task.

↪ **Set** env_type **on the overall control panel to** STD_POSNER **(Apply). Do** View, EVENTS **to see how the task is represented.**

There are three *groups* of events shown here, which correspond to a Neutral cue (no cue), a Valid cue,

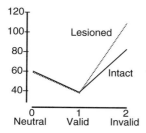

Figure 8.27: Graph log results for both the intact and lesioned network on the Posner spatial cuing task. The lesioned case shows a specific slowing on the invalid trials.

and an `Invalid` cue. There is just one event for the neutral case, which is the presentation of the target object in the left location. For the valid case, the first event is the cue presented on the left, followed by a target event with the target also on the left. The invalid case has the same cue event, but the target shows up on the right (opposite) side of space. The network's activations are not reset between the cue and target events within a group, but they are reset at the end of a group (after the target). Thus, residual activation from the cuing event can persist and affect processing for the target event, but the activation is cleared between different trial types.

↪ Turn the network display back on (it was turned off automatically by the previous batch run). `Clear` the graph log, and then `Step`. Note how the network responds to each of the three conditions of the Posner task as you continue to `Step` through these cases. Press `Batch` on the `attn_ctrl` control panel to run a batch of 10 runs.

Your graph log should resemble figure 8.27. Note that it is impossible to add the "neutral," "valid," and "invalid" labels to the graph in the simulator, so you will have to remember that these are associated with the 0, 1 and 2 (respectively) points on the X axis, as is shown in the figure.

Question 8.9 (a) *By what mechanism does the spatial cue influence the subsequent processing of the target in the valid and invalid cases?* **(b)** *How is this influence reflected in the settling time (report results from the batch run)?*

Typical reaction times for young adults (i.e., college students) on this task are roughly: neutral, 370 ms; valid 350 ms; invalid 390 ms, showing about 20 ms on either side of the neutral condition for the effects of attentional focus. These data should agree in general with the pattern of results you obtained, but to fit the data precisely you would have to add a constant offset of roughly 310 ms to the number of cycles of settling for each trial type. This constant offset can be thought of as the time needed to perform all the other aspects of the task that are not included in the simulation (e.g., generating a response). Note also that one cycle of settling in the network corresponds with one millisecond of processing in humans. Of course, this relationship is not automatic — we adjusted the time constant for activation updating (`vm_dt`) so that the two were in agreement in this particular experiment.

Now let's explore the effects of the `wt_scale` parameters on the network's performance, which helps to illuminate how the network captures normal performance in this task. First, let's try reducing `spat_obj` from 2 to 1, which reduces the influence of the spatial system on the object system.

↪ Do a `Batch` run with `spat_obj` set to 1.

You should find that the network settling time for the invalid condition has decreased from roughly 83 cycles for the standard network to roughly 75 cycles for this case. This faster settling for the invalid trials is just what one would expect — because there is less of a spatial attention effect on the object system, the invalid cue does not slow it down as much. The effects on the other trial types are less interesting, and involve some technical effects of the `wt_scale` parameters on processing speed in the network.

↪ Set `spat_obj` back to 2.

Now let's try reducing the influence from the V1 layer to the spatial representations by reducing the value of `v1_spat` from 2 to 1.5 and then to 1.

↪ Do a `Batch` for `v1_spat` of 1.5 and then 1.

Again the interesting effect is in the invalid trials, where the network takes an average of roughly 91 and 115 cycles for `v1_spat` values of 1.5 and 1, respectively. As V1 has less effect on the spatial pathway, it becomes more and more difficult for input in a novel location (e.g., the target presented on the opposite side

	Valid	Invalid	Diff
Adult Normal	350	390	40
Elderly Normal	540	600	60
Patients	640	760	120
Elderly normalized (*.65)	350	390	40
Patients normalized (*.55)	350	418	68

Table 8.3: Reaction times for the Posner spatial cuing task for various populations as shown. The normalized scores enable the elderly and patient data to be compared with the adult normals, revealing that the patients have a larger invalid-valid difference than would be expected just by their overall slowing.

of the cue) to overcome the residual spatial activation in the cued location. This shows that the spatial pathway needs to have a balance between sensitivity to bottom-up inputs and ability to retain a focus of spatial attention over time. This network allows this balance to be set separately from that of the influence of the spatial pathway on the object pathway (controlled by the `spat_obj` parameter), which is not the case with the Cohen et al. (1994) model.

↪ Set `v1_spat` back to 2 before continuing.

One additional manipulation we can make is to the eccentricity (visual distance) of the cue and target. If they are presented closer together, then one might expect to get less of an attentional effect, or even a facilitation if the nearby location was partially activated by the cue.

↪ This can be tested by setting `env_type` in the control panel to `CLOSE_POSNER` (Apply). Run this case.

You will see that an overlapping set of spatial representations is activated, and a `Batch` run reveals that there is no longer a significant slowing for the invalid case relative to the neutral case (but the validity effect remains).

↪ Switch the `env_type` back to `STD_POSNER` before continuing.

Effects of Spatial Pathway Lesions

As we mentioned earlier, Posner et al. (1984) showed that patients who had suffered lesions in one hemisphere of the parietal cortex exhibit differentially impaired performance on the invalid trials of the Posner spatial cuing task. Specifically, they are slower when the cue is presented on the side of space processed by the intact hemisphere (i.e., ipsilateral to the lesion), and the target is then processed by the lesioned hemisphere. The patients showed a 120 ms difference between invalid and valid cases, with a validly cued RT of roughly 640 ms, and an invalidly cued RT of 760 ms. These data can be compared to matched (elderly) control subjects who showed a roughly 60 ms invalid-valid difference, with a validly cued RT of 540 ms and an invalidly cued RT 600 ms (table 8.3).

You should notice that, as one might expect, older people are slower than the young adult normals, and older people with some kind of brain damage are still slower yet, due to generalized effects of the damage. In this case, we are interested in the specific involvement of the parietal lobes in these attentional phenomena, and so we have to be careful to dissociate the specific from the generalized effects. To determine if the patients have a specific attentional problem, we must first find a way of *normalizing* the data so that we can make useful comparisons among these different groups (including the model). We normalize by dividing the elderly control's data by a constant factor to get the same basic numbers reported for the adult normals (or the model). If there is a specific effect of the brain damage, we should find that the pattern of reaction times is different from the adult normals even when it is appropriately normalized.

To find the appropriate scaling factors, we use the ratio between the valid RT's for the different groups. Ideally, we would want to use the neutral case, which should be a good measure of the overall slowing, but only the valid and invalid trial data are available for the patients and elderly controls. So, to compare the elderly controls with the adult normals, we take the adult valid RT's of 350 ms, and divide that by the elderly control subjects valid RT's of 540 ms, giving a ratio of .65. Now, we multiply the elderly controls invalid RT's (600 ms) by this factor, and we should get something close to the adult normals invalid RT's (390 ms). Indeed, the fit is perfect – 600 ∗ .65 = 390. The elderly controls thus appear to behave just like the adult normals, but with a constant slowing factor.

However, when we apply this normalizing procedure to the patient's data, the results do not fit well. Thus, we again divide 350 ms by the the 640 ms valid RT's, giving a ratio of .55. Then, we do $760 * .55 = 418$, which is substantially slower than the 390 ms invalid times for the adult normals (table 8.3). This makes it clear that the patients are specifically slower in the invalid trials even when their overall slowing has been taken into account by the normalizing procedure. This differential slowing is what led to the hypothesis that these patients have difficulty disengaging attention.

Now, we lesion the model, and see if it simulates the patient's data. However, because the model will not suffer the generalized effects of brain damage (which are probably caused by swelling and other such factors), and because it will not "age," we expect it to behave just like a adult subject that has only the specific effect of the lesion. Thus, we compare the model's performance to the normalized patient values. Although we can add in the 310 ms constant to the models' settling time to get a comparable RT measure, it is somewhat easier to just compare the difference between the invalid and valid cases, which subtracts away any constant factors (see the Diff column in table 8.3).

↪   To lesion the model, press `Lesion` in the `attn_ctrl` control panel, and select `SPAT1_2` to lesion both levels of spatial representations, and `HALF` and `HALF` to lesion one half of the locations, and 1 out of the 2 spatial units in each location. Select `r.wt` and confirm that these units (the back 2 units on the right for `Spat1`, and the back right unit for `Spat2`) have their weights zeroed out. `Batch` run the lesioned network.

Question 8.10 (a) *Report the resulting averages.* **(b)** *Compute the invalid-valid difference, and compare it with the patient's data, and with the intact network.* **(c)** *Turn the network display back on, select* `act`, *and* `Step` *through the events. Explain why the lesioned model is slower on the invalid trials in terms of the activation dynamics of the network.*

You should have found that you can simulate the apparent disengage deficit without having a specific "disengager" mechanism. One additional source of support for this model comes from the pattern of patient data for the opposite configuration of the cuing task, where the cue is presented in the lesioned side of space, and the invalid target is thus presented in the intact side. Interestingly, data from Posner et al. (1984) clearly show that there is a very reduced invalid-valid reaction time difference for this condition in the patients. Thus, it appears that it is easier for the patients to switch attention to the intact side of space, and therefore less of an invalid cost, relative to the normal control data. Furthermore, there appears to be less of a valid cuing effect for the patients when the cue and target are presented on the damaged side as compared to the intact side. Let's see what the model has to say about this.

↪   Set `env_type` to `REVERSE_POSNER` (and `Apply`), and do a `Batch` run for this case.

You should see that the network shows a reduced difference between the valid and invalid trials compared to the intact network (an average of roughly 55 cycles for valid, 61 for invalid, for a difference of only around 6 compared to around 41 for the intact network). Thus, the cue has less of an effect — less facilitation on valid trials and less interference on invalid ones. This is exactly the pattern seen in the Posner et al. (1984) data. In the model, it occurs simply because the stronger intact side of space where the target is presented has less difficulty competing with the damaged side of space where the cue was presented. In contrast, the disengage theory would predict that the lesioned network on the reverse Posner task should perform like the intact network on the standard Posner task. Under these conditions, any required disengaging abilities should be intact (either because the network has not been lesioned, or because the cue is presented on the side of space that the lesioned network should be able to disengage from).

As mentioned previously, additional lesion data comes from *Bálint's syndrome* patients, who suffered from *bilateral* parietal lesions. The most striking feature of these patients is that they have *simultanagnosia* — the inability to recognize multiple objects presented simultaneously (see Farah, 1990 for a review). The more complex spatial attention model described in the next section will provide a more useful demonstration of this aspect of the syndrome. Interestingly, when such subjects were tested on the Posner task (e.g., Coslett & Saffran, 1991), they exhibited a *decreased* level of attentional effects (i.e., a smaller invalid-valid difference). As emphasized by Cohen et al. (1994), these data provide an important argument against the *disengage* explanation of parietal function offered by Posner and colleagues, which would instead predict bilateral slowing for invalid trials (i.e., difficulty disengaging). The observed pattern of data falls naturally out of the model we have been exploring.

↪ To simulate this condition, first set `env_type` back to `STD_POSNER` (and `Apply`), and then do another `Lesion`, but this time do a `FULL` lesion (specified by the `locations` parameter) of `HALF` (`n_units_per_loc`) the `SPAT1_2` units.

↪ `Batch` run the bilaterally lesioned network.

Question 8.11 (a) *Report the results of the* `Batch` *run for the bilaterally lesioned network.* **(b)** *Explain how and why these results differ from those of the unilaterally lesioned network.*

Finally, we can explore the effects of a more severe lesion to the parietal spatial representations, which might provide a better model of the syndrome known as *hemispatial neglect* (typically referred to as just *neglect*). As described previously, neglect results from unilateral lesions of the parietal cortex (usually in the right hemisphere), which cause patients to generally neglect the lesioned side of space. We simulate neglect by doing a similar lesion to the unilateral one we did before, but by doing `FULL` for `n_units_per_loc` to lesion both of the units in each location.

↪ Specifically, do `Lesion` with `SPAT1_2`, `locations = HALF`, `n_units_per_loc = FULL`. Now, set `env_type` back to the `MULTI_OBJ` case (`Apply`). Do `Run` in the overall control panel (if it was too hard to see, `Step` through again).

Observe that even when the more salient object is in the lesioned side of space, the network still focuses attention on the intact side. Thus, it is specifically neglecting this lesioned side. In the first case, this causes the network to activate the cue object representation, which does not stop the network settling, resulting in a full 200 cycles of settling.

↪ Now set `env_type` to `STD_POSNER`, and then do a `Run` again (or `Step`).

You will see a similar neglect phenomenon, which makes the network completely incapable of switching attention into the damaged side of space to detect the target (again resulting in the full 200 cycles of settling for the invalid case).

Interestingly, if one does the `REVERSE_POSNER` case, then all attentional effects are completely eliminated, so that the settling times are relatively similar in all three conditions (roughly around 67 cycles). This is not because the network is incapable of processing stimuli in the damaged side of space — by looking at the activations in the network you can see that it does process the cue. Instead, the target presented to the good side of space has no difficulty competing with the weak residual representation of the cue in the damaged side. Competition can explain the general tendency for neglect on the grounds that it is very rare to actually have no other competing stimuli (which can be relatively weak and still win the competition), coming into the intact side of space, so that attention is usually focused on the intact side.

The smaller level of damage that produces the slowed target detection times in the Posner task may be more closely associated with the phenomenon of **extinction**, in which patients with unilateral parietal lesions show neglect only when there is a relatively strong competing visual stimulus presented to the good side of space (e.g., the cue in the invalid trials of the Posner task). Thus, the model may be able to account for a wide range of different spatial processing deficits associated with parietal damage, depending on both the severity and location of damage.

Temporal Dynamics and Inhibition of Return

Another interesting aspect of the Posner spatial cuing task has to do with the temporal dynamics of the attentional cuing effect. To this point, we have ignored these aspects of the task by assuming that the cue activation persists to the point of target onset. This corresponds to experimental conditions when the target follows the cue after a relatively short delay (e.g., around 100 ms). However, the Posner task has also been run with longer delays between the cue and the target (e.g., 500 ms), with some interesting results. Instead of a facilitation effect for the valid trials relative to the invalid ones, the ordering of valid and invalid trials actually reverses at the long delays (e.g., Maylor, 1985). This phenomenon has been labeled *inhibition of return*, to denote the idea that there is something that inhibits the system from returning attention to the cued location after a sufficient delay.

Our model can be used to simulate at least the qualitative patterns of behavior on the Posner task over different delays. This is done by varying the length of cue presentation (a variable delay event could have been inserted, but residual activation would persist anyway, and varying the cue length is simpler), and turning on the accommodation current, which causes neurons that have been active for a while to "fatigue" (see section 2.9 in chapter 2 for details). Thus, if the cue activation persists for long enough, those spatial representations will become fatigued, and if attention is subsequently directed there, the network will actually be slower to respond. Also, because the spatial activations have fatigued, they no longer compete with the activation of the other location for the invalidly cued trials, eliminating the slowing.

Now, let's see this in the model.

↪ First, press the `Defaults` button to restore the default parameters, and then un-lesion the network by doing `Lesion` and selecting `NO_LESION` for the `lesion_lay` parameter. Next, set `env_type` to `STD_POSNER`. Then, set `accom` to `ACCOMMODATE` in the control panel (`Apply`). Next, let's choose a cue duration that, even with the accommodation channels active, still produces the original pattern of results. Set `cue_dur` to 75. Now, do a `Batch` run.

You should observe the now-familiar pattern of a valid facilitation and an invalid slowing.

↪ `Batch` run with increasing durations (change using the `cue_dur` field) in increments of 25 from 75 to 200.

You should see that the valid-invalid difference decreases with increasing duration, equalizes at 125 epochs, and by 150 epochs, the validly cued condition is actually *slower* than the invalidly cued one, which is the hallmark of the inhibition of return phenomenon (figure 8.28).

↪ `Step` through the running of the network with `cue_dur` at 150.

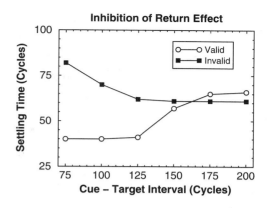

Figure 8.28: Inhibition of return effect seen with long interstimulus intervals between the cue and target (175–200 cycles) as a result of accommodation of the spatial representations. Here the network is slower to respond to the validly cued location compared to the invalidly cued one.

Question 8.12 *Report in detail what happens on the valid and invalid trials that produces the inhibition of return effect.*

Object-Based Attentional Effects

So far, we have explored spatially mediated attentional effects. However, the very same mechanisms (and model) can be used to understand object-based attentional effects. For example, instead of cuing one region of space, we can cue one object, and then present a display containing the cue object and another different object, and determine which of the two objects is processed more readily. By analogy with the Posner spatial cuing paradigm, we would expect that the cued object would be processed more readily than the non-cued one. Of course, one would have to use different, but similar cue and target objects to rule out a target detection response based on the cue itself.

Because a simple object recognition task is problematic, the object-based attention studies that have been run experimentally typically involve a comparison between two operations (e.g., detecting a small visual target) on one object versus two operations on two different objects. If the spatial distances associated with these operations are the same in the two conditions, any difference in reaction time would indicate a cost for switching attention between the two objects. Such an object cost has been found in a number of studies (Duncan, 1984; Vecera & Farah, 1994; Mozer et al., 1992).

In the simulator, we can run the simpler cuing experiment analogous to the Posner task because we have transparent access to the internal representations, and can measure the object processing facilitation directly.

↪ Set env_type to OBJ_ATTN. Then do View, EVENTS to see what the network will experience.

The first event is a control condition, where we present two objects without any prior cuing. Note that, as in the MULTI_OBJ case, the target object is more strongly activated than the cue object, so the network will process the target object. The next event is a cuing event, where the cue object is presented in the central location. Then, within the same group so that activations persist, the next event presents the two objects just as in the first event. Thus, if the prior object cue is effective, it should be able to overcome the relatively small difference in bottom-up salience between the two objects, so that the network processes the cue object and not the target. Finally, the next two events are for the case where the two objects appear in the same location. Recall that before, the network was unable to select either object for processing in this case, because they are spatially overlapping. Perhaps now, with the object-based attentional cue, the network will be able to focus on the cue object.

↪ Press Defaults. Then Step (you may also need to turn the network display on). Note how the network responds to each of the three task conditions as you continue to Step through these cases.

You should observe that the prior object cue is indeed capable of influencing subsequent processing in favor of the same object. Note also that the spatial system responds to this in the appropriate manner — it activates the spatial location associated with the cued object. Finally, note that the top-down object cue is sufficient to enable the system to select one object (even the less active one) when the two objects are presented overlapping in the same location.

↪ Go to the PDP++Root window. To continue on to the next simulation, close this project first by selecting .projects/Remove/Project_0. Or, if you wish to stop now, quit by selecting Object/Quit.

8.5.3 Summary and Discussion

Perhaps the most important lesson from this simulation is that attentional effects are the direct consequence of some of the basic principles developed in the first part of this book: inhibitory competition, bidirectional interactive processing, and multiple constraint satisfaction. This has some important implications. First, it suggests that we should expect to find attention-like effects throughout the cortex, consistent with some recent views (Desimone & Duncan, 1995; Allport, 1989). Second, as emphasized by Cohen et al. (1994), understanding attention in terms of more basic neural information processing principles can result in a simpler conceptual model that avoids the need for things like a disengage mechanism. Third, it suggests that by studying attentional effects, we are observing these fundamental principles in action, and we could potentially use detailed behavioral data to further constrain our model's implementation of these principles. For example, the detailed time-course of cue presentation, delay periods, and the measured attentional cuing and inhibition of return effects should provide specific constraints.

There are a number of important spatial attention effects that we have not addressed in our model, but that are addressed by other models based on similar principles (e.g., Mozer & Sitton, 1998). For example, it appears that spatial attention can be expressed in a variety of different shapes and sizes. Using the popular "spotlight" analogy, the spotlight of attention can range from narrow and intense to wide and diffuse, and it can also be discontinuous. These kinds of phenomena could potentially be addressed in an expanded version of the present model by scaling up the spatial and object representations to allow for much more complex patterns of activity to develop.

There are also detailed neurophysiological recordings of attentional phenomena in monkeys that could potentially be simulated using something like the model we explored here (e.g., Moran & Desimone, 1985;

Motter, 1993). These recordings show that stimulus-specific neural firing in V4 is reduced when visual processing ("attention") is directed toward other stimuli within the receptive field of the neuron, but not when this attention is directed outside the receptive field. Such attentional effects could result directly from lateral inhibitory connectivity (i.e., competition) among V4 neurons, but it is also possible that interactions between the spatial and object pathways could be important for explaining these and other similar effects.

Our model has some important limitations. For example, because we focused specifically on the contribution of the dorsal cortical spatial processing pathway to attention, other potentially important contributors were not represented. In particular, the thalamus has often been discussed as playing an important role in attention (e.g., LaBerge, 1990; Crick, 1984). Although a complete discussion of the role of the thalamus is beyond the present scope, it is worth noting that a model based on many of the same principles we just explored is consistent with much of the biological and behavioral data on thalamic attention (Wager & O'Reilly, submitted).

One concern that readers may have about the present model is the simplicity of the object representations. Clearly, it is highly unrealistic to assume that there is a unique one-to-one mapping between low-level visual features and object representations. How much is this simplification contributing to the observed results? The next section helps to address this concern by using the detailed object recognition system described previously in conjunction with a spatial processing pathway.

8.6 Spatial Attention: A More Complex Model

The simple model we just explored provides a useful means of understanding the basic principles of spatial attention as it interacts with object processing. However, the model does not really address one of the main motivations for having spatial attention in the first place — to avoid the binding problem when perceiving displays containing multiple objects. The next simulation basically combines both of the previous two models, the full-fledged object recognition model and the simple spatial attention model. The resulting model can use spatial attention to restrict the object processing path-

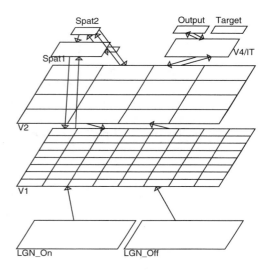

Figure 8.29: Object recognition model with interactive spatial representations that enable sequential processing of multiple objects.

way to one object at a time, enabling it to successfully perform in an environment containing multiple objects. Because all of the essential ideas have been covered in the discussion of the previous models, we proceed directly into the exploration of this model.

8.6.1 Exploring the Complex Attentional Model

[*Note: this simulation requires a minimum of 128Mb of RAM to run.*]

↪ **Open the project** `objrec_multiobj.proj.gz` **in** `chapter_8` **to begin.**

You will notice that the network is essentially the same as in the object recognition model, except for the addition of two spatial processing layers, `Spat1` and `Spat2` (figure 8.29). These two layers are laterally interconnected with V1 and V2, respectively, and amongst themselves, providing the interactions that give rise to spatially mediated attentional effects. There is also a `Target` layer next to the output layer, which does not interact with the network, but is useful because it displays the identities of the objects presented to the network. Thus, the output activation should correspond to one of the active target units.

↪ Do `BuildNet` in the `objrec_ctrl` control panel to build and connect the network. Then, load trained weights by doing `LoadNet`. Select `r.wt` in the network window, and examine the connectivity patterns for the spatial layers.

These spatial layers have a similar spatial extent as their corresponding object pathway representations. However, there is just one unit per unique location in the spatial system, because unlike the object processing system, there is no need to represent multiple features at each location. Note also that there is an excitatory self-connection in the `Spat1` layer, which helps to ensure that a contiguous region of spatial representations is activated, as opposed to having multiple blobs of activity. This encourages the system to focus completely on one object, instead of on parts of two different objects.

The main test of this model involves presenting multiple objects in different locations, and letting the spatial representations focus processing on one of these objects, which should then be recognized by the object recognition pathway. Thus, this is essentially the same task as the `MULTI_OBJS` environment in the previous model. However, unlike that environment, we present both objects with equal activation and let the network select which to focus on. Small differences in the strengths of the weights for the different features of the objects will result in one being slightly more active than another.

We present the network with patterns composed of two objects in random locations. To fit two objects into the relatively small input region with enough space in between to clearly distinguish them, we present the objects in the smallest of the sizes used in the previous object recognition model, even though this size is just at the lower limit of the resolution of the network (and thus causes more errors).

↪ To run this test, press `StepTest` in the control panel.

You will see two objects presented to the network, with the activations updated every 5 cycles of settling. Notice that in the first few updates, the V1 representations for both of the objects are activated, but shortly thereafter, the spatial pathway settles on one of the two locations where the objects are present. This then provides a top-down bias on the V1 system, that results in

only the features for one of the two objects remaining active. Thus, it is only these features that drive further processing in the subsequent object-processing layers (V2 and V4/IT). From the object processing pathway's perspective, it is as if only one object had been presented (except for the transient activation of both object's features, which can confuse the network somewhat).

In this particular case, the network should recognize the object in the lower right hand corner (object number 12 in figure 8.12). Notice that the unit active in the output layer is one of the two possibilities activated in the `Target` layer, indicating it has correctly identified one of the two possible objects. We can record the network's performance in a testing grid log.

↪ Do `View`, `TEST_LOG` to open the testing grid log. Then do `StepTest` again.

When the settling has completed, you should notice that the grid log is updated. The `sum_Outp_wrng` column in this log contains the output of a "wrong on" statistic — it gives a 1 if the unit in the output is not one of the possibilities in the target layer (i.e., the output unit was wrongly active), and a 0 otherwise. Note that a standard squared-error statistic would not be useful in this case, because the network never activates both outputs, and it chooses the object to activate essentially at random, so a single-unit target could not be anticipated. Also shown in the log are the actual output activations, and the targets.

↪ You can continue to `StepTest` through the other patterns in the environment.

Notice that the network makes errors (i.e., `sum_Outp_wrng` values of 1) with some frequency. There are several reasons for this. First, as we mentioned, the objects are small and relatively difficult for the network to recognize even when presented singly. Second, the initial activation of all features in V1 appears to confuse the network somewhat — when one of the two possible spatial locations is activated at the start of settling, the rate of errors is reduced by two thirds. This latter version may be more representative of human visual experience, where spatial attention is directed in a more top-down manner as one actively explores an environment. However, it is a much more interesting demonstration of the network's dynamics when the spatial representation is not clamped in advance.

To test how much the spatial processing pathway contributes to performance, we can reduce its level of influence over the object processing pathway.

↪ Set the `fm_spat1_scale` parameter to .01 instead of 1.

This will reduce the impact of the spatial pathway significantly, and should render the network incapable of focusing processing on individual objects. This may provide a useful model of the object recognition deficits (simultanagnosia) observed in patients with bilateral parietal lobe lesions (Bálint's syndrome patients), who presumably have lost the equivalent of the spatial pathway in our model. These patients cannot recognize objects when multiple are present in the field at once, but can recognize individually-presented objects (just like our earlier object recognition model without a spatial pathway).

↪ Do `InitTest` and then `StepTest` again.

Question 8.13 *Describe the effects of this manipulation on the patterns of activation in the network, and the consequences thereof for the network's ability to tell one object from another.*

↪ Set `fm_spat1_scale` back to 1 before continuing.

Note that although we want the spatial input to have a strong impact on the object processing pathway, we do not want this spatial input to be strong enough to produce activation in the object pathway all on its own. Instead, spatial attention should have an essentially *modulatory* role, which favors some activations over others, but does not directly activate features all by itself. Competitive inhibition produces this modulatory effect in the model, because those units that receive activation from both the spatial representations and the bottom-up featural inputs will win the competition over other units that just receive activation from only one of these sources.

Although spatial attention is useful for enabling an object processing pathway to focus on a single object in an multi-object environment, it would be even more useful if attention could be sequentially directed to the different objects present in the scene. We can implement a simple version of this kind of attention switching

by taking advantage of the accommodation ("fatigue") properties of neurons used in the previous simulation to capture the inhibition of return effect (see section 2.9 for details). After a given object has been processed by the network, the currently active neurons will fatigue due to accommodation, and a new set of neurons can then become activated. Presumably these new neurons will be those that represent another object present in the environment.

↪ Set `accommodate` field to `ACCOMMODATE` in the control panel (`Apply`).

This will turn on the accommodation channels that let potassium ions out after a unit has been active for some period of time. It will also extend the maximum settling time so that the activation dynamics have time to play out.

↪ Now, do `InitTest` and `StepTest` on the process control panel.

You will see the same first event. But notice that after it has correctly recognized the object in the lower right, the focus of activation moves gradually over to the object in the upper left, which is also correctly recognized. Note that the spatial attention actually seems to move continuously across space, and takes a little while to settle over the second object. Thus, the output is momentarily confused in the middle of this transition before it correctly recognizes this second object. This continuous movement of the spatial focus is probably due in part to the self connections within the spatial system, which tend to favor the activation of nearby locations.

Although this demonstration is interesting and illustrates the potential of the network's emergent activation dynamics to achieve sensible-looking attention switching, it is not a very reliable mechanism. Thus, if you continue running on subsequent events, it does not achieve correct recognition of both objects with particularly high frequency. It is likely that better performance on this kind of task will require the explicit training of a control system that provides top-down activation of the spatial representations to direct attention toward different objects. Nevertheless, this kind of accommodation mechanism is probably helpful in allowing attention to be switched.

↪ Before continuing, set `accommodate` to `DONT_ACCOMMODATE` (or hit `Defaults`).

This model could be used to account for some of the phenomena in the extensive literature on **visual search** (e.g., Duncan & Humphreys, 1989; Treisman, 1996). The typical visual search paradigm involves searching for a target shape among a field of distractors. If the target is distinct enough from the distractors, and if the distractors themselves are relatively homogeneous, then this search process can be quite rapid (i.e., it does not appear to depend very much on the number of distractors). This rapid search has been described as taking place in parallel. In contrast, when the distractors are similar to the target, and/or there are multiple different distractor shapes, search goes more slowly, and the time seems to depend on the number of distractor stimuli. This has been characterized as serial search (i.e., searching sequentially through the display items until the target is located). In reality, the simple parallel/serial distinction appears to be more of a continuum that depends on a number of factors (e.g., Duncan & Humphreys, 1989). See Mozer and Sitton (1998) for a visual search model that has some key properties in common with the one we have been exploring, which addresses some of these subtleties.

Finally, we can replicate the object-based attentional cuing that we demonstrated in the previous model. As before, we present one object in the center of the display, and then present two objects on either side, and see if the network processes the cued object. We also cue with the object that the network would not otherwise choose to process on its own as before, so that we can be sure that the cuing is driving the effect. We will do this by working with the underlying process control panel that runs the testing that we've been doing, giving you a better sense of the "guts" of the system.

↪ Do `View, TEST_PROCESS_CTRL` on the overall (`objrec_ctrl`) control panel, to bring up the `SequenceEpoch` process control panel that controls the testing process. Change the `environment` field on the process control panel. Just click on the current value (should be `vis_sim_test`), and then go down to the bottom of the menu under `ScriptEnv`, where you should find `obj_attn_test`. Apply this change, and then `ReInit` (equivalent to `InitTest`) and `Step` (equivalent to `StepTest`).

You will see the network process object number 17 and identify it correctly.

↪ Then, `Step` again.

You will see two objects (12 and 17) presented (this is just the first event from the prior explorations). The network processes the cued object this time, even though in previous cases it has processed object 12 preferentially. Note that, to ensure that the spatial representations do not contribute to the effect, we have reinitialized them between the cue and subsequent inputs. Thus, this demonstration shows that object-based attentional cuing effects can be found even in this more realistic object recognition model.

↪ To stop now, quit by selecting `Object/Quit` in the `PDP++Root` window.

8.6.2   Summary and Discussion

This model shows that the principles we developed regarding the interaction between spatial and object attention scale up well to a more complex and realistic model of object recognition. More generally, this model demonstrates how spatial attention can help solve the binding problem by restricting object-recognition processing to only one object's features at a time. Spatial attention is effective in this case because objects are spatially contiguous.

8.7   Summary

The visual system entails a sequence of processing stages, starting in the retina, continuing to the **LGN** of the **thalamus**, and into area **V1** in the cortex. V1 has **topographically** organized **retinotopic** representations that encode the visual world according to **oriented edges**, providing a relatively efficient means of encoding the visual form of objects. These V1 receptive field properties arise naturally in a self-organizing model using Hebbian learning on natural visual scenes, and can thus be understood as representing the basic **correlational structure** present in visual scenes.

Beyond V1, visual processing is divided into two major pathways. The **object recognition** or **"what"** pathway involves areas in the **ventral** stream of processing from **V2**, **V4**, to **IT**. A model of this pathway developed **spatially invariant** representations that collapse across differences in spatial location and size, while retaining the distinctions between different objects. These representations formed gradually over sequential layers of processing. The network **generalized** the invariance transformation, learning about novel objects in a subset of locations and sizes and recognizing them in a large number of novel locations and sizes.

The other major visual processing pathway is the **spatial** or **"where"** pathway in the **dorsal** stream of processing in the **parietal** cortex. We explored the ability of this pathway to influence the allocation of **attention** to spatial locations. Spatial attention can interact with and facilitate processing in the object recognition pathway, enabling multiple objects to be processed by sequentially focusing attention to these objects. We also explored spatial attention in the Posner spatial cuing task. Our lesioned model simulated the performance of **neglect** patients (with lesions in one parietal hemisphere), who exhibit slowed processing of targets represented in the lesioned hemisphere.

8.8 Further Reading

Mozer and Sitton (1998) presents a comprehensive treatment of many different attentional (and object recognition) phenomena using many of the same computational principles employed in the models described in this chapter.

For a comprehensive and influential discussion of attention, see Desimone and Duncan (1995).

Behrmann and Tipper (1994) discuss many of the phenomena from neuropsychological studies of neglect.

Farah (1990) gives a compact treatment of higher-level vision from a neuropsychological perspective, and her new book is also good (Farah, 1999).

The following are some particularly useful papers on the neural basis of object recognition and visual processing more generally: Desimone and Ungerleider (1989); Ungerleider and Haxby (1994); Goodale and Milner (1992); Tootell, Dale, Sereno, and Malach (1996); Logothetis and Sheinberg (1996); Tanaka (1996).

Chapter 9

Memory

Contents

9.1   Overview 275

9.2   **Weight-Based Memory in a Generic Model of Cortex** **277**

    9.2.1   Long-Term Priming *278*

    9.2.2   AB–AC List Learning *282*

9.3   **The Hippocampal Memory System** **287**

    9.3.1   Anatomy and Physiology of the Hippocampus *287*

    9.3.2   Basic Properties of the Hippocampal Model   *289*

    9.3.3   Explorations of the Hippocampus *293*

    9.3.4   Summary and Discussion *296*

9.4   **Activation-Based Memory in a Generic Model of Cortex** **298**

    9.4.1   Short-Term Priming *298*

    9.4.2   Active Maintenance *299*

    9.4.3   Robust yet Rapidly Updatable Active Maintenance *303*

9.5   **The Prefrontal Cortex Active Memory System** . . **305**

    9.5.1   Dynamic Regulation of Active Maintenance   *306*

    9.5.2   Details of the Prefrontal Cortex Model . . . *307*

    9.5.3   Exploring the Model *310*

    9.5.4   Summary and Discussion *312*

9.6   **The Development and Interaction of Memory Systems** **314**

    9.6.1   Basic Properties of the Model *314*

    9.6.2   Exploring the Model *315*

    9.6.3   Summary and Discussion *317*

9.7   **Memory Phenomena and System Interactions** . . **318**

    9.7.1   Recognition Memory *318*

    9.7.2   Cued Recall *319*

    9.7.3   Free Recall *319*

    9.7.4   Item Effects *320*

    9.7.5   Working Memory *320*

9.8   **Summary** **320**

9.9   **Further Reading** **321**

9.1   Overview

Memory can be very broadly defined as any persistent effect of experience. This definition is much broader than the layperson's conception of memory as the ability to explicitly remember facts, figures, events, names, and faces. The popular conception of memory is also narrow in failing to appreciate the diversity of brain areas and representations that participate in the encoding of any given "memory." This notion of a unitary memory system was also a popular scientific conception, at least until relatively recently. In this chapter we provide a broad perspective on memory that emphasizes the contributions of several different brain areas and the ways in which these areas may have become specialized for different types of memory.

Consistent with our emphasis on understanding the neural mechanisms underlying cognitive phenomena, we focus on a mechanistic account of memory phenomena. Thus, instead of describing the kinds of memories subserved by different parts of the brain according to memory *content* (e.g., implicit, declarative, spatial, visual, etc.), we distinguish the different components of memory according to the properties of their underlying *mechanisms* (e.g., how effects of prior experience are physically maintained in the neural network, and how differences in neural network properties can result in different kinds of representations).

Persistent effects of experience can take one of two general forms in a neural network — changes in the weights (**weight-based memory**) or persistent activity (**activation-based memory**). Because weight-based memories result from weight changes, we typically view them as the product of the kinds of learning mechanisms discussed in chapters 4–6. Similarly, the architectural properties that determine how activation flows through the network (chapter 3) play an important role in our understanding of the nature of activation-based memories. Thus, you have already learned a great deal about memory without necessarily realizing it! This chapter builds on these earlier foundations by applying principles of learning and activation propagation toward understanding a range of memory phenomena in humans and other animals.

The learning and processing principles developed to this point are intended to apply generally to the cortex. Thus, our first goal is to explore the general memory capacities of a generic cortical model. We will see that this cortical model of memory seems to apply more specifically to the posterior areas, and not necessarily to the frontal lobe. Thus, we will use our generic model to characterize the *posterior-cortical memory system* (as discussed in chapter 7).

The representations that result from the integrated effects of learning over many experiences comprise perhaps the most important form of memory exhibited by the posterior cortical system. These memories have traditionally been characterized as *semantic* and *procedural memory*, emphasizing the extent to which they capture stable aspects of the environment ("semantics"), or often-repeated task components ("procedures"). For example, the object recognition model in chapter 8, employing the basic learning principles developed in chapters 4–6, can be said to have developed semantic memories for the different objects it can recognize.

Short-term and *long-term priming* are two other important and related memory phenomena that the posterior memory system can subserve. Priming refers to a facilitory effect on processing items from prior pro-

cessing of similar items (just as priming a pump facilitates subsequent pumping). We can understand short-term priming in terms of the residual activation of immediately prior processing, while long-term priming reflects the weight changes resulting from prior processing. This latter form of priming is relatively long-term due to the persistence of the underlying weight changes, whereas the residual activation underlying short-term priming dissipates relatively rapidly. Interestingly, long-term priming can be understood using the same underlying mechanisms that ultimately lead to semantic/procedural memories — the difference is that priming results from single "tweaks" of the weights, while semantic/procedural memories require the accumulation of many incremental weight changes over a relatively long period of time.

Although the posterior-cortical system has powerful learning and activation mechanisms and provides the foundation for many memories, it has some important limitations that necessitate the use of additional, specialized memory systems. In the domain of weight-based memories, we will see that our generic cortical model can suffer from a *catastrophic* level of *interference* from subsequent learning, such that almost everything the network learned about one list of items is lost due to interference from a second list of similar items. People show some level of interference on such tasks, but not nearly as much as our generic cortical model. As mentioned in chapter 7, we suggest that this discrepancy is due to an intrinsic tradeoff between the long-term learning of semantic representations and the ability to learn rapidly arbitrary information such as a list of words. The hippocampus and related structures (which we refer to simply as the hippocampus) seem specialized for this latter form of rapid arbitrary learning, while the cortex slowly accumulates semantic/procedural representations based on many experiences with the environment.

Hippocampally mediated memories have been characterized as *episodic* (representing the contents of episodes or events; Tulving, 1972), *declarative* (representing explicitly accessible information; Squire, 1992), or *spatial* (representing locations in space; O'Keefe & Nadel, 1978). We instead emphasize the underlying mechanisms that enable the hippocampal system to learn rapidly without suffering undue interference, specifically the use of *sparse conjunctive* representations. Such representations result in *pattern separation*, so that information is encoded very distinctly (separately), which reduces interference. The conjunctive nature of the representations can also *bind* together many different features, enabling entire episodes to be recalled from partial cues, for example.

In the domain of activation-based memory, the generic posterior cortex model is challenged by *working memory* tasks, such as mental arithmetic (e.g., multiplying 42 times 7). Such tasks typically involve both *rapid updating* of information (e.g., rapidly storing the partial products of $7x2$ and $7x4$) and *robust maintenance* of this information (e.g., not forgetting 14 while computing $7x4$). We will see that our generic cortical model cannot satisfy both of these demands because they are mutually contradictory. Thus, we suggest that the posterior cortex is supplemented by the specialized *frontal cortex* (and more specifically the *prefrontal cortex*), which has a *dynamic gating* mechanism that can dynamically switch between rapid updating and robust maintenance.

When the dynamic frontal gating mechanism is "closed," the frontal cortex maintains activation patterns with little interference from outside activity, and when it "opens," the frontal cortex can be rapidly updated. We show how such a gating mechanism can be implemented by the neuromodulatory substance *dopamine* under the control of the temporal-differences learning algorithm described in chapter 6. Thus, our frontal cortex model can learn when it is appropriate to maintain and when it is appropriate to update based on task demands.

We divide our exploration of memory according to the broad mechanisms of weight- and activation-based memory, and begin by exploring weight-based priming in our generic cortical model (i.e., the posterior cortex). We then challenge this model to rapidly learn lists of arbitrary but overlapping items, where we encounter catastrophic interference. This motivates the need for the hippocampal memory system — we will see that our model of the hippocampus is much more capable of rapid learning of arbitrary information. We next move on to activation-based memories, first by exploring short-term priming in the generic cortical model. We then challenge this model to perform more demanding working memory tasks, where we see that it cannot both robustly maintain and rapidly update information. This motivates the need for the frontal memory system – we will see that our frontal model is much more capable of handling working memory tasks. Then, we explore the development and interaction of both activation-based and weight-based memory mechanisms in a model of the A-not-B ($A\overline{B}$) task. Finally, we summarize some of the ways that the basic mechanisms developed in this chapter can be applied to explain a wider range of memory phenomena.

9.2 Weight-Based Memory in a Generic Model of Cortex

In previous chapters we explored the formation of representations that capture the structure of the environment (*model learning*) and the structure of tasks (*task learning*). Chapters 4-6 discussed the basic principles behind these types of learning, and how these principles can be implemented by changes in weights (synaptic efficacies) on the connections between neurons. Chapter 7 discussed in general terms how multiple layers of neurons organized into multiple processing streams in the cortex can produce complex transformations of input signals, which emphasize some distinctions and deemphasize or collapse across others. Chapter 8 showed how this works in the case of spatially invariant object recognition, where the network collapsed across distinctions in the spatial locations of objects, while retaining distinctions between different objects.

We can now summarize these earlier chapters as explorations into the ways that semantic/procedural memories are formed over long-term exposure to, and interaction with, the environment. The formation of such representations (and their use in constraint-satisfaction style processing) is perhaps the most important contribution of the posterior cortex to cognition. In the following section, we explore another manifestation of memory in the posterior cortex, *long-term* or *weight-based* priming. This form of memory is manifest after single exposures to stimuli, and results in our model from the same kinds of weight changes that, over a longer time scale, result in the formation of semantic/procedural memories (McClelland & Rumelhart, 1986). Thus, these priming effects provide a behavioral window into the neural mechanisms of learning, in addition to playing an important role in cognition by providing a trace of recent experience.

Importantly, many forms of long-term priming are intact (at normal levels) even in patients with hippocampal system lesions (Graf, Squire, & Mandler, 1984), which supports the idea that this priming does indeed reflect cortical learning, and not learning in the hippocampus. Thus, although one might have expected based on our previous characterization that the hippocampus is *solely* responsible for rapid learning effects, intact long-term priming in hippocampally lesioned patients suggests that the effects of a single stimulus presentation can in fact be mediated by the relatively small weight changes in the cortex that are consistent with the slow overall acquisition of semantic/procedural knowledge.

9.2.1 Long-Term Priming

The term *priming* generally refers to any facilitory effect of prior processing on subsequent processing. For example, if people read a list of words out loud and then read that same list of words again, they will be faster the second time around. Interestingly, priming can also be seen across semantically related words, so that reading "bread" facilitates the reading of "butter," for example. Many different forms of priming have been described (Schacter, 1987), but from our mechanistic perspective we will consider three cross-cutting dimensions for delineating different types of priming: (1) duration, (2) content, and (3) similarity. The duration dimension has been discussed already, and involves the distinction between short-term (activation-based) and long-term (weight-based) priming. We will discuss activation-based priming at greater length in section 9.4, and focus on weight-based priming here. The content dimension reflects the nature of the representations involved, for example including visual, lexical (word-based), and semantic representations.

The similarity dimension reflects the similarity between the prior *prime* stimulus and the subsequent *probe* stimulus. A special case of this dimension is called *repetition* priming, where the prime and the probe are identical (e.g., the example of reading a list of words and then reading those same words again a second time more rapidly). More generally, similarity-based priming involves the spread of activation along associative links (e.g., along semantic associations, or according to visual similarity), resulting in facilitation for probes that are similar to the prime (e.g., bread priming butter). This spreading activation can also produce weight changes, so that one might expect both short-term and long-term priming in this case. Indeed, long-term priming of this form has been recently demonstrated and explained using just this type of model (Becker, Moscovitch, Behrmann, & Joordens, 1997). In what follows, we will focus on the simpler case of repetition priming in the lexical content dimension, but we assume that the same basic principles apply across all examples of long-term priming.

One of the main behavioral methodologies for studying long-term repetition priming is *stem completion*, in which participants first study a list of words, and they are then presented with a list of initial word fragments (stems) and asked to generate words that complete these stems. Unbeknownst to the subjects, many of these stems can be completed with the previously studied words. For example, a participant might read "reason" initially, and then later be asked to complete the stem "rea___." Because the stems are constructed to have several possible completions and are pre-tested to ensure these possible completions are roughly equally likely to be produced, any increased probability of coming up with the studied word (relative to the pre-test levels) can be taken as an indication of some residual effects of processing the word. In other words, the initial studying of the word has *primed* the subsequent processing of that word. The fact that the list study is separated from the stem completion task by a relatively long time period (tens of minutes) and the study list contains more words than could be maintained in active memory suggests that a relatively long-lasting mechanism is at work (i.e., *long-term priming*, as compared to the much more transient short-term priming produced by residual activations).

One way of conceptualizing the stem completion task for modeling purposes is as a *one-to-many mapping*, because one stem input can be completed with many different possible words. A related priming paradigm that makes this one-to-many mapping even more explicit is the *homophone* task used by Jacoby and Witherspoon (1982). Homophones are two words that have the same pronunciation but different spelling. Participants in this task were primed with one homophone (e.g., "Name a musical instrument that uses a *reed*"), and were later asked (by spoken instruction) to spell the critical word (e.g., "Spell the word /r$\bar{e}$d/," where /r$\bar{e}$d/ is the phonetic representation of the pronunciation of both spellings). The input is the ambiguous pronunciation, and the output is one of the two possible spellings. The behavioral result is that participants produce the primed spelling more frequently than a control group who have not been primed.

The model we will explore next simulates this one-to-many mapping paradigm by learning to associate two different output patterns with a given input pattern. For simplicity, we use random distributed patterns for the input and output patterns. An initial period of slow training allows the network to acquire the appropriate associations (i.e., to simulate the subject's prior lifelong experience that results in the relevant knowledge about homophones and their spellings). One can think of this initial training as providing the semantic memory for the network, so that on any given trial the network produces one of the two appropriate outputs in response to the input pattern.

Training is followed by a testing phase in which the network is presented with one particular association of a given input, and then tested to see which word it will produce for that input. We will see that a single trial of learning, at exactly the same learning rate and using the same learning mechanisms that enabled the network to acquire the semantic information initially, results in a strong bias toward producing the primed output. Thus, this model simulates the observed behavioral effects and shows that long-term priming can be viewed as simply a natural consequence of the same slow learning processes that establish cortical representations in the first place.

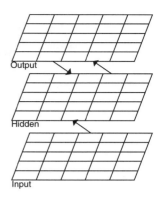

Figure 9.1: Network for exploring weight-based (long-term) priming. Two different output patterns are associated with each input pattern.

Exploring the Model

↪ Open the project `wt_priming.proj.gz` in `chapter_9` to begin.

Notice that the network has a standard three layer structure, with the input presented to the bottom and output produced at the top (figure 9.1).

↪ Press `View`, `EVENTS` in the `wt_prime_ctrl` control panel.

You will see an environment view with 6 events shown (figure 9.2). For each event, the bottom pattern represents the input and the top represents the output. As you should be able to tell, the first set of 3 events and the second set of 3 events have the same set of 3 input patterns, but different output patterns. The names of the events reflect this, so that the first event has input pattern number 0, with the first corresponding output pattern (labeled a), so it is named 0_a. The fourth event has this same input pattern, but the second corresponding output pattern (labeled b), so it is named 0_b. The environment actually contains a total of 13 different input patterns, for a total of 26 input-output combinations (events).

↪ Now you can iconify this environment window.

First, we will train the network using the standard combination of Hebbian and error-driven learning as developed in chapters 4–6.

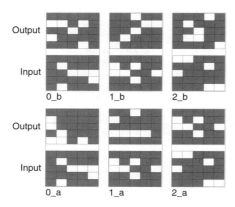

Figure 9.2: Six sample input (bottom) – output (top) patterns for training. Events 0_a and 0_b have the same input pattern, but map to two different output patterns, producing a one-to-many (two) mapping.

↪ First, do View, TRAIN_LOG to get a graph log of training progress. Do Train in the control panel to start training — you can see the network being trained on the patterns. Then, turn off the Display in the network speed the process.

The graph log shows two statistics of training. As with the Reber grammar network from chapter 6 (which also had two possible outputs per input), we cannot use the standard sum_se error measure (which target would you use when the network can validly produce either one?). Instead, we use a *closest event* statistic to find which event among those in the training environment has the closest (most similar) target output pattern to the output pattern the network actually produced (i.e., in the minus phase). This statistic gives us three results, only one of which is useful for this training phase, but the others will be useful for testing so we describe them all here: (a) the distance dist from the closest event (thresholded by the usual .5), which will be 0 if the output exactly matches one of the events in the environment; (b) the name of the closest event ev_nm, that does not appear in the graph log because it is not a numerical value, but it will appear on our testing log used later; (c) sm_nm that is 0 if this closest event has the same name as that of the event currently being presented to the network (i.e., it is the "correct" output),

and 1 otherwise (think of it as a binary distance or error measure computed on the names).

The sum of the closest event distances over the epoch of training is plotted in yellow in the graph log. As the network starts producing outputs that exactly match valid outputs in the environment (though not necessarily the appropriate outputs for the given input pattern), this should approach zero. Instead of plotting the sm_nm statistic, the graph log shows both_err, plotted in blue. Like sm_nm, this compares the closest event name with the actual input name, but this one looks only at the part of the event name that identifies the input pattern (i.e., the portion of the name before the _ character). Thus, it gives a 1 if the output is wrong for *both* possible outputs. This, too, should approach zero as the network trains.

As something of an aside, it should be noted that the ability to learn this one-to-many mapping task depends critically on the presence of the kWTA inhibition in the network — standard backpropagation networks will learn to produce a *blend* of both output patterns instead of learning to produce one output or the other (cf. Movellan & McClelland, 1993). Inhibition helps by forcing the network to choose one output or the other, because both cannot be active at the same time under the inhibitory constraints. We have also facilitated this one-to-many mapping by adding in a small amount of noise to the membrane potentials of the units during processing, which provides some randomness in the selection of which output to produce. Finally, Hebbian learning also appears to be important here, because the network learns the task better with Hebbian learning than in a purely error driven manner. Hebbian learning can help to produce more distinctive representations of the two output cases by virtue of different correlations that exist in these two cases. O'Reilly and Hoeffner (in preparation) provides a more systematic exploration of the contributions of these different mechanisms in this priming task.

Having trained the network with the appropriate "semantic" background knowledge, we are now ready to assess its performance on the priming task.

↪ Iconify the training graph log. Press View on the wt_prime_ctrl control panel and select TEST_LOGS.

This will bring up two text logs to display the results of testing. We will perform two different kinds of tests. First, we will assess any biases that may exist to respond to the input patterns with either the a or b outputs. This assessment of the *baseline* responses is done with learning turned off. Second, we will turn learning on and train the network to alternately produce the a output (i.e., present the a output in the plus phase and adjust the weights just as was done during training) and then the b output. When compared with the baseline, we will be able to see if one trial of learning to produce a particular output will have a substantial effect on the probability of producing that output.

First, let's collect the baseline values without learning. The `wt_update` parameter in the control panel, which should be set to `TEST`, determines that we will not do any learning at this point.

↪ Do `Test` in the control to present one epoch of events.

You can see in the `Event` column of the larger text log that the events were presented in sequential order, with all the a outputs presented first and then all the b outputs. Because we are only testing now, the outputs were not actually presented (i.e., no plus phase was run, only a minus phase where only the input pattern is presented), which means that the first half of the list is basically the same as the second half, because it is the same input patterns in both halves. This order of event presentation will make more sense when we turn on the training. Any differences in the two halves at this point are due to the noise added to the unit membrane potentials.

The other columns to pay attention to in the larger text log are `ev_nm` and `Outp_sm_nm`. The first is the closest event name for the actual output produced by the network as described previously. Because it will generally be producing one of the two correct outputs, the critical issue is whether it is an a or b response. You should see that there is a fairly random set of output responses. To determine how many times the network produced the output pattern corresponding to the particular target output for the current event, you can look at the `Outp_sm_nm` column (which we will refer to as simply `sm_nm`). There is a 0 every time the same name as the event was produced (i.e., the same output pattern), and a 1 otherwise. You should observe that roughly 50 percent of the time it produces the same name as the current event. The smaller log shows you this result by summing the `sm_nm` column, and also summing the `both_err` column just to monitor the actual accuracy of the network in producing one of the two correct outputs. Note also that the `dist` statistic is not perfect, but most of the errors are less than 1 in magnitude.

↪ Look at the summary statistics in the smaller text log.

You should have observed that the network always produced a valid response (a or b) and produced the a response roughly 50 percent of the time. Given that the network was trained equally often to produce the a and b responses, this is just the kind of baseline performance that we would expect.

Now, let's turn learning on, and see if there are any obvious effects of one trial of learning on a given input pattern for subsequent performance on that same input.

↪ Set `wt_update` to `ON_LINE` in the control panel, to learn (update the weights) after each event (and `Apply` that change). Then, press `Test` again in the process control panel.

Now, because we are learning after each event, there is a plus phase following the minus phase, where the a output is trained in the first half of the inputs, and the b output is trained in the second half. Note that the evaluation of the network's output is all done in the minus phase, *before* this plus phase training is provided, so it reflects the prior state of the network.

As a result of having seen the a output associated with a particular input pattern in the first half of the list of events, we would expect that the network would be more likely to produce this a output when it comes to that input pattern again in the second half. Thus, unlike in the baseline case, you should observe a systematic difference in the responses of the network in the two halves of the patterns (figure 9.3).

Question 9.1 (a) *What do you notice about the probability of the network producing the a output in the second half of the events (i.e., the second time through the same inputs patterns)?* **(b)** *How does this affect the* sm_nm *statistic (i.e., what is the summary value for*

trial	Event	sum_se	Outp_dist	ev_nm	sm_nm	both_err
0	0_a	5.22935	0	0_b	1	0
1	1_a	6.48608	0	1_b	1	0
2	2_a	7.77501	0.273233	2_b	1	0
3	3_a	7.64788	0	3_b	1	0
4	4_a	5.41569	0.551383	4_b	1	0
5	5_a	0	0	5_a	0	0
6	6_a	10.2454	0	6_b	1	0
7	7_a	8.33851	0	7_b	1	0
8	8_a	5.64973	2.61438	8_b	1	0
9	9_a	10.2408	0	9_b	1	0
10	10_a	3.21385	1.06278	10_b	1	0
11	11_a	2.82117	2.42077	11_b	1	0
12	12_a	4.69916	0.253711	12_b	1	0
13	0_b	6.68981	0	0_a	1	0
14	1_b	5.40769	0.330821	1_a	1	0
15	2_b	7.51547	0	2_a	1	0
16	3_b	7.73557	0	3_a	1	0
17	4_b	1.94789	1.94789	4_b	0	0
18	5_b	0.414954	0.414954	5_b	0	0
19	6_b	10.5514	0	6_a	1	0
20	7_b	8.79166	0	7_a	1	0
21	8_b	9.64561	0	8_a	1	0
22	9_b	10.2245	0	9_a	1	0
23	10_b	3.53423	0.766472	10_a	1	0
24	11_b	7.46935	0	11_a	1	0
25	12_b	5.72054	0	12_a	1	0

Figure 9.3: Text log output showing weight-based priming effects — the network responds with the b outputs (shown in the ev_nm column) to the a inputs (shown in the Event column), and vice-versa, as a result of prior exposure.

---

this)? **(c)** *Now,* Test *again, and report what happens for both the first and second time the events are presented.* **(d)** *Explain why this behavior occurs, and relate it to the priming results for humans described earlier.*

↪ Go to the PDP++Root window. To continue on to the next simulation, close this project first by selecting .projects/Remove/Project_0. Or, if you wish to stop now, quit by selecting Object/Quit.

Summary and Discussion

The relatively simple model we just explored provides a reasonable in-principle account of the mechanistic basis for long-term priming. Specifically, it shows that the same learning mechanisms used to construct representations over long periods of exposure to an environment (i.e., semantic memories) can also be used to explain the effects of single exposures to particular items (Mc-Clelland & Rumelhart, 1986). By demonstrating this in the context of a one-to-many mapping task (e.g., stem completion or homophone disambiguation), it was easy

to observe the preference for producing a given output over the other possibilities. It is also possible to observe priming effects on reaction time latencies using a similar single-learning-mechanism model (Becker et al., 1997).

These results suggest that in addition to learning powerful semantic representations, the posterior cortex can exhibit memory-like effects based on single item presentations. We will discuss in section 9.7 how these priming kinds of memory effects can play a role in more complex memory phenomena by providing a *familiarity* signal. Furthermore, in chapter 10 we explore a model of inflectional morphology in language production that takes advantage of the priming and competition exhibited in the present model to explain some previously thorny phenomena in that domain.

9.2.2   AB–AC List Learning

We have seen that a simple model of the cortex can use slow learning to both develop new representations (over many learning trials), and show priming-like effects after single exposures to familiar items (i.e., those items having existing representations). However, one is often faced with the task of having to rapidly encode novel information on the basis of only a few learning trials (e.g., learning someone's name, the definition of a new word, where one's car is parked, a phone number). The priming-like phenomenon in the cortex does not appear to be capable of this kind of task (e.g., just look at how long it took for the network to learn the input-output associations in the previous exploration). Thus, we have reason to be pessimistic that the cortex will succeed at all memory tasks.

In this section we will explore a commonly used experimental task that demands rapid learning of novel associations, and see that the basic cortical model does not in fact succeed. This task is particularly challenging because there is a high level of overlap between the novel associations to be learned — this overlap is ecologically valid, however, because we are often required to remember information about very similar things (e.g., where one's car is parked today as opposed to previous days). The task is commonly known as the AB–AC *paired associates* list learning task (e.g.,

Barnes & Underwood, 1959), where A represents one set of words that are associated with two different sets of other words, B and C. For example, the word *window* will be associated with the word *reason* in the AB list, and then *window* will be associated with *locomotive* on the AC list. After studying the AB list of associates, subjects are tested by asking them to give the appropriate B associate for each of the A words. Then, subjects study the AC list (often over multiple iterations), and are subsequently tested on both lists for recall of the associates after each iteration of learning the AC list. Although subjects do exhibit some level of interference on the initially learned AB associations as a result of learning the AC list, they still remember a reasonable percentage (see figure 9.4 for representative data).

McCloskey and Cohen (1989) tried to get a standard backpropagation network to perform this AB–AC list learning task and found that the network suffered from what they described as **catastrophic interference**. A comparison of typical human data with the network's performance is shown in figure 9.4. Whereas human performance goes from 100 percent correct recall on the AB list immediately after studying it to roughly 60 percent after learning the AC list, the network immediately drops to 0 percent recall well before the AC list is learned. In the model we explore here, we start by replicating this catastrophic interference effect in a standard cortical network like that used to model long-term priming in the previous section. However, instead of just concluding that neural networks are not good models of human cognition (as McCloskey & Cohen, 1989 did), we will explore how a few important parameters can affect the level of interference. By understanding these parameters and their consequences, we will gain further insight into some of the tradeoffs involved in learning and memory.

The original catastrophic interference finding has inspired a fair amount of subsequent research (e.g., Kortge, 1993; French, 1992; Sloman & Rumelhart, 1992; McRae & Hetherington, 1993), much of which is consistent with the basic idea that interference results from the re-use of the same units (and weights) to learn different associations. After learning one association with a given set of weights, the subsequent weight changes made to learn a different association tend to undo the

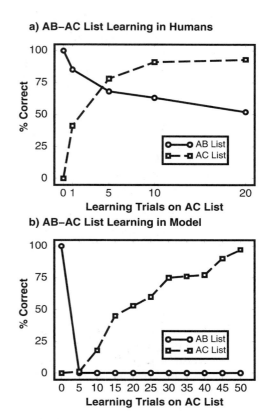

Figure 9.4: Human and model data for AB–AC list learning. a) Humans show some interference for the AB list items as a function of new learning on the AC list items. b) Model shows a catastrophic level of interference. (data reproduced from McCloskey & Cohen, 1989).

previous learning. This will happen any time shared weights are sequentially used to learn different, incompatible associations (e.g., two different locations for where one's car is parked, or the two different associates (B and C) for the A words in the AB–AC task).

There are two different ways of avoiding this kind of interference: (1) have different units represent the different associations, or (2) perform slow *interleaved* learning, allowing the network to shape the weights over many repeated presentations of the different associations in such a way as to accommodate their differences (e.g., as was done in the initial training of the

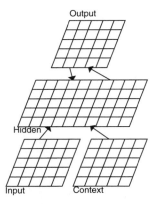

Figure 9.5: Network for the AB–AC list learning task, with the `Input` layer representing the A stimulus, the `Context` input representing the list context, and the `Output` being the B or C word associate, depending on the list context.

long-term priming network from the previous section). Although the second option is compatible with our basic cortical model, it does not address the situation that we are interested in here, where one needs to rapidly and sequentially learn novel information. Therefore, we will explore the first option. However, as we have stressed previously, this solution conflicts with the use of overlapping distributed representations, where the same units participate in the representation of many different items.

We will see that we can either have a set of parameters that result in overlapping distributed representations (in which case we get catastrophic interference), or we can have a set of parameters which result in **sparser** (having fewer units active) **separated** representations, where we can reduce interference, but give up the benefits of overlapping distributed representations. In section 9.3 below, we will explore a model of the hippocampus (and related structures), which appears to resolve this dilemma by providing a specialized memory system based on sparse separated representations that can subserve rapid learning without suffering undue interference.

Exploring the Model

The basic framework for implementing the AB–AC task is to have two input patterns, one that represents the A stimulus, and the other that represents the "list context" (figure 9.5). Thus, we assume that the subject develops some internal representation that identifies the two different lists, and that this serves as a means of disambiguating which of the two associates should be produced. These input patterns feed into a hidden layer, which then produces an output pattern corresponding to the B or C associate. As in the previous simulation, we use a distributed representation of random bit patterns to represent the word stimuli.

↪   Open `ab_ac_interference.proj.gz` in `chapter_9` to begin.

You will see the network as described previously. First, let's look at the training environment.

↪ Press the `View, EVENTS_AB` button to view the distributed input/output patterns for the AB list. Do `View, EVENTS_AC` to see the AC items.

The bottom patterns for each event are the A item and the list context, and the upper pattern is the associate. Note that the first item in the AB list (`0_b`) has the same A pattern as the first item in the AC list (`0_c`). This is true for each corresponding pair of items in the two lists. The list context patterns for all the items on the AB list are all similar random variations of a common underlying pattern, and likewise for the AC items. Thus, the list context patterns are not identical for each item on the same list, just very similar (this reflects the fact that even if the external environmental context is constant, the internal perception of it fluctuates, and other internal context factors like a sense of time passing change as well). Go ahead and iconify these windows.

Now, let's see how well the network performs on this task.

↪   Do `View, TRAIN_GRAPH_LOG` to get a graph log of training performance. Then, do `Run` on the control panel.

You will see the graph log being updated as the network is trained, initially on the AB list, and then on the AC list. The red line shows the error expressed as the number of list items incorrectly produced, with the criterion for correct performance being all units on the right side of .5. This red line error is plotted for the training set (AB then AC), and the yellow line shows the error for testing *always on the AB list*. Note that the red and yellow lines start out being roughly correlated with each other, but are not identical because testing (yellow line) occurs after each epoch of training, and so the weights are different than when each item was presented during the training epoch (red line).

When the red line (training error) gets to zero (or if 50 epochs pass without getting to zero), the network automatically switches to training on the AC list. Thus, you will see the red line for the training set jump up immediately for this new set of training events. However, replicating the McCloskey and Cohen (1989) results (figure 9.4), you will also see the yellow line for testing the AB list jump up immediately as well, indicating that learning on the AC list has interfered catastrophically with the prior learning on the AB list. Let's collect some statistics by running a batch of training runs.

↪ Do View, BATCH_TEXT_LOG to get a log of the results. Then run a batch of 5 "subjects" with Batch.

The summary average statistics taken at the end of the AC list training for each "subject" will appear in the batch text log after the 5 subjects have been run. avg_sum_se shows the average training error, which should be 0, and avg_tst_se shows the average testing error on the AB list.

Question 9.2 (a) *Report the average testing statistic (avg_tst_se) for a batch run of 5 simulated subjects.* (b) *How do these results compare to the human data presented in figure 9.4?* (c) *Looking at the training graph log, roughly how many epochs does the network take to reach its maximum error on the AB list after the introduction of the AC list?*

Having replicated the basic catastrophic interference phenomenon, let's see if we can do anything to reduce the level of interference. Our strategy will be to retain the same basic architecture and learning mechanisms while manipulating certain key parameters. The intention here is to illuminate some principles that will prove important for understanding the origin of these interference effects, and how they could potentially be reduced — though we will see that they have relatively small effects in this particular context.

↪ Turn on the Display in the network, do a Run.

Notice how overlapping the distributed hidden unit representations are — many of the same units are active across multiple input patterns.

↪ To see this overlap more clearly, view act_avg in the network display — this shows the average unit activations across patterns (computed using a running average). A subset of the units have relatively high (near 50%) activation averages, indicating that they are disproportionately active across patterns.

This overlap seems obviously problematic from an interference perspective, because the AC list will activate and reuse the same units from the AB list, altering their weights to support the *C* associate instead of the *B*. Thus, by reducing the extent to which the hidden unit representations overlap (i.e., by making them *sparser*), we might be able to encourage the network to use separate representations for learning these two lists of items.

↪ Let's test this idea by reducing the hid_kwta parameter in the ab_ac_ctrl panel to 4 instead of 12.

This will allow only 4 units to be active at a time in the hidden layer, which should result in less overlapping distributed representations.

↪ Clear the graph log and run a Batch with this reduced hidden layer activity (don't forget to turn the Display off in the network).

Question 9.3 (a) *Report the resulting average testing statistic (avg_tst_se).* (b) *Describe any effects that this manipulation has on the number of epochs it takes for the network to reach its maximum error on the AB list after the introduction of the AC list.* (c) *How do these results compare to the human data presented in figure 9.4?*

The network may not have performed as well as expected because nothing was done to encourage it to use *different* sets of 4 units to represent the different associates. One way we can encourage this is to increase the variance of the initial random weights, making each unit have a more quirky pattern of responses that should encourage different units to encode the different associates.

↪ Thus, change wt_var from .25 to .4.

Another thing we can do to improve performance is to enhance the contribution of the list context inputs relative to the A stimulus, because this list context disambiguates the two different associates.

↪ Do this by changing `fm_context` from 1 to 1.5.

This increases the weight scaling for context inputs (i.e., by increasing the r_k (`wt_scale.rel`) parameter in equation 2.17). We might imagine that strategic focusing of attention by the subject accomplishes something like this.

Finally, increased amounts of Hebbian learning might contribute to better performance because of the strong correlation of all items on a given list with the associated list context representation, which should be emphasized by Hebbian learning. This could lead to different subsets of hidden units representing the items on the two lists because of the different context representations.

↪ Do this by setting `hebb` to .05 instead of .01.

↪ `Clear` the graph log and run a `Batch` with all of these new parameters.

Question 9.4 (a) *Report the average testing error* (`avg_tst_se`) *for the batch run, and the number of epochs it takes the network to reach its maximum error on the AB list after the introduction of the AC list.* **(b)** *Informal testing has shown that this is basically the best performance that can be obtained in this network — is it now a good model of human performance?*

Although the final level of interference on the AB list remains relatively high, you should have observed that these manipulations have significantly slowed the onset of this interference. Thus, we have some indication that these manipulations are having an effect in the right direction, providing some support for the principle of using sparse, non-overlapping representations to avoid interference.

One important dimension that we have not yet emphasized is the speed with which the network learns — it is clearly not learning as fast (in terms of number of exposures to the list items) as human subjects do. Further, the manipulations we have made to improve interference performance have resulted in even longer training times (you can see this if you don't clear the log

between runs with default and these new parameters). Thus, we could play with the `lrate` parameter to see if we can speed up learning in the network.

↪ Keeping the same "optimal" parameters, set the lrate to .1, and do a `Batch`.

Although the increase in learning rate successfully speeded up the learning process, repeated testing of this faster versus slower learning rates shows that the faster learning rate produces substantially more interference! This makes sense, because the larger learning rate produces larger weight changes that undo the AB list learning faster on the AC list. This should help you appreciate how impressive the fast, relatively interference-free human performance is.

We will see in the next section that achieving the level of separation necessary to learn rapidly requires a specialized neural architecture — our simple cortical model is just not up to the task.

↪ Go to the `PDP++Root` window. To continue on to the next simulation, close this project first by selecting `.projects/Remove/Project_0`. Or, if you wish to stop now, quit by selecting `Object/Quit`.

Summary and Discussion

We have seen that we can improve the rapid, arbitrary learning performance of a simple cortical network by moving away from distributed, overlapping representations toward sparser, separated representations. However, what we ended up with in the above exploration was really an awkward compromise network that was trying to learn sparse, separated representations, but was unable to achieve sufficient levels of pattern separation to really work effectively. Thus, this simple cortical architecture seems to work best with the slow, interleaved learning strategy that is so effective for most other forms of cortical learning.

Instead of trying to achieve all forms of learning within the cortical system, the brain appears to have developed two specialized systems (McClelland et al., 1995). One system, the posterior cortex, uses slow interleaved learning, and produces the kinds of powerful overlapping distributed representations that we have discussed and explored throughout the text. The other system, the hippocampus, uses an extreme form of sparse, pattern separated representations to enable rapid sequential learning of arbitrary associations without suffering from the kinds of interference problems we just observed. This system is the topic of the next section.

9.3 The Hippocampal Memory System

The preceding explorations have set the stage for the hippocampal memory system by demonstrating the strengths and limitations of the cortical memory system. Thus, we can understand the function of the hippocampus and related structures in terms of a tradeoff discovered in the standard cortical model — learning new things rapidly requires that different, non-overlapping sets of units be used to minimize interference, which is contrary to the need for distributed, overlapping representations to efficiently represent the underlying structure of the environment. A considerable amount of data supports this distinction between the hippocampus and the cortex (McClelland et al., 1995; Squire, 1992). In this section, we will see how a model that incorporates many important biological properties of the hippocampus can perform rapid learning while suffering from significantly less interference than a distributed, cortical-like network. The model is based on the implementation developed by O'Reilly, Norman, and McClelland (1998) and O'Reilly and Rudy (in press).

9.3.1 Anatomy and Physiology of the Hippocampus

As described in chapter 7, the hippocampus sits on top of the cortical hierarchy, receiving a wide range of different types of information from various cortical areas (see e.g., Squire et al., 1989 and figure 9.6). Thus, the hippocampus receives inputs that represent essentially the entire cortical state at one time (e.g., the cortical representation of the current state of the environment). To serve its role as a memory system, the hippocampus must then encode this input pattern so that some fraction of the original pattern can be used to retrieve the original whole. Critically, this retrieval, which occurs initially in the hippocampus, can spread back out to the cortex, resulting in the reinstatement of the original cortical representation.

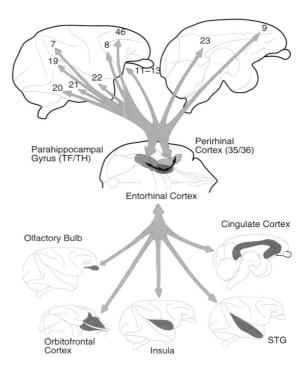

Figure 9.6: Bidirectional connectivity between the hippocampus, specifically the entorhinal cortex (EC), and a wide range of other cortical areas. Adapted from Squire et al. (1989).

Figure 9.7 shows a drawing of the anatomical structure of the hippocampus, and figure 9.8 shows a simplified schematic of the principal areas and patterns of connectivity, including the **dentate gyrus (DG)**, the fields of Ammon's Horn including the **CA3**, and **CA1**, as well as the **entorhinal cortex (EC)**, which serves as the primary cortical input/output pathway for the hippocampus. The **subiculum** is another input/output area, that likely plays a similar role to the EC, perhaps with a greater emphasis on subcortical and motor representations.

Anatomically, each area in the hippocampus has the same basic excitatory and inhibitory structure as described for the cortex in chapter 3, with the exception of the feedback projections — the hippocampal connectivity is mostly just feedforward. The ability of the

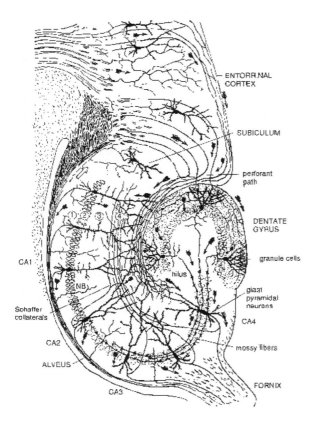

Figure 9.7: Anatomical structure of the hippocampal formation. Reproduced from Shepherd (1990).

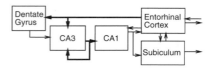

Figure 9.8: Schematic diagram of the principal areas and patterns of connectivity of the hippocampal formation.

	Rat		Model	
Area	Neurons	Pct Act	Units	Pct Act
EC	200,000	7.0	144	25.0
DG	1,000,000	0.5	625	1.0
CA3	160,000	2.5	240	5.0
CA1	250,000	2.5	384	9.4

Table 9.1: Rough estimates of the size of various hippocampal areas and their expected activity levels in the rat (data from Squire et al., 1989; Boss et al., 1987; Boss et al., 1985; Barnes et al., 1990). Also shown are corresponding values for the model.

inhibitory neurons to regulate activity levels in the hippocampal system plays an essential role in our model, as we will see. Also, the same kinds of learning mechanisms are probably at work in the cortex and hippocampus (indeed, the hippocampus is where most of the research on synaptic modification has been done).

The rough sizes and activity levels of the hippocampal layers in the rat are shown in table 9.1. Note that the DG seems to have an unusually sparse level of activity (and is also roughly 4–6 times larger than other layers), but CA3 and CA1 are also less active than the EC input/output layer.

A fair amount is known about the detailed patterns of connectivity within the hippocampal areas (e.g., Squire et al., 1989). Starting with the input, the EC has a

columnar structure, and there are topographic projections to and from the different cortical areas (Ikeda, Mori, Oka, & Watanabe, 1989; Suzuki, 1996). The *perforant path* projections from EC to DG and CA3 are broad and diffuse, but the projection between the DG and CA3, known as the mossy fiber pathway, is sparse, focused, and topographic. Each CA3 neuron receives only around 52–87 synapses from the mossy fiber projection in the rat, but each synapse is widely believed to be significantly stronger than the perforant path inputs to CA3.

The lateral (recurrent) projections within the CA3 project widely throughout the CA3, and a given CA3 neuron will receive from a large number of inputs sampled from the entire CA3 population. Similarly, the Schaffer collaterals, which go from the CA3 to the CA1, are diffuse and widespread, connecting a wide range of CA3 to CA1. Finally, the interconnectivity between the EC and CA1 is relatively point-to-point, not diffuse like the projections from EC to DG and CA3 (Tamamaki, 1991).

Physiological recordings of neural activity in the hippocampus reveal some very important properties of the representations in different hippocampal areas. For ex-

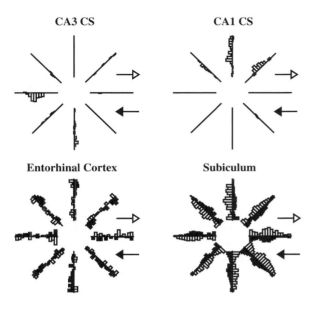

CA3 CS **CA1 CS**

Entorhinal Cortex **Subiculum**

Figure 9.9: Patterns of firing for neurons in the CA3, CA1, EC, and subiculum in an eight-arm radial maze, with the amount of firing shown according to the rat's location and direction of travel within the maze. The cortical-like neurons in the EC and subiculum have highly distributed activity patterns. In contrast, the CA3 and CA1 neurons are highly sparse and conjunctive, firing in only one or two specific locations.

ample, figure 9.9 shows the patterns of neural firing on an eight-arm radial maze, where the neurons in the CA3 fire only in a particular location on a particular arm in only one direction. This specificity can be explained if the CA3 neurons can only be activated by particular *conjunctions* of sensory features that are only present in specific locations. This and a wealth of similar data suggests that the CA3, and to a lesser extent the CA1, has sparse conjunctive representations, which will be very important for our model. In contrast, the input/output areas (EC and subiculum) have a much more distributed, overlapping character that is typical of the cortex.

9.3.2 Basic Properties of the Hippocampal Model

Our model is based on what McNaughton has termed the "Hebb-Marr" model of hippocampal function

(Hebb, 1949; Marr, 1969, 1970, 1971; McNaughton & Morris, 1987; McNaughton & Nadel, 1990). This model provides a framework for associating functional properties of memory with the biological properties of the hippocampus. Under this model, the two basic computational structures in the hippocampus are the feedforward pathway from the EC to area CA3 (via DG), which is important for establishing the encoding of new memories, and the recurrent connectivity within CA3, which is primarily important for recalling previously stored memories.

In light of the position of the hippocampus on top of the cortical hierarchy (figure 9.6), our overall conception of the role of the hippocampus in memory is one of **binding** together disparate cortical representations as belonging together in a particular memory. The detailed "content" of the memory resides out in the cortex, and the hippocampus is simply the binder, grouping together subsets of cortical representations. Thus, the hippocampus does not store *semantic* information, which is instead represented by the dense interconnectivity and overlapping distributed representations of the cortex (though it can bind together pieces of semantic information as isolated "facts" — e.g., "there is a 30% chance of rain today").

Hippocampal memories can be characterized as **episodic** — the memory associated with a particular episode (Tulving, 1972). For example, hippocampal memories would encode the episode when you heard the weather report for today. This tendency to represent specific episodes in the hippocampus makes sense if we think that its representations are separated out so that most every "slice" of time gets stored in its own separate representation. Of course, this is an extreme view, and it is likely that hippocampal representations can combine multiple episodes of experience. We also do not imagine that the hippocampus has a complete record of all prior "slices" of experience, because these representations will fade into oblivion if not reinstated and reinforced periodically.

Because the hippocampus and cortex are so highly interdependent, many interesting phenomena can be explained in terms of their interactions. For example, associations between cortical representations initially encoded in the hippocampus can be gradually incorporated into the aggregation learned by the cortex itself, through the standard slow learning process. This phenomenon is known as **consolidation**, and it can explain some interesting properties of memory loss (amnesia) that occurs when the hippocampus is damaged.

Consider the phenomenon of **retrograde amnesia**, where the most recent memories up to the point of the hippocampal damage are lost, while memories from the more distant past are preserved. This goes against the usual time course of forgetting, where memories get worse as more time passes. Retrograde amnesia can be explained if these distant memories were consolidated into the intact cortical system, whereas more recent memories remained dependent on the now-damaged hippocampus. For a more detailed treatment of this set of ideas and issues, see McClelland et al. (1995). We will cover other examples of hippocampal-cortical memory interactions in section 9.7.

In what follows, we describe the critical functional properties of the hippocampal system in terms of two competing mechanisms: **pattern separation** and **pattern completion**. Pattern separation leads to the formation of different, relatively non-overlapping representations in the hippocampus. As discussed previously, when different subsets of units are used to encode different memories, there is no interference because different sets of weights are involved. Pattern completion enables *partial cues* to trigger the activation of a complete, previously encoded memory. Thus, pattern separation operates during the *encoding* of new memories, and pattern completion operates during the *retrieval* of existing memories.

Encoding and Retrieval

We can summarize the basic operations of the model by explaining how the encoding and retrieval of memories works in terms of the areas and projections of the hippocampus. The general scheme for encoding is that activation comes into the EC from the cortex, and then flows to the DG and CA3, forming a pattern separated representation across a sparse, distributed set of units that are then bound together by rapid Hebbian learning within the recurrent collaterals (also, learning in the feedforward pathway helps to encode the representa-

tion). Simultaneously, activation flows from the EC to the CA1, forming a somewhat pattern separated but also *invertible* representation there — that is, the CA1 representation can be inverted to reinstate the corresponding pattern of activity over the EC that originally gave rise to the CA1 pattern in the first place (McClelland & Goddard, 1996). An association between the CA3 and CA1 representations is encoded by learning in the connections between them.

Having encoded the information in this way, retrieval from a partial input cue can occur as follows. Again, the EC representation of the partial cue (based on inputs from the cortex) goes up to the DG and CA3. Now, the prior learning in the feedforward pathway and the recurrent CA3 connections leads to the ability to complete this partial input cue and recover the original CA3 representation. Pattern completion in the CA3 works much like the exploration from chapter 3. This completed CA3 representation then activates the corresponding CA1 representation, which, because it is invertible, is capable of recreating the complete original EC representation.

If, on the other hand, the EC input pattern is novel, then the weights will not have been facilitated for this particular activity pattern, and the CA1 will not be strongly driven by the CA3. Even if the EC activity pattern corresponds to two components that were previously studied, but not together, the conjunctive nature of the CA3 representations will prevent recall (O'Reilly et al., 1998).

Pattern Separation

The main mechanism that the hippocampus uses to achieve pattern separation is to make the representations *sparser* (having fewer units active). This is the principle we tried to exploit in our "cortical" model of AB–AC list learning in section 9.2.2, with relatively small effects (but in the right direction) — as we summarized previously, the hippocampus employs sparseness on a fairly dramatic scale in the DG, CA3 and CA1 areas, which consequently has much larger effects.

To understand why sparse representations lead to pattern separation, first imagine a situation where the hippocampal representation is generated at random with

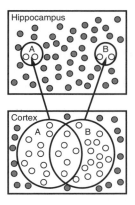

Figure 9.10: Illustration of pattern separation in the hippocampus. Small gray circles represent units. Circles A and B in the cortex and hippocampus indicate two sets of representations composed of patterns of active units. In the cortex, they are overlapping, and encompass relatively large proportions of active units. In the hippocampus, the representations are sparser as indicated by their smaller size, and thus overlap less (more pattern separation). Units in the hippocampus are conjunctive and are activated only by specific combinations of activity in the cortex.

some fixed probability of a unit getting active. In this case, if you have fewer units active, the odds that the same units will be active in two different patterns will go down (figure 9.10). For example, if the probability of getting active for one pattern (i.e., the sparseness) is .25, then the probability of getting active for both patterns would be $.25^2$ or .0625. If the patterns are made more sparse so that the probability is now .05 for being active in one pattern, the probability of being active in both patterns falls to .0025. Thus, the pattern overlap is reduced by a factor of 25 by reducing the sparseness by a factor of 5 in this case. However, this analysis assumes that units are activated at random, ignoring the fact that they are actually driven by weighted connections with the input patterns.

A more complete understanding of pattern separation can be achieved by considering the concept of a unit's *activation threshold* — how much excitation it requires to overcome the inhibitory competition from other units (Marr, 1969; O'Reilly & McClelland, 1994). To produce sparse representations, this threshold must be rel-

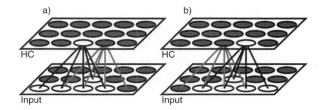

Figure 9.11: Conjunctive, pattern-separated representations result from sparseness. The extreme case where only one receiving unit (in the upper layer, representing the hippocampus) is allowed to be active is shown here for simplicity. Each receiving unit has roughly the same number of randomly distributed connections from the input units. The two shown here have overlapping input connections, except for one unique unit each. Thus, two very similar input patterns sharing all the overlapping units and differing only in these unique units (shown in panels a and b) will get completely non-overlapping (separated) memory representations. Thus, the conjunctive memory representation resulting from sparseness produces pattern separation.

atively high (e.g., because the level of inhibition is relatively strong for a given amount of excitatory input). Figure 9.11 shows how a high inhibitory threshold leads simultaneously to both pattern separation and **conjunctive representations**, which are representations that depend critically on the entire conjunction of active units in the input. The central idea is that sensitivity to the conjunction of activity in the input produced by a high threshold leads to pattern separation because even if two input patterns share a relatively large number of overlapping inputs, the overall *conjunction* (configuration) of input activity can be different enough to activate different hippocampal units.

A high threshold leads to conjunctive representations because only those units having the closest alignment of their weight patterns with the current input activity pattern will receive enough excitation to become activated. In other words, the activation a unit receives must be a relatively high proportion of the total number of input units that are active, meaning that it is the specific combination or conjunction of these inputs that are responsible for driving the units. Figure 9.11 illustrates this effect in the extreme case where only the most excited receiving unit gets active. In reality, multiple (roughly

1–5%) units are activated in the hippocampus at any given time (table 9.1), but the same principle applies.

For pattern separation to work optimally, it is important that different receiving units are maximally activated by different input patterns. This can be achieved by having a high level of variance in the weights and/or patterns of partial connectivity with the inputs. We implemented this idea in the simple AB–AC list learning model by increasing the variance of the random initial weights, which reduced interference somewhat. In the hippocampus, the perforant pathway has diffuse, random connectivity, which ensures that individual DG and CA3 neurons are maximally excited by different input patterns, facilitating pattern separation in these areas.

Pattern Completion

Pattern completion is as important as pattern separation for understanding hippocampal function. If only pattern separation were at work, then any time you wanted to retrieve previously stored information using anything other than exactly the same original input activation pattern, the hippocampus would instead store a new pattern separated version of the input instead of recognizing it as a retrieval cue for an existing memory. Thus, to actually use the memories stored in the hippocampus, the countervailing mechanism of pattern completion is needed.

There is a fundamental tension between pattern separation and pattern completion. Consider the following event: a good friend starts telling you a story about something that happened to her in college. You may or may not have heard this story before, but you have heard several stories about this friend's college days. How does your hippocampus know whether to store this information as a new memory and keep it separate (using pattern separation) from the other memories, or to instead complete this information to an existing memory and reply "you told me this story before?" In one case, your hippocampus has to produce a completely new activity pattern, and in the other it has to produce a completely old one. If you have perfect memory and the stories are always presented exactly the same way each time, this problem has an obvious solution. However, imperfect memories and noisy inputs (friends) require

a judgment call. Thus, there is a basic tradeoff operating within the hippocampus itself between pattern separation and completion. Optimizing this tradeoff can actually be used to understand several features of the hippocampal biology (O'Reilly & McClelland, 1994).

Details of the Model

We now describe further details about the model that are generally based on the biology, but are also shaped by the necessity of having a reasonably simple working model. These details include the sizes and activity levels of the model layers, the structure of the EC input representations, and the implementation of the invertible CA1-EC mapping.

Figure 9.12 shows the structure of the model, and an example activation pattern. Table 9.1 shows that the model layers are roughly proportionately scaled based on the anatomy of the rat, but the activation levels are generally higher (less sparse) to obtain sufficient absolute numbers of active units for reasonable distributed representations given the small total number of units. The activity levels are implemented using the basic kWTA inhibition function. We use just CPCA Hebbian learning here because it is sufficient for simple information storage, but it is likely that the hippocampus can also take advantage of error-driven learning in more complex tasks (O'Reilly & Rudy, in press).

The EC input representations incorporate the topographic and columnar characteristics of the EC by having different cortical areas and/or sub-areas represented by different *slots*, which can be loosely thought of as representing different feature dimensions of the input (e.g., color, font, semantic features, etc.). Our EC has 36 slots with four units per slot; one unit per slot is active, with each unit representing a particular "feature value." There are two functionally distinct layers of the EC, one that receives input from cortical areas and projects into the hippocampus (superficial or EC_in), and another that receives projections from the CA1 and projects back out to the cortex (deep or EC_out). Although the representations in these layers are probably different in their details, we assume that they are functionally equivalent, and use the same representations across both for convenience.

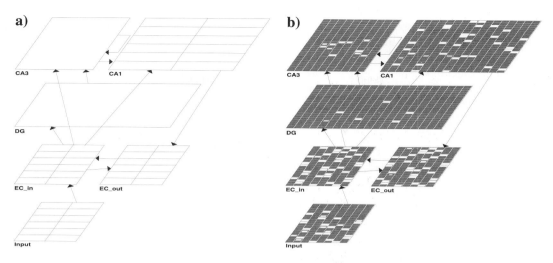

Figure 9.12: The hippocampus model. **a)** The areas and connectivity, and the corresponding columns within the Input, EC, and CA1. **b)** An example activity pattern. Note the sparse activity in the DG and CA3, and intermediate sparseness of the CA1.

We argued above that the CA1 translates the pattern-separated CA3 representations back into activation patterns on the EC during pattern completion using invertible representations. At the same time it must also achieve some amount of pattern separation to minimize interference in the learning of CA3-CA1 mappings. Indeed, this pattern separation in CA1 may explain why the hippocampus actually has a CA1, instead of just associating CA3 directly back with the EC input. These two functions of the CA1 are in conflict, because invertibility requires a systematic mapping between CA1 and EC, and pattern separation requires a highly nonlinear (nonsystematic) mapping. The model achieves a compromise by training the CA1-EC mapping to be invertible in pieces (referred to as *columns*), using pattern-separated CA1 representations. Thus, over the entire CA1, the representation can be composed more systematically and invertibly (without doing any additional learning) by using different combinations of representations within the different columns, but within each column, it is conjunctive and pattern separated (McClelland & Goddard, 1996).

In the model, the CA1 columns have 32 units each, so that the entire CA1 is composed of 12 such columns. Each column receives input from 3 adjacent EC slots (i.e., 12 EC units), which is consistent with the relatively point-to-point connectivity between these areas. The weights for each CA1 column were trained by taking one such column with 9.4 percent activity level and training it to reproduce any combination of patterns over 3 `EC_in` slots (64 different combinations) in a corresponding set of 3 `EC_out` slots. Thus, each CA1 has a conjunctive, pattern separated representation of the patterns within the 3 EC slots. The cost of this scheme is that more CA1 units are required (32 vs 12 per column in the EC), which is nonetheless consistent with the relatively greater expansion in humans of the CA1 relative to other hippocampal areas as a function of cortical size (Seress, 1988). A further benefit is that only certain combinations of active CA1 units (within a column) correspond to valid EC patterns, allowing invalid combinations (e.g., due to interference) to be filtered out. In the real system, slow learning can develop these CA1 invertible mappings in all the columns separately over time.

9.3.3 Explorations of the Hippocampus

[Note: this model requires at least 64Mb of RAM to run.]

In this exploration of the hippocampus model, we will use the same basic AB–AC paired associates list learning paradigm as we used in the standard cortical network previously. The hippocampus should be able to learn the new paired associates (AC) without causing undue levels of interference to the original AB associations, and it should be able to do this much more rapidly than was possible in the cortical model.

↪ Open project `hip.proj.gz` in `chapter_9` to begin.

You should recognize the network structure as that shown in figure 9.12. As with other large models, this one is stored as a skeleton that needs to be built.

↪ Press the `BuildNet` button on the overall control panel. Also, open up a log to monitor training by doing `View, TRAIN_TRIAL_LOG`.

First, we will observe the process of activation spreading through the network during training.

↪ Do `StepTrain` in the control panel.

You will see an input pattern from the AB training set presented to the network. This input pattern is composed of three parts, the first two representing the two associate items, and the third representing the list source/context information. As before, the list context is slightly different for each item.

During training, all three parts of the input pattern are presented. For testing, the second associate is omitted, requiring pattern completion in the hippocampus to fill it in based on the partial cue of the A stimulus and the context. You will see that activation flows from the `EC_in` layer through the DG, CA3 pathway and simultaneously to the CA1, so that the sparse CA3 representation can be associated with the invertible CA1 representation, which will give back this very `EC_in` pattern if later recalled by the CA3.

At the end of settling, you should notice that all of the active units in the network are selected (i.e., outlined with a white, dotted line). They will remain selected during the settling on the next pattern, allowing you to easily compare the representations for subsequent events.

↪ `StepTrain` through several more (but fewer than 10) events, and observe the relative amount of pattern overlap between subsequent events on the `EC_in`, DG, CA3, and CA1 layers.

You should have observed that the `EC_in` patterns overlap the most, with CA1 overlapping the next most, then CA3, and finally DG overlaps the least (on some monitors it can be somewhat difficult to make out the selected units and thus the overlap).

Question 9.5 *Using the explanation given earlier about the pattern separation mechanism, and the relative levels of activity on these different layers, explain the overlap results.*

Each epoch of training consists of the 10 list items, followed by testing on 3 sets of testing events. The first testing set contains the AB list items, the second contains the AC list items, and the third contains a set of novel *lure* items to make sure the network is treating novel items as such. The network automatically switches over to testing after each pass through the 10 training events. Before we get to this testing, we need to open some logs.

↪ Do `View, TEST_LOGS`, which will bring up two logs — a text log and a graph log.

↪ Set `train_updt` in the control panel to `NO_UPDT` (and `Apply`). Then, do `Run` on the train process and monitor the training text log until the 10th event has been presented (`trial` number 9).

At this point the network display should again start updating with the first test event. We will wait until the network has been trained for 2 more epochs before we do a detailed examination of testing, but you can observe some of the testing process at this point. You will notice that the input pattern presented to the network is missing the middle portion, which corresponds to the second associate (B or C), and that as the activation proceeds through the network, it is sometimes capable of filling in this missing part in the EC layers (pattern completion) as a result of activation flowing up through the CA3, and back via the CA1 to the `EC_out`.

↪ After watching this for a bit, set `test_updt` to `NO_UPDT` (`Apply`) and let the network continue processing until it stops after 3 epochs of training and testing.

Now, we will go through the testing process in detail by stepping one event at a time.

↪ First, set `test_updt` to `CYCLE_UPDT` to see activation propagation in the network on a cycle-by-

epc_ctr	trial	Event	stm_err_on	stm_err_off	rmbr
0	0	i0_i0_c0i0_	0.0555556	0.0833333	1
0	1	i1_i1_c0i1_	0.416667	0.555556	0
0	2	i2_i2_c0i2_	0.166667	0.555556	0
0	3	i3_i3_c0i3_	0.111111	0.194444	1
0	4	i4_i4_c0i4_	0.0277778	0.0833333	1
0	5	i5_i5_c0i5_	0.0833333	0.166667	1
0	6	i6_i6_c0i6_	0.0833333	0.222222	1
0	7	i7_i7_c0i7_	0.0833333	0.138889	1
0	8	i8_i8_c0i8_	0.277778	0.555556	0
0	9	i9_i9_c0i9_	0.0833333	0.25	1
1	0	i0_i10_c1i0_	0	0	1
1	1	i1_i11_c1i1_	0.0555556	0.194444	1
1	2	i2_i12_c1i2_	0.0277778	0.0555556	1
1	3	i3_i13_c1i3_	0	0.0277778	1
1	4	i4_i14_c1i4_	0	0.0277778	1
1	5	i5_i15_c1i5_	0	0.25	1
1	6	i6_i16_c1i6_	0	0.194444	1
1	7	i7_i17_c1i7_	0	0.166667	1
1	8	i8_i18_c1i8_	0.111111	0.333333	1
1	9	i9_i19_c1i9_	0.0555556	0.0833333	1
2	0	i20_i20_c2i0_	0.388889	0.777778	0
2	1	i21_i21_c2i1_	0.472222	0.833333	0
2	2	i22_i22_c2i2_	0.166667	0.916667	0
2	3	i23_i23_c2i3_	0.444444	0.611111	0
2	4	i24_i24_c2i4_	0.361111	0.777778	0
2	5	i25_i25_c2i5_	0.416667	0.666667	0
2	6	i26_i26_c2i6_	0.555556	0.722222	0
2	7	i27_i27_c2i7_	0.666667	0.805556	0
2	8	i28_i28_c2i8_	0.166667	0.916667	0
2	9	i29_i29_c2i9_	0.527778	0.611111	0

Figure 9.13: Text log display for testing the hippocampal network. Shows results after training on both AB and AC lists, with 70 percent remember responses for the AB list and 100 percent for the AC list.

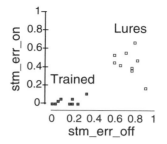

Figure 9.14: Composite graph log display for testing the hippocampal network, showing two kinds of errors — units that should be off but were erroneously on (stm_err_on), and units that should be on but were erroneously off (stm_err_off). The training items have relatively few of both types of errors, and the lure items are mostly inactive (high stm_err_off.

cycle basis. Then, let's `Clear` the testing text log (`Trial_1_TextLog`). Then, do `StepTest`.

You will see the first testing event in the EC_in layer, which corresponds to a studied A stimulus, an empty gap where the B stimulus would be, and a list context representation for the AB list. Since this was studied, it is likely that the network will be able to complete the pattern, which you should be able to see visually as the gap in the EC activation pattern gets filled in.

When the network has stopped settling on this pattern, you can compare the activity pattern produced over EC_out with the original stored activity pattern.

↪ To do so, press the `targ` button in the network window.

You should see that there is a target pattern (which is only used for our comparison purposes) for this layer, and because the active units are selected, you can relatively easily compare these two (alternatively, you can compare by switching back and forth between `act` and `targ`).

Now, look at the first line of the testing text log (figure 9.13). The two critical columns here are

stim_err_on and stim_err_off. The first shows the proportion of units that were erroneously activated in EC_out (i.e., active but not present in the `targ` pattern), and the second shows the proportion of units that were erroneously *not* activated in EC_out (i.e., not active but present in the `targ` pattern). When both of these measures are near zero, then the network has correctly recalled the original pattern. A large stim_err_on indicates that the network has *confabulated* or otherwise recalled a different pattern than the cued one. This is relatively rare in the model (O'Reilly et al., 1998). A large stim_err_off indicates that the network has failed to recall much of the probe pattern. This is common, especially for the novel lure items in the last testing set (as we will see).

Now, look at the graph log just to the right of this testing text log (`Trial_1_GraphLog`, figure 9.14). This shows the stim_err_on plotted on the Y axis against stim_err_off on the X axis, with each event showing up as a dot at a particular location. To the extent that these dots are in the lower left hand corner, the network is recalling accurately. This log is automatically cleared before each new testing set, so you can be sure all the dots are for one particular testing environment. To code discrete responses from the network, we need to set thresholds for these statistics. The following thresholds were somewhat arbitrarily chosen to provide reasonable performance: if `stim_err_on` is less than .2, and `stim_err_off` is less than .4, then we say that the hippocampus has remembered the item. This is shown in the `rmbr` column in the text log, with a 1 for successful remembering. Ignore the other columns at this point, because they are not relevant to this simulation.

↪ Continue to `StepTest` for a few more patterns.

Make sure you understand the relationship between the network's performance and the statistics in the logs.

↪ Then, turn `test_updt` back to `NO_UPDT` (or `TRIAL_UPDT` if you want to see the end state of recall for each event), and continue to step until all 10 studied items have been tested. Then, `StepTest` again.

You will see that the `epc_ctr` field in the testing text log increments from 0 to 1. Now we are presenting the very same "A" stimulus, but with the list context for the second (AC) pairing of items (which has yet to be trained). Thus, we expect that the network will not successfully recall these items, because it has not learned of them yet.

↪ `StepTest` for the next 10 items, the AC list.

The network should not `rmbr` any of them, but you might notice that the `stim_err_off` values are somewhat smaller than you might expect for items that the network has not been trained on, which is caused by the similarity of these probes to the studied items (they overlap 50%). The next set of testing events is a completely novel set of lure items (i.e., "DE"), to which the network should give high `stim_err_off` values indicating lack of prior exposure to any aspect of these items.

↪ `StepTest` for the next 10 items, the Lure list.

Question 9.6 *Report the total number of* `rmbr` *responses from your testing text log for the first, second, and third testing environments* (`Test_AB`, `Test_AC`, *and* `Lure`, *respectively*).

Now, having trained on the AB associates, and tested the resulting performance, we will train the network for two epochs on the AC associates, and then examine the testing log as the network is automatically tested after this training epoch, looking for signs of interference.

↪ Set the `train_epcs` field to 5 instead of 3. Then, set `train_env` to `TRAIN_AC` instead of `TRAIN_AB`.

Then `Run` the process. Monitor the training and testing text logs as the network is trained and tested.

Question 9.7 (a) *Again report the total number of* `rmbr` *responses from your testing text log for the first, second, and third testing environments* (`Test_AB`, `Test_AC`, *and* `Lure`, *respectively*) *after each epoch of training on AC.* **(b)** *Do you find evidence of any interference from learning AC on the testing results for AB?* **(c)** *Compare and contrast the performance of this hippocampus model with that of the cortical model and the human data of this same basic task from section 9.2.2, paying particular attention to both interference and number of epochs necessary to learn.*

↪ Go to the `PDP++Root` window. To continue on to the next simulation, close this project first by selecting `.projects/Remove/Project_0`. Or, if you wish to stop now, quit by selecting `Object/Quit`.

9.3.4 Summary and Discussion

We have seen that the pattern separation capabilities of the hippocampal formation as captured in our model enable it to rapidly and sequentially learn arbitrary information (e.g., the AB–AC paired associate lists) without suffering from massive levels of interference. This unique ability suggests that the hippocampal system plays a complementary role to the slow-learning cortical system that forms richly overlapping distributed representations based on task and model learning principles. Importantly, although this story is supported and motivated by relevant behavioral and neuroscience data, it is founded on basic computational principles.

For example, we can understand interference in terms of the shared use of units and weights for different associations, which makes it clear that pattern separation is critical for avoiding interference. However, pattern separation is incompatible with the pattern overlap in distributed representations that is useful for generalization, similarity-based reasoning, and efficient encoding of high-dimensional, complex environments. This tradeoff between sparse, pattern-separated representations and overlapping distributed representations, in addition to the constraint that cortical learning requires slow, interleaved learning, motivates the idea that there are two specialized memory systems, instead of one system that tries to achieve a compromise.

Going down a level of detail, the notion of pattern separation fits quite well with the detailed biological properties of the hippocampal formation, providing further support for the idea that this structure is specialized for the pattern separation function. In short, there is considerable synergy here between computational principles and behavioral and neuroscience data.

Although we find the present model of hippocampal function compelling, there is considerable controversy in the literature regarding the best way to characterize the functional role of the hippocampus. For example, a number of researchers support the notion originally developed by O'Keefe and Nadel (1978) that the hippocampus implements a spatial map, and is used primarily for spatial navigation. One stimulus for this model was the discovery that hippocampal neurons in the rat seem to encode specific spatial locations (e.g., figure 9.9). We have seen that this kind of specific, conjunctive firing can be explained in terms of the more general function of forming sparse, pattern separated representations. Furthermore, there is little evidence that there is any kind of topography to the hippocampal representations, calling into question its role as a map. Instead, it might be better viewed as producing episodic memories of spatial locations (i.e., binding together all the features present in a given location), without necessarily encoding much about the spatial relationships among different locations (e.g., McNaughton & Nadel, 1990).

Another body of literature dealing with the function of the hippocampus comes from animal learning paradigms such as conditioning and discrimination learning. Sutherland and Rudy (1989) proposed that the hippocampus is necessary to learn nonlinear problems that require a configuration or conjunction of stimuli to be formed (we explored this kind of problem using the "impossible" task in chapter 5). For example, in the *negative patterning* problem, rats have to learn that stimulus A leads to reward ($A+$), as does stimulus B ($B+$), but that both A and B together do not ($AB-$) (this is the same as the XOR task studied by Minsky & Papert, 1969; Rumelhart et al., 1986a). Rats without a hippocampus are impaired on learning this prob-

lem, suggesting that the hippocampus might be useful in learning that the conjunction of A and B is different than the two stimuli individually. This view is consistent with the idea suggested above that the sparse, pattern separated representations in the hippocampus are also *conjunctive*, in that they bind together different stimulus elements.

Subsequent experimentation with cleaner hippocampal lesions has shown that the hippocampus is not always (or even usually) necessary to learn nonlinear problems (Rudy & Sutherland, 1995). These findings are consistent with the idea that the cortex can learn complex tasks through error-driven learning (as explored in chapter 5), but that this learning must be slow — even intact rats take many iterations to learn complex nonlinear problems, as would be expected of cortical learning. The balance between pattern separation and pattern completion is also relevant here, because it is likely that an intact hippocampus will be doing task-inappropriate pattern completion in these complex nonlinear tasks, with many epochs of error-driven learning necessary to achieve the appropriate hippocampal representations. O'Reilly and Rudy (in press) contains an implemented model (based on the hippocampal model we just explored) and fuller discussion of these phenomena.

The hippocampus has been a popular target of computational modeling, and there are a large number of other models in the literature, many of which share basic ideas in common with our model (e.g., Treves & Rolls, 1994; Hasselmo & Wyble, 1997; Moll & Miikkulainen, 1997; Alvarez & Squire, 1994; Levy, 1989; Burgess, Recce, & O'Keefe, 1994; Samsonovich & McNaughton, 1997), but some that make very different claims about the role of the hippocampus in learning. For example, two models (Schmajuk & DiCarlo, 1992; Gluck & Myers, 1993) claim that only the hippocampus is capable of performing error-driven learning, and is used to "teach" the cortex. Such models are inconsistent with recent data showing that children with very early hippocampal lesions nevertheless acquire semantic information normally, while still suffering from significant episodic (i.e., hippocampal) memory deficits (Vargha-Khadem et al., 1997).

Some of the computational models of the hippocampal anatomy and physiology have provided quantitative estimates of potential storage capacity of the hippocampal system (e.g., Treves & Rolls, 1994; Moll & Miikkulainen, 1997). Other models have emphasized the role of neuromodulators in memory storage and retrieval (e.g., Hasselmo & Wyble, 1997). The issue of storage of sequential information (e.g., for sequential locations visited within an environment) has been addressed in several models (e.g., Levy, 1989; Burgess et al., 1994; Samsonovich & McNaughton, 1997). This rich computational literature has played a critical role in shaping ideas about hippocampal function ever since the early ideas of Marr (1971), and constitutes one of the great successes of computational modeling in cognitive neuroscience.

9.4 Activation-Based Memory in a Generic Model of Cortex

Having explored weight-based memories in the cortex and hippocampus, we now turn to activation-based memories. A good example of a simple form of activation-based memory can be found in the attentional model from chapter 8. In this model, residual activation from processing a cue stimulus affects subsequent processing of a target, leading to either faster processing (when the cue and target are in the same location) or slower processing (when they are in different locations). In this section we will explore how this kind of residual activation can result in an *activation based* or *short-term priming* effect, similar to the weight-based one but lasting only as long as these residual activations. This activation-based priming is a basic property of the simple cortical model, just like weight-based priming.

After exploring the priming effects of residual activation, we will challenge our basic cortical model with more demanding forms of active memory, where information must be maintained for relatively longer periods of time and also updated rapidly.

9.4.1 Short-Term Priming

As discussed in section 9.2.1, priming can be divided into the three dimensions of duration, content, and similarity. The distinction between weight-based and activation-based priming is one of duration, in that the activation state typically decays within a couple of seconds, whereas weight changes can last for long periods of time. As we saw in chapters 4–6, learning is based on activation values, so activation-based and weight-based priming are similar on the other dimensions (content and similarity). This has recently been supported in the case of semantic priming (Becker et al., 1997), which was previously thought to occur only in an activation-based form.

In the following exploration, we will use the same basic paradigm as the previous weight-based priming exploration. Thus, the network is trained to perform a one-to-many mapping as in a stem-completion or homophone-priming task. However, in this case, we will turn off any weight changes during the priming test and just observe the effects of residual activation on subsequent network performance. Note that in reality one cannot just turn off learning in this way, so the mechanistic basis of a given priming effect (i.e., weights or activations) is not as clear as it is in our models. Thus, behavioral experimentalists must resort to other techniques of telling the two apart. One way to do this is to pit the two types of priming against each other, so that prior, but not immediately preceding, experience builds up the weights to favor one response, but immediate experience favors another. We will explore this idea in greater detail in the context of the $A\overline{B}$ phenomenon in section 9.6.

Exploring the Model

↪   Open the project `act_priming.proj.gz` in `chapter_9` to begin.

This is essentially just the same simulation as the weight priming one, so we will assume you are already familiar with the network and environment. We begin by loading a pre-trained network, and opening up the test logs.

↪   Do `LoadNet` in the control panel, followed by `View`, `TEST_LOGS`.

Let's test this network (using a somewhat different setup than last time) to obtain a baseline measure of performance.

trial	Event	sum_se	Outp_dist	ev_nm	sm_nm	both_err
0	0_a	0	0	0_a	0	0
1	0_b	1.7529	1.7529	0_b	0	0
2	1_a	0	0	1_a	0	0
3	1_b	2.18947	2.06997	1_a	1	0
4	2_a	0	0	2_a	0	0
5	2_b	5.43822	0.467382	2_a	1	0
6	3_a	0	0	3_a	0	0
7	3_b	1.05335	1.05335	3_b	0	0
8	4_a	0	0	4_a	0	0
9	4_b	6.26163	0.663053	4_a	1	0
10	5_a	0	0	5_a	0	0
11	5_b	4.02698	2.36882	5_a	1	0
12	6_a	0	0	6_a	0	0
13	6_b	5.74102	2.00435	6_a	1	0
14	7_a	0	0	7_a	0	0
15	7_b	8.85609	0	7_a	1	0
16	8_a	0	0	8_a	0	0
17	8_b	9.4205	0.444151	8_a	1	0
18	9_a	0	0	9_a	0	0
19	9_b	7.888	1.64196	9_a	1	0
20	10_a	0	0	10_a	0	0
21	10_b	5.20613	0.337607	10_a	1	0
22	11_a	0	0	11_a	0	0
23	11_b	6.4702	1.40431	11_a	1	0
24	12_a	0	0	12_a	0	0
25	12_b	5.32969	0.33391	12_a	1	0

Figure 9.15: Text log output showing activation-based priming effects — the network responds with the a outputs (shown in the ev_nm column) to the b inputs (shown in the Event column), as a result of the immediately prior input.

↪ Press Test in the control panel.

This test has the "a" and "b" responses to a given input being presented one after another, which allows us to determine the immediate impact of seeing the "a" case on the response to "b." When the "a" case is presented, we clamp the output response pattern to the "a" value. When the "b" case is then presented, only the input pattern is presented, so the "b" output response just serves as a comparison pattern for the actual output produced by the network given the input. You should observe that the network produces the "a" response for the "b" trials about half the time. However, this is not an indication of priming, because we are completely resetting the activations after each event is presented! Thus, this roughly 50 percent "a" response reflects the random biases of the trained network.

The act_decay parameter in the act_prime_ctrl overall control panel controls the extent to which the activations are decayed (reset) after each event is processed. Let's observe the effects of keeping the activations completely intact from one trial to the next.

↪ Change the act_decay parameter to 0 instead of 1. Press Apply and Test again.

You should notice an increased tendency for the network to respond with "a" in the "b" trials (figure 9.15).

Question 9.8 (a) *Report the number of times the network responded "a" instead of "b" for the "b" test trials.* (b) *Explain why* act_decay *has this effect on performance.*

In summary, this simulation replicates our earlier weight-based priming results using residual activations instead of weight changes, and illustrates a simple form of activation-based memory that our model of the cortex naturally exhibits.

↪ Go to the PDP++Root window. To continue on to the next simulation, close this project first by selecting .projects/Remove/Project_0. Or, if you wish to stop now, quit by selecting Object/Quit.

9.4.2 Active Maintenance

In addition to simple priming, it would be useful to have a form of activation-based memory that persists for longer periods of time, and that can maintain information even in the face of noise or interference from activity elsewhere in the network. This kind of memory would be useful for things like holding on to information that is needed for ongoing processing, as in the case of mental arithmetic as mentioned previously (e.g., computing $42 * 7$). In this task, one needs to keep track of intermediate results and also where one is in the sequence of steps necessary to solve the problem. Maintaining this information in an active form (i.e., **active maintenance**) is useful because it needs to be *rapidly updated* (i.e., as you move on to subsequent steps), and it also needs to be *readily accessible* to ongoing processing — having active representations of the relevant information achieves these goals in a way that more passive weight-based memories cannot. This kind of activation-based memory is typically referred to as **working memory** (Baddeley, 1986).

The most obvious neural network mechanism for achieving active maintenance is recurrent bidirectional excitatory connectivity, where activation constantly circulates among active units, refreshing and maintaining

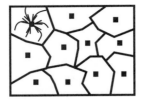

Figure 9.16: Attractor states (small squares) and their basins of attraction (surrounding regions), where nearby activation states are attracted to the central attractor state. Each stable attractor state could be used to actively maintain information over time. Note that the two-dimensional activation space represented here is a considerable simplification of the high-dimensional activation state over all the units in the network.

their activation (Braver, Cohen, & Servan-Schreiber, 1995; Dehaene & Changeux, 1989; Zipser, Kehoe, Littlewort, & Fuster, 1993). One can think of the effects of these recurrent connections in terms of an *attractor*, where the activation pattern of the network is attracted toward a stable state that persists over time as discussed in chapter 3 (figure 9.16). An attractor is useful for memory because any perturbation away from that activation state is pulled back into the attractor, allowing in principle for relatively robust active maintenance in the face of noise and interference from ongoing processing.

The area around the attractor where perturbations are pulled back is called the *basin of attraction*. For robust active maintenance, one needs to have attractors with wide basins of attraction, so that noise and other sources of interference will not pull the network out of its attractor. When there are many closely related representations linked by distributed connections, the basin of attraction around each representation is relatively narrow (i.e., the network can easily slip from one representation into the next). Thus, densely interconnected distributed representations will tend to conflict with the ability to maintain a specific representation actively over time.

It is important to understand why active maintenance specifically demands wide attractor basins where on-line processing may not. During on-line processing (e.g., of sensory inputs), there is external input that can bias activation states in an appropriate way. In contrast, we assume that the actively maintained representation is solely responsible for the information it represents,

so that it cannot rely on external biasing inputs. Putting this somewhat more generally, one can afford to activate related information when the original information is externally available, but when required to accurately maintain the original information itself, one does not want to activate related information because of the risk of losing track of the original information.

For example, if one sees smoke, it is reasonable to activate the representation of fire as an *inference* based on a visible input, as long as this visible input is always present to constrain processing and clearly delineate perceptual truth from inference. However, if one has to actively maintain a representation of smoke in the absence of further sensory input, this kind of *spreading activation* of related representations can be problematic. In essence, one wants the active maintenance system to serve like an external input — it should veridically maintain information that is used to constrain processing elsewhere. Thus, one can either see or remember seeing smoke and use either the sensory input or the actively maintained smoke information to infer fire, but one should not then either hallucinate or falsely remember seeing fire (note that this problem gets much worse when the inferences are less certain than smoke $\rightarrow$ fire).

The distinction between inferential processing and active maintenance points to a tradeoff, in that one wants to have spreading activation across distributed connections for inference, but not for active maintenance. This is one reason why one might want to have a specialized system for active maintenance (i.e., the frontal cortex), while the generic (posterior) cortex is used for inference based on its accumulated semantic representations, as discussed further in section 9.5.

In what follows we explore the impact of connectivity and attractor dynamics on active maintenance by first examining a model where there are a set of features that can participate equally in different distributed representations. This model effectively has no attractors, and we will see that it cannot maintain information over time in the absence of external inputs — the activation instead spreads across the distributed representations, resulting in a loss of the original information. When we introduce distributed representations that sustain attractors, active maintenance succeeds, but not in the presence of significant amounts of noise — wider attractor

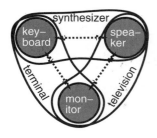

Figure 9.17: Three related items (television, terminal, synthesizer) represented in an overlapping, distributed fashion as two out of three common features.

basins are necessary. These wider basins are present in the final configuration we explore, where the units are completely *isolated* from each other. This completely prevents activation spread and yields very robust active maintenance (O'Reilly et al., 1999a), but at the loss of the ability to perform inference via activation spread.

To explore these ideas, we use the simple overlapping distributed representations of a *television*, *synthesizer*, and *terminal* in terms of the features of *keyboard*, *speaker*, and *monitor*, as shown in figure 9.17. This is the same example that we explored in chapter 3, in the context of a similar kind of problem with activation spread in distributed representations. Note that in this earlier case, the problem was solved by using inhibition. That will not help here because, unlike before, there will be no external inputs to favor the activation of the appropriate units.

Exploring the Model

↪ Open the project act_maint.proj.gz in chapter_9 to begin.

You will see that the network has three hidden units representing the three features (figure 9.18). The input units provide individual input to the corresponding hidden unit. In an active maintenance context, one needs to have the individual features of a distributed representation mutually support each other via excitatory connections.

↪ View r.wt in the network window and select the different hidden units to view their weights.

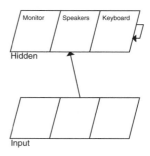

Figure 9.18: Network for exploring active maintenance.

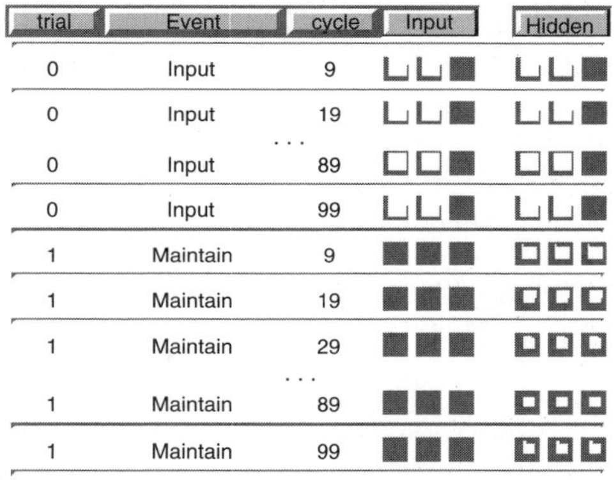

trial	Event	cycle	Input	Hidden
0	Input	9	⊔⊔■	⊔⊔■
0	Input	19	⊔⊔■	⊔⊔■
0	Input	89	☐☐■	☐☐■
0	Input	99	⊔⊔■	⊔⊔■
1	Maintain	9	■■■	☐☐☐
1	Maintain	19	■■■	☐☐☐
1	Maintain	29	■■■	☐☐☐
1	Maintain	89	■■■	☐☐☐
1	Maintain	99	■■■	☐☐☐

Figure 9.19: Grid log showing spreading activation and loss of maintained information with distributed interconnectivity among the hidden units.

You should see the bidirectional excitatory connections among the three hidden units, which in theory might enable them to actively maintain the representations even after the input pattern is turned off.

There are two "events" in the environment, one where an input pattern is presented to the network, and another where the input is zeroed out (not presented). We are interested in how well the information in the hidden units is maintained during this second event.

↪ Return to viewing act in the network, and then press the Run button.

You will see the network presented with inputs and the units respond, but it will probably be too quick to get a clear idea of what happened.

↪ Do View, GRID_LOG, and then Run again.

The grid log shows the activity of the input and hidden units during the first event (input is present) and the second event (input is removed). You should see that when the two features are active in the input, this activates the appropriate hidden units corresponding to the distributed representation of *television*. However, when the input is subsequently removed, the activation does not remain concentrated in the two features, but spreads to the other feature (figure 9.19). Thus, it is impossible to determine which item was originally present. This spread occurs because all the units are interconnected.

Perhaps the problem is that the weights are all exactly the same for all the connections, which is not likely to be true in the brain.

↪ Set the wt_mean parameter in the control panel to .5 (to make room for more variance) and then try a range of wt_var values (e.g., .1, .25, .4). Be sure to do multiple runs with each variance level.

Question 9.9 *Describe what happened as you increased the amount of variance. Were you able to achieve reliable maintenance of the input pattern?*

The activation spread in this network occurs because the units do not mutually reinforce a particular activation state (i.e., there is no attractor) — each unit participates in multiple distributed patterns, and thus supports each of these different patterns equally. Although distributed representations are defined by this property of units participating in multiple representations, this network represents an extreme case. To make attractors in this network, we can introduce *higher-order* representations within the distributed patterns of connectivity.

A higher-order representation in the environment we have been exploring would be something like a *television* unit that is interconnected with the *monitor* and *speakers* features. It is higher-order because it joins together these two lower-level features and indicates that they go together. Thus, when *monitor* and *speakers* are active, they will preferentially activate *television*, which will in turn preferentially activate these two feature units. This will form a mutually reinforcing attractor that should be capable of active maintenance.

↪ To test out this idea, set net_type to HIGHER_ORDER instead of DISTRIBUTED, and Apply. A new network window will appear.

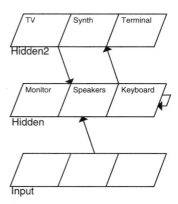

Figure 9.20: Network for exploring active maintenance, with higher-order units in Hidden2 that create mutually reinforcing attractors.

You can see that this network has an additional hidden layer with the three higher-order units corresponding to the different pairings of features (figure 9.20).

↪ First hit Defaults to restore the original weight parameters, and then do a Run with this network.

You should observe that indeed it is capable of maintaining the information without spread. Thus, to the extent that the network can develop distributed representations that have these kinds of higher-order constraints in them, one might be able to achieve active maintenance without spread. Indeed, given the multilayered nature of the cortex (see chapter 3), it is likely that distributed representations will have these kinds of higher-order constraints.

To this point, we have neglected a very important property of the brain — *noise*. All of the ongoing activity in the brain, together with the somewhat random timing of individual spikes of activation, produces a background of noise that we have not included in this simulation. Although we generally assume this noise to be present and have specifically introduced it when necessary, we have not included it in most simulations because it slows everything down and typically does not significantly change the basic behavior of the models. However, it is essential to take noise into account in the context of active maintenance because noise tends to accumulate over time and degrade the quality of maintained information — the active maintenance system must be capable of overcoming this degradation.

↪ To add noise (we just add it to the membrane potential on each time step), set the `noise_var` parameter on the control panel to .01. Do several `Run`s.

You should have observed that in the presence of noise, even the higher-order distributed representations cannot prevent the spread of activation. The explanation is relatively straightforward — the noise was sufficiently large to move the network outside of the original attractor basin and into that of another representation. This indicates that the higher-order distributed representations may not have sufficiently wide attractor basins for robust active maintenance.

A parameter that should play an important role in this network is the strength of the recurrent weights. For example, if these weights were made sufficiently weak, one would expect that the network would be incapable of active maintenance. At the other extreme, it might be the case that very strong recurrent weights would produce a more robust form of active maintenance that better resists noise. The strength of the recurrent weights is determined by the `wt_scale` parameter in the control panel, which has been set to 1.

↪ Set this now to .05 (and keep the noise set to .01), and do a couple of `Run`s.

You should observe that the network is now no longer capable of maintaining information once the input goes away.

↪ Now let's see if making the recurrent weights stronger improves the ability to overcome noise. Try `wt_scale` values of 2 and 5 with multiple `Run`s each.

Question 9.10 **(a)** *Does this seem to improve the network's ability to hold onto information over time?* **(b)** *Explain your results, keeping in mind that the recurrent weights interconnect all of the hidden units.*

Although some kinds of distributed representations could exhibit sufficiently robust active maintenance abilities, there is another type of representation that is guaranteed to produce very robust active maintenance. This type of representation uses *isolated* units that do not have distributed patterns of interconnectivity, and thus that have very wide basins of attraction. Because

there is no interconnectivity between units, it is impossible for activation to spread to other representations, resulting in perfect maintenance of information even in the presence of large amounts of noise. These isolated units can be self-maintaining by having an excitatory self-connection for each unit.

↪ To explore this kind of representation, set `net_type` to `ISOLATED` (`Apply`). You can verify the connectivity by using `r.wt`. Set the `wt_scale` back to 1, but keep the `noise_var` at .01, and then `Run` several times.

You should observe that the network is now able to maintain the information without any difficulty, even with the same amount of noise that proved so damaging to the previous network. However, this isolated network no longer has the ability to perform any of the useful computations that require knowledge of which features go together, because each unit is isolated from the others. Nevertheless, the posterior cortex can represent all of this relationship information via overlapping distributed representations, so it should be okay for a specialized active maintenance system to use more isolated representations, given their clear advantages in terms of robustness. We will explore this idea further in section 9.5.

9.4.3 Robust yet Rapidly Updatable Active Maintenance

In addition to the basic need for maintaining information over time (without the kind of activation spreading that we saw above), activation-based working memory representations also need to meet two potentially conflicting needs: they sometimes need to be maintained in the face of ongoing processing, while at other times they need to be updated as a function of current information. For example, when doing mental arithmetic, one needs to maintain some partial products while at the same time computing and updating others.

The following simple task, which is similar in many respects to the continuous performance tasks (CPT) often used to test working memory (Servan-Schreiber, Cohen, & Steingard, 1997; Rosvold, Mirsky, Sarason, Bransome, & Beck, 1956), provides a clear demonstration of working memory demands. Stimuli (e.g., letters) are presented sequentially over time on a computer display. If a particular *cue* stimulus is shown (e.g., an A), then the subject has to remember the *next* stimulus, and determine if it matches the one that comes two stimuli after that. After *every* stimulus presentation, a button must be pressed — one button if a match event has just occurred, and another button otherwise. Thus, whether one wants to encode a stimulus into active memory or not depends dynamically on preceding stimuli, and cannot be determined as a function of the specific stimulus itself. Further, once encoded, the stimulus must be maintained in the face of the two intervening stimuli.

Because of this need both to maintain robustly and update rapidly, the working memory system cannot adopt a consistent strategy for active maintenance — it cannot always make the active memories robust by making them insensitive to their inputs, because this would preclude updating. Similarly, if the active memories are easily updatable as a function of their inputs, they will not be robustly maintained in the face of irrelevant information on these inputs.

In this section we will see that the kind of simple active memory system that we have been exploring is missing the kind of dynamic switching between maintenance and updating that seems to be necessary. Thus, the need for this kind of dynamic regulation system provides one more reason to believe that there is a specialized neural system for supporting activation-based working memory. We will explore some ideas regarding the nature of this specialized system and its dynamic regulation in section 9.5.

Exploring the Model

↪ Continue to use project `act_maint.proj.gz` (or open it). Press the `Defaults` button to reset to default parameters if already open.

We are now going to explore an environment that starts out by presenting an input pattern and then removing that input (as before), and then a new input pattern will be presented and then removed. Under some circumstances, we can imagine that the network would want to update the active memory representations to reflect the second input, but in other circumstances, this input may be irrelevant and should be ignored. It should be clear at the outset that the same network with the

same parameters cannot achieve both of these objectives. Thus, we will explore how the parameters can be manipulated to alter the network's tendency to maintain or update.

↪ To select this new environment, set `env_type` on the overall `act_maint_ctrl` control panel to `MAINT_UPDT` instead of `MAINT`.

We also want to use the `ISOLATED` network as explored previously, because it provides the best active maintenance performance.

↪ Set `net_type` to `ISOLATED` (if it is not already).

To add realism and ensure that the basic maintenance task is not completely trivial, let's also add noise.

↪ Set the `noise_var` parameter to .01. View the `GRID_LOG` (if not already open), and then `Run` the network.

The first part is the same as before, but then the `Input2` input is presented, followed by the `Maint2` maintenance period. Note that the grid log will scroll, such that at the end of the run, only this last set of events is shown. You can use the VCR-style arrow buttons at the top of the log to scroll back and forth to view the entire sequence.

You should observe in this case that the network updates its internal representation upon the `Input2` input pattern presentation. If the task context at this point called for the active maintenance of this new input (e.g., in the CPT-like task described previously, `Input1` would be the cue stimulus in this case), then this would be desirable behavior. However, it is also possible that `Input2` could be a transient bit of information that should not be maintained (e.g, one of the two intervening stimuli in the CPT-like task). In this latter case, the network's behavior would be inappropriate.

The obvious parameter to manipulate to determine whether the network robustly maintains or rapidly updates is the relative strength of the recurrent self-maintenance connections compared to the input connections. The `wt_scale` parameter in the control panel lets us adjust this, by determining the relative strength of the recurrent self-maintenance connections.

↪ Try setting the `wt_scale` parameter to 2 instead of the default of 1, and `Run` a couple of times.

Question 9.11 (a) *Describe what happens when the* Input2 *pattern is presented.* **(b)** *Now try a* wt_scale *of 3 instead of 2. What happens with* Input2*?* **(c)** *Explain why changing* wt_scale *has the observed effects.*

You should have observed that by changing the relative strength of the recurrent weights compared to the input weights, you can alter the network's behavior from rapid updating to robust maintenance. This suggests that if the relative strength of these connections could be dynamically controlled (e.g., by a specialized controller network as a function of prior input stimuli), then an activation-based memory system could satisfy the unique demands of working memory (i.e., robust maintenance *and* rapid updating).

↪ Go to the PDP++Root window. To continue on to the next simulation, close this project first by selecting .projects/Remove/Project_0. Or, if you wish to stop now, quit by selecting Object/Quit.

9.5 The Prefrontal Cortex Active Memory System

The preceding explorations have established a set of specializations that we would expect an activation-based working memory system to have relative to our generic model of the posterior cortex, namely: relatively wide attractor basins (e.g., through the use of more isolated self-maintaining connectivity) and dynamic control of rapid updating versus robust maintenance. There is a growing body of evidence that supports the idea that the prefrontal cortex (and perhaps the entire frontal cortex) does have these kinds of specializations. Furthermore, it has been relatively well established using a variety of methodologies that the prefrontal cortex plays a central role in working memory (e.g., Fuster, 1989; Goldman-Rakic, 1987; Miller et al., 1996; O'Reilly et al., 1999a). Thus, there is converging evidence that the prefrontal cortex is a specialized area for activation-based working memory. In this section, we review some of the relevant evidence, and then explore a simple model of the frontal activation-based working memory system.

At an anatomical level, the frontal cortex seems to have a fairly distinctive "striped" pattern of connectivity (Levitt, Lewis, Yoshioka, & Lund, 1993). These stripes define regions of interconnectivity among groups of prefrontal neurons that appear to be relatively isolated from other such groups. These stripes are generally consistent with the idea explored previously that the frontal representations might achieve wide attractor basins by being more isolated. Furthermore, the recurrent interconnectivity within a stripe would obviously be important for active maintenance.

Recent electrophysiological evidence from direction-coding neurons in delayed-response tasks further supports this notion, suggesting that the frontal cortex is composed of small groups (*microcolumns*) of neurons that all encode the same directional information (*iso-coding* neurons) (Rao, Williams, & Goldman-Rakic, 1999). This suggests that these neurons are tightly interconnected with each other, and presumably less influenced by the surrounding microcolumns of neurons that encode other directions. Such a pattern of activity is exactly what would be expected from the isolated representations idea. However, it is not exactly clear at this point how to reconcile this data with the anatomical stripes, which appear to be at a larger scale.

Physiological evidence from recordings of neurons in monkeys performing tasks that require information to be maintained over time suggests that the prefrontal cortex supports working memory (e.g., Fuster & Alexander, 1971; Kubota & Niki, 1971). For example, in the *delayed response* task, food is hidden in one of two wells, and then covered during a delay period. Then, after the delay (which can vary, but is typically between 2 and 20 seconds), the monkey is allowed to choose which well to uncover. Thus, the location of the food must be maintained over the delay. Recordings of frontal neurons show the persistent activation of location-coding representations over the delay. Furthermore, frontal lesions cause impairments on delayed response tasks (Fuster, 1989; Goldman-Rakic, 1987).

Neural recording data from Miller et al. (1996) more specifically identifies the prefrontal cortex as the location where activation-based memories can be maintained in the face of possible interference from ongoing processing (i.e., robust active maintenance). In these studies, monkeys saw sequences of stimuli and had to respond when the first stimulus in the sequence was repeated. If we label the stimuli with letters (they were actually pictures presented on a computer monitor), such a sequence would be: $ABCDA$, where the second A should trigger a response. Miller et al. (1996) found that neurons in the inferior-temporal cortex (IT) only represented the most recently presented stimulus. Interestingly, these IT neurons did exhibit a reliable difference in activation when the initial stimulus was repeated, which can be attributed to the weight-based priming mechanism discussed previously (section 9.2). Thus, performance in this task could conceivably be mediated either by this weight-based memory, or by activation-based memory.

To force the use of activation-based memories, Miller et al. (1996) used an $ABBA$ variant of the task, where the intermediate stimuli could also have repeats. They found that monkeys initially tended to respond to the second internal repeat (i.e., the second B), but that with training they could learn to use the frontal activation-based memory of the initial stimulus to respond only when this stimulus repeated. Thus, this series of experiments nicely captures the differences between the posterior and frontal cortex. The posterior cortex (e.g., IT) can do simple weight-based priming, but not robust active maintenance, whereas the prefrontal cortex can do the robust active maintenance of stimuli in the face of ongoing processing.

Active maintenance has also been localized to the prefrontal cortex in humans using functional magnetic resonance imaging (fMRI) as subjects performed a working memory task (Cohen, Perlstein, Braver, Nystrom, Noll, Jonides, & Smith, 1997). Importantly, this study was specifically able to show that the prefrontal cortex was active during the maintenance period, not just at the start and end of it, which corroborates the findings of sustained frontal activation in the monkey recordings. Much of the other evidence for working memory in the prefrontal cortex comes from more complex tasks, that will be discussed in the context of higher-level cognition in chapter 11. In the next section, we focus on evidence suggesting that the prefrontal cortex can dynamically regulate between robust maintenance and rapid updating based on task demands.

9.5.1 Dynamic Regulation of Active Maintenance

There is substantial evidence to suggest that the neuromodulatory substance dopamine (DA) plays an important role in regulating the frontal active memory system (O'Reilly et al., 1999a; Cohen et al., 1996). DA agonists (i.e., drugs that mimic or enhance the effect of dopamine) have been found to improve memory performance in humans (Luciana, Depue, Arbisi, & Leon, 1992), and DA antagonists (i.e., drugs that block the effects of DA) interfere with performance in delayed-response tasks in monkeys (Sawaguchi & Goldman-Rakic, 1991), and directly affect frontal neuronal activity (Williams & Goldman-Rakic, 1995). DA in the frontal cortex typically synapses in combination with other inputs, enabling it to modulate the efficacy of these inputs (Lewis, Hayes, Lund, & Oeth, 1992; Williams & Goldman-Rakic, 1993), and has been shown electrophysiologically to potentiate both afferent excitatory and inhibitory signals (Chiodo & Berger, 1986; Penit-Soria, Audinat, & Crepel, 1987). Finally, DA has played an important role in explaining frontal deficits associated with schizophrenia (Cohen & Servan-Schreiber, 1992).

On the basis of the preceding evidence, Cohen et al. (1996) proposed that the midbrain nuclei that send dopamine to the frontal cortex (i.e., the *ventral tegmental area, VTA*), under control of descending cortical projections, enable the frontal cortex to actively regulate the updating of its representations by controlling the release of dopamine in a strategic manner. Specifically, they proposed that the afferent connections into the frontal cortex from other brain systems are usually relatively weak compared to stronger recurrent excitation, but that DA enhances the strength of these afferents at times when rapid updating is necessary. Thus, DA serves as a dynamic *gating* mechanism, such that when DA is firing, the "gate" into the active memory representations is open (leading to rapid updating), but otherwise is closed (leading to robust maintenance). Note that this dynamic regulation of the relative strength of the input versus the recurrent maintenance connections is just the kind of mechanism that we explored in the previous simulations by manually adjusting the weight scaling parameter. Hochreiter and Schmidhuber (1997) have also provided purely computational motivations in favor of such a gating mechanism.

One consequence of this DA regulation idea is that the VTA should exhibit a burst of (phasic) firing at those times when the frontal cortex needs to be updated. Schultz et al. (1993) have found that indeed, the VTA exhibits transient, stimulus-locked activity in response to stimuli that predicted subsequent meaningful events (e.g., reward or other cues that then predict reward). Further, this role of DA as a gating mechanism is synergistic with its role in reward-based learning, as explored in chapter 6. As we will see in chapter 11, this kind of learning mechanism enables the network to adaptively control the updating and maintenance of working memory representations as a function of task demands. This avoids the apparent "homunculus" (small "man" inside the brain) that would otherwise be required to control working memory in a useful fashion.

Although we focus on the role of the VTA in this model, it is also possible that the *basal ganglia* play an important role in controlling frontal active memory. As discussed in chapter 7, the basal ganglia appear to be specialized for high-threshold detection and initiation of "actions." In the cognitive domain, the action that basal ganglia firing may initiate is the gating in of memories in the frontal cortex. This could be effected by the disinhibition of cortico-thalamic loops via the connections from the basal ganglia to the regions of the thalamus that are interconnected with the frontal cortex. One advantage of the basal-ganglia system over the VTA is its potential for much finer resolution in determining which regions of frontal cortex to update, and which *not* to update. Although we are currently exploring these ideas, the present model focuses on the VTA because it is much simpler and the potential advantages of the basal ganglia system are not relevant to the simple task explored here.

9.5.2 Details of the Prefrontal Cortex Model

The model we will explore in this section incorporates the specializations discussed earlier, enabling us to simulate the role of the prefrontal cortex in active maintenance. Specifically, we include a dynamic gating mechanism (based on the dopamine system) that regulates

Trial	Input	Maint	Output
1	STORE-A	A	A
2	IGNORE-B	A	B
3	IGNORE-C	A	C
4	IGNORE-D	A	D
5	RECALL	A	A

Table 9.2: A sequence of trials in the simple active maintenance task modeled in this section, showing the input (control cue and stimulus), what should be maintained in active memory, and what should be output.

the strength of the connections in the prefrontal cortex, and we make the prefrontal representations isolated and self-maintaining (as we did in a previous simulation). Because the dopaminergic gating system is driven by the reinforcement learning mechanisms developed in chapter 6, the model instantiates the important synergy between reinforcement learning mechanisms and the learned control of active maintenance.

As discussed in chapter 6, we can think of the prefrontal cortex as playing the role of a *context* representation in a simple recurrent network (SRN), which is consistent with the general view of the prefrontal cortex as providing an internal representation of task context (Cohen & Servan-Schreiber, 1992). When we add in the dynamic dopamine-based gating mechanism, this context representation can become much more flexible than that of a standard SRN, which always performs a simple copy operation after each trial. To harness this flexibility, the gating mechanism must learn when to update working memory — this is where the dopamine-based reinforcement learning mechanisms discussed in chapter 6 are used. If you have not yet read section 6.7 you might want to do so now before continuing — it will enable you to understand the model in greater detail. Otherwise, you should still be able to get the main ideas from the presentation here.

To explore the basic principles of active maintenance in the model, we will use a simple task that requires information to be stored and maintained over time in the face of other distracting inputs, and then recalled. These are the basic task requirements of the working memory span tasks commonly used to measure working memory capacity (Daneman & Carpenter, 1980;

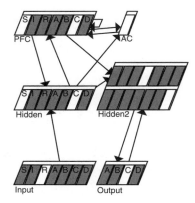

Figure 9.21: The prefrontal cortex active maintenance model. The input contains task control units (S=store, I=ignore, R=recall) and stimulus units (A-D). The output contains the stimulus units. The hidden (posterior cortex) and prefrontal cortex (PFC) have simple one-to-one representations of the input stimuli. The AC unit and the output hidden layer learn the significance of the cues for task performance, and how to produce the appropriate outputs.

Shah & Miyake, 1996). In our version, explicit cues are presented that mark each input as something to be stored, ignored, or recalled. The network must learn to use these cues to dynamically control the updating and maintenance of active memory. There are four stimuli that we will label A–D, any of which can serve as something to be maintained and later recalled, or as something to be ignored. After each stimulus presentation, the network is required to produce an output, which is always just the stimulus being presented on the input, except in a recall trial, where it is the previously stored stimulus. Thus, the "ignore" stimuli cannot be completely ignored if a correct output is to be produced on ignore trials — they are just ignored from the perspective of the frontal active maintenance system. It is this need to maintain some information while at the same time processing other information that lies at the heart of the notion of working memory as distinct from simple short-term memory, and is the main thing tested by the working memory span tasks.

An example sequence of trials in the task is shown in table 9.2, and figure 9.21 shows the model for this task. The input representation has three units for the control cues (S, I, and R for store, ignore, and recall, respectively), and four units for the four stimuli. The output has the four stimuli units. The hidden (posterior cortex) and prefrontal cortex (PFC) representations are simple one-to-one copies of the input representations. The adaptive critic (AC) unit, which represents the dopamine controlling system, learns to control when to update and maintain information in the PFC on the basis of rewards delivered as a function of whether it produces the correct output on recall trials. Specifically, a "positive" reward of 1 is provided to the AC if the originally stored stimulus is produced on the output, and a "negative" reward of 0 is given otherwise. The second hidden layer (Hidden2) learns to map the hidden and PFC representations to the correct outputs — it does this using standard error-driven learning (under the assumption that the correct answer is provided).

The central feature of the model is how it captures the interaction between dopamine and the prefrontal cortex, based on the dynamics of the adaptive critic unit. The AC unit learns to predict future reward on the basis of presently available stimuli using the *temporal differences* (TD) algorithm (Sutton, 1988). The change in activation of this AC unit (i.e., the temporal-difference) provides a model of the stimulus-driven changes in dopamine release relative to its constant baseline (*tonic*) level (Schultz et al., 1997; Montague et al., 1996). Thus, when the AC's activation increases (signaling an increase in expected future rewards), this corresponds to an extra pulse of dopamine release, and when its activation decreases, there is a decrease or gap in the level of dopamine release. This AC unit corresponds to the neural system (which may be located in the prefrontal cortex itself) that controls the firing of the dopaminergic neurons in the VTA.

The model uses this dopaminergic signal to modulate the strength of the connections in the PFC. Specifically, when there is an increase in dopamine release, all the connections coming from the posterior cortex into the PFC are transiently strengthened by a uniform modulatory *gain* factor (implemented in the simulator by dynamically changing the wt_scale.abs parameters that govern the strength of different projections, see section 2.5.1). This will update the representations in the PFC as a function of the current inputs.

There are three different qualitative directions of AC change (increase, no change, and decrease) that have corresponding effects on the PFC. If the AC unit predicts that the current inputs will lead to future reward, it will encode these inputs in the active maintenance of the PFC. If there is no change in AC activity (i.e., no increase or decrease in expected rewards), then the modulatory gain on the PFC inputs is low, so that the information maintained in the PFC is undisturbed by ongoing processing (e.g., the "ignore" stimuli). If there is a decrease in dopamine (negative change in AC activity), then the modulatory gain on the input weights remains low, and the modulatory gain on the recurrent weights that implement maintenance in the PFC is also decreased, so that information in the PFC is deactivated. As reviewed previously, there is at least suggestive evidence for these kinds of effects of dopamine on the PFC.

The AC–PFC relationship is formalized in the model with the following equations for the absolute weight scale terms s_{in} (the weight scaling of the PFC inputs) and s_{maint} (the weight-scaling of the PFC self-maintenance connections):

$$s_{in} = b_{in} + \delta + \nu \qquad (9.1)$$

$$s_{maint} = b_{maint} + \delta + \nu \qquad (9.2)$$

where δ is the change in AC activation (see equation 6.5), and ν is a random noise value that allows for random trial-and-error exploration during the initial phases of learning. The base-level parameters b_{in} and b_{maint} determine the basic level of each weight-scaling (gain) parameter, and are typically set to 0 and 1, respectively. Both of the weight-scaling terms are bounded between 0 and 1.

As discussed in chapter 6, the temporal-difference algorithm that is used to train the AC unit depends critically on having a representation of prior input information at the point at which reward is received. It uses this information to learn which stimuli occurring earlier in time reliably predict reward later in time. An important feature of the present model is that this prior input information is actually maintained in active memory (and not via a contrivance like the CSC used in chapter 6), so it should be available at the point of reward.

However, the fact that this information is maintained *in the PFC* causes the following catch-22 problem. The

AC controls when the PFC gets updated by detecting when a given stimulus is predictive of reward. At the time of reward, the stimulus is represented in the PFC, and the AC learns that this PFC representation is predictive of reward. However, at the start of any subsequent trials involving this rewarded stimulus, the stimulus is only present in the *input* and not in the PFC, because the inactive AC unit needs to be activated to get the stimulus into the PFC. Thus, the PFC needs to be updated with the current input for the AC to recognize the input as predictive of reward, but the AC unit needs to recognize the input as predictive of reward for the stimulus to get into the PFC in the first place!

One possible solution to this problem would be to ensure that the hidden layer always represents the contents of the PFC (e.g., by having relatively strong top-down projections). However, this is incompatible with the need to use the hidden layer for ongoing processing — in the present task, the hidden layer needs to represent the intervening "ignore" stimuli between the storage event and the recall event to be able to produce the correct outputs on these trials.

The solution that we have adopted is to generalize the same dopaminergic gain modulation mechanism used for the inputs to the PFC to the outputs from the PFC. Thus, at the point when reward is received (or anticipated), the PFC will drive the hidden units with sufficient strength that they will reflect the information stored in the PFC, and the AC will learn that these hidden representations are predictive of reward. Then, at the start of a subsequent storage trial, the hidden units will trigger the firing of the AC and enable the PFC to be updated with the appropriate information. To implement this, we introduce a new dynamic weight-scaling term, s_{out}, that is updated just as in equation 9.2. Further computational motivations for the use of output gating can be found in Hochreiter and Schmidhuber (1997).

Another possible solution to the catch-22 problem is to have the PFC always represent the current input in addition to whatever information is being maintained. This way, the input-driven PFC representations can directly trigger the AC system, which then fires a dopamine signal to "lock in" those representations, which are thus the same ones that will be active later when reward is delivered. The problem with this solution is that network-based active maintenance mechanisms (e.g., recurrent activation) cannot easily tell the difference between representations that are transiently active and those that should be maintained — once a set of units becomes active, recurrent connectivity will automatically maintain them.

One attractive solution to this problem would be if there were a biophysical switch where an additional excitatory current is activated for those neurons that should be maintaining information, but not for the transiently active neurons. When the input signals go away, those neurons with this extra current will dominate and thereby maintain information. Dopamine could then play a role in throwing this switch. Interestingly, there is some evidence for exactly this set of mechanisms in the PFC (Yang & Seamans, 1996) and considerably more evidence in the basal ganglia (e.g., Surmeier, Baras, H. C. Hemmings, Narin, & Greengard, 1995; Surmeier & Kitai, 1999), with several computational models exploring this kind of mechanism (Camperi & Wang, 1997; Fellous, Wang, & Lisman, 1998; Dilmore, Gutkin, & Ermentrout, 1999). Furthermore, frontal recordings have shown that inputs transiently control neural firing there, but that the maintained activation pattern subsequently re-emerges (Miller et al., 1996).

We have implemented the present model using the intrinsic current switch mechanisms, and although it works better in some respects than the recurrent-activation based model, these mechanisms are somewhat more complex and less contiguous with previous models. Thus, we explore the version where maintenance depends entirely on recurrent activation here.

9.5.3 Exploring the Model

↪ Open the project `pfc_maint_updt.proj.gz` in `chapter_9` to begin.

You should see the network depicted in figure 9.21.

↪ As usual, use `r.wt` to view the network connectivity.

You should see that the hidden and prefrontal cortex (PFC) layers have one-to-one connectivity, and the PFC has isolated self-connectivity to enable it to maintain information without activation spread. The AC unit receives from the hidden and PFC layers — these are the connections that will enable it to predict subsequent reward. Also, the PFC receives a "dummy" connection from the AC — this does not actually send any activation, and is there to enable the PFC to read the δ signal from the AC unit, which is used to set the gating modulation of the PFC connections. The second hidden layer (`Hidden2`) receives from the first hidden layer and the PFC, and is trained by standard error-driven (and Hebbian) learning to produce the appropriate output on the output layer.

Now, let's step through some trials to see how the task works.

↪ Switch back to viewing activations (`act`). Do `Step` in the `pfc_ctrl` control panel.

In the input, you can see that the store input cue unit (labeled S) and one of the stimuli units are activated. This activation has spread to the corresponding hidden layer units, and the `Hidden2` layer has computed a guess as to the correct output (at random at this point). Thus, this is a standard minus activation phase. As explained in chapter 6, the AC unit is actually clamped to its prior value in the minus phase. Similarly, we also clamp the PFC representations to their prior values in the minus phase. Thus, these are both zero at this point.

↪ Press `Step` again.

The subsequent plus phase happens, where the correct output value is presented. It is also during this time that the AC unit is free to settle into whatever activation state its inputs dictate, or if an external reward was provided on this trial, then the AC unit would instead be clamped to that reward value. Because the proper setting of the modulation of the PFC weights depends on the difference between the plus and minus activation states of the AC unit, we then have to run a second plus phase where the PFC units are updated with the gain parameters set appropriately. In reality, these two plus phases need not be so discretely separated, and can instead be viewed as two aspects of a single plus phase.

↪ Press `Step` again to see the second plus phase.

Nothing will happen, because there was no reward, and so the difference in AC activations was 0, and thus the modulation of the weights going into the PFC is at the base level (which is 0 in this case). However, as we will see, sometimes the gating noise ν will be sufficient to allow the PFC units to become activated.

The next trial should be an "ignore" trial, where the I input is activated in conjunction with another stimulus unit.

↪ Step through the three phases of this trial and those of any subsequent "ignore" trials, until you see the R input unit activated.

This signals a recall trial. In the minus phase of this trial, the network should have activated the output unit of the stimulus that was originally stored. Because it was not stored (and because the Hidden2 layer wouldn't know how to produce the right activation even if it was), the output unit is likely wrong.

↪ Step into the first plus phase.

The AC unit will have a reward value clamped on it — in this case, the reward will be 0 (actually a very small number, $1e - 12$, as an actual 0 indicates the absence of any reward information at all) because it did not get the correct output. Thus, not much progress was made on this sequence, but it does provide a concrete instantiation of the task.

↪ Continue to Step through trials until you see a couple of cases where the random gating noise causes the network to update the PFC representations (i.e., you see the PFC units become activated).

This can happen on any type of trial. This random exploration of what information to hold on to is an essential characteristic of this model, and of reinforcement-based learning mechanisms in general. We will discuss this aspect of the model later.

Note that after the network receives an external reward signal, it will automatically reset the AC unit, and this will deactivate any active PFC representations. This is due to the absorbing reward mechanism discussed in chapter 6. This resetting mechanism is obviously necessary to allow the network to gate in new information on subsequent trials. We know from neural recording studies that PFC active memory representations are deactivated just after they are needed (e.g., Fuster, 1989; Goldman-Rakic, 1987), but exactly how this deactivation takes place at a biological level is not known. This model would suggest that it might be a reflection of the absorbing reward mechanism.

The initial phase of training in the network serves mainly to train up the Hidden2 layer to produce the correct output on the store and ignore trials. However,

on some occasions, the contents of a store trial will be encoded in the PFC, and the network will produce the correct output, just by chance. When this happens, the weights into the AC unit are incremented for those units that were active. Let's watch the progress of learning.

↪ Do View, EPOCH_LOG to open a log for monitoring learning performance. Then, press r.wt and select the AC unit, so we can watch its weights learn. Then, do Run and watch the weights.

You will see them increment slowly — notice that, after an initial increase on the R units, the weight from the S units in both the hidden and PFC layers increment the most. This is because although different stimuli can be stored, the S cue is always going to be present on a successful storage trial, and will have its weights incremented proportionally often. As the Hidden2 layer gets better at interpreting the (randomly) stored PFC representations, correct outputs on the recall trials will be produced more frequently, and the frequency of weight updates will increase.

After every epoch of 25 store-ignore-recall sequences, the graph log will update. The red line shows the standard sum-squared-error for the outputs the network produces. The yellow line shows a count of the number of "negative" rewards given to the network on recall trials (i.e., trials where the correct output was not produced). Thus, both of these error measures will be high at the start, but should decrease as the network's performance improves.

After continued training, something important happens — the weights from the S (store) unit in the Hidden layer to the AC unit get strong enough to reliably activate the AC unit when the store unit is active. This means that the stimulus information will be reliably stored in active maintenance in the PFC on each trial, and this will clearly lead to even better performance and tuning of both the AC unit and Hidden2 layer weights. This improvement is reflected in the yellow line of the graph log plot, which rapidly accelerates downwards, and should reach zero within 6 or so epochs. Training will stop automatically after two epochs of perfect recall trial performance.

Now, let's examine the trained network's performance in detail.

↪ Do View, GRID_LOG, and return to viewing act in the network.

You should see a grid log that shows the activations of the main layers in the network for each phase of processing.

↪ Press Clear on this grid log. Then, Step through an entire store-ignore-recall sequence.

You should observe that the activation pattern on the store trial (the S unit and the stimulus) are stored in active memory in the PFC, and maintained in the face of the intervening "ignore" trials, such that the network is able to produce the correct output on the recall trial.

Question 9.12 (a) *Describe what happens to the AC unit on the store trial, and then throughout the remainder of the sequence.* **(b)** *Explain how the AC unit accurately predicts future reward, and at what point it does so (note that the external reward is visible as the activation state of the AC unit on the first plus phase of the recall trial).*

You might have also noticed that the hidden units corresponding to those active in the PFC were not strongly activated on the correct recall trial, even though we have a mechanism for causing the PFC units to activate the hidden units to avoid the catch-22 problem described earlier. Recall that these output weights from the PFC are only activated by a positive AC phase difference (temporal differences) signal — when the network accurately predicts reward, this signal is 0, and therefore these weights are not enhanced, and the hidden units do not reflect the PFC activation. Thus, this model makes an interesting prediction regarding the reactivation of information maintained in the PFC when the task is being performed correctly. This is only one of a number of similar such predictions that this model makes regarding neural activations in various parts of the system as a function of the progression of learning. Thus, neural recording data in monkeys performing similar such tasks could provide important tests of the basic ideas in this model.

↪ Go to the PDP++Root window. To continue on to the next simulation, close this project first by selecting .projects/Remove/Project_0. Or, if you wish to stop now, quit by selecting Object/Quit.

9.5.4 *Summary and Discussion*

This model has shown how there can be an important synergy between reinforcement learning mechanisms and the learned control of active maintenance. The model brings together biological data on the role of dopamine in the prefrontal cortex with computational constraints that motivate the need for dynamic control over updating and maintenance in the active working memory system. That there appears to be a good synergy between these different levels of analysis is encouraging, but definitive support for these ideas is not yet available.

Another source of encouragement for these ideas comes from the work of Braver and Cohen (2000), who present a model of the AX-CPT (continuous performance task) based on largely the same principles as the model just we explored. This AX-CPT task involves maintaining stimulus information over sequential trials to detect certain target sequences (e.g., A followed by X) as distinguished from other non-target sequences (e.g., A followed by Y, or B followed by X, or B followed by Y). This task has been extensively studied in behavioral and neuroimaging studies (e.g., Servan-Schreiber et al., 1997; Barch, Braver, Nystrom, Forman, Noll, & Cohen, 1997), and the model explains a number of patterns in the data in terms of dynamically controlled active memory mechanisms.

Although many of the ideas regarding the way the prefrontal cortex is specialized are speculative and go beyond existing data, they point to the importance of using a computational approach toward understanding brain function. The computational models we have explored have highlighted a set of constraints that the prefrontal cortex likely must satisfy in one way or another. This provides a unique source of insight into the role of specific aspects of the biology of the frontal cortex (e.g., why it has such an intimate relationship with the dopamine system), and into the role of the frontal cortex within the larger cognitive system (e.g., by contrasting the role of spreading activation in the frontal and the posterior cortex). In short, we think the underlying motivations and computational constraints we have identified will outlive any specific details that may not hold up over time.

This prefrontal cortex model has extended our repertoire of basic neural mechanisms by relying heavily on *neuromodulation*, specifically by dopamine. We have seen that the network can achieve contradictory objectives (e.g., maintenance and updating) by dynamically modulating the strengths of different sets of connections. There are other models in the literature that have exploited neuromodulators to achieve other contradictory objectives (e.g., storage versus recall in the hippocampus based on the neuromodulator acetylcholine; Hasselmo & Wyble, 1997). We think that the use of neuromodulation plays an essential role in transforming the fairly static and passive network models of information processing (e.g., where an input is simply mapped onto a corresponding output) into more dynamic and flexible models that more closely approximate the behavior of real organisms.

Of course, any time we introduce new mechanisms such as neuromodulation, we must question whether they are really essential, or rather constitute a kind of "hack" or easy solution to a problem that could perhaps be more elegantly or parsimoniously resolved with a more careful or judicious application of existing mechanisms. We are sensitive to this concern. For example, in the case of our model of the hippocampus, we did not find it necessary to include the neuromodulatory mechanisms proposed by Hasselmo and Wyble (1997). This was in part because the natural dynamics of the network actually end up resolving some of the problems that Hasselmo and Wyble (1997) had used neuromodulation for. Nevertheless, we do think that neuromodulation plays an important role in the hippocampus, especially as it is used in a more dynamic, controlled-processing context (see chapter 11 for more discussion).

Another important development reflected in this model is the use of reinforcement learning for something that is typically considered to be a high-level cognitive function, working memory. Thus, reinforcement learning may have a much wider application beyond its prototypical role in relatively low-level classical conditioning. Interestingly, the more discrete, trial-and-error nature of reinforcement learning seems to resonate well with the more explicit, deliberate kinds of learning strategies that are often associated with higher-level cognition (e.g., problem solving).

Nevertheless, successful learning in this model (specifically in the Hidden2 layer) also depended critically on the kind of incremental, gradient-based learning that our previous models have emphasized. Thus, we can see an indication here of how both of these kinds of learning can cooperate and interact in interesting ways in the acquisition of complex behaviors. Perhaps one of the most important examples of this learning has to do with the shaping of the frontal representations themselves, which is likely a product of both gradient-based and more discrete reinforcement mechanisms. Again, we will follow up on these ideas more in chapter 11.

Finally, we should note that this model raises as many questions as it answers (if not more). For example, is it really possible to explain all updating of active memory in terms of differences in predicted future reward, as is the case in this model? Perhaps this basic mechanism has been coopted and generalized (especially in humans?) to allow for dynamic working memory updating in a manner that is not so directly tied to reward prediction?

In addition to this basic functional-level issue, the model raises a number of questions about the biological mechanisms involved. As we mentioned previously, the basal ganglia could provide an alternative source of gating instead of, or in addition to, the VTA. Also, we discussed two possible solutions to the catch-22 problem for learning when to update the active memory representations — which of these solutions is actually employed by the brain (or is it some other as-yet-unimagined solution)?

Some other questions raised by the model include: where exactly is the neural system that controls the firing of the VTA? It must be much more complex than the simple AC unit in our model — how does that complexity affect the learning and performance of the network? An important objective of this kind of computational model is to focus empirical research on questions such as these.

9.6 The Development and Interaction of Memory Systems

In this section, we explore the development and interaction of activation- and weight-based memory. Whereas previous sections focused on these forms of memory separately, here we consider cases where changes in the weights and persistent activity interact in the same system, and sometimes support competing responses. This competition can arise when the weights have been enhanced (primed) for one response pathway in the network (e.g., as a result of repeated practice), but the persistent activity from recent processing favors a competing pathway. In addition to exploring these interactions, this model provides an introduction to important issues in the study of development. Neural network models provide an important tool for understanding how experience and maturational/genetic factors can interact in producing the patterns of changes that take place as an organism develops into adulthood (Elman et al., 1996).

The $A\overline{B}$ ("A-not-B") paradigm (Piaget, 1954), which has been studied extensively in human infants and several animal species, provides a good example of competition between activation- and weight-based memory (Munakata, 1998). In the $A\overline{B}$ task, subjects watch an experimenter hide a toy in one location (A). They are typically allowed to search for the object after a short delay, and this procedure is repeated. Subjects then watch the experimenter hide the object in a new location (B). Following a short delay, human infants often search perseveratively at A, making the $A\overline{B}$ error. Weight-based memory may support perseverative reaching to A while persistent activity — dependent on the development of the prefrontal cortex — can direct correct reaching to B. Consistent with this, lesions of the prefrontal cortex impair infant and adult rhesus monkeys' performance on the $A\overline{B}$ task (Diamond & Goldman-Rakic, 1989, 1986).

It is important to note that many researchers have criticized Piagetian tests such as the $A\overline{B}$ task for underestimating infants' knowledge, because they require "performance" factors (such as reaching) to demonstrate an underlying "competence" (such as a concept of object permanence); infants may have the underlying compe-

tence but fail Piagetian tasks due to performance limitations. Under this assumption, researchers have designed clever experiments that demonstrate earlier signs of competence. For example, a reduced production of perseverative errors has been observed in *gaze* and *expectation* variants of the $A\overline{B}$ task. Hofstadter and Reznick (1996) found that when infants' looking and reaching behaviors differ in this task, the looking response is more accurate. And, infants make fewer errors in gaze variants of the $A\overline{B}$ task in which they observe hidings at A and B without ever reaching (Hofstadter & Reznick, 1996; Matthews, 1992; Lecuyer, Abgueguen, & Lemarie, 1992). Finally, in violation-of-expectation variants of the $A\overline{B}$ task, 8- to 12-month-old infants look longer when a toy hidden at B is revealed at A than when it is revealed at B, following delays at which they would nonetheless search perseveratively at A (Ahmed & Ruffman, 1998; Baillargeon & Graber, 1988; Baillargeon, DeVos, & Graber, 1989).

These demonstrations of sensitivity to an object's new hiding location are commonly treated as evidence that infants "know" where toys are hidden in the $A\overline{B}$ task, but search perseveratively due to deficits external to their knowledge representations, such as deficits in inhibitory control. However, as we shall see, we can understand these findings in terms of the competition between activation- and weight-based memory in the neural network framework without needing to invoke notions of reified knowledge and ancillary deficits.

9.6.1 Basic Properties of the Model

In this model we explore the ways in which activation- and weight-based memory can support competing responses in the $A\overline{B}$ task. Weight-based memory is implemented as standard CPCA Hebbian learning that occurs as a function of the activity of the units in the network. Activation-based memory is implemented by having recurrent connections among representations in the network, much like those discussed in the prefrontal-style active memory system in the previous section. Note that in the original model (Munakata, 1998) and the exercises presented here, these recurrent weights are increased by hand to simulate the effects of development; however, the potential role of experience in shaping such weights has been demonstrated elsewhere (Munakata, McClelland, Johnson, & Siegler, 1997).

The input representations for the model are based on the idea that spatial location and object identity are processed in separate pathways, as discussed in chapter 8. Thus, one pathway represents the location of the hidden toys, while another represents the identities of the toy(s) and the lids that cover the toys when hidden. These feed into a hidden layer that represents the locations, but which also receives input from the object representations. This hidden layer, which has self-recurrent connections to each representation of a given location, represents a prefrontal-like active memory system.

The model has two output layers (for reaching and gaze/expectation); the single difference between them is the frequency of their responses (i.e., the updating of the unit activity) during the $A\overline{B}$ task. The gaze/expectation layer responds to every input, while the reaching layer responds only to inputs corresponding to a stimulus within "reaching distance." This updating constraint on the output layers is meant to capture the different frequencies of infants' reaching and gaze/expectation during the $A\overline{B}$ task. Reaching is permitted at only one point during each trial – when the apparatus is moved to within the infant's reach. In contrast, nothing prevents infants from forming expectations (which may underlie longer looking to impossible events) throughout each trial. Similarly, although infants' gaze is sometimes restricted during $A\overline{B}$ experiments, infants nonetheless have more opportunities to gaze than to reach. As we shall see in the simulations, more frequent responses can change the dynamic between active and weight-based traces, resulting in dissociations between looking and reaching.

The network's initial connectivity includes a bias to respond appropriately to location information, e.g., to look to location A if something is presented there. Infants appear to enter $A\overline{B}$ experiments with such biases.

9.6.2 Exploring the Model

↪ Open the project `ab.proj.gz` in `chapter_9`.

Let's examine the network first (figure 9.22). Notice that there are three location units corresponding to lo-

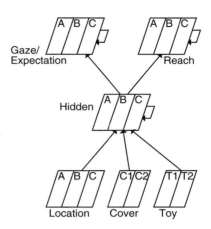

Figure 9.22: The $A\overline{B}$ network, with location, cover, and toy inputs, and gaze/expectation and reach outputs. The internal hidden layer maintains information over the delay while the toy is hidden using recurrent self-connections, and represents the prefrontal cortex (PFC) in this model.

cations A, B, and C, represented in the location-based units in the network. Also, there are two cover (lid) input units corresponding to C1, the default cover type, and C2, a different cover type, and two toy units corresponding to T1, the default toy, and T2, a different toy type.

↪ Now, click on `r.wt` and observe the connectivity.

Each of the three input layers is fully connected to the hidden layer, and the hidden layer is fully connected to each of the two output layers. You can see that there is an initial bias for the same locations to be more strongly activating, with weights of .7, while other locations have only a .3 initial connection weight. Connections from the toy and cover units are relatively weak at .3. The hidden and output layers have self-recurrent excitatory connections back to each unit, which are initially of magnitude .1, but we can change this with the `rec_wts` parameter in the control panel. Stronger weights here will improve the network's ability to maintain active representations. We are starting out with relatively weak ones to simulate a young infant that has poor active maintenance abilities.

Now, we can examine the events that will be presented to the network.

↪ Click on `View`, `EVENTS` in the `ab_ctrl` control panel.

There are three types of trials, represented by the three rows of events that you see in this window: pretrials (corresponding to the "practice" trials provided at the start of an experiment to induce infants to reach to *A*), *A* trials, and *B* trials. Each of these trial types can be repeated multiple times, as can the events within the trial. In the version we will be running, the $A\overline{B}$ task will consists of four pretrials, two *A* trials, and one *B* trial. Each trial consists of four segments, corresponding to the experimental segments of an $A\overline{B}$ trial as follows: (1) *start*, covers sit in place on the apparatus before the experimenter draws infant's attention to a particular location; (2) *presentation*, experimenter draws the infant's attention to one location in apparatus; (3) *delay*, the apparatus sits with covers in place; and (4) *choice*, the experimenter presents the apparatus with covers in place for the infant's response (reaching permitted only during this segment). During each segment, patterns of activity are presented to the input units corresponding to the visible aspects of the stimulus event; all other input units have no activity. The levels of input activity represent the salience of aspects of the stimulus, with more salient aspects (e.g. a toy that the experimenter waves) producing more activity.

Now, let's run the network. It is much easier to tell what is going on in the network by looking at a grid log display, rather than viewing each trial of activation separately.

↪ Iconify the events, then do `View`, `GRID_LOG`. Then press the `Run` button (which does a `ReInit` and `Run` of the training process).

When you do this, the network will run through an entire $A\overline{B}$ experiment, and record the activations and weights in the grid log (figure 9.23), which is not updated dynamically during processing since the `Display` button is turned off.

We can simply jump to specific points in the experiment using the buttons in the control panel.

↪ Press `ViewPre` to see the pretrials.

The main columns of interest for now are the `Event` column, which tells you which event is being presented, and the next column over from that, which shows a miniature rendition of the activations in the network af-

ter each event. The other columns show the weights, which can be somewhat more difficult to interpret at this point, so we will postpone that.

You should notice that when the toy is presented during the `p-toy-pres` events, the corresponding hidden *A* location is also activated and the network "looks" toward this location in the gaze/expectation layer. Because Hebbian learning is taking place after each trial, those units that are coactive experience weight increases, which in this case increases the propensity of the network to activate the *A* location representations.

↪ Next press `ViewA`.

You will see the *A* testing trials, where the network's tendency to reach to the *A* location is assessed. Note that as a result of the Hebbian learning, the hidden and output units are more active here than in the pretrials.

↪ Now press `ViewB`.

Question 9.13 (a) *Describe what happens to the network's internal representations and output (gaze, reach) responses over the delay and choice trials. You should observe the network making the $A\overline{B}$ error.* (b) *Explain why the network is performing as it is in terms of the interactions between the weights learned from prior experience on* A *trials, and the recurrent activity within each representation.*

↪ Now increase the `rec_wts` parameter to .75 from the default of .3, and `Run` and `ViewB` again.

Question 9.14 (a) *Describe how the network responds (i.e., in the gaze and reach outputs) this time.* (b) *Given that the experience-based weights learned during the experiment are basically the same in this and the previous case, explain why the network performs differently.*

↪ Now decrease the `rec_wts` parameter to an intermediate value of .47, and `Run` and `ViewB` again.

Question 9.15 (a) *What happens on the* B *trial this time?* (b) *Explain why the network exhibits these different responses, simulating the dissociation observed in infants.*

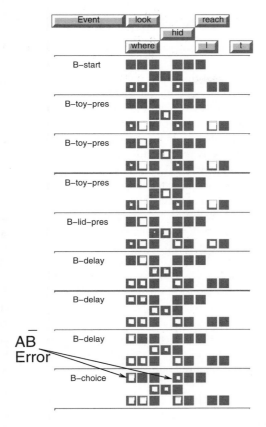

Figure 9.23: The grid log display for the $A\overline{B}$ task, showing the activations of units in the network over time. Shown are the B trials, where the network makes the $A\overline{B}$ error.

Infants typically perform better (making fewer $A\overline{B}$ errors) when there is a shorter delay between hiding and when they can reach.

↪ To simulate this, set the delay field to 1 (the default delay has been 3). Keep the recurrent weights at .47. Then Run and ViewB. Then, try a Delay of 5 and Run and ViewB (note that you will need to manually scroll the grid log to see the last parts of the trial).

Question 9.16 (a) *What happens on the B trials with those two delays?* (b) *Explain these effects of delay on the network's behavior.*

Finally, there is an interesting effect that can occur with very weak recurrent weights, which do not allow

the network to maintain the representation of even the *A* location very well on *A* trials. Because the weight changes toward *A* depend on such maintained activity of the *A* units, these weight-based representations will be relatively weak, making the network perseverate less to *A* than it would with slightly stronger recurrent weights.

↪ To see this effect, Set delay back to 3, and then reduce the rec_wts to .15, Run, and look at the activations of the units in the *B* choice trial. Then compare this with the case with rec_wts of .3.

You should be able to see that there is a less strong *A* response with the weaker recurrent weights, meaning a less strong $A\overline{B}$ error (and further analysis has confirmed that this is due to the amount of learning on the *A* trials).

↪ To stop now, quit by selecting Object/Quit in the PDP++Root window.

9.6.3 Summary and Discussion

This model has brought together some of the threads of this chapter and shown how some of the complexities and subtleties of behavior can be explained in terms of interactions between different kinds of memory traces. Instead of postulating inert, canonical knowledge representations that sit like statements printed in a book, waiting to be read by some kind of homunculus, the view of knowledge that emerges from this kind of model is embedded, dynamic, graded, and emergent (Munakata et al., 1997). Within this framework, perseveration and inhibition arise through the basic dynamics of network processing, rather than through a specific inhibition system (in the same way that attention deficits arose from such dynamics rather than through a specific disengage mechanism in chapter 8). Explicit computational models play a central role in developing this perspective, by taking what would otherwise sound like vague handwaving and grounding it in the principles of neural networks.

An important virtue of the kind of neural network model we just explored is that it takes advantage of the task dependency in many different kinds of behavior. The fact that behavior can vary significantly with sometimes seemingly minor task variations can either be treated as a nuisance to be minimized and ignored, or as a valuable source of insight into the dynamics of cognition. Within an intrinsically dynamic neural network framework, these task variations amount to just that much more data that can be used to test and constrain models. Although important for understanding all aspects of cognition, such models are particularly important for studying the dynamics of development, which is all about changes over time.

9.7 Memory Phenomena and System Interactions

In this final section we will extend the ideas developed to this point by discussing how a range of different memory phenomena can be explained in terms of the underlying neural mechanisms explored in this chapter. Specifically, we will focus on the three specialized brain areas described earlier: posterior cortex, frontal cortex (and specifically the prefrontal cortex), and the hippocampus and related structures. We will sketch how these areas and their computational properties could contribute to some well-known memory phenomena, but we will not explore explicit models.

To provide a context for this discussion, it is important to understand the nature of the traditional memory models that have been developed largely from a cognitive, functional perspective (e.g., Hintzman, 1988; Gillund & Shiffrin, 1984; Anderson, 1983). For the most part, these models present a monolithic view of memory where there is a single type of system that contains all of the memory traces, and there is typically a single canonical representation of a given memory within the system. In contrast, our framework stipulates that there are multiple interacting memory systems, each having different characteristics and emphasizing different types of information.

This multiple memory systems view has been advocated by a number of researchers (e.g., Schacter, 1987; Squire, 1987), and is becoming increasingly popular (Schacter & Tulving, 1994). However, the increased complexity that comes with this multiple systems view seems to have thwarted the development of explicit computational models that instantiate it. Thus, although still in the early stages of development, the framework outlined in this chapter can be seen as a first step toward providing a computationally explicit model that captures the multiple memory systems view.

9.7.1 Recognition Memory

Recognition memory refers to the ability to discriminate recently experienced stimuli from novel or less recently experienced stimuli. In the psychological laboratory, this is typically operationalized by showing participants a list of words (or pictures), and then testing them after some delay with some of those "old" words and new *lure* words that were not on the previous list. At test, the participants are asked to say whether a given word is "old" or "new," and sometimes they are also asked on what basis they think the word is "old," for reasons that will be clear in a moment.

O'Reilly et al. (1998) have used the hippocampus model described in this chapter to account for the contribution of the hippocampus to a range of recognition memory phenomena. The hippocampus can enable the subject to *recollect* the experience of having seen an item before, thus subserving recognition. Thus, if an input stimulus triggers a strong activation pattern in the hippocampus that reinstates on the entorhinal cortex both the input item representation and possibly some representation of the original study context, the subject can be reasonably confident in making an "old" judgment.

Indeed, O'Reilly et al. (1998) found that the hippocampus model produced a relatively high-threshold, high-quality recollective response to test items. The response from the hippocampus is "high-threshold" in the sense that studied items sometimes trigger the recollection of the probe item, but lures never do so. The response is "high-quality" in the sense that, most of the time, the recollection signal consists of part or all of a single studied pattern, as opposed to a blend of studied patterns. The high-threshold, high-quality nature of recollection can be explained in terms of the conjunctivity of hippocampal representations: Insofar as recollection is a function of whether the features of the test probe were encountered *together* at study, lures (which contain many novel feature conjunctions, even if their constituent features are familiar) are unlikely to trigger recollection. Furthermore, the activity patterns that are recalled are likely to belong together because they were encoded conjunctively.

In addition to the hippocampus, recognition can be subserved by the posterior cortex in the form of a priming-like *familiarity* signal. The idea here is that one can be sensitive to the effects of small weight changes resulting from experiencing an item, such that at test the studied items can be discriminated from the new items on the basis of being "primed." Note that even though we think the underlying priming mechanism is the same for familiarity and other kinds of perceptual or semantic priming, the representational content is probably different (i.e., the weight changes are localized in different cortical areas). Considerable evidence suggests that familiarity judgments are subserved by the entorhinal and other cortical areas (rhinal cortex) surrounding the hippocampus (e.g., Aggleton & Brown, 1999; Miller & Desimone, 1994). Thus, we think of familiarity as weight-based priming localized in the rhinal cortex areas, which are likely to have high-level representations of stimuli that combine together a range of stimulus and context features. Such representations can provide a more unique, stimulus-specific basis for familiarity than lower level representations.

Familiarity-based recognition memory likely has very different properties from hippocampally mediated recollection, as one would expect if it was based on our generic cortical model. Rather than being "high threshold," the familiarity of a stimulus appears to be a graded function of overlap among input patterns, and is thus more susceptible to false alarms. Traditional monolithic memory models may provide a reasonable characterization of familiarity, insofar as these models make recognition judgments based on the *global match* (i.e., graded level of pattern overlap) between the test probe and studied items.

In short, we conceive of recognition memory as a function of both hippocampally mediated recollection and familiarity mediated by the rhinal cortex. This computationally and biologically motivated framework is consistent with behaviorally motivated dual-process models of recognition memory (Yonelinas, 1994; Jacoby, Yonelinas, & Jennings, 1997), which posit that subjects consult a familiarity signal when recollection fails. By having an explicit computational model of these processes, we can begin to explain the huge range of behavioral data in recognition memory.

Some of the key behavioral phenomena such a model must address are: the *list length effect*, where increasing the number of items on a list results in worse recognition memory; the *repetition effect*, where items repeated more times on a list (*strong* items) are recognized better than items repeated fewer times (*weak* items); and the *null list strength effect*, where the recognition of weak items on a *mixed* list having both weak and strong items is equivalent to recognition of weak items on a list comprised entirely of weak items (*pure weak*), meaning that the strengthening of some list items does not interfere with the recognition of weak list items. Interestingly, it appears that this null list strength effect is more a property of the familiarity system than of the recollection system (Norman & Schacter, submitted).

9.7.2 Cued Recall

Cued recall is a paradigm for studying memory where a partial cue is presented, and the subject is required to recall the entire original memory associated with this cue. This is the paradigm that we have already simulated in the context of the AB–AC list learning task, where the input cue was the A word plus the list context, and the subject is required to then produce the corresponding B or C word. We saw in section 9.3 that the hippocampus is ideally suited for performing this kind of memory, by virtue of its *pattern completion* capabilities. Although the hippocampus is undoubtedly responsible for cued recall memory for rapidly learned, relatively arbitrary information, the cortex should certainly be capable of performing pattern completion for information that has been encoded there. Thus, the cortex is likely involved when performing cued recall of well-learned semantic information (e.g., "What is the name of the place where the president lives?").

9.7.3 Free Recall

Another paradigm for studying memory is free recall, where no cues are given to the subject, who must then generate previously learned information. For example, a subject will study a list of words, and, after a delay, be asked to recall the entire list of words. Of course, the initial prompt to recall the list serves as a minimal cue, but nothing is provided to support the retrieval of each individual word from the list. Based on everything we have learned in this chapter, it seems clear that the hippocampus is primarily responsible for encoding arbitrary information such as words on a list. However, the prefrontal cortex also plays a critical role in free recall by virtue of its ability to organize information during encoding and recall, and implement a temporally extended sequence of strategic steps necessary to retrieve the information from the hippocampus. We will discuss more about this kind of strategic processing in the prefrontal cortex in chapter 11.

Two of the key behavioral phenomena to be explained in a model of free recall are: *serial position effects*, where words studied at the beginning and ending of a list are recalled better than ones in the middle (Burgess, 1995 presents a neural network model of these effects). The standard explanation of such effects is that the last items are retained in active memory (i.e., the prefrontal cortex), while the first items are encoded better in long-term memory (i.e., the hippocampus); and *chunking effects*, where items that can be grouped ("chunked") together (e.g., along semantic dimensions) are recalled better than ungroupable lists. Data from frontally lesioned patients indicates that the prefrontal cortex is responsible for strategic grouping in free recall (Gershberg & Shimamura, 1995).

9.7.4   *Item Effects*

In addition to the kind of task used to probe memory (i.e., recognition, cued, and free recall), another important aspect of memory that has been studied is the effects of different item properties. For example, are distinctive items recalled better than less distinctive items? What about high versus low frequency items? In general, our computational framework for understanding memory provides a rich source of explanation for such effects. Items can differ in the nature of their representations in each of the three main areas (posterior cortex, hippocampal system, and frontal cortex), and in the extent to which they depend on these different areas. Thus, some item effects can be explained by the differential involvement of different areas, whereas others can be explained by the effects of item representations

on encoding within a given area. Although we will not elaborate these ideas at this point, we point to it as an important area for future research.

9.7.5   *Working Memory*

As mentioned previously, working memory refers to the active use of memory for cognitive processing. As we saw, the prefrontal cortex appears to be specialized for a kind of robust, rapidly updating active memory that fits many people's description of what working memory is. However, we also think that working memory can be subserved in many cases by the hippocampal system, which can encode conjunctions of information during processing for later recall. For example, as one is reading a series of paragraphs (such as these), there is simply too much information to keep all of it online in an active state in the prefrontal cortex. Thus, the active representations that emerge from sentence processing (see chapter 10 for relevant models) can be encoded in the hippocampus, and then accessed as necessary during the processing of subsequent text. In addition to the hippocampus, we also think that the posterior cortex plays an important role in working memory, by facilitating the activation of appropriate representations according to rich semantic links, for example. Thus, working memory is a sufficiently general construct as to involve virtually the entire cognitive apparatus. For more discussion of how the framework developed in this text can be applied to understanding working memory, see O'Reilly et al. (1999a).

9.8   Summary

Starting with a simple distinction between **weight-based** and **activation-based** memory, based on the properties of individual neurons, we have developed a more complex overall picture of memory as a product of interacting neural systems, each with their own distinctive properties. We focused on the three major components of the cognitive memory system: the **posterior cortex**, the **frontal cortex**, and the **hippocampal system**.

In the domain of weight-based memory, **interference** from the **rapid learning of arbitrary informa-**

tion (e.g., the AB–AC list learning task) causes problems for our generic posterior-cortical model because of its **overlapping, distributed representations**. The hippocampus can be seen as a complementary memory system that uses **sparse, pattern separated representations** to avoid this interference. By using two specialized systems, the benefits of each are still available — overlapping distributed representations in the cortex can be used for **inferential processing** of **semantic** information, while the sparse pattern separated representations of the hippocampus are used for rapidly encoding arbitrary information.

In the domain of activation-based memory, the unique demands of **rapid updating** and **robust maintenance** imposed by many **working memory** tasks requires specialized neural mechanisms that appear to be characteristic of the prefrontal cortex, and are also in conflict with overlapping distributed representations characteristic of the posterior cortex, which tend to cause **excessive spreading activation**.

We saw how each of the memory components contributes to specific memory phenomena. The posterior cortex supports a relatively simple form of memory called **priming**, where prior processing results in the facilitation of subsequent processing. Priming has both weight-based (**long-term**) and activation based (**short-term**) aspects. The hippocampus supports relatively interference-free rapid arbitrary learning, as in the AB–AC list learning task. The prefrontal cortex can learn to dynamically control its robust, rapidly updatable active maintenance in a working memory task. The memory components can also interact in a wide range of other memory phenomena.

We find it notable that the cognitive architecture can be differentiated according to memory — because memory is so tightly integrated with processing in a neural network, it makes sense that qualitative distinctions in memory representations underlie the distinctions between different types of processing in the cognitive architecture.

9.9 Further Reading

Schacter (1996) provides a very readable introduction to the cognitive neuroscience of memory.

Squire (1992) and Cohen and Eichenbaum (1993) have been influential and cover a lot of data on hippocampal function.

McClelland and Chappell (1998) presents a unified neural-network based treatment of a number of human memory phenomena.

O'Reilly and Rudy (in press) presents a detailed treatment and models of the role of the hippocampus and cortex in animal learning phenomena.

Miller et al. (1996) gives a very detailed treatment of influential studies on the neurophysiology of activation-based memory in the frontal cortex.

Miyake and Shah (1999) provide a very recent collection of articles on working memory, mostly from the human behavioral perspective.

Chapter 10

Language

Contents

10.1 Overview 323
10.2 The Biology and Basic Representations of Language 325
   10.2.1 Biology *325*
   10.2.2 Phonology *327*
10.3 The Distributed Representation of Words and Dyslexia 329
   10.3.1 Comparison with Traditional Dual-Route Models *330*
   10.3.2 The Interactive Model and Division of Labor 331
   10.3.3 Dyslexia *331*
   10.3.4 Basic Properties of the Model *333*
   10.3.5 Exploring the Model *335*
   10.3.6 Summary and Discussion *341*
10.4 The Orthography to Phonology Mapping 341
   10.4.1 Basic Properties of the Model *343*
   10.4.2 Exploring the Model *344*
   10.4.3 Summary and Discussion *349*
10.5 Overregularization in Past-Tense Inflectional Mappings 350
   10.5.1 Basic Properties of the Model *352*
   10.5.2 Exploring the Model *353*
   10.5.3 Summary and Discussion *357*
10.6 Semantic Representations from Word Co-occurrences and Hebbian Learning 358
   10.6.1 Basic Properties of the Model *360*
   10.6.2 Exploring the Model *361*
   10.6.3 Summary and Discussion *365*
10.7 Sentence-Level Processing 365
   10.7.1 Basic Properties of the Model *367*
   10.7.2 Exploring the Model *370*
   10.7.3 Summary and Discussion *375*
10.8 Summary 376
10.9 Further Reading 377

10.1 Overview

Language plays an important role in many cognitive phenomena, and represents a major point of divergence between human cognition and that of even our closest animal relatives. The nature of the relationship between cognition and language (e.g., does one require the other?) has been much debated. Neural network models can provide a useful perspective in this debate, instantiating mechanistic principles that suggest a rich and interesting relationship between cognition and language.

Specifically, language can be viewed as a set of specialized but interacting processing pathways in perceptual, motor, and association areas. These pathways interact with other pathways in these areas, via learned associations, to produce human cognition. For example, verbal input can activate perceptual and nonverbal motor representations, and vice versa. Over time, learning is shaped by influences both of language on cognition and of cognition on language.

The issue of how words are represented in the brain is obviously central to understanding language, and it provides a central organizing theme of this chapter. The repository of word-level representations is referred to as the **lexicon**, and many traditional approaches have assumed that there is a centralized, canonical lexicon in the brain where each word is uniquely represented. In contrast, our basic principles of representation (chapter 7) suggest that word-level representations should be distributed across a number of different pathways specialized for processing different aspects of words.

This idea of a **distributed lexicon** has been championed by those who model language from the neural network perspective (e.g., Seidenberg & McClelland, 1989; Plaut, 1997). We begin this chapter with a model instantiating this idea, where **orthographic** (written word forms), **phonological** (spoken word forms), and **semantic** (word meaning) representations interact during basic language tasks such as reading for meaning, reading aloud, speaking, and so forth. The orthographic and phonological pathways constitute specialized perceptual and motor pathways, respectively, while the semantic representations likely reside in higher-level association areas. In this model, activation in any one of these areas can produce appropriate corresponding activation in the other areas. Furthermore, interesting dependencies develop among the pathways, as revealed by damage to one or more of the pathways. Specifically, by damaging different parts of this model, we simulate various forms of acquired **dyslexia** — disorders in reading that can result from brain damage.

Another theme of the chapter concerns the many regularities in human language, which can be conceived of as obeying rules. However, rarely are these rules absolute — there always seem to be exceptions. From a symbolic, computer-metaphor perspective, one would implement such a system as a set of rules augmented with a lookup-table of what to do with the exceptions. In contrast, the dedicated, content-specific nature of neural network representations does not require a formal separation between the processing of regularities and exceptions — the network will automatically process a given input pattern according to its specific interactions with the learned weight patterns. If the input aligns with a regular mapping weight pattern, the appropriate mapping units will be automatically engaged; exception inputs will similarly automatically engage their appropriate mapping units (and many mapping units are

shared between regulars and exceptions in a rich distributed representation). Thus, neural network models can allow more parsimonious accounts of the often complex web of regularities and exceptions in language by modeling them with a unified set of principles (Plaut et al., 1996; Seidenberg, 1997).

Our basic distributed lexicon model is elaborated throughout the chapter using more detailed models that focus on subsets of pathways. One extension of our distributed lexicon model explores the mapping between orthography and phonology in greater detail. The visual word perception pathway appears to be located within the ventral object recognition pathway, and can be viewed as a specialized version of object recognition. Thus, we apply the basic principles of visual object recognition from chapter 8 to this model. We focus on the model's ability to *generalize* its knowledge of the orthography–phonology mapping to the pronunciation of *nonwords* (e.g., "nust," "mave"), according to the regularities of the English language. These generalization tests reveal the model's ability to capture the complex nature of these regularities.

Another extension of the distributed lexicon model explores the production of properly *inflected* verbs in the mapping from semantics to phonological speech output. These inflections alter words to explicitly indicate or *mark* specific types of grammatical contrasts such as singular/plural or present/past tense, and the like. We focus on the *past-tense* inflectional system, which has played a large role in the application of neural networks to language phenomena. Developmentally, children go through a period where they sometimes *overregularize* the regular past-tense inflection rule (i.e., add the suffix *-ed*), for example producing *goed* instead of *went*. Overregularization has been interpreted as evidence for a rule-based system that overzealously applies its newfound rule. However, neural networks can simulate the detailed pattern of overregularization data, so a separate rule-based system is unnecessary. We will see that the correlational sensitivity of Hebbian learning, combined with error-driven learning, may be important for capturing the behavioral phenomena.

A third extension of the distributed lexicon model explores the ultimate purpose of language, which is to convey meaning (semantics). We assume that semantic representations in the brain involve the entirety of the associations between language representations and those in the rest of the cortex, and are thus complex and multifaceted. Language input may shape semantic representations by establishing co-occurrence relationships among different words, such that words that co-occur together are likely to be semantically related. Landauer and Dumais (1997) have shown that a Hebbian-like PCA-based mechanism can develop useful semantic representations from word co-occurrence in large bodies of text, and that these representations appear to capture common-sense relationships among words. We explore a model of this idea using the CPCA Hebbian learning developed in chapter 4.

Although we focus primarily on individual words, language clearly involves higher levels of processing as well — sequences of words must somehow be integrated over time to produce representations of the meaning of larger-scale structures such as phrases, sentences, and paragraphs. Similarly, complex internal representations must be translated into a sequence of simpler expressions during speech production or writing. Thus, temporally extended sequential processing, as developed in chapter 6, is critical for understanding these aspects of language. The specialized memory systems of the hippocampus and frontal cortex as discussed in chapter 9 are also likely to be important.

The temporally extended structures of language are characterized by **syntax**, and we will see how networks can learn to process sentences constructed according to simple syntactic rules. Behavioral data suggest that, despite having regularities, natural language syntax is highly case-specific, because the interpretation of a given sentence often depends on the specific meanings of the words involved. Again, this is easy to account for with the specialized, dedicated representations in a neural network. We explore this interaction between semantics and syntax in a replication of the *sentence gestalt* model of St. John and McClelland (1990).

We end this introduction with a broad perspective on language as a metaphor for how distributed representations can provide such a powerful mechanism for encoding information. The fundamental source of power in language comes from the ability to flexi-

bly recombine basic elements into novel configurations (phonemes into words, words into sentences, sentences into paragraphs, paragraphs into sections, etc.). The meaning of these novel combinations emerges as a distributed entity existing over time, and is not localizable to any specific piece. Similarly, distributed representations exist as novel combinations of more basic unit-level pieces that convey meaning as an emergent property of the whole. Indeed, we do not think this similarity is accidental: language is the way we unpack distributed representations in our brains and communicate them to another person via a serial communications channel, with the hope that a corresponding distributed representation will be activated in the receiver's head.

10.2 The Biology and Basic Representations of Language

Language involves a range of different cortical areas. To situate the models that follow, we first identify some of the main brain areas and their potential interactions. We also discuss relevant aspects of the input/output modalities of language. We assume that everyone is familiar with the visual properties of words, and so focus on the details of phonology. Most people are not explicitly familiar with these details, even though they obviously have extensive implicit familiarity with them (as evidenced by their ability to produce and comprehend speech).

10.2.1 Biology

The biological basis of language, specifically the anatomical specializations of different cortical areas for different language functions, is difficult to study for several reasons. First, because nonhuman animals do not have full-fledged language abilities, we cannot perform invasive electrical recording studies of language function (and if other animals did have language function, we probably wouldn't stick electrodes in their brains!). Thus, we must rely on "natural experiments" that produce brain damage in humans (i.e., neuropsychology) and on neuroimaging. Although some progress has been made using neuropsychological and neuroimaging methods to identify specific relationships between corti-

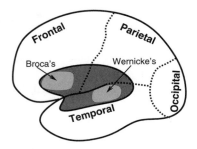

Figure 10.1: General areas of the cortex that appear to be specialized for language (dark shading), containing Broca's and Wernicke's areas as indicated.

cal areas and language functions, one overriding finding has been that these relationships can be rather variable across individuals.

We actually find this variability reassuring, because it suggests that the kinds of general-purpose learning mechanisms used in our models play an important role in shaping the biological substrates of language. Clearly, learning plays a large role in language acquisition — we spend years gradually acquiring the structure of our native tongue. Furthermore, we can be relatively confident that the biological substrates specialized for the written aspects of language are not genetically pre-specified, because writing was developed well after evolutionary selection could have developed a genetic basis specifically for it. Nevertheless, as discussed in chapter 4, there can be many complex interactions between genetic predispositions or biases and the learning process, and it seems reasonable that there may be some genetic specializations that facilitate language learning.

With the important caveats of individual variation in mind, we describe some very general aspects of the cortical specializations for language. Most students of psychology are probably familiar with the two brain areas most commonly described as important for language: **Broca's** and **Wernicke's**. Broca's area is located in the posterior prefrontal cortex (Brodmann's areas 44 and 45, figure 10.1) on the left side of the brain, and is apparently responsible for the production of speech output, including higher order grammatical and syntactic aspects. Patients with damage to Broca's area, who are said to have Broca's **aphasia**, primarily have deficits

in speech production (but can also have comprehension deficits as well). Specifically, they are unable to produce fluent speech, and often omit function words and other aspects of grammatical structure. This pattern of deficits makes sense if you think of Broca's area as a supplementary and higher-level area for controlling (sequencing, organizing into grammatical forms) the motor outputs of the speech production musculature.

Wernicke's area, located right at the junction between the superior temporal lobe and the parietal and occipital corticies (Brodmann's area 22, see figure 10.1), is apparently involved in accessing semantic information via language. Patients with damage to Wernicke's area, who are said to have Wernicke's aphasia, exhibit impairments in speech comprehension, and also produce semantically incomprehensible speech, but they do so fluently (though they do also make grammatical errors). This pattern also makes sense, given that Wernicke's area is probably important for associating language processing representations in the temporal lobe with other semantic information encoded in the occipital lobe (e.g., visual semantics) and the parietal lobe (e.g., spatial and functional semantics).

Thus, Broca's and Wernicke's can be thought of as complementary deficits, in the "surface" properties of speech production and in the "deep" semantic properties of language comprehension and production, respectively. The first model we examine expresses a similar set of complementary deficits when damaged in different places, but in the domain of reading instead of speech (also observed behaviorally). Thus, the model deals with **alexia** or **dyslexia** (these terms are often used interchangeably to refer to deficits in reading ability).

Another very simplified way of thinking about the distinction between Broca's and Wernicke's aphasias is that Broca's involves a deficit in *syntax* and Wernicke's involves a deficit in *semantics*. We will see in section 10.7 that the frontal cortex location for Broca's area is consistent with the need for actively maintained context information to perform syntactic processing.

Although these distinctions between Broca's and Wernicke's aphasia have some degree of validity, it is important to emphasize that they fall short of explaining all of the neuropsychological data. For example, the idea that Broca's area is responsible for syntax fails to account for the dissociations between syntactic deficits in production and comprehension observed in people with Broca's area damage (Berndt, 1998). Although this data is damaging for theorists who posit a strictly modular distinction between syntax and semantics (e.g., Berndt & Caramazza, 1980), we see it as consistent with the kind of variability that occurs through general cortical learning mechanisms discussed previously. In a neural network framework, specialization is typically a matter of degree.

The neural basis of semantic representations is a very complicated and contentious issue, but one that neural network models have made important contributions to, as we will discuss in more detail in section 10.6. Part of the complication is that semantic information is only partially language-specific — for example, there are visual, auditory, and functional semantics that are most likely associated with the cortical areas that process the relevant kind of information (e.g., visual cortex for visual semantics). The result is that virtually every part of the cortex can make a semantic contribution, and it is therefore very difficult to provide a detailed account of "the" neural basis of semantics (e.g., Farah & McClelland, 1991; Damasio, Grabowski, & Damasio, 1996). Certainly, Wernicke's area is only a very small part of the semantics story.

There are a number of other brain areas that typically produce language impairments when damaged, but we won't discuss them in detail here. A useful generalization that emerges from the locations of these areas is that language seems to be localized in the areas surrounding the superior part of the temporal cortex, including the adjacent parietal, frontal, and occipital cortex (figure 10.1). Further, language function appears to be typically localized in the left hemisphere, often even in left-handed individuals. Although right-hemisphere damage often leads to measurable effects on language abilities, these are not as catastrophic as left-hemisphere damage. For more detailed overviews of the neural basis of language, see Alexander (1997), Saffran (1997), and Shallice (1988).

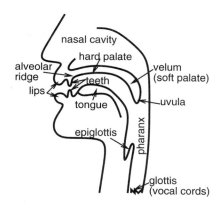

Figure 10.2: Major features of the vocal tract, which is responsible for producing speech sounds.

10.2.2 Phonology

Phonology is all about the sounds of speech, both in terms of speech *production* and the physiological/acoustic characteristics of the human sound producing hardware, and speech *comprehension* of the resulting sound waves by the auditory system. Clearly, there is a relationship between the two, because differences in the way a phoneme is produced will typically yield corresponding differences in its auditory characteristics. We focus on the productive aspect of phonology, because our models focus on speech production in the context of reading aloud.

The human speech production system is based on vibrating and modulating air expelled from the lungs up through the vocal cords (also known as the *glottis*) and out the mouth and nose. This pathway is called the *vocal tract* (figure 10.2). If the vocal cords are open, they do not vibrate when air passes through them. For speech sounds made with open cords, the phoneme is said to be *unvoiced*, whereas it is *voiced* if the cords are closed and vibrating. Changing the positions of things like the tongue and lips affects the acoustic properties of the (vibrating) air waves as they come up from the lungs. The different phonemes are defined largely by the positions of these parts of the system. In our discussion we will gloss over many of the details in such distinctions between phonemes; the critical characterization of the phonemic representations for our models

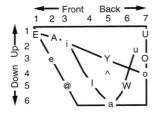

Figure 10.3: Two-dimensional organization of the vowels according to the position of the tongue: front or back and up or down.

Phon	Examples	F/B	U/D	Rnd/Flt	Sht/Lng
/E/	keep, heat	1	1	flat	long
/i/	hit	3	2	flat	short
/A/	make	2	1	flat	long
/e/	bed, head	2	3	flat	short
/@/	cat	3	5	flat	short
/U/	boot	7	1	round	long
/u/	put, bird	6	2	round	short
/O/	hope	7	3	round	long
/o/	dog, call	7	4	round	short
/a/	pot, father	5	6	flat	short
/∧/	cup, ton, the	5	4	flat	short
/I/	bike	4	5	flat	short
/W/	now, shout	6	5	flat	short
/Y/	boy, toil	5	3	round	short

Table 10.1: Representations for vowels, using the PMSP phoneme labels, with features based on location of tongue (front/back and up/down) and the lip position (round or flat) and short versus long. Note that the long vowels are represented by capital phoneme letters, and capitals are also used to represent the diphthongs (/I/, /W/, /Y/).

is a distributed representation that roughly captures the similarity structure among different phonemes.

The two general categories of phonemes, *vowels* and *consonants,* have their own sets of phonological characteristics that we will discuss in turn. Although there is an international standard labeling system for the different phonemes (a phonetic alphabet), we will not use these labels here because they require nonalphabetic symbols, and sometimes take more than one character to represent. Things are much simpler for the models and programs that operate on them if we can use standard English letters to represent the phonemes. We adopt such a phonemic alphabet from Plaut, McClelland, Seidenberg, and Patterson (1996) (hereafter known as PMSP).

Vowels

Vowels form the central "core" of a word or syllable, are always voiced, and provide a means for letting air escape as a word is said. You can sing a vowel sound for a while, but the same is not usually true of consonants. Vowels vary along four different dimensions as captured in our representations. Figure 10.3 shows two of these dimensions, based on the position of the tongue along both the front-back and up-down dimensions within the mouth. The other two dimensions are the positions of the lips (either rounded or flat) and the "length" of the vowel sound (either short or long). A long vowel is typically made with the vocal apparatus more "tensed" than a similar short vowel. Table 10.1 shows each vowel with an example for you to try out, and its values along each of these dimensions.

The activity pattern corresponding to a vowel in our network contains 1 unit active out of a group of 7 representing front/back, 1 out of 6 for up/down, and then 1 out of 4 representing one of the four possible combinations of round/flat and short/long. This coding was designed to avoid features that are active 50 percent of the time, which would be inconsistent with the sparse representations the network itself develops.

Consonants

Unlike the vowels, the consonants are typically produced by *restricting* airflow, which causes a distinctive sound depending on where the restriction occurs, the way in which it is done (called the *manner*), and whether it is voiced. For example, the /s/ sound is made by pushing unvoiced air through a small opening produced by pushing the tongue up against the gums (also known as the *alveolar ridge*). The /z/ sound is just the same, except that it is voiced (the vocal cords are closed). Thus, the three critical features in our consonant representations are the location at which the airflow is restricted, the manner, and voicing.

Phon	Examples	Loc	Mnr	Vce
/p/	pit	lb	ps	−
/b/	bit	lb	ps	+
/m/	mit	lb	ns	+
/t/	tip	al	ps	−
/d/	dip	al	ps	+
/n/	nick	al	ns	+
/k/	cat	vl	ps	−
/g/	get	vl	ps	+
/N/	ring	vl	ns	+
/f/	fat	ld	fr	−
/v/	very	ld	fr	+
/s/	sit	al	fr	−
/z/	zip	al	fr	+
/T/	thin	dt	fr	−
/D/	this	dt	fr	+
/S/	she	pl	fr	−
/Z/	beige	pl	fr	+
/C/	chin	vl	fr	−
/j/	urge	vl	fr	+
/l/	lit	dt	lq	+
/r/	rip	al	lq	+
/y/	yes	al	sv	+
/w/	whip	lb	sv	+
/h/	hip	gl	fr	−

Table 10.2: Representations for consonants, using the PMSP phoneme labels, with features based on location of restriction (lb=labial=lips, ld=labio-dental=lips-teeth, dt=dental=teeth, al=alveolar=gums, pl=palatal=palate, vl=velar=soft palate, gl=glottal=epiglottis), manner (ps=plosive, fr=fricative, sv=semi-vowel, lq=liquid, ns=nasal), and voicing (yes or no).

Airflow can be restricted by the lips (called labial or lb), lips and teeth (labio-dental or ld), teeth (dental, dt), gums (alveolar, al), palate (roof of the mouth, pl), soft palate (velum, vl), and the epiglottis (gl) (figure 10.2). Restrictions can be made in the following manners: A *plosive* restriction is like the phoneme /p/ as in "push" — the air is restricted and then has an "explosive" burst through the restriction. A *fricative* restriction is a constant "friction" sound, like the phoneme /s/. A *semi-vowel* (also known as *glide*) is a consonant that is produced a lot like a vowel, without much restriction, such as the phoneme /y/ as in "yes." A *liquid* is smooth and

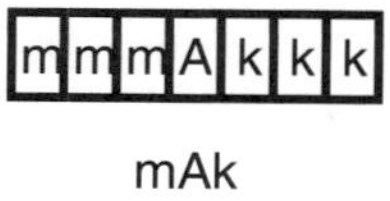

mAk

Figure 10.4: Phonological representation of a word (in this case "make"), which is vowel-centered with repeating consonants in the onset and coda slots.

"liquid" sound, like the phoneme /l/ in "lit." Finally, a *nasal* restriction involves a complete blockage of the air out the mouth, so that the nose becomes the primary outlet (e.g., in the phoneme /n/ as in "nun"). See table 10.2 for a full listing of the consonants and their features.

Words

We use a specific scheme for combining individual phonemes into a representation of a whole word. The representation is *vowel centered*, with slots on each side for the *onset* and *coda* consonants that surround the word. This scheme is sufficient for the monosyllabic words used in all the models in this chapter. Within the onset and coda, the slots are filled with repeats of the consonant in cases where there are fewer different consonants than slots (figure 10.4). An alternative to this repetition scheme would be to insert a "blank" phoneme in the extra slots, but this has the drawback of making these blanks very high frequency, which can impede learning. The repetition also enables a somewhat more systematic orthographic to phonological mapping to be developed, because words share onset and coda syllables, but not in every position. For example, ground and god would not overlap in the onset or coda at all using blanks (/-grWnd-/ vs. /-gad-/), but do overlap using repetition (/ggrWndd/ vs. /gggaddd/).

10.3 The Distributed Representation of Words and Dyslexia

The number of separable representational systems (different brain areas) potentially involved in representing some aspect of a given word is probably quite large. If we restrict our focus to those areas essential for read-

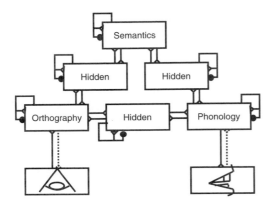

Figure 10.5: For the purposes of reading, words are represented in a distributed fashion across orthographic (visual word recognition), phonological (speech output), and semantic areas. The direct route for reading goes directly from orthography to phonology, while the indirect route goes via semantics.

ing aloud, then this number becomes more manageable, consisting principally of *orthographic* (i.e., visual word recognition) representations, *phonological* (i.e., speech output) representations, and *semantic* representations (e.g., Seidenberg & McClelland, 1989; Van Orden, Pennington, & Stone, 1990). In this section, we explore a model (based on one developed by Plaut & Shallice, 1993) that demonstrates the interaction between these three different areas, with complete bidirectional connectivity between them (figure 10.5). Thus, the model provides an instantiation of the *distributed lexicon* idea.

The model has two different pathways leading from orthographic input to phonological output. The **direct pathway** goes directly from orthography to phonology, while the **indirect** or **semantic pathway** goes via semantics. The presence of these two pathways gives rise to many interesting phenomena in reading, and touches on some important theoretical issues that have been much debated in the literature. We review this debate in the following section. The subsequent section discusses a novel mechanism for explaining the behavioral effects of brain damage that arises in an interactive, multipathway neural network model such as ours. Our model can potentially address a number of relevant behavioral and clinical reading phenomena — we focus on understand-

ing the effects of brain damage on reading ability, as are reviewed in the third section below. Then, we go on to explore the model.

10.3.1 Comparison with Traditional Dual-Route Models

Traditional, symbolic, rule-based accounts of reading aloud posit two *routes* for reading, a direct route based on explicit rules for mapping orthography to phonology, and a "lexical" route containing a word-based lookup table (or similar such mechanism) of exceptions to these rules (Pinker, 1991; Coltheart, Curtis, Atkins, & Haller, 1993; Coltheart & Rastle, 1994). Note that other traditional dual-route theories focused on lexical access (i.e., reading for meaning, not reading aloud) use the term "direct" to refer to the orthographic to lexical/semantic pathway, and "indirect" to refer to an indirect route via phonology to the "lexicon" — we have adopted the terminology of Plaut et al. (1996), which is more appropriate for reading aloud. Although traditional dual-route accounts may seem at great odds with our interactive, distributed model (and advocates of the two approaches have engaged in contentious debate), there is actually quite general agreement about the existence of the two basic pathways discussed: the direct orthography to phonology pathway, and the more indirect pathway via semantics. Thus, the central issue in the debate is not so much about dual versus single routes, but rather about the nature of the processing mechanisms taking place within each of these routes.

The real contrast between the traditional and neural network models is in the use of explicit, formal rules in the direct pathway of the traditional model compared with a neural network that is sensitive to the systematicity of mappings. This contrast has implications for understanding the way that the two routes divide up the reading task, and the extent to which there is a sharp dividing line between the two. The neural network model of the direct pathway is sensitive to both systematicity (regularity) *and frequency*, whereas the rule-based system is only concerned with regularity. Thus, the direct pathway in a neural network will learn the regular pronunciations, *and the high-frequency irregulars*, whereas the low-frequency irregulars will rely more on the semantic pathway (because the semantics-to-phonology mapping lacks the overwhelming regularities of the orthography-to-phonology pathway, it can more easily support low frequency irregulars).

In contrast, the rule-based system would not be expected to handle the high-frequency irregulars. Further, instead of having a discrete switch between the two routes, the network approach involves simultaneous, interactive processing and a much *softer* division of labor. See Plaut et al. (1996) (PMSP) for discussion of the empirical evidence supporting the neural network view.

Interestingly, even exception words (e.g., "blown," which does not rhyme with the regulars "clown," "down," etc.) exhibit systematicities in the orthography to phonology mapping (e.g., rhyming with "grown"), posing a challenge to the traditional account of a simple lookup table for exceptions (see section 10.4 for specific examples and more discussion). Instead, such systematicities suggest that the exception mapping appears to take into account subregularities. The neural network system naturally handles these subregularities in much the same way it captures the systematicities of the regular mapping. In contrast, proponents of the traditional account have had to revise their models to include a neural network for performing the exceptional mappings (Pinker, 1991). Given that there is really a continuum between the regular and exception mappings, and that a neural network can handle both the regular and exception mappings, it seems strange to continue to maintain a sharp mechanistic distinction between these mappings.

Because the present model uses a small number of words and is focused more on capturing the broadest level relationships among the different types of dyslexias, it is not really capable of addressing the frequency and regularity effects that play such an important role in the debate about the nature of processing in the direct pathway. We will revisit these issues with the subsequent model (section 10.4) where we explore a much more elaborated and realistic instantiation of the direct pathway based on the PMSP model. The results from this model show that a neural network implementation of the direct pathway does indeed learn the high frequency irregulars in addition to the regulars.

10.3.2 The Interactive Model and Division of Labor

The interactive (bidirectionally connected) nature of the model leads to some important phenomena. Regardless of where the activation originates (orthography, semantics, or phonology), it will flow simultaneously through the direct and indirect pathways, allowing both to contribute to the activation of the other representations. These dual interacting pathways allow a *division of labor* for processing different types of words to emerge over learning. For example, if the direct pathway reliably produces the correct phonological activations for high-frequency words, then the indirect pathway will experience less pressure (i.e., less error-driven learning) to acquire the ability to produce these phonological activations itself.

Unless one of these pathways becomes damaged, it may be relatively difficult to see effects of this division of labor. Thus, the model can exhibit complex effects of damage arising from the premorbid division of labor of certain classes of words on different pathways. This division of labor can extend beyond basic parameters like frequency and regularity to include factors such as the relative richness of the semantic representations for different words. Thus, the interactive neural network approach provides a novel and parsimonious explanatory mechanism for patterns of behavior under damage that can otherwise appear rather puzzling, requiring improbably complex patterns of coincident damage to various specialized pathways to explain within traditional models.

10.3.3 Dyslexia

Dyslexia is a generic term for a reading problem. Many different types or categories of reading problems have been identified, with the type best known in popular culture being *developmental* dyslexia. We focus on three main categories of *acquired* dyslexia (i.e., acquired as a result of brain damage, not developmental factors): **phonological**, **deep**, and **surface** dyslexia.

People with phonological dyslexia have a selective deficit in reading pronounceable nonwords (e.g., "nust") compared with reading real words. In terms of our distributed lexicon model (figure 10.5), phonological dyslexia can be understood as a lesion to the direct pathway connecting orthography and phonology, so that preserved reading goes via semantics, which does not have representations for nonwords. In contrast, in the intact system, the quasi-regular mappings between word spelling and pronunciation are learned by the direct pathway, enabling nonwords to be pronounced. As with all brain lesions, there can be varying degrees of damage and thus varying degrees of impairment in reading nonwords among people with phonological dyslexia.

People with deep dyslexia are like those with phonological dyslexia in that they cannot read nonwords, but they also exhibit significant levels of *semantic errors,* in which they mistakenly read words as semantically related words (e.g., reading "dog" as "cat"). People with deep dyslexia also make *visual errors* (e.g., reading "dog" as "dot"), and sometimes even make combined visual and then semantic errors (e.g., "sympathy" read as "orchestra," presumably via "symphony"). Note that it is difficult to distinguish visual and phonological errors, so we count these as the same (and the distinction is not relevant for our model). They also tend to make more errors on abstract words (e.g., "truth") compared to more concrete words (e.g., "chair"), which may reflect something about the richness and robustness of the semantic representations for these items.

One explanation of deep dyslexia involves a direct pathway lesion as in phonological dyslexia to account for nonword reading impairments, with additional damage in the semantic pathway to account for semantic errors (Plaut & Shallice, 1993; Plaut, 1999). Alternatively, a somewhat more parsimonious account can be given based on the learned division of labor phenomenon described in the previous section. In this account, deep dyslexia results just from more severe damage to the direct pathway than that which leads to phonological dyslexia (see also, Friedman, 1996). Because the semantic pathway comes to depend on the direct pathway to produce correct phonological outputs during learning, a severe direct pathway lesion can reveal this underlying dependence by eliminating the direct pathway contribution. We expect that the newly independent semantic pathway would make errors (which would have otherwise been prevented by the direct pathway) based on similarities among semantic representa-

tions (i.e., semantic errors), which is the key characteristic of deep dyslexia. We will see that our model instantiates this alternative account of deep dyslexia (as well as the original one studied by Plaut & Shallice, 1993).

Surface dyslexia, in contrast with both phonological and deep dyslexia, is characterized by the preserved ability to read nonwords, but impairments in retrieving semantic information from written words, and difficulty in reading exception words, especially *low-frequency* ones like "yacht." People with surface dyslexia also make visual errors, but do not make semantic errors. Thus, we can interpret surface dyslexia as resulting from damage to the semantic pathway in our distributed lexicon model (figure 10.5), with preserved ability to use the direct orthography to phonology pathway for reading nonwords, regular words, and high-frequency exception words.

The learned division of labor phenomenon is necessary to explain the low-frequency exception word reading impairment in surface dyslexia, as demonstrated by the PMSP model. Because the pronunciation of exception words does not follow regularities present in other words, it is easier to learn this exceptional mapping via semantics instead of directly in the orthographic to phonological representations. Thus, the direct pathway will come to depend relatively heavily on the indirect pathway for the pronunciation of these low-frequency exceptions. High frequency exceptions are learned in the direct pathway simply because the high levels of exposure to these words will drive learning in the direct pathway. Thus, when the semantic pathway is damaged, the underlying dependence of low-frequency exceptions on this pathway is revealed. Note that PMSP did not actually simulate the full set of pathways. Instead, they simulated the effect of a semantic pathway by providing partial correct input to the appropriate phonological representations during training of their direct pathway model, and then removed these inputs to simulate semantic damage.

In the simulation exercises below, we will see how these forms of dyslexia — phonological, deep and surface — emerge from just these kinds of damage.

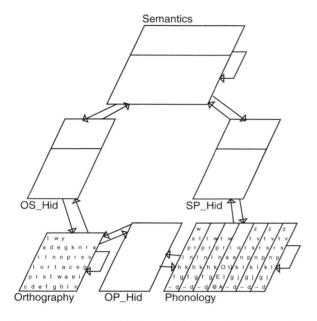

Figure 10.6: The model, having full bidirectional connectivity between orthography, phonology, and semantics.

10.3.4 Basic Properties of the Model

Our model is based directly on one developed to simulate deep dyslexia (Plaut & Shallice, 1993; Plaut, 1995). We use the same set of words and roughly the same representations for these words, as described below. However, the original model had only the pathways from orthography to semantics to phonology, but not the direct pathway from orthography to phonology. This pathway in the original model was assumed to be completely lesioned in deep dyslexia; further damage to various other parts of the original model allowed it to simulate the effects seen in deep dyslexia. Our model includes the direct pathway, so we are able to explore a wider range of phenomena, including surface and phonological dyslexia, and a possibly simpler account of deep dyslexia.

Our model looks essentially identical to figure 10.5, and is shown in figure 10.6. There are 49 hidden units in the direct pathway hidden layer (OP_Hid), and 56 in each of the semantic pathway hidden layers. Plaut and Shallice (1993) emphasized the importance of *at-*

Conc	Phon	Abst	Phon
tart	tttartt	tact	ttt@ktt
tent	tttentt	rent	rrrentt
face	fffAsss	fact	fff@ktt
deer	dddErrr	deed	dddEddd
coat	kkkOttt	cost	kkkostt
grin	grrinnn	gain	gggAnnn
lock	lllakkk	lack	lll@kkk
rope	rrrOppp	role	rrrOlll
hare	hhhArrr	hire	hhhIrrr
lass	lll@sss	loss	lllosss
flan	fllonnn	plan	pll@nnn
hind	hhhIndd	hint	hhhintt
wave	wwwAvvv	wage	wwwAjjj
flea	fllE---	plea	pllE---
star	sttarrr	stay	sttA---
reed	rrrEddd	need	nnnEddd
loon	lllUnnn	loan	lllOnnn
case	kkkAsss	ease	---Ezzz
flag	fll@ggg	flaw	fllo---
post	pppOstt	past	ppp@stt

Table 10.3: Words used in the simulation, with 20 concrete and 20 abstract words roughly matched on orthographic similarity. Also shown is the phonological representation for each word.

tractor dynamics (chapter 3) to encourage the network to settle into one of the trained patterns, thereby providing a *cleanup* mechanism that cleans up an initially "messy" pattern into a known one. This mechanism reduces the number of "blend" responses containing components from different words. We implemented this cleanup idea by providing each of the main representational layers (orthography, semantics, and phonology) with a recurrent self-connection.

To train the network, we used largely the same representations developed by Plaut and Shallice (1993) for the orthography, phonology, and semantics of a set of 40 words, and taught the network to associate the corresponding representations for each word. Thus, we seem to be somewhat implausibly assuming that the language learning task amounts to just associating existing representations of each type (orthography, phonology, and semantics). In reality, these representations are likely developing at the same time as the mappings are being learned (see section 10.6 for a model of the development of semantic representations). Furthermore, people usually learn the semantic and phonological representations for words before they learn the corresponding orthography (and illiterate people never learn the orthography). Thus, the model does not accurately capture many aspects of language acquisition. Nevertheless, the trained model does appear to provide a reasonable approximation to the distributed nature of word representations in a literate adult.

Twenty of the 40 words in our training corpus were *concrete* nouns (i.e., referring to physical objects), and 20 were more *abstract*. As mentioned above, people with deep dyslexia treat these two types of words differently. Specifically, they make more semantic errors on abstract words than concrete ones, presumably because the semantic representations of concrete words are richer and more robust to damage. The two sets of words were closely matched on orthographic features (table 10.3).

The semantic representations developed by Plaut and Shallice (1993) capture the concrete/abstract distinction by having different numbers of semantic feature units. There are 67 such features for the concrete words (e.g., *main-shape-3d, found-woods, living*), and 31 for the abstract ones (e.g., *has-duration, relates-location, quality-difficulty*). The concrete words have an average of 18.05 features active per word, while the abstract words have an average of only 4.95 features active. These are obviously "cartoon" semantics that fail to capture the full subtlety of the real thing, but the similarity in activation patterns between words does a reasonable job of capturing general intuitions, as shown in a cluster plot (figure 10.7). We retain the distinction between concrete and abstract words in the semantic hidden layers by dividing the units into two groups, corresponding to concrete semantic features (35 units) and abstract semantic features (21 units).

We slightly modified the Plaut and Shallice (1993) representations of orthography and phonology for our model, adopting consistent, simple representations for both. These simplifications are appropriate for the simplified, small-scale nature of this model; subsequent models will use more realistic representations. The

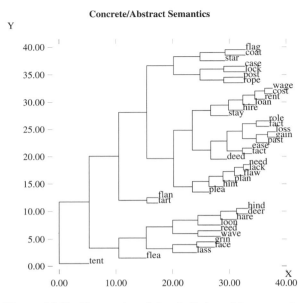

Figure 10.7: Cluster plot of the similarity of the semantic representations for the 40 different words, where the abstract words occupy the central cluster, surrounded by two main branches of the concrete words, which correspond roughly to living versus synthetic things.

Plaut and Shallice (1993) orthographic representations were distributed at both the word and letter level. We eliminated the letter-level distributedness by using individual units to represent a letter, but retained the word-level distributedness by constructing words as combinations of letter-level activations across 4 slots in left-to-right order. The letter-level distributed features were not actually used for any relevant aspect of the model, and the localist letter units are more consistent with the original phonological representations.

The Plaut and Shallice (1993) phonological representations had 7 slots of localist phoneme units, with "blank" units for unused slots. We instead use our standard repeating phonology representations described previously in section 10.2.2, which are consistent with those used for subsequent simulations. However, instead of using distributed features for each phoneme (as we do in subsequent models), we just used individual units to represent each phoneme (as in the original model).

The network is trained by randomly selecting (on each trial) one of the three main representational layers to act as the "input" layer, and then setting the others as targets. Thus, the network learns to take any one aspect of a word's representation and map it onto the other corresponding representations. Standard parameters were used, with 25 percent hidden unit activity.

10.3.5 Exploring the Model

↪ Open the project `dyslex.proj.gz` in `chapter_10` to begin.

You should see that the network is not constructed — it is stored as a skeleton to keep the project file relatively small. Because the network takes some time to train (for 250 epochs), we will just load in a pre-trained network to begin with.

↪ Do `LoadNet` in the overall `dyslex_ctrl` control panel.

Normal Reading Performance

For our initial exploration, we will just observe the behavior of the network as it "reads" the words presented to the orthographic input layer. Note that the letters in the input are ordered left-to-right from the bottom to the top.

↪ Press `View` on the overall control panel and select `TEST_LOGS`, to bring up two testing logs (`Trial_2_TextLog`, and `Epoch_2_TextLog`). Then do `StepTest` to test the first item.

You will see the activation flow through the network, and it should settle into the correct pronunciation and semantics for the first word, "tart."

In the large square `Trial_2_TextLog`, you should see a record of the network's performance on this word, including the name of the input word (in column `Event`), and the name of the word that was closest to the phonemic output produced by the network (in column `ev_nm`). In this case, this should be the same as the input word, because it pronounced it correctly. The distance between the actual network phonemic output and this closest event is shown in the column just before `ev_nm` (column `min_Phon_dst`, which should show a 0). The fact that this closest output is the same

name as the input is reflected by a zero in the `sm_nm` column (a 1 here would indicate error when the two names were not the same). As you step through the patterns, you should monitor these values to make sure the network is reading correctly. As you step through the words, also pay attention in the network display to the timing of the initial activation of the phonological representations.

↪ Continue to `StepTest` through the words.

Question 10.1 (a) *Do you think the initial phonological activation is caused by the "direct" input via orthography or the "indirect" input via semantics?* **(b)** *Check for any cases where this initial phonological pattern is subsequently altered when the later input arrives, and describe what you find.* **(c)** *Discuss what this might imply about the behavior of the network under damage to either of these pathways.*

Reading with Complete Pathway Lesions

We next explore the network's ability to read with one of the two pathways to phonology removed from action. This relatively simple manipulation provides some insight into the network's behavior, and can be mapped onto two of the three dyslexias. Specifically, when we remove the semantic pathway, leaving an intact direct pathway, we reproduce the characteristics of surface dyslexia, where words can be read but access to semantic representations is impaired and visual errors are made. When we remove the direct pathway, reading must go through the semantic pathway, and we reproduce the effects of deep dyslexia by finding both semantic and visual errors. Note that phonological dyslexia is a milder form of deep dyslexia, which we explore when we perform incremental amounts of partial damage instead of lesioning entire pathways.

We begin by lesioning the semantic pathway.

↪ Set `lesion_path` on the overall control panel to `SEMANTICS`, and `Apply`.

This does not actually remove any units or other network structure; it just flips a "lesion" flag that (reversibly) deactivates an entire layer. Note that by removing an entire pathway, we make the network rely on the intact one. This means that the errors one would

trial	Event	min_Phon_dist	ev_nm	sm_nm	con_vis	abs_vis
0	tart_tttartt	0.554259	tact_ttt@ktt	1	1	0
1	tent_tttentt	0	tent_tttentt	0	0	0
2	face_fffAsss	0.309112	face_fffAsss	0	0	0
3	deer_dddErrr	0	deer_dddErrr	0	0	0
4	coat_kkkOttt	0	coat_kkkOttt	0	0	0
5	grin_grrinnn	0	grin_grrinnn	0	0	0
6	lock_lllakkk	0	lock_lllakkk	0	0	0
7	rope_rrrOppp	0	rope_rrrOppp	0	0	0
8	hare_hhhArrr	0	hare_hhhArrr	0	0	0
9	lass_lll@sss	0	lass_lll@sss	0	0	0
10	flan_fllonnn	0	flaw_fllo---	1	1	0
11	hind_hhhIndd	0	hind_hhhIndd	0	0	0
12	wave_wwwAvvv	0	wave_wwwAvvv	0	0	0
13	flea_fllE---	0	flea_fllE---	0	0	0
14	star_sttarrr	0	stay_sttA---	1	1	0
15	reed_rrrEddd	0	need_nnnEddd	1	1	0
16	loon_lllUnnn	0	loon_lllUnnn	0	0	0
17	case_kkkAsss	0	case_kkkAsss	0	0	0
18	flag_fll@ggg	0	flaw_fllo---	1	1	0
19	post_pppOstt	0.375283	past_ppp@stt	1	1	0
20	tact_ttt@ktt	0	tact_ttt@ktt	0	0	0
21	rent_rrrentt	0	rent_rrrentt	0	0	0
22	fact_fff@ktt	0	fact_fff@ktt	0	0	0
23	deed_dddEddd	0	need_nnnEddd	1	0	1
24	cost_kkkostt	0.292739	coat_kkkOttt	1	0	1
25	gain_gggAnnn	0	grin_grrinnn	1	0	1
26	lack_lll@kkk	0	lock_lllakkk	1	0	1
27	role_rrrOlll	0	role_rrrOlll	0	0	0
28	hire_hhhIrrr	0.422775	hare_hhhArrr	1	0	1
29	loss_lllosss	0.293549	lass_lll@sss	1	0	1
30	plan_pll@nnn	0	plan_pll@nnn	0	0	0
31	hint_hhhintt	0	hint_hhhintt	0	0	0
32	wage_wwwAjjj	0	wage_wwwAjjj	0	0	0
33	plea_pllE---	0	plea_pllE---	0	0	0
34	stay_sttA---	0	stay_sttA---	0	0	0
35	need_nnnEddd	0	need_nnnEddd	0	0	0
36	loan_lllOnnn	0.528279	loon_lllUnnn	1	0	1
37	ease_---Ezzz	0	ease_---Ezzz	0	0	0
38	flaw_fllo---	0	flaw_fllo---	0	0	0
39	past_ppp@stt	0	past_ppp@stt	0	0	0

Figure 10.8: Text log output from complete semantic pathway lesion, showing selected columns with relevant data. 1's in the sm_nm column indicate errors (output name not the same as input), con_vis shows where these errors were automatically scored as visual for the concrete words, and abs_vis shows visual errors for abstract words.

expect are those associated with the properties of the *intact* pathway, not the lesioned one. For example, lesioning the direct pathway makes the network rely on semantics, allowing for the possibility of semantic errors to the extent that the semantic pathway doesn't quite get things right without the assistance of the missing direct pathway. Completely lesioning the semantic pathway itself does *not* lead to semantically related errors — there is no semantic information left for such errors to be based on!

Now, let's test the network and look at the results in the Trial_2_TextLog (figure 10.8).

↪ Do RunTest (you will probably want to toggle the network Display off for increased speed, and just rely on the text log output).

Question 10.2 (a) *How many times did the network with only the direct pathway make a reading mistake overall (you can count the number of 1's in the* sm_nm *column, or look at the* Epoch_2_TextLog *which has counted them for you)? Notice that the* min_Phon_dst *column was always less than 1, indicating that the phonological output closely matched a known word — if it were larger than 1 (a threshold we arbitrarily chose) we would score the output as a* novel *blend of phonological features that does not correspond closely to any of the 40 words in the training set.* **(b)** *What does the lack of blends say about the cleanup properties of the network?*

For each of the errors, compare the word the network produced (ev_nm) with the input word (Event). If the produced word is very similar orthographically (and phonologically) to the input word — this is called a *visual* error, because the error is based on the visual properties instead of the semantic properties of the word. The simulation automatically scores errors as visual if the input orthography and the response orthography (determined from the response phonology) overlap by two or more letters. To see the network's automatic scoring, you need to scroll the Trial_2_TextLog over so you can see the columns on the right-hand side of the log, especially con_vis and abs_vis, which show the visual errors for the concrete and abstract words, respectively (note that these have been extracted and other columns removed in figure 10.8).

↪ Use the scroll bar at the bottom of the Trial_2_TextLog to scroll the log horizontally so you can see the columns on the right hand side of the log.

Question 10.3 *How many of the semantically lesioned network's errors were visual, broken down by concrete and abstract, and overall?*

Now, let's try the direct pathway lesion and retest the network (text log results shown in figure 10.9).

↪ Set lesion_path to DIRECT this time. Again, RunTest through the words.

Question 10.4 (a) *What was the total number of errors this time, and how many of these errors were visual?* **(b)** *For the remainder of the errors, use your*

trial	Event	min_Phon_dist	ev_nm	sm_nm	con_vis	con_sem	abs_vis	abs_visem	abs_sem
0	tart_tttartt	0	grin_grrinnn	1	0	0	0	0	0
1	tent_tttentt	0	tent_tttentt	0	0	0	0	0	0
2	face_fffAsss	0	face_fffAsss	0	0	0	0	0	0
3	deer_dddErrr	0	deer_dddErrr	0	0	0	0	0	0
4	coat_kkkOttt	0	rope_rrrOppp	1	0	0	0	0	0
5	grin_grrinnn	0	stay_sttA---	1	0	0	0	0	0
6	lock_lllakkk	0	loan_lllOnnn	1	1	0	0	0	0
7	rope_rrrOppp	0	tact_ttt@ktt	1	0	0	0	0	0
8	hare_hhhArrr	0	tart_tttartt	1	1	0	0	0	0
9	lass_lll@sss	0	star_sttarrr	1	0	0	0	0	0
10	flan_fllonnn	0	loan_lllOnnn	1	1	0	0	0	0
11	hind_hhhIndd	0	hind_hhhIndd	0	0	0	0	0	0
12	wave_wwwAvvv	0	case_kkkAsss	1	1	0	0	0	0
13	flea_fllE---	0	tact_ttt@ktt	1	0	0	0	0	0
14	star_sttarrr	1.86154	flag_fll@ggg	1	0	0	0	0	0
15	reed_rrrEddd	0	reed_rrrEddd	0	0	0	0	0	0
16	loon_lllUnnn	0	loon_lllUnnn	0	0	0	0	0	0
17	case_kkkAsss	0	flag_fll@ggg	1	0	1	0	0	0
18	flag_fll@ggg	0	flag_fll@ggg	0	0	0	0	0	0
19	post_pppOstt	0	rope_rrrOppp	1	0	1	0	0	0
20	tact_ttt@ktt	0	tact_ttt@ktt	0	0	0	0	0	0
21	rent_rrrentt	0	rent_rrrentt	0	0	0	0	0	0
22	fact_fff@ktt	0	hint_hhhintt	1	0	0	0	0	0
23	deed_dddEddd	0	deed_dddEddd	0	0	0	0	0	0
24	cost_kkkostt	0	cost_kkkostt	0	0	0	0	0	0
25	gain_gggAnnn	0	gain_gggAnnn	0	0	0	0	0	0
26	lack_lll@kkk	0	need_nnnEddd	1	0	0	0	0	1
27	role_rrrOlll	0	rent_rrrentt	1	0	0	0	0	0
28	hire_hhhIrrr	0	hire_hhhIrrr	0	0	0	0	0	0
29	loss_lllosss	0	cost_kkkostt	1	0	0	1	1	1
30	plan_pll@nnn	0	need_nnnEddd	1	0	0	0	0	1
31	hint_hhhintt	0	hint_hhhintt	0	0	0	0	0	0
32	wage_wwwAjjj	0	wage_wwwAjjj	0	0	0	0	0	0
33	plea_pllE---	0	plea_pllE---	0	0	0	0	0	0
34	stay_sttA---	0	stay_sttA---	0	0	0	0	0	0
35	need_nnnEddd	0	reed_rrrEddd	1	0	0	1	0	0
36	loan_lllOnnn	0	loan_lllOnnn	0	0	0	0	0	0
37	ease_---Ezzz	0	lock_lllakkk	1	0	0	0	0	0
38	flaw_fllo---	0	need_nnnEddd	1	0	0	0	0	1
39	past_ppp@stt	0	past_ppp@stt	0	0	0	0	0	0

Figure 10.9: Text log output from complete direct pathway lesion, showing selected columns with relevant data. In addition to those from the previous figure, con_sem and abs_sem show semantic errors for concrete and abstract, and abs_visem shows visual and semantic errors for abstract words. There were also blend and other errors that are not shown.

"common sense" judgment and the cluster plot in figure 10.7 (which usually agrees with common sense, but not always) to determine if there is a semantic similarity between the response and the input word (i.e., semantic errors) — count the number of cases for which you think this is true.

The simulation also does automatic coding of semantic errors, but they are somewhat more difficult to code because of the variable amount of activity in each pattern. We use the criterion that if the input and response semantic representations overlap by .4 or more as measured by the **cosine** or **normalized inner product** between the patterns, then errors are scored as semantic. The formula for the cosine is:

$$d = \frac{\sum_i a_i b_i}{\sqrt{(\sum_j a_j^2)(\sum_j b_j^2)}} \qquad (10.1)$$

which goes from 0 for totally non-overlapping patterns to 1 for completely overlapping ones. The value of .4 does a good job of including just the nearest neighbors in the cluster plot shown in figure 10.7. Nevertheless, because of the limited semantics, the automatically coded semantic errors do not always agree with our intuitions.

338   CHAPTER 10. LANGUAGE

No.	Layer(s) lesioned	Dyslexia Type
0	OS_Hid	Surface
1	SP_Hid	Surface
2	OP_Hid	Phono
3	OS_Hid + Comp Dir	Deep
4	SP_Hid + Comp Dir	Deep
5	OP_Hid + Comp Sem	Surface

Table 10.4: Types of lesions performed automatically by the simulator. The lesion number (No.) corresponds to the batch counter variable in the simulator. *Comp Dir* is a complete lesion of the direct pathway (in addition to partial lesions of indicated layer), and *Comp Sem* is similarly an additional complete semantic pathway lesion. The dyslexia type indicates which type of dyslexia the lesion simulates.

The text log also has columns for blend responses (when the distance to the closest valid output pattern is greater than 1), and a catch-all *other* column when none of these criteria apply (due to space constraints, neither of these are shown in the figures, 10.8 and 10.9).

To summarize the results so far, we have seen that a lesion to the semantic pathway results in purely visual errors, while a lesion to the direct pathway results in a combination of visual and semantic errors. To a first order of approximation, this pattern is observed in surface and deep dyslexia, respectively. As simulated in the PMSP model, people with surface dyslexia are actually more likely to make errors on low-frequency irregular words, but we cannot examine this aspect of performance because frequency and regularity are not manipulated in our simple corpus of words. Thus, the critical difference for our model is that surface dyslexia does not involve semantic errors, while the deep dyslexia does. Visual errors are made in both cases.

Reading with Partial Pathway Lesions

We next explore the effects of more realistic types of lesions that involve partial, random damage to the units in the various pathways, where we systematically vary the percentage of units damaged. The simulation is configured to automatically step through a series of six different lesion types, corresponding to damaging different layers in the semantic and direct pathways as shown in

table 10.4. For each type of lesion, we remove units in increments of 10 percent from the layer in question, observing the effects on reading performance.

The first two lesion types damage the semantic pathway hidden layers (OS_Hid and SP_Hid), to simulate the effects of surface dyslexia. The next type damages the direct pathway (OP_Hid), to simulate the effects of phonological dyslexia, and at high levels, deep dyslexia. The next two lesion types damage the semantic pathway hidden layers again (OS_Hid and SP_Hid) but with a simultaneous complete lesion of the direct pathway, which corresponds to the model of deep dyslexia explored by Plaut and Shallice (1993). Finally, the last lesion type damages the direct pathway hidden layer again (OP_Hid) but with a simultaneous complete lesion of the semantic pathway, which should produce something like an extreme form of surface dyslexia. This last condition is included more for completeness than for any particular neuropsychological motivation.

↪ To set up the simulation for the lesioning tests, iconify the current text logs, set lesion_path back to NO_LESION, and do View, LESION_LOGS from the overall control panel.

You will see two graph logs appear. The graph on the left (RepiBatch_3_GraphLog) displays the automatically-scored error types as a function of level of damage of a given type. The graph on the right (LesAmtBatch_3_GraphLog) displays the results from the last lesion level (90%) for each different type of lesion. The lesion types are numbered across the X axis as in table 10.4.

↪ Do LesionTest to run the lesion test.

The network display will flash and update several times at the beginning of each lesion (even if the Display is turned off), with only the final of these flashes corresponding to the actual lesion (the others occur as the network is rebuilt, reconnected, and reloaded between each lesion). Then, all the items will be "read" by the network, and scored (you probably want to keep Display off for this). You will be able to see the lesioned units in the network, but don't be confused by the fact that several of the layers in the intact network (figure 10.6) have "missing" units compared to the square layer box (this was done to better organize the units in meaningful groups within the layers).

The graph will display the results (though you can't really see the first point). Note that the first level of damage is 0 percent (i.e., an intact network), and so is not very interesting. However, the next time the network display is updated, you should notice that several units from the OS_Hid layer are missing — this reflects the partial damage, which will increase in severity next time through. You should notice that the left graph begins to reflect the presence of visual errors on both concrete and abstract words by around 30 percent damage levels (X axis value of 3).

After one iteration up through 90 percent damage levels (X axis value of 9 in the left graph), the lesion sequence will proceed to the next layer as shown in table 10.4 (i.e., the SP_Hid layer this time), and so on until all the lesion types have been performed. When complete, a picture of the damage effects at the 90 percent level will be evident in the LesAmtBatch_3_GraphLog on the right.

Unfortunately, you probably will not be able to make much sense of the results you obtain in your graphs because of the random nature of the lesion — you would need to average over many different instances of each lesion type to get reliable statistics about the expected types of errors from each lesion type. The process you just ran was configured to just run one instance of each lesion type, but it can be run with more repetitions (using the SetN function in the control panel). We ran the lesion battery with 25 repetitions for each lesion, and produced some easier-to-read graphs of the main results.

Figure 10.10 shows the results for the different lesions of the semantic pathway with an intact direct pathway (i.e., lesion types 0 and 1), with concrete and abstract plotted separately. Like the network with the completely lesioned semantic pathway, this network makes almost exclusively visual errors, which is generally consistent with surface dyslexia, as expected. It is somewhat counterintuitive that semantic errors are not made when lesioning the semantic pathway, but remember that the intact direct pathway provides orthographic input directly to the phonological pathway. This input generally constrains the phonological output to be something related to the orthographic input, and it prevents any visually unrelated semantic errors from creeping in. In other words, any tendency toward semantic errors due to damage to the semantic pathway is preempted by the direct orthographic input. We will see that when this direct input is removed, semantic errors are indeed made.

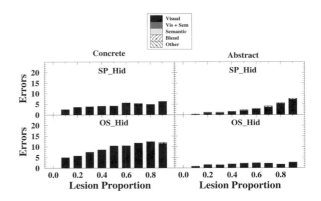

Figure 10.10: Error types for semantic pathway lesions with an intact direct pathway. $N = 25$ for each point.

ing in. In other words, any tendency toward semantic errors due to damage to the semantic pathway is preempted by the direct orthographic input. We will see that when this direct input is removed, semantic errors are indeed made.

Interestingly, lesions of the semantic layer itself produce more errors for *concrete* versus abstract words — this is (also) somewhat counterintuitive. This finding can be understood by considering the division of labor that develops when the semantic system is much better able to process concrete words compared with abstract ones. The direct pathway will then have to take up more of the responsibility for processing abstract words. The effects of damage can be understood in two complementary ways. From the perspective of dependence on the damaged semantic pathway, concrete words suffer more because they depend more on this damaged pathway. From the perspective of dependence on the intact direct pathway, abstract words suffer less because they depend more on this intact pathway. This result shows that there can be general effects of semantic variables even though the network does not make specific confusions among words with similar semantics (i.e., semantic errors). However, we are not aware of data from people with surface dyslexia that would substantiate the existence of this effect in humans, and it is possible that other factors such as frequency and regularity would swamp this effect.

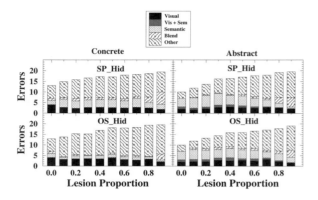

Figure 10.11: Error types for semantic pathway lesions in conjunction with a completely lesioned direct pathway. $N = 25$ for each point.

Figure 10.11 shows the same semantic pathway lesions as the previous figure, in conjunction with a complete lesion of the direct pathway (i.e., lesion types 3 and 4). This corresponds to the type of lesion studied by Plaut and Shallice (1993) in their model of deep dyslexia. For all levels of semantic pathway lesion, we now see semantic errors, together with visual errors and a relatively large number of "other" (uncategorizable) errors. This pattern of errors is generally consistent with that of deep dyslexia, where all of these kinds of errors are observed. Comparing figure 10.11 with the previous figure, we see that the direct pathway was playing an important role in generating correct responses, particularly in overcoming the semantic confusions that the semantic pathway would have otherwise made.

Question 10.5 *Compare the first bar in each graph of figure 10.11 (corresponding to the case with only a direct pathway lesion, and no damage to the semantic pathway) with the subsequent bars.* **(a)** *Does additional semantic pathway damage appear to be necessary to produce the semantic error symptoms of deep dyslexia?* **(b)** *Explain why the direct pathway lesion leads to semantic errors.*

Figure 10.11 also shows the relative number of semantic errors for the concrete versus abstract words. One characteristic of deep dyslexia is that patients make

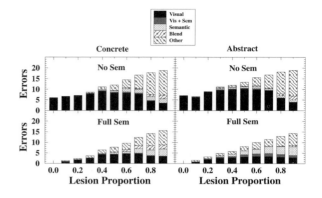

Figure 10.12: Error types for direct pathway lesions, with both an intact semantic pathway *(Full Sem)*, and with a complete semantic pathway lesion *(No Sem)*.

more semantic errors on abstract words relative to concrete words.

Question 10.6 **(a)** *Is there evidence in the model for a difference between concrete and abstract words in the number of semantic errors made?* **(b)** *Explain why this occurs in terms of the nature of the semantic representations in the model for these two types of words (recall that concrete words have richer semantics with more overall units).*

Figure 10.12 shows the effects of direct pathway lesions, both with (lesion type 2) and without (lesion type 5) an intact semantic pathway. Let's focus first on the case with the intact semantic pathway (the *Full Sem* graphs in the figure). Notice that for smaller levels of damage (i.e., about 40% and below), relatively few or no semantic errors are produced, with most of the errors being visual. This pattern corresponds well with phonological dyslexia, especially assuming that this damage to the direct pathway interferes with the pronunciation of nonwords, which can presumably only be read via this direct orthography to phonology pathway. Unfortunately, we can't test this aspect of the model because the small number of training words provides an insufficient sampling of the regularities that underlie successful nonword generalization, but the large-scale model of the direct pathway described in the next section produces nonword pronunciation deficits with even relatively small amounts of damage.

Interestingly, as the level of damage increases, the model makes increasingly more semantic errors, such that the profile of performance at high levels of damage (e.g., 90%) provides a good fit to deep dyslexia, which is characterized by the presence of semantic and visual errors, plus the inability to pronounce nonwords. The semantic errors result from the learning-based division of labor effect as described previously (section 10.3.2). Furthermore, we see another aspect of deep dyslexia in this data, namely a greater proportion of semantic errors in the abstract words than in the concrete ones (especially when you add together semantic and visual + semantic errors).

Finally, the last case of direct pathway damage with a completely lesioned semantic pathway produces mostly visual and "other" errors.

↪ Go to the `PDP++Root` window. To continue on to the next simulation, close this project first by selecting `.projects/Remove/Project_0`. Or, if you wish to stop now, quit by selecting `Object/Quit`.

10.3.6 Summary and Discussion

This model illustrates how words can be represented in a distributed fashion across a set of different specialized areas (layers), and how damage to various of these layers produces behavioral results similar to those observed in different types of dyslexia. The general framework for the interactions between orthographic, semantic, and phonological representations instantiated by this model will be elaborated in subsequent models.

One general conclusion that can be drawn from these results is that it can be difficult to localize damage based just on patterns of error. For example, certain levels of both direct and semantic pathway lesions produce only visual errors —- only with larger direct pathway lesions do semantic errors start to appear. Thus, purely behavioral approaches to cognitive neuroscience are often underconstrained, and require converging evidence from additional methodologies, including computational models like these (see also, Plaut & Shallice, 1993; Plaut, 1995).

10.4 The Orthography to Phonology Mapping

The next model explores the important issues of regularities and exceptions in the orthography to phonology mapping. A much larger number of words is needed to establish what counts as a regularity, especially given the complexity of the nature of this mapping in English, as described below. The mapping from written word spelling orthography to phonology has been studied extensively for roughly 3,000 English monosyllabic words in a series of influential models (Seidenberg & McClelland, 1989; Plaut et al., 1996). These models confront two central issues: (1) the relationship between the processing of regular versus exception words, specifically whether a single system can process both; (2) the ability to simulate the systematic performance of skilled human readers in pronouncing novel nonwords, which depends on properly encoding the often subtle regularities that govern how letter strings are typically pronounced.

To understand these issues, we must first understand the nature of regularities and exceptions. A **regularity** can be defined as a mapping (between a letter and a phoneme) that is present in a relatively large number of examples from the language. For example, consider the pronunciation of the vowel *i* in the words *mint*, *hint*, and *flint*. In every case, it is pronounced the same way (as a *short* vowel), making this the regular pronunciation. The group of words that define a regularity like this is called a **neighborhood**. In contrast, the word *pint* is pronounced differently (with a *long* vowel), making it an **exception** word. Note that the regular pronunciation is *context dependent* because it depends on other letters in the word, particularly for the vowels. For example, the words *mind*, *hind*, and *find* form another neighborhood of regular pronunciation, but with the long form of the vowel this time. Another neighborhood of long vowels comes from the familiar "rule" regarding the effects of a final *e*, as in *mine*, *fine*, and *dine*.

Thus, as many non-native learners of English are probably painfully aware, the regularities in English are not simple (Rosson, 1985). A single system may be well suited to perform this mapping, because many factors need to be considered simultaneously to determine what the "regular" response is. Furthermore, the irregulars can be thought of as extreme examples of context dependency where the pronunciation is dependent on the configuration of the entire word. Thus, there is a continuum between regularity and irregularity. A neural network with appropriately trained weights can deal with this continuum very naturally by taking all the appropriate contingencies into account in making its response. In contrast, the traditional rule-based account of the direct spelling-to-sound pathway requires an elaborate and improbable collection of "rules" to deal with the properties of this mapping (e.g., Coltheart et al., 1993).

Given the existence of regularities like those described above, it makes sense that proficient English speakers pronounce a novel nonword like *bint* just like *mint* and not like *pint*. Given the complex nature of the regularities, this systematic behavior must be appropriately sensitive to conjunctions of letters in some cases (e.g., so that *bine* is pronounced like *mine* while *bint* is pronounced like *mint*), but also appropriately insensitive to these conjunctions so that the initial *b* can be pronounced the same way independent of the other letters. Thus, the correct generalization performance for nonwords depends critically on representations that are both *conjunctive* (depending on letter conjunctions like *-int* and *-ine*), and *combinatorial* (allowing arbitrary combinations, like the initial *b* being combined with *-int* and *-ine*). One goal of neural network models of reading is to show how such appropriate representations can develop through learning to pronounce the known English words.

Seidenberg and McClelland (1989) developed a neural network model of reading that learned to perform the orthography to phonology mapping for nearly 3,000 monosyllabic English words (hereafter the SM89 model). However, due to an unfortunate choice of input/output representations, this model did not generalize to pronounceable nonwords very well, failing to produce the same kinds of systematic pronunciations that people produce for the same word inputs.

The representations in the SM89 model were called *wickelfeatures*, due to their conjunctive nature inspired by the ideas of Wickelgren (1979). Each wickelfeature represented a conjunction of three letters or phonemes. An entire word input was represented by the activa-

tion of all wickelfeatures (including an initial and final "blank" represented by _) contained in the word. For example, _think_ was represented by _th thi, hin, ink, and nk_. Although the conjunctive nature of these representations was useful for capturing the interdependence of pronunciation on other letters as discussed above, it did not allow for combinatorial representations of letters (e.g., the representation of the *b* in *bank* was completely different from that of the *b* in *blank*). This lack of combinatoriality would obviously impair the network's ability to generalize to novel words properly.

The model developed by Plaut et al. (1996) (the PMSP model) corrected the problems with the SM89 representations by having single units represent letters and phonemes regardless of their surrounding context (i.e., combinatorial representations). Specifically, they divided the word into three parts, the *onset*, *vowel*, and *coda*, with one set of letter/phoneme representations for each of these parts. For example, the word think would be represented by the t and h units in the onset (plus one other unit as described below), the i unit in the vowel, and the n and k, units in the coda. This makes the mapping between letter and pronunciation very systematic because the same representations are reused over and over again regardless of their surrounding context.

However, one could imagine that the extreme combinatoriality in PMSP would lead to confusion over the exact nature of the word, because order information within a given part is not actually encoded in the input (i.e., think and htikn are represented identically). This isn't much of a problem in English (as evident in this example) because there aren't many different words that differ only in letter order within one of the three parts (onset, vowel, coda). The PMSP model also added some conjunctive representations that have very specific pronunciation consequences, such as th, sh, and ch, because here the order is quite significant for pronunciation (this conjunctive unit is the extra one active in think referred to above). A similar scheme was developed for the output phonology, combining combinatorial and conjunctive elements.

In short, the PMSP model used hand-tuned representations that significantly simplified and regularized the orthography to phonology mapping. Although the success of this model provides a useful demonstration of the importance of appropriate representations, the fact that these representations had to be specially designed by the researchers and not learned by the network itself remains a problem. In the model we present here, we avoid this problem by letting the network discover appropriate representations on its own. This model is based on the ideas developed in the invariant object recognition model from chapter 8.

From the perspective of the object recognition model, we can see that the SM89 and PMSP models confront the same tradeoff between position invariant representations that recognize objects/features in multiple locations (as emphasized in the PMSP model) and conjunctive representations that capture relations among the inputs (as accomplished by the wickelfeatures in SM89 and the conjunctive units in PMSP). Given the satisfying resolution of this tradeoff in the object recognition model through the development of a hierarchy of representations that produce both increasingly invariant and increasingly more featurally complex representations, one might expect the same approach to be applicable to word reading as well. As alluded to above, visual word recognition is also just a special case of object recognition, using the same neural pathways and thus the same basic mechanisms (e.g., Farah, 1992). Thus, we next explore a reading model based on the object recognition model.

10.4.1 Basic Properties of the Model

The basic structure of the model is illustrated in figure 10.13. The orthographic input is presented as a string of contiguous letter activities across 7 letter slots. Although distinct letter-level input representations are used for convenience, these could be any kind of visual features associated with letters. Within each slot, there are 26 units each representing a different letter plus an additional "space" unit.[1] Words were presented in all of the positions that allowed the entire word to fit (without wraparound). For example, the word think was presented starting at the first, second, or third slot.

---

[1]This was not used in this simulation, but is present for generality and was used in other related simulations.

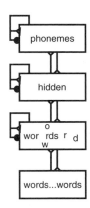

Figure 10.13: Basic structure of the orthography to phonology reading model. The orthographic input has representations of words appearing at all possible locations across a 7 letter position input. The next hidden layer receives from 3 of these slots, and forms locally invariant but also somewhat conjunctive representations. The next hidden layer uses these representations to map into our standard 7 slot, vowel-centered, repeating consonant phonological representation at the output.

These position changes are analogous to the translating input patterns in the object recognition model, though the number of different positions in the current model is much smaller (to keep the overall size of the model manageable).

The next layer up from the input, the Ortho_Code layer, is like the V2 layer in the object recognition model — it should develop locally invariant (e.g., encoding a given letter in any of the 3 slots) but also conjunctive representations of the letter inputs. In other words, these units should develop something like the hand-tuned PMSP input representations. This layer has 5 subgroups of units each with a sliding window onto 3 out of the 7 letter slots. The next hidden layer, which is fully connected to both the first hidden layer and the phonological output, then performs the mapping between orthography and phonology. The phonological representation is our standard 7 slot, vowel-centered, repeating consonant representation described in section 10.2.2.

We used the PMSP corpus of nearly 3,000 monosyllabic words to train this network, with each word presented according to the square root of its actual fre-

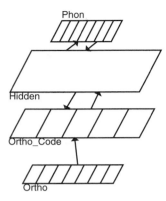

Figure 10.14: The actual network, in skeleton view. There are 7 slots of 3x9 (27) input units (total of 189), 5x84 or 420 units in the first hidden layer (Ortho_Code), 600 units in the second hidden layer, and 7 slots of 2x10 (20) phonology output units (140 total).

quency. This square root compression of the frequency (also used in some of the PMSP models) enables the network to train on the low-frequency words in a reasonable amount of time (it takes several weeks as it is). PMSP demonstrated qualitatively similar results with actual and square-root compressed frequencies. Because each word could appear in any of the positions in the input such that the entire word still fit within the 7 slots, shorter words appeared in more different positions than longer ones. However, the word itself, and not the word-position combination, was subject to the frequency manipulation, so shorter words did not appear more often.

The activity constraints were set to 15 percent activity in the hidden layers, and the proportion of Hebbian learning was set to .0005 — this value was necessarily small to prevent the constant pressure of the Hebbian component from swamping the error term and preventing successful learning of the corpus. Further, as with the object recognition model and other large networks, the learning rate was reduced after 300 epochs (from .01 to .001) to prevent "thrashing" (i.e., where subsequent weight changes cause undue interference with previous ones). All other parameters were standard. These nonstandard parameters (15% activity instead of 25%, smaller Hebbian learning, and learning

rate decrease over time) are all characteristic of larger networks trained on large corpora.

10.4.2 Exploring the Model

[Note: this simulation requires a minimum of 128Mb of RAM to run.]

↪ Open the project ss.proj.gz (ss stands for spelling-to-sound) in chapter_10 to begin.

Again, this very large network, which looks just like that shown in figure 10.14, is not constructed. We will build and load a trained network (which took a couple of weeks to train!).

↪ Do LoadNet in the overall ss_ctrl control panel.

Reading Words

First, we will see that the network can read words that are presented to it, using a standard list of probe words developed by Taraban and McClelland (1987).

↪ Do StepTest in the overall control panel.

The first word the network reads is "best," presented at the left-most edge of the input. You can read this word from the input pattern by identifying individual letters within each of the 4 activated 3x9 slots. Each of these 3x9 slots corresponds to one location and contains 26 units corresponding to one of the 26 letters of the alphabet (with one extra unit). The slots begin with the "a" unit in the lower left, "b" to the right of "a," and "c" to the right of "b," then "d," "e," and "f" above them, and so on. To familiarize yourself with the layout of the input patterns, verify that "best" is in fact the pattern presented. The output pattern produced, /bbbestt/ is the correct pronunciation. To verify this, we can view the phonology patterns and then compare each phoneme slot's output with the appropriate patterns.

↪ Press View on the ss_ctrl overall control panel, and select CONSONANTS.

The initial 3 slots (i.e., the onset) should all have /b/'s, which we can find by examining the corresponding phonological pattern.

↪ Click on the b button in the consonant window.

You should see that this pattern matches that in the first 3 slots of the output. Next, let's look at the coda, which should have an /s/ and 2 /t/s.

Code	Meaning	Example
HRC	High freq regular consistent	best
HRI	High freq regular inconsistent	bone (c.f., done)
HAM	High freq ambiguous	brown (c.f., blown)
HEX	High freq exception	both (c.f., cloth)
LRC	Low freq regular consistent	beam
LRI	Low freq regular inconsistent	brood (c.f., blood)
LAM	Low freq ambiguous	blown (c.f., brown)
LEX	Low freq exception	bowl (c.f., growl)

Table 10.5: Codes for the probe words used to test the network and its settling times. *Regular consistent* means there are no other inconsistent pronunciations, whereas *regular inconsistent* words have other inconsistent versions (examples given). *Ambiguous* is where there is no clear regularity, and *exceptions* are the exceptions to the regularities.

env	trial	Event	sum_se	lst_cycles	ph_out	epoch
0	0	best_best_bbbestt_HRC	0	40	bbbestt	410
0	1	best_best_bbbestt_HRC	0	42	bbbestt	410
0	2	best_best_bbbestt_HRC	0	46	bbbestt	410
0	3	best_best_bbbestt_HRC	0	39	bbbestt	410
0	4	big_big_bbbiggg_HRC	0	63	bbbiggg	410
0	5	big_big_bbbiggg_HRC	0	41	bbbiggg	410
0	6	big_big_bbbiggg_HRC	0	47	bbbiggg	410
0	7	big_big_bbbiggg_HRC	0	44	bbbiggg	410
0	8	big_big_bbbiggg_HRC	0	62	bbbiggg	410
0	9	came_kAm_kkkAmmm_HRC	0	49	kkkAmmm	410
0	10	came_kAm_kkkAmmm_HRC	0	40	kkkAmmm	410
0	11	came_kAm_kkkAmmm_HRC	0	42	kkkAmmm	410
0	12	came_kAm_kkkAmmm_HRC	0	40	kkkAmmm	410
0	13	class_kl@s_kll@sss_HRC	0	45	kll@sss	410
0	14	class_kl@s_kll@sss_HRC	0	37	kll@sss	410
0	15	class_kl@s_kll@sss_HRC	0	41	kll@sss	410
0	16	dark_dark_dddarkk_HRC	0	41	dddarkk	410
0	17	dark_dark_dddarkk_HRC	0	40	dddarkk	410
0	18	dark_dark_dddarkk_HRC	0	45	dddarkk	410

Figure 10.15: `Trial_1_TextLog` showing the output of the network as it reads a series of words in different locations.

↪ Click on the `t` button in the consonants window, and then scroll down to the `s` button (it's number 11), and select it with the middle button (or shift-left button).

The patterns should match those produced by the network. Next, we can examine the vowel /e/.

↪ Select `View`, `VOWELS`. Then click on the `e` button.

You should see that this pattern matches the central vowel slot pattern.

Fortunately, you don't need to go through this pattern matching process every time, because the simulator can do it for you, with the results shown in a text log.

↪ Iconify the consonant and vowel windows, and then do `View`, `TEST_LOG`, which will bring up the `Trial_1_TextLog` window. Do `StepTest` again.

Now we will go through the contents of the text log (figure 10.15). The word input to the network is shown in the `Event` column (e.g., `best_best_bbbestt_HRC`), and has four components: the orthography (`best`), the phonemes (`best`), the repeated consonant phonology (`bbbestt`), and a special status code (`HRC`, see table 10.5). The pronunciation that the network actually produced is shown in the `ph_out` column, which should show that the correct output was produced. Note that this output may occasionally contain an "X," indicating that the phoneme in this position did not exactly match one of the valid phoneme patterns. Also shown are the number of cycles it took for the network to settle, the training epoch, and the `sum_se` error.

Let's continue to observe the network's reading performance, observing specifically the translation invariance property.

↪ `StepTest` several more times.

You should notice that the "best" input appears in successively more rightward positions in the input. Despite these differences in input location, the network produces the correct output. This spatial invariance coding, like the one we explored in chapter 8, requires the network to both maintain some information about the local ordering of the letters (so it pronounces "best" instead of "steb," for example), but also treat the entire pattern the same regardless of where it appears. We will see in a moment that this network developed the same general solution to this problem as the object recognition network, using a combination of locally spatially invariant and yet conjunctive encoding.

You can continue to observe the network's performance, and speed up the process by controlling the rate at which the network display is updated.

↪ To switch the network updating to only update after each trial, instead of each cycle, set `net_updt` to `TRIAL_UPDT` instead of `CYCLE_UPDT`. Continue to `StepTest`.

Although you may observe an occasional error (especially as the items get lower in frequency and more irregular), the network should pronounce most words correctly — no small feat itself given that there are nearly 3,000 words presented in as many as 4 different locations each!

Network Connectivity and Learning

Now, let's explore the connectivity and weights of the trained network.

↪ Click on `r.wt` and click on some units on the left hand side of the `Ortho_Code` layer.

Notice that these units receive from the left-most portion of the orthography input. We can use a trick of viewing nothing in the NetView to see the "skeleton" of the network as shown in figure 10.14, and see how these connections align with the orthography slots.

↪ Click on the `r.wt` button using the middle mouse button (or `Shift` plus the left mouse button) to unselect it and see the skeleton, and then toggle back and forth by reselecting `r.rwt`.

You should see that the left-most `Ortho_Code` units are receiving from the left-most 3 letter slots, where each letter slot is a $3x9$ group of units. You should also see that the other groups of units as you progress to the right within `Ortho_Code` receive from overlapping groups of 3 letter slots.

↪ Click back to viewing `r.wt` with the left button, and click on `Ortho_Code` units all throughout the layer.

As you click on these `Ortho_Code` units, pay attention to the patterns of weights. You should notice that there are often cases where the unit has strong weights from the same input letter(s) across two or three of the slots. We have preselected some examples of different patterns of connectivity that we can step through now.

↪ Press `PickUnit` on the `ss_ctrl` control panel, and then select `OC_I1`.

This unit (the one selected toward the right side of the `Ortho_Code` layer) is a good example of a single-letter invariant unit. It clearly represents the letter "i" in all 3 slots, thus providing a locally spatially invariant representation of the letter "i," much like the units in the V2 layer of the object recognition model from chapter 8. When the network's hidden layer learns about the pronunciation consequences associated with the letter "i" in a particular position using a representation like this, this learning will automatically generalize to all 3 locations of the letter "i". This invariant coding is just the kind of thing that the PMSP hand-tuned input representations were designed to accomplish, and we can see that this network learned them on its own.

We can trace the link from this `Ortho_Code` "i" unit up to the hidden layer to see how it is processed there. We will view the weights of a hidden unit that the 'i' unit projects strongly to.

↪ Select `PickUnit` again and select `HID_I`.

In addition to viewing the weights into the hidden unit, the original `Ortho_Code` 'i' unit, plus another we will examine in a moment, are selected (highlighted with a dashed white border). You can see that this hidden unit is strongly driven by the `Ortho_Code` unit that we were just viewing, and also that it receives a very clear pattern in the central vowel slot from the phonological output layer. Because the weights in the network are generally symmetric, we can often interpret what a unit projects to by looking at what it receives from. However, to be sure, let's also look at the sending weights.

↪ Select `s.wt`, which will show the sending weights.

By switching back and forth between `s.wt` and `r.wt`, you can see that they are generally, but not exactly, symmetric (the Hebbian learning component is only approximately symmetric, but the error-driven is always symmetric).

To interpret the phonological output pattern that this hidden unit wants to produce, we need to again look at the vowel phonology.

↪ Do `View`, `VOWELS`. Then, click on the `i` button and then scroll down and middle-click (or shift-click) on the `I` button.

You should see that this particular hidden unit wants to produce either an /i/ or /I/ sound, which are the two main pronunciations of the letter 'i', just as we would expect from the input to this unit from the invariant 'i' detector in the `Ortho_Code` layer. Further, we can also see that this hidden unit receives from other units in `Ortho_Code` that also code for the letter "i."

↪ Do `PickUnit` again and select `OC_I2`, and then click back to viewing `r.wt` instead of `s.wt`.

Now you can see the weights of the unit in the middle of the `Ortho_Code` layer that is strongly interconnected with the hidden layer unit — this unit also represents the letter "i" in any of 3 input locations. You can also go back to `HID_I` and verify that the other `Ortho_Code` units that this hidden unit receives strongly from also have invariant "i" representations.

↪ Do `PickUnit` again and select `HID_I`, and then click on the left-most `Ortho_Code` unit that has a strong (yellow) weight value.

We will explore a somewhat more complex example of invariant coding now, where an `Ortho_Code` unit represents two different letters, "o" and "w," across different locations.

↪ `PickUnit OC_OW`.

Although the connections are somewhat more faint (because they are distributed more widely), you should be able to see that this unit receives most strongly from the letter "o" in all 3 of the ending locations, and the letter "w" in the last two locations. Now, let's trace the strongest connection from this unit to the hidden layer.

↪ `PickUnit HID_OW`.

You should see that the hidden unit projects most strongly to a single feature in the vowel slot — as we will see, this feature is shared by the /u/ /W/ vowel phonemes.

↪ Verify this by doing `View` on `VOWELS` and selecting u and W, while comparing with the `HID_OW` weights.

This mapping from 'o' and 'w' to the /W/ vowel is obviously relevant for the regular mapping from words like *how* → /hW/, and the activation of the /u/ phoneme makes sense if this unit is also activated by other `Ortho_Code` units that should activate that pronunciation (you can find evidence for this in the weights, but the connections are not as strong and are thus harder to see). This last set of units demonstrates that more complex *conjunctions* of input letters are represented in the network as well, which is also reminiscent of layer V2 units in the object recognition model, and of the wickelfeatures of the SM89 model and the hand-tuned conjunctive units in the PMSP model.

There are several important lessons from this exercise in tracing the weights. First, the network seems to learn the right kinds of representations to allow for good generalization. These representations are similar to those of the V2 layer of the object recognition model in that they combine spatial invariance with conjunctive feature encoding. Second, although we are able to obtain insight by looking at some of the representations, not all are so easily interpretable. Further, once the network's complex activation dynamics are figured into the picture, it is even more difficult to figure out what is happening in

the processing of any given input. As we know from the nature of the mapping problem itself, lots of subtle countervailing forces must be balanced out to determine how to pronounce a given word. Finally, the fact that we can easily interpret some units' weights is due to the use of Hebbian learning, which causes the weights to reflect the probabilities of unit co-occurrence.

↪ Poke around some more at the network's weights, and document another relatively clear example of how the representations across the `Ortho_Code` and `Hidden` layers make sense in terms of the input/output mapping being performed.

Question 10.7 (a) *Specify what* `Ortho_Code` *units you have chosen, what letters those* `Ortho_Code` *units encode, how the hidden unit(s) combine the* `Ortho_Code` *units together, and what phonemes the hidden unit(s) produce on the output.* **(b)** *Relate your analysis to the need for both spatial invariance and conjunctive encoding.*

Nonword Pronunciation

We next test the network's ability to *generalize* by pronouncing nonwords that exploit the regularities in the spelling to sound mapping. A number of nonword sets exist in the literature — we use three sets that PMSP used to test their model. The first set of nonwords is comprised of two lists, the first derived from regular words, the second from exception words (Glushko, 1979). The second set was constructed to determine if nonwords that are homophones for actual words are pronounced better than those which are not, so the set is also comprised of two lists, a control list and a homophone list (McCann & Besner, 1987). The third set of nonwords were derived from the regular and exception probe word lists that we used to test the network earlier (Taraban & McClelland, 1987).

↪ Do `PickTest` and select `GLUSHKO`. Then `StepTest` (don't forget to click back on `act` in the network).

Looking at the `Trial_1_TextLog`, we can see that network correctly pronounced the nonword "beed" by producing /bbbEddd/.

Nonword Set	Model	PMSP	People
Glushko regulars	95.3	97.7	93.8
Glushko exceptions raw	79.0	72.1	78.3
Glushko exceptions alt OK	97.6	100.0	95.9
McCann & Besner ctrls	85.9	85.0	88.6
McCann & Besner homoph	92.3	n/a	94.3
Taraban & McClelland	97.9	n/a	100.0[1]

Table 10.6: Summary of nonword reading performance. The raw values for the Glushko are for only the single provided output, whereas *alt OK* shows the results when alternative outputs that are consistent with the training corpus are allowed. 1. Human accuracy for the Taraban & McClelland set was not reported but was presumably near 100 percent (the focus of the study was on reaction times).

Regular Nonwords

Word	Phon	Repi	Output	Comment
mune	myUn	myyUnnn	mmmUnnn	
wosh	waS	wwwaSSS	wwwoSSS	alt: os → /o/

Exception Nonwords

Word	Phon	Repi	Output	Comment
blead	blEd	bllEddd	blleddd	alt: bread → /bred/
bood	bUd	bbbUddd	bbbuddd	alt: good → /gud/
bost	bost	bbbostt	bbbOstt	alt: host → /hOst/
cose	kOz	kkkOzzz	kkkOsss	alt: dose → /dOs/
domb	dam	dddammm	ddd∧mmm	alt: numb → /d∧m/, some → /s∧m/
doot	dUt	dddUttt	dddXttt	X = phoneme error
grook	grUk	grrUkkk	grrukkk	alt: book → /buk/
wone	wOn	wwwOnnn	www∧nnn	alt: done → /d∧n/
wull	w∧l	www∧lll	wwwulll	alt: full→/ful/

Table 10.7: Errors on the Glushko (1979) regular and exception nonwords. *Phon* is the phonological representation, *Repi* is the repeating consonant phonology, *Output* is the actual output produced by the network (an X indicates uninterpretable phoneme output), and *Comment* provides explanation of network output in terms of the training corpus, alt = valid alternative pronunciation produced by network.

↪ Continue to `StepTest` through some more items on this and the other two testing lists (using `PickTest` to switch to a different list).

The total percentages for both our model, PMSP (where reported) and the comparable human data are shown in table 10.6. Clearly, the present model is performing at roughly the same level as both humans and the PMSP model. Thus, we can conclude that the network is capable of extracting the often complex and subtle underlying regularities and subregularities present in the mapping of spelling to sound in English

Control Nonwords

Word	Phon	Repi	Output	Comment
gurst	gurst	gggurst	gggurtt	
dawp	dop	dddoppp	ddd@ppp	ap → /@p/ (lap, etc.)
phoyce	fYs	fffYsss	fffOsss	final e = long vowel
shret	Sret	Srrettt	Trrettt	also output sret
tolph	tolf	tttolff	tttOlTT	coda ph low freq, → th
zupe	zUp	zzzUppp	yyyUppp	
snocks	snaks	snnakss	snnakkk	inflected form?
goph	gaf	gggafff	gggappp	ph low freq in coda
lokes	lOks	lllOkss	lllekss	vowel migration
broe	brO	brrO—	brrU—	
faije	fAj	fffAjjj	fffAzzz	no err: no j in coda
zute	zUt	zzzUttt	yyyUttt	cute → kyUt
yome	yOm	yyyOmmm	yyy∧mmm	some → s∧m
zope	zOp	zzzOppp	nnnOppp	z low freq, nope
jinje	jinj	jjjinjj	jjjInzz	no err: no j in coda

Homophone Nonwords

Word	Phon	Repi	Output	Comment
stawp	stop	sttoppp	stt@ppp	e = long vowel
shooze	SUz	SSSUzzz	sssOzzz	
golph	golf	gggolff	gggOlTT	coda ph low freq, → th
phocks	faks	fffakss	fffekss	
coph	kaf	kkkafff	kkkaSSS	coda ph low freq, → sh
fownd	fWnd	fffWndd	fffXndd	X = phoneme error
bawx	boks	bbbokss	bbbosss	also output bok
waije	wAj	wwwAjjj	wwwAzzz	no err: no j in coda
muel	myUl	myyUlll	yyyUlll	also output mUl
binje	binj	bbbinjj	bbbinss	no err: no j in coda

Table 10.8: Errors on the McCann & Besner (1987) control and homophone nonwords. Columns are as in table 10.7.

Word	Phon	Repi	Output	Comment
bood	bUd	bbbUddd	bbbuddd	alt: good → gud

Table 10.9: Errors on the Taraban & McClelland (1987) nonwords. Columns are as in table 10.7.

monosyllables, and applying these to nonwords.

For your convenience, the errors for all the nonword lists are summarized in tables 10.7 through 10.9. The full log of network responses is available in `ss.resp` in the directory where the project is. To pick one response across all the different locations of a given word, we just picked a correct response if there was one, and if not, we picked an informative error if there was any variation.

As indicated in the Comment column in tables 10.7 through 10.9, we tried to determine for each error why the network might have produced the output it did. In many cases, this output reflected a valid pronunciation present in the training set, but it just didn't happen to be the pronunciation that the list-makers chose. This

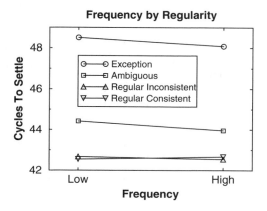

Figure 10.16: Settling time as a function of frequency and consistency of words. Greater frequency and consistency both result in faster settling, but there is an interaction — frequency does not matter for consistent words. This captures pattern seen in human reading latencies.

was particularly true for the Glushko (1979) exception list (for the network and for people); table 10.6 lists the original "raw" performance and the performance where alternate pronunciations are allowed. Also, the McCann and Besner (1987) lists contain two words that have a "j" in the coda, which never occurs in the training set. These words were excluded by PMSP, and we discount them here too. Nevertheless, the network did sometimes get these words correct, though not on the specific testing trial reported here.

Question 10.8 *Can you explain why the present model was sometimes able to pronounce the "j" in the coda correctly, even though none of the training words had a "j" there? (Hint: Think about the effect of translating words over different positions in the input.)*

Naming Latencies

One final aspect of the model that bears on empirical data is its ability to simulate naming latencies as a function of different word features. The features of interest are word *frequency* and *consistency* (as enumerated in table 10.5). The empirical data shows that, as one might expect, higher frequency and more consistent words

are named faster than lower frequency and inconsistent words. However, frequency interacts with consistency, such that the frequency effect decreases with increasing consistency (e.g., highly consistent words are pronounced at pretty much the same speed regardless of their frequency, whereas inconsistent words depend more on their frequency). The PMSP model shows the appropriate naming latency effects (and see that paper for more discussion of the empirical literature).

We assessed the extent to which our model also showed these naming latency effects by recording the average settling time for the words in different frequency and consistency groups (table 10.5). The results are shown in figure 10.16, showing the appropriate main effects of frequency and regularity, plus the critical interaction, whereby the most consistent words do not exhibit a frequency effect. Although the qualitative patterns are correct in our model, the quantitative patterns differ somewhat from those produced by PMSP. For example, exception words are differentially slower in our model relative to the PMSP.

↪ Go to the `PDP++Root` window. To continue on to the next simulation, close this project first by selecting `.projects/Remove/Project_0`. Or, if you wish to stop now, quit by selecting `Object/Quit`.

10.4.3 Summary and Discussion

This model has expanded and elaborated the direct route between orthography and phonology explored previously in the simpler model from section 10.3. Specifically, we have seen how the complex regularities of the spelling to sound mapping in English can be effectively represented using the same representational principles as the invariant object recognition model from chapter 8. Thus, the model places visual word processing within the larger context of visual object recognition.

This model used a single pathway for processing both regular and exception words, in direct contradiction to the traditional dual-route theories. These theories hold that the direct mapping between spelling and sound should only occur for regular words via the application of explicit rules. Nevertheless, this model exhibits significantly poorer performance for low frequency irregulars than other word categories. Thus, if this model

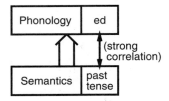

Figure 10.17: Semantics to phonology mapping, showing separable inflectional component that maps a semantic representation of "past tense" onto the regular phonological inflection of "add -ed." The regularity of this mapping produces a strong correlation between these two features.

were incorporated together with an indirect route via semantics, these low frequency irregulars should come to depend more on the indirect route than the direct route represented in this model. This is exactly what was demonstrated in the PMSP model through the use of a simulated semantic pathway. For more discussion of the single versus dual-route debate, see PMSP.

10.5   Overregularization in Past-Tense Inflectional Mappings

In this section we explore a model of the mapping between semantics and phonological output — this is presumably the mapping used when verbally expressing our internal thoughts. For monosyllabic words, the mapping between the semantic representation of a word and its phonology is essentially random, except for those relatively rare cases of onomotopoeia. Thus, the semantics to phonology pathway might not seem that interesting to model, were it not for the issue of **inflectional morphology**. As you probably know, you can change the ending or inflection of a word to convey different aspects of meaning. For example, if you want to indicate that an event occurred in the past, you use the *past tense* inflection (usually adding "-ed") of the relevant verb (e.g., "baked" instead of "bake"). Thus, the semantic representation can include a "tense" component, which gets mapped onto the appropriate inflectional representation in phonology. This idea is illustrated in figure 10.17.

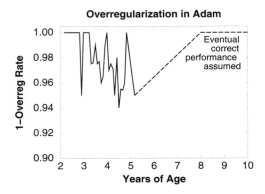

Figure 10.18: U-shaped curve of irregular past-tense inflection production in the child "Adam." The Y axis shows 1 minus the overregularization rate, and the X axis his age. In the beginning, Adam makes no overregularizations, but then, right around age three, he starts to overregularize at a modest rate for at least 2.5 more years. We must assume that at some point he ceases to overregularize with any significant frequency, as represented by the dotted line at the end of the graph.

As in the reading model in the previous section, exceptions to the general rule of "add -ed" exist for the past tense inflection (e.g., "did" instead of "doed," "went" instead of "goed"). Thus, similar issues regarding the processing of the regulars versus the irregulars come up in this domain. These regular and irregular past-tense mappings have played an important and controversial role in the development of neural network models of language.

U-Shaped Curve of Overregularization

At the heart of the controversy is a developmental phenomenon known as the **U-shaped curve** of irregular past-tense inflection due to **overregularization**. In a U-shaped curve, performance is initially good, then gets *worse* (in the middle of the "U"), and then gets better. Many children exhibit a U-shaped curve for producing the correct inflection for irregular verbs — initially they correctly produce the irregular inflection (saying "went," not "goed"), but then they go through a long period where they make overregularizations (inflecting an irregular verb as though it were a regular, "goed" instead of "went"). Finally, they learn to treat the irregulars as irregulars again.

Figure 10.18 shows the overregularization pattern for one of the children (Adam) in the *CHILDES* database of samples of children's speech (MacWhinney & Snow, 1990), which serves as the primary documentation of this phenomenon. As this figure makes clear, the overregularization is not an all-or-nothing phenomenon, as some have mistakenly assumed. Instead, it occurs sporadically, with individual verbs being inflected correctly one moment and overregularized the next, and overall rates of overregularization varying considerably at different points in time (Marcus, Pinker, Ullman, Hollander, Rosen, & Xu, 1992). Nevertheless, at least in a subset of cases, there is clearly an early correct period before any overregularization occurs, and a mature period of subsequent correct performance, with an intervening period where overregularizations are made. We will see that the model behaves in a similar fashion.

Existing Neural Network Models

The overregularization phenomenon was originally interpreted as the result of a rule-based system that gets a bit overzealous early in language acquisition. Then, Rumelhart and McClelland (1986) developed a neural network model that showed a U-shaped overregularization curve, and they argued that it did so because networks are sensitive to regularities in the input-output mapping, and will have a tendency to overregularize. However, Pinker and Prince (1988) pointed out several problems with the Rumelhart and McClelland (1986) model. Perhaps the most troubling was that most of the U-shaped effect was apparently due to a questionable manipulation in the training set. Specifically, a large number of lower-frequency regular words were suddenly introduced after the network had learned a smaller number of high-frequency words that were mostly irregulars. Thus, this sudden onslaught of regular words caused the network to start treating the irregular words like regulars — overregularization.

Although a number of network models of past tense learning have been developed since (Plunkett & Marchman, 1993, 1991; Hoeffner, 1997, 1992; Daugherty & Seidenberg, 1992; Hare & Elman, 1992; MacWhin-

ney & Leinbach, 1991), none has been entirely successful in capturing the essential properties of the U-shaped curve directly in terms of the properties of the network itself, without the need for introducing environmental or other questionable manipulations that do most of the work. For example, the Plunkett and Marchman (1993) model is widely regarded as a fully satisfactory account, but it has several limitations. First, it depends critically on a manipulation of the training environment, which starts out much as in the original Rumelhart and McClelland (1986) model with a small number of high frequency, mostly irregular verbs. Then, instead of adding new verbs all at once, they continuously add them to the training set. This continuous adding of new, mostly regular verbs triggers the overregularization in the network, and does not change the basic problem that the network itself is not driving the overregularization. Furthermore, Hoeffner (1997) was unable to replicate their original results using a more realistic corpus based on English, as opposed to the artificial corpus used in the original model.

One can distinguish two different levels of analysis for understanding the origin of the past-tense U-shaped developmental curve (O'Reilly & Hoeffner, in preparation):

Mechanistic: What kinds of learning/processing mechanisms naturally give rise to a U-shaped learning curve, and more specifically, do neural network models naturally produce such curves, or do they require environmental or "external" manipulations to produce them?

Environmental: What are the actual statistical properties of the linguistic environment that surround this U-shaped learning curve, and is it in fact reasonable to explain this phenomenon largely in terms of these statistics, in conjunction with a relatively generic learning mechanism sensitive to such statistics, (e.g., a neural network).

It should be clear that explanations at either or both of these levels of analysis could potentially account for the observed U-shaped curve phenomenon, but this has not generally been appreciated in the literature, leading to arguments that confuse issues across these levels. Existing neural network models have tended to focus on the environmental level of analysis, while the critiques of these models have emphasized the mechanistic level.

In this section, we explore a model that more directly addresses the critiques by showing that certain mechanistic neural network principles naturally lead to the U-shaped overregularization phenomenon. Specifically, these mechanistic principles are the familiar ones that we have explored throughout this text, including interactivity (bidirectional connectivity), inhibitory competition, and Hebbian learning.

A Competitive, Priming-Based Model

The central intuition behind this approach is that the regular and irregular mappings of a given irregular form are in a state of competition, with the explicit training on the irregular item favoring the irregular form, and all of the training on regular forms conspiring to support the regular inflection. In the presence of interactive, competitive activation dynamics, the regular and irregular mappings can compete as two mutually-exclusive activation states on the time scale of an individual production trial. This activation-based competition makes the network susceptible to priming-like effects (e.g., as explored in chapter 9), where random variations in the prior training history can favor the production of one form over another. For example, a string of regular productions will tend to favor the production of an overregularization for a subsequent irregular form.

The simulations demonstrate that an interactive, competitive network is highly sensitive to these priming-like effects, and by extension show that this results in a high rate of past-tense overregularization in a model of inflectional morphology. Interactivity plays an important role by producing attractor dynamics (chapter 3), where the regular and irregular mappings are two separate attractors, and small changes in the network weights can make relatively large changes in the attractor landscape, leading to an overregularization. These ideas were first developed in small-scale networks such as the weight-priming model explored in chapter 9, and then in the large scale model that we explore here.

Interestingly, almost all previous past-tense models have used standard feedforward backpropagation networks, which lack both interactivity and competition

(see box 5.2 for a summary of the standard feedforward backpropagation algorithm). Such networks react to the competition between the regular and irregular mappings strictly at the level of the weight changes, and not in the activation dynamics taking place on individual trials. These weight changes are slow to accumulate and tend to produce "blends" of two mutually exclusive alternatives instead of choosing discretely between them on a trial-by-trial basis.

Furthermore, the backpropagation learning mechanism is explicitly designed to perform gradient-descent in error, which should produce a monotonically improving, not U-shaped, learning curve for the past tense (Hoeffner, 1997). Thus, when the slowly accumulating weight-based competition is combined with the gradient-descent nature of purely error-driven learning, the backpropagation network's weights tend to monotonically resolve the competition in favor of the explicitly trained irregular form. This results in a monotonically decreasing level of overregularizations, and not a U-shaped curve.

We explore these ideas in a model that instantiates the past tense mapping illustrated in figure 10.17. We compare the results using Leabra with those of a standard backpropagation network to test the idea that Leabra's distinctive features (especially interactivity and inhibitory competition) are important for producing a more realistic U-shaped curve.

10.5.1 Basic Properties of the Model

The model has a semantic input projecting through a hidden layer to the phonological output layer (figure 10.19). The general structure and approach for this model are based on the work of Hoeffner (1997, 1992), which also provided the initial corpus of words for this model. The network is trained to produce the appropriate pronunciation of 389 different monosyllabic English verbs (90 irregulars and 299 regulars) in the past tense and the four other types of inflection in the English verb inflection system, for a total of 1945 training items.

The five different English verb inflections are shown in table 10.10. These inflections convey extra semantic information about each verb. Thus, the semantic input for the model has two main components (fig-

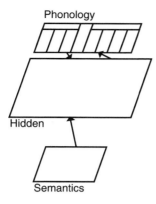

Figure 10.19: Past tense network, mapping from semantics to phonology.

Inflection	Reg sfx	Regular/Irregular examples
Base	–	I walk to the store daily.
		I go to the store daily.
Past	-ed	I walked to the store yesterday.
		I went to the store yesterday.
3rd pers sing	-s	She walks to the store daily.
		She goes to the store daily.
Progressive	-ing	I am walking to the store now.
		I am going to the store now.
Past participle	-en	I have walked to the store before.
		I have gone to the store now.

Table 10.10: The five inflectional forms of English verbs.

ure 10.17), a "core" semantic pattern that represents the basic meaning of the verb that is constant across all the inflections (e.g., the basic conception of walking), and an inflectional component that represents one of the five senses of the verb. No attempt was made to accurately represent the core semantics, because the mapping between them and phonology is largely random anyway. Thus, random bit patterns are used across the first 100 units of the semantic layer to encode the core pattern, and sequential groups of 4 units are used to represent each of the 5 inflections over the next 20 units, for a total of 120 semantic input units.

The phonology representations are the standard vowel-centered repeating consonant ones described in

section 10.2.2, with one additional slot at the end to accommodate an additional inflectional phoneme when needed. To highlight the inflectional component for the purposes of human decoding of output, we also included four extra phonemes to represent the inflections that occurred in this last slot — /D/ for -ed (same features as /d/), /G/ for -ing (combination of /n/ and /g/), /Z/ (same features as /z/) for the 3rd person singular when it sounds more like a /z/ (e.g., changes), and /P/ (past participle) for -en (same features as /n/).

As in the previous simulation, the words are presented with the square root of their actual Francis and Kučera (1982) frequency. There are 400 hidden units, with 7.5 percent percent active at a time. This level of sparseness is useful for learning the arbitrary mapping between semantics and phonology, due to the need to keep the different patterns relatively separate (as we saw in chapter 9, sparseness produces pattern separation). The Hebbian learning magnitude is .001. We also ran a network with pure error-driven learning and a generic backpropagation network for comparison, as discussed later.

10.5.2 Exploring the Model

[Note: this simulation requires a minimum of 64Mb of RAM to run.]

↪ Open the project `pt.proj.gz` in `chapter_10` to begin.

Again, the project is large and takes a long time to train, so it is stored with the network in skeleton form, and we have to build it and load pretrained weights.

↪ Do `LoadNet` in the `pt_ctrl` overall control panel.

This network has already been through the U-shaped overregularization period and is generally producing correct outputs for all the words.

To start, we will just observe the network as it produces phonological outputs from semantic patterns.

↪ Do `StepTest`.

You can see the semantic input being presented, and the network settling produces an activation pattern over the phonological output. This is the word "be" in the base form, but you wouldn't know that just by looking at the activations. We can open up a text log to see the translation of the input/output patterns.

↪   Do `View`, `TEST_LOG`, which brings up the `Trial_1_TextLog`. Press the full-forward (>|) VCR button on the top to see the previous trial.

The translation of the actual output produced is shown in the `output` column, and the identity of the input pattern is shown in column `Event`.

The event is coded by an initial number representing the index (0 to 388) of the verb, followed by its target pronunciation, followed by a code indicating inflection type (1–5 in the order of table 10.10) and the regularity status of the verb (1 = irregular, 2 = regular). Thus, the 11 here represents the base inflection of an irregular verb. You can also see that there were no errors (`sum_se` is 0), and that the network took 30 cycles to produce the output.

Looking back at the network, notice the 4 active units next to each other in the second to last row of the semantic input. These 4 units indicate that the base inflection is to be produced. When you step to the next word, you will see that the 4 units adjacent to the previous 4 are now activated, indicating the past inflection is to be produced (i.e., "was" in this case).

↪ `StepTest` to "was," and then continue to `StepTest` through the remaining inflections of this verb ("is," "being," and "been").

Now, let's skip to a regular word, "care" (/kAr/), and see all five of its inflections (i.e., "care," "cared," "cares," "caring," and "cared").

↪   Press the `GoTo` button and enter in 600. Then, `StepTest` through the 5 inflections.

Now that we can see that the network has learned the task, let's try to analyze some of the connectivity to determine how it is working. Because we are most interested in the past-tense mapping, we will focus on that first. To find out which hidden units are most selective for the past-tense inflectional semantics, we will look at the sending weights from the past-tense inflectional semantics units to the hidden layer.

↪ Click on `s.wt` in the network (sending weights), and then click on the first past-tense inflectional semantics unit (fifth unit from the left in the second-to-last row).

One interesting question is whether there is consistency in these weights across all 4 past-tense inflection units — we would expect this from Hebbian learning, but not necessarily in a purely error-driven network that

does not produce consistent weight patterns (chapter 6).
↪ Click on the 3 adjacent past-tense units to the right of the previous one.

You should observe that indeed the sending weight patterns are quite consistent. You can also check that the other inflectional semantics units consistently tend to activate a different set of hidden units (except the past participle seems to activate a subset of the same units activated by the past-tense units).

↪ Click on all the other inflectional semantics units and observe the sending weight patterns to the hidden layer.

Now, let's go back to the first past tense inflectional unit and mark the most strongly connected hidden units for subsequent probing. We do this by selecting units according to the strength of the weights.

↪ Press `Selections/Select Units` in the network window (right hand side menu). In the popup window, type in `s.wt` for the `variable`, select > for the relationship (`rel`), and .5 for the comparison value (`cmp_val`).

You should see the three "brightest" hidden units are now selected. We will try to interpret the weights for one of these units.

↪   Click on the second from the left of the three selected hidden units.

You can now see the sending weights for this unit — you should see that this unit doesn't favor any particular onset phonemes (all are uniformly weighted), but it has a clear pattern of weighting for particular coda phonemes. Let's try to interpret the pattern of weighting for the last non-inflection coda slot (second from the last slot, where each slot is 2 columns wide), which is where the regular past-tense inflection ("-ed," pronounced with either a /t/ or /d/ phoneme) is expressed. We can compare the consonant patterns for these phonemes with the weight pattern.

↪ Press `View` button on the `pt_ctrl` control panel, and select `CONSONANTS`. Click on the `t` and then with the middle button (or shift and left button) on `d` and `n`.

You should see that the pattern of weights is consistent with the idea that this past-tense hidden unit produces the regular "-ed" inflection. It is not immediately clear why the /n/ phoneme is also supported by the weights, but it could just be because it is very similar overall to the /t/ and /d/ phonemes. Next, we can look at the final inflectional phoneme slot.

↪ Press `View` again and select `INFLECTIONS`. Click on the `D` event button (for the /D/ inflectional phoneme) on the left side of the window, and also the `-` button for the blank pattern.

By comparing these patterns with the weights in the last slot, you can see that the unit codes for either the `D` inflection (equivalent to `d`) or the blank. Therefore, it is very clear that this unit plays an important role in producing the regular past tense inflection. Presumably, other units that compete with these units get more activated by the irregular words, and thus are able to suppress the regular inflection. It is the sensitive dynamics of this kind of competition as the network settles that contributes to a relatively strong U-shaped overregularization curve, as we will see.

↪ Analyze the production of the progressive *-ing* inflection, using using the same technique we just used for the past tense inflection (the *-ing* inflectional semantics start at the third unit from the left in the last row).

Question 10.9 (a) *Do the most active units code for the appropriate inflectional phonological pattern?* **(b)** *Describe the steps you took to reach this answer.*

Although it is interesting to see something about how the network has learned this task, the most relevant empirical data is in the time-course of its overregularizations during training. We automatically scored the phonological output from the network for each trial as it learned, looking for overregularizations of irregular past tense words, in addition to a number of other patterns of output that are not discussed here (see the files `pt_all.css` and `pt_words_all_full.list` for details).

Figure 10.20 shows the plot of overregularizations for both the Leabra network we have just been exploring and a standard feedforward backpropagation network (Bp) run on the same task. Note that, following convention, overregularization is plotted as 1 minus the proportion of overregularization errors, which gives the characteristic U-shape that is evident in the graph. The plots also show the proportion of phonologically valid responses that the network made for past-tense verbs, which is important for evaluating when overregularizations occur relative to any period of early correct responding.

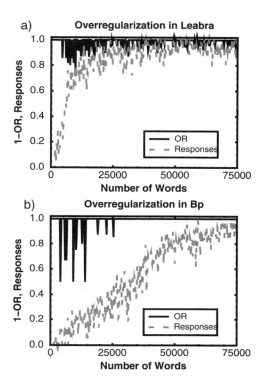

Figure 10.20: Plot of overregularizations and total responses as the network learns for (a) Leabra and (b) backpropagation (Bp). In Leabra there is a clear initial period where overregularizations are absent, but the network is producing valid responses for up to 50 percent of the past-tense verbs, but this is not present in the Bp network. Then, overregularization in Leabra (plotted as 1 minus the number of overregularizations) begins and continues at a low sporadic rate for an extended period, whereas overregularization in Bp is resolved relatively quickly. Thus, the Leabra network, but not Bp, provides a reasonable fit to the developmental data.

There are two critical U-shaped curve features that are evident in the comparison between the Leabra and Bp networks. First, the Leabra network achieves a substantial level (around 50%) of responding prior to the onset of overregularization. Thus, the network demonstrates an early-correct period of irregular verb production, where irregular verbs are being produced without overregularization errors. This is the critical aspect of the empirical data that previous models have failed to capture without questionable manipulations of the training corpus or other parameters. These other models look more like the Bp network in the figure, with overregularization beginning quite early relative to the level of responding. Furthermore, increasing the learning rate in Bp uniformly advances both responding and overregularization, preserving the same basic relationship.

The second critical feature is the overall level of overregularization and its tendency to continue on at a low, sporadic rate over an extended period of time, which is an important characteristic of the human data. The Leabra network shows this characteristic, but the Bp network exhibits a rapidly resolving overregularization period, consistent with the purely gradient-descent nature of Bp. The extended overregularizations in Leabra can be attributed to a dynamic competition between the regular and irregular mappings that is played out on each settling trial, and is affected by small weight changes that effectively prime the regular mapping (O'Reilly & Hoeffner, in preparation). Thus, during a protracted period of learning, the Leabra network is dynamically balanced on the "edge" between the regular and irregular mappings, and can easily shift between them, producing the characteristic low rate of sporadic overregularizations.

To provide a more representative quantitative assessment of these two critical features, O'Reilly and Hoeffner (in preparation) ran 25 random networks through the early correct period and recorded the number of valid responses to past-tense irregulars prior to the first and second overregularization (figure 10.21). Again, a standard backpropagation (Bp) network was compared with Leabra, with three different levels of Hebbian learning: none (H0), .001 (as explored above), and .005. The results confirm that Leabra exhibits a significantly more substantial early correct period compared to Bp, and further shows that Hebbian learning has little effect either way.

O'Reilly and Hoeffner (in preparation) also ran 5 of each type of network for a full 300 epoch period and counted the total number of overregularizations produced (figure 10.22). This also confirms our previous single-network results — the interactivity and inhibitory competition in Leabra facilitate a dynamic

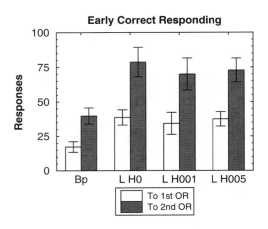

Figure 10.21: Total number of phonologically valid responses made by the network ($N = 25$) to past-tense irregulars prior to the first and second overregularization, for four different networks: backpropagation (Bp) and Leabra (L) with three levels of Hebbian learning, none (H0), .001, and .005. This provides a measure of the extent of the early correct period prior to the onset of overregularization. The interactivity and inhibitory competition in Leabra appear to contribute significantly relative to a generic backpropagation network (Bp), but Hebbian learning does not seem to have a strong effect either way.

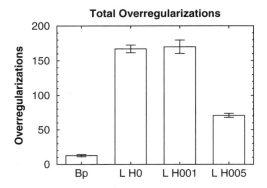

Figure 10.22: Total number of overregularizations made over training for same networks as in the previous figure ($N = 5$). As before, there is a main effect of Leabra versus backpropagation (Bp), with Leabra producing a substantially larger number of overregularizations. Too much Hebbian learning (.005) reduces the overregularization in Leabra, but smaller amounts have no effect.

priming-like overregularization phenomenon that is absent in the feedforward backpropagation network (Bp). Again, Hebbian learning does not increase the effect, and here we find that with a larger Hebbian level (.005), overregularization is actually decreased.

The null or detrimental effects of Hebbian learning in this large-scale model are somewhat inconsistent with smaller-scale models of the dynamic competition and priming account of overregularization as explored by O'Reilly and Hoeffner (in preparation). Nevertheless, it is clear that the major effect here is in the activation dynamics that facilitate the competition between the irregular and regular mappings, and although Hebbian learning does not facilitate the effects, it does facilitate our ability to interpret the network's weights as we did above. The impairment in overregularizations with larger amounts of Hebbian learning (.005) can be attributed to its tendency to differentiate (cluster separately, see chapter 4) the irregular and regular mappings such that overregularization becomes less likely.

↪ Go to the `PDP++Root` window. To continue on to the next simulation, close this project first by selecting `.projects/Remove/Project_0`. Or, if you wish to stop now, quit by selecting `Object/Quit`.

10.5.3   *Summary and Discussion*

This exploration shows that two important mechanistic principles of activation flow incorporated into the Leabra model, interactivity and inhibitory competition, produce a reasonable account of the developmental U-shaped overregularization curve in terms of competition between the irregular and regular mappings and priming-like effects from the regular mapping that lead to overregularizations (O'Reilly & Hoeffner, in preparation). The Leabra network exhibits both a more substantial early correct responding period, and a much more extended overregularization period with many more total overregularizations, as compared to the kind of feedforward backpropagation network used in most previous models.

However, despite these encouraging findings, a more detailed and rigorous evaluation of the model's fit to the human data is complicated by several factors. First, the human data are woefully underspecified, with lon-

gitudinal data available for only a handful of cases, and recording starting well after the onset of language production. Thus, it is difficult to determine if a U-shaped curve is truly universal, or is just seen in a subset of individuals (Hoeffner, 1997).

Second, it is difficult to achieve a valid mapping between network learning rates and human learning rates. The network is completely focused on acquiring the semantics to phonology mapping on each trial, and it learns exceedingly rapidly compared with children. For example, the network achieved well over 90 percent valid responding to irregular pasts after only 25,000 trials of training.

It is difficult to know how to map the model's trials onto a child's learning experience. For example, if we assume that the child is exposed to at most 8 minutes of speech per day (at a rate of one word per second) that contributes to their learning of semantics to phonology, the equivalent time period to achieve 90 percent valid responding for the child would amount to only 52 days! The entire time span of the U-shaped curve in the network, and complete mastery of the corpus (roughly 75,000 trials), would be just 156 days, rather than the years observed empirically. Although one could apply some kind of generic scaling to the network's performance, it is likely that a major part of the difference is due to the complexity and subtlety of the larger language acquisition task that the child is performing. Thus, it is probably premature to expect these relatively simple models to provide a detailed chronological picture.

Finally, one advantage of the above model relative to others in the literature is that it uses a completely static training environment. The network's gradual learning of this environment results in a gradual expansion of its productive vocabulary, which is a nice contrast to the external imposition of this expansion by the researcher. Nevertheless, a child's semantic representations are gradually developing during this same time period, and this may place important constraints on the learning process that are not reflected in our static model.

Thus, probably the best interpretation of this model is that it demonstrates that a network with a static environment *can* exhibit a U-shaped curve, and that it does so

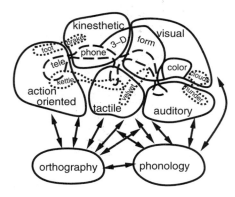

Figure 10.23: Illustration of how semantic information might be distributed across a number of more specific processing pathways, represented here by different sensory modalities. Linguistic representations (orthography, phonology) are associated with corresponding distributed activation patterns across semantics. Figure adapted from Allport, 1985.

using the mechanistic principles in Leabra that are well motivated for a number of other reasons. The complexity of the model and the task(s) it performs may need to be increased to better fit the human data.

10.6 Semantic Representations from Word Co-occurrences and Hebbian Learning

Our next model explores the development of the semantic representation component of the distributed lexicon framework based on statistical properties of the linguistic inputs. As discussed in chapter 7, semantic representations, like word representations, are viewed as distributed throughout various specialized brain areas. This notion of distributed semantics is well captured by figure 10.23, adapted from Allport (1985), which shows the representations of various items (a telephone, velvet, etc.) across several different specialized processing pathways. Although these pathways are represented only by sensory modality in the figure, a number of other types of specializations (e.g., chronological, sequential, task-oriented, episodic, etc.) probably also contribute to the overall distributed representation of an item. Indeed, essentially any pattern of activity anywhere in the brain that contributes some item-specific

information could be considered a semantic representation.

One influential neural network model of human semantic representations (Farah & McClelland, 1991) used basic neural network principles to explain a somewhat puzzling pattern of dissociations across patients with different kinds of semantic deficits. The dissociations involve selective deficits for knowledge about living things versus nonliving things. Different groups of patients have deficits in one of these categories, but are relatively spared in the other (i.e., a *double-dissociation*; Warrington & Shallice, 1984; Warrington & McCarthy, 1983, 1987). One natural conclusion from this data is that human semantic information is organized according to the kinds of taxonomic categories that one might use in playing 20 questions: e.g., animal, vegetable, or mineral/man-made (Hillis & Caramazza, 1991).

Alternatively, as first proposed by Warrington and colleagues and subsequently elaborated by Farah and McClelland (1991), category-specific semantic deficits might arise based on the *sensory* versus *functional* associations with living versus nonliving things. People predominantly list sensory features when describing living things (e.g., "brown," "large" for a bear), and functional features when describing tools and other artifacts (e.g., "used for pounding in nails" for a hammer) (Farah & McClelland, 1991). Thus, the living-thing deficit could be explained by damage to sensory semantic areas, and the nonliving-thing deficit could be explained by damage to functional semantic areas. This account is much more consistent with the kind of distributed semantics envisioned in figure 10.23, which builds off of the well-known specialization of brain areas for different sensory modalities.

The simulation of this sensory–functional idea not only captured the basic dissociation between living and nonliving things, it also resolved an apparent difficulty for this approach quite naturally. Specifically, the verbal (non-implemented) sensory–functional account appeared to mistakenly predict that patients with the living-thing deficit should still show intact functional semantics for living things (whereas patients with the nonliving-thing deficit should still show intact sensory semantics for nonliving things). This pattern does not appear to hold in the patients, however. The model implementing the sensory–functional idea demonstrated that the kinds of mutual support dynamics that emerge from bidirectionally connected neural networks (chapter 3) can account for this effect: after the functional semantics associated with living things lost their mutual support from the previously stronger sensory semantics representations, they became much more difficult to activate and therefore showed an impairment, even though the functional representations themselves were intact. In summary, the Farah and McClelland (1991) model showed how distributed semantic representations can exhibit counterintuitive dynamics under damage, in a manner consistent with the observed neuropsychological data.

The Farah and McClelland (1991) model is consistent with all the basic principles of our framework, but it does not address the question of how semantic representations develop from experience in the first place, and it cannot be easily probed using our own common-sense intuitions about semantics because it used random semantic patterns (much like we did above in the past-tense model). Therefore, we instead explore a model that implements just one piece of the larger distributed semantic network but allows us to see how semantic representations can develop in the first place, and to explore the properties of these representations using our own familiar intuitions about semantic meaning.

The semantic representations in our model emerge from simply accumulating information about which words tend to occur together in speech or reading. This model is based on the ideas of Landauer and Dumais (1997), who have developed a method they call *latent semantic analysis* or *LSA* that is based on computing the principal components (using a variant of PCA; see chapter 4) of word co-occurrence statistics. They have shown that just this co-occurrence information can yield semantic representations that do a surprisingly good job at mimicking human semantic judgments.

For example, an LSA system trained on the text of a psychology textbook was able to get a passing grade on a multiple choice exam based on the text. Although the performance (roughly 65–70% correct) was well short of that of a good student, it is nonetheless surprising that a simple automated procedure can perform as well as it does. LSA has also been used to perform automated essay grading, by comparing the semantic representation of a student's essay with those of various reference essays that have received different human grades. The correlation between grades assigned by LSA and those of human graders was the same as that between different human graders.

The word co-occurrence approach captures word *association* semantics, not just *definitional* semantics. For example, the definition of the word "bread" has nothing to do with the word "butter," but these two words are highly linked associationally. It appears that these associational links are important for capturing the structure of human semantic memory. For example, in semantic priming studies, the word "butter" is read faster when preceded by the word "bread" than when preceded by an unrelated word (e.g., "locomotive").

As you might expect from chapter 4, Hebbian model learning provides a natural mechanism for learning word co-occurrence statistics. Indeed, CPCA Hebbian learning is closely related to the the sequential principal components analysis (SPCA) technique that the LSA method is based on. Interestingly, the network and training we use here are essentially identical to those used in the Hebbian model of receptive field development in the early visual system, as described in chapter 8. In both of these models, the network extracts the reliable correlations from naturalistic input stimuli using a simple Hebbian learning mechanism.

This type of learning requires a sufficiently large sample of text for the extraction of useful statistics about which words tend to co-occur. A particularly convenient source of such text is this textbook itself! So, we trained a simple CPCA Hebbian network by having it "read" an earlier draft of this textbook paragraph-by-paragraph, causing it to represent the systematic patterns of co-occurrence among the words. In the following exploration, we then probe the resulting network to see if it has captured important aspects of the information presented in this text.

One of the most important themes that emerges from this exploration, which is highly relevant for the larger distributed semantics framework, is the power of distributed representations to capture the complexity of semantic information. We will see that the distributed and

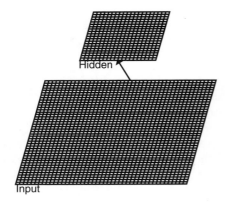

Figure 10.24: Semantic network, with the input having one unit per word. For training, all the words in a paragraph of text are activated, and CPCA Hebbian learning takes place on the resulting hidden layer activations.

competitive activation dynamics in the network can perform multiple constraint satisfaction to settle on a pattern of activity that captures the meaning of arbitrary groups of words, including interactions between words that give rise to different shades of meaning. Thus, the combinatorics of the distributed representation, with the appropriate dynamics, allow a huge and complex space of semantic information to be efficiently represented.

10.6.1   Basic Properties of the Model

The model has an input layer with one unit per word (1920 words total), that projects to a hidden layer containing 400 units (figure 10.24). On a given training trial, all of the units representing the words present in one individual paragraph are activated, and the network settles on a hidden activation pattern as a function of this input. If two words reliably appear together within a paragraph, they will be semantically linked by the network. It is also possible to consider smaller grouping units (e.g., sentences) and larger ones (passages), but paragraph-level grouping has proven effective in the LSA models. After the network settles on one paragraph's worth of words, CPCA Hebbian learning takes place, encoding the conditional probability that the input units are active given that the hidden units are. This process is repeated by cycling through all the para-

graphs in the text multiple times.

The development of effective semantic representations in the network depends on the fact that whenever two similar input patterns are presented, similar hidden units will likely be activated. These hidden layer representations should thus encode any reliable correlations across subsets of words. Furthermore, the network will even learn about two words that have similar meanings, but that do not happen to appear together in the same paragraph. Because these words are likely to co-occur with similar other words, both will activate a common subset of hidden units. These hidden units will learn a similar (high) conditional probability for both words. Thus, when each of these words is presented alone to the network, they will produce similar hidden activation patterns, indicating that they are semantically related.

To keep the network a manageable size, we filtered the text before presenting it to the network, thereby reducing the total number of words represented in the input layer. Two different types of filtering were performed, eliminating the least informative words: high-frequency noncontent words and low frequency words. The high-frequency noncontent words primarily have a syntactic role, such as determiners (e.g., "the," "a," "an"), conjunctions ("and," "or," etc.), pronouns and their possessives ("it," "his," etc.), prepositions ("above," "about," etc.), and qualifiers ("may," "can," etc.). We also filtered transition words like "however" and "because," high-frequency verbs ("is," "have," "do," "make," "use," and "give"), and number words ("one," "two," etc.). The full list of filtered words can be found in the file `sem_filter.lg.list` (the "lg" designates that this is a relatively large list of high-frequency words to filter) in the `chapter_10` directory where the simulations are.

The low-frequency filtering removed any word that occurred five or fewer times in the entire text. Repetitions of a word within a single paragraph contributed only once to this frequency measure, because only the single word unit can be active in the network even if it occurs multiple times within a paragraph. The frequencies of the words in this text are listed in the file `eccn_lg_f5.freq`, and a summary count of the number of words at the lower frequencies (1–10) is given in the file `eccn_lg_f5.freq_cnt`. The actual filtered text itself is in `eccn_lg_f5.cln`, providing a sense of the "telegraphic" nature of the input the network receives.

In addition, the network has no sense of word order or any other syntactic information, so it is really operating at the level of the "gist." That the network is operating on such minimal input makes its performance all the more impressive. Nevertheless, achieving substantially better levels of comprehension will likely require a substantially more complex network that processes more of the information available in real texts.

10.6.2 Exploring the Model

[Note: this simulation requires a minimum of 128Mb of RAM to run.]

↪ Open the project `sem.proj.gz` in `chapter_10` to begin.

As before, the network is a skeleton, and must be built and trained weights loaded.

↪ Do `LoadNet` on the `sem_ctrl` control panel.

Individual Unit Representations

To start, let's examine the weights of individual units in the network.

↪ Select `r.wt`, and then select various hidden units at random to view.

You should observe sparse patterns of weights, with different units picking up on different patterns of words in the input. However, because the input units are too small to be labeled, you can't really tell which words a given unit is activated by. The `GetWordRF` button (get receptive field in terms of words) on the `sem_ctrl` control panel provides a work-around to this problem.

↪ View the weights for the lower-leftmost hidden unit, and then hit the `GetWordRF` button.

A `String_Array` window will pop up, containing an alphabetized list of the words that this hidden unit receives from with a weight above the `rf_thresh` of .5 (table 10.11). You can resize this window to see more of the words at one time, and you can use the middle mouse button to scroll the text within one field.

One of the most interesting things to notice here is that the unit represents multiple roughly synonymous

act activation activations algorithm allow already approaches arbitrary areas argue artificial aspect assess atoms balance based basic behavior bias biological biologically biology bit body calcium called capable categories cell channel channels charge chl closed cognition combination combine complicated components computational compute computed concentrations conductance confused consider consistent constantly contain continuous correlations corresponding cpca critical cross current currents demands derivative described detailed detector detectors determined difference different diffusion discussed divide division electrical electricity emphasize encoded enter environment equal equation etc exceeds excitatory explain extent family fast favor fires firing flow follow forces form function functioning generally generec hand hebbian help hypothesis identify imagine implement implementing important include including inconsistent indicated individual influence information inhibitory input inputs integrates integrating integration interactivity interested ion ions kind labor language largely last later leak learning leaving let level likelihood liquid magnitude major manner matches mathematically matter mechanisms membrane memories minus model modeling models modification movement name need negative net network networks neural neuron neurons non notice now number numbers occur open opened opposite oriented parallel pass pattern phase phonology picture plus positive possibly potassium potential practical prevents principles processing properties purposes put rapid rate reasons recall referred reflected reflects relevant remains research responding result rule same saw say see sends separate showed shown sign simple slow soft special specific specifically states strongest suggested summarized summary survival synaptic textbook things think threshold time times towards tradeoff turn type types typically understanding updated variable versa version via vice voltage vowel weights work world writing

Table 10.11: List of words with weights > .5 for the lower-leftmost hidden unit, as produced by the `GetWordRF` button.

terms. For example, you should see the words "act," "activation," and "activations," in the fields numbered 0–2 in the window. By scrolling through this list you should see many more examples of this.

Question 10.10 *List some other examples of roughly synonymous terms represented by this unit.*

This property of the representation is interesting for two reasons. First, it indicates that the representations are doing something sensible, in that semantically related words are represented by the same unit. Second, these synonyms probably do not occur together in the same paragraph very often. Typically, only one version of a given word is used in a given context. For example, "The activity of the unit is..." may appear in one paragraph, while "The unit's activation was..." may appear in another. Thus, for such representations to develop, it must be based on the similarity in the general contexts in which similar words appear (e.g., the co-occurrence of "activity" and "activation" with "unit" in the previous example). This generalization of the semantic similarity structure across paragraphs is essential to enable the network to transcend rote memorization of the text itself, and produce representations that will be effective for processing novel text items.

↪ View the `GetWordRF` representations for several other units to get a sense of the general patterns across units.

Although there clearly is sensible semantic structure at a local level within the individual-unit representations, it should also be clear that there is no single, coherent theme relating all of the words represented by a given unit. Thus, individual units participate in representing many different clusters of semantic structure, and it is only in the aggregate patterns of activity across many units that more coherent representations emerge. This network thus provides an excellent example of distributed representation.

Distributed Representations via Sending Weights

A more appropriate technique for exploring the nature of the distributed semantic representations is to look at the sending weights from a given word to the hidden layer. This will show the pattern of hidden units that represent that word, and by doing this for multiple different words, we can get a sense of how many hidden units the words have in common. In other words, we can look at distributed pattern overlap as a measure of the similarity structure (as discussed in chapter 3).

↪ Press `SelWord` on the `sem_ctrl` control panel. Enter "attention" as the word, and click both the `view` and `selwts` buttons on.

This will allow us to view the weights for the input unit corresponding to the word "attention," and it will select all of the hidden units which have a weight value greater than the `rf_thresh` of .5.

↪ You have to select `s.wt` in the network to actually view the sending weights.

You should see a pattern of hidden units that have strong weights from this word unit, with the strongest units selected (indicated by the white dashed line surrounding the unit). By itself, this pattern is not very meaningful. However, we can now compare the pattern with that of another, related word.

↪ Do `SelWord` again, but enter in "binding" as the word this time, and click the `selwts` button off.

Event	attenti	binding	dyslexi
attention	1	0.415	0.090
binding	0.415	1	0.118
dyslexia	0.090	0.118	1

Table 10.12: Cosine matrix of the hidden representations for the words "attention," "binding," and "dyslexia".

By turning `selwts` off, we ensure that the previously selected units from "attention" will remain so. Now, you should be able to see that in several cases, the strong weights for "binding" overlap with those of the selected units from "attention." Thus, these overlapping units represent both of these concepts, as one might expect given that they have a clear semantic relationship. Now let's see what a more unrelated word looks like.

↪ Do `SelWord` again, and enter "dyslexia" as the word, and keep the other buttons as they are.

You should now observe considerably less overlap among the strong weights from "dyslexia" and the selected units from "attention," which is appropriate given that these words are not as closely related.

The `SelWord` process can be performed automatically for two different words by using the `PairProbe` button. The first word's weights will be selected, and the second word's weights will be viewed as color values.

↪ Do some `PairProbe`s for other word pairs that you expect to be semantically related in this textbook, and pairs that you expect to be unrelated.

Summarizing Similarity with Cosines

Instead of just eyeballing the pattern overlap, we can compute a numerical measure of similarity using *normalized inner products* or *cosines* between pairs of sending weight patterns (see equation 10.1 from the dyslexia model in section 10.3). The `WordMatrix` button does this computation automatically for a list of words (separated by spaces), producing a matrix of all pairwise cosines, and a cluster plot of this distance matrix.

↪ Do `WordMatrix`, and enter "attention binding dyslexia" as the words.

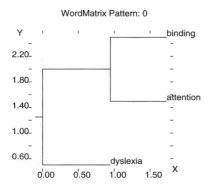

Figure 10.25: Cluster plot of the similarity structure for attention, binding, and dyslexia as produced by the `WordMatrix` function.

You should replicate the same basic effect we saw above — attention and binding are more closely related to each other than they are to dyslexia. This can be seen in the cluster plot (figure 10.25) by noting that attention and binding are clustered together. The cosine matrix appears in the terminal window where you started the program (it should look like table 10.12). Here, you can see that the cosine between "attention" and "binding" is .415, (relatively high), while that of "attention" and "dyslexia" is only .090, and that between "binding" and "dyslexia" is only .118.

↪ Do a `WordMatrix` for several other words that the network should know about from "reading" this textbook.

Question 10.11 (a) *Report the cluster plot and cosine matrix results.* **(b)** *Comment on how well this matches your intuitive semantics from having read this textbook yourself.*

Distributed Representations via Activity Patterns

To this point we have only used the patterns of weights to the hidden units to determine how similar the semantic representations of different words are. We can also use the actual pattern of activation produced over the hidden layer as a measure of semantic similarity. This is important because it allows us to present multiple word inputs at the same time, and have the network choose a hidden layer representation that best fits this combination of words. Thus, novel semantic representations can be produced as combinations of semantic representations for individual words. This ability is critical for some of the more interesting and powerful applications of these semantic representations (e.g., multiple choice question answering, essay grading, etc.).

The `ActProbe` function can be used to do this activation-based probing of the semantic representations.

↪ Select `act` in the network window. Press `ActProbe` on the `sem_ctrl` control panel, and you will be prompted for two sets of words. Let's start with the same example we have used before, entering "attention" for the first word set, and "binding" for the second.

You should see the network activations updating as the word inputs are presented. The result pops up in a window, showing the cosine between the hidden activation patterns for the two sets of words. Notice that this cosine is lower than that produced by the weight-based analysis of the `WordMatrix` function. This can happen due to the activation dynamics, which can either magnify or minimize the differences present in the weights.

Next, let's use `ActProbe` to see how we can sway an otherwise somewhat ambiguous term to be interpreted in a particular way. For example, the term "attention" can be used in two somewhat different contexts. One context concerns the implementational aspects of attention, most closely associated with "competition." Another context concerns the use of attention to solve the binding problem, that is associated with "invariant object recognition." Let's begin this exploration by first establishing the baseline association between "attention" and "invariant object recognition."

↪ Do an `ActProbe` with "attention" as the first word set, and "invariant object recognition" as the second.

You should get a cosine of around .302. Now, let's see if adding "binding" in addition to "attention" increases the hidden layer similarity.

↪ Do an `ActProbe` with "attention binding" as the first word set, and "invariant object recognition" again as the second.

The similarity does indeed increase, producing a cosine of around .326. To make sure that there is an interaction between "attention" and "binding" producing this increase, we need to test with "binding" alone.

↪ Do an `ActProbe` with "binding" as the first word set, and "invariant object recognition" again as the second.

The similarity drops back to .288. Thus, there is something special about the combination of "attention" and "binding" together that is not present by using each of them alone. Now if we instead probe with "attention competition" as compared to "invariant object recognition," we should activate a different sense of attention, and get a smaller cosine.

↪ Do an `ActProbe` with "attention competition" as the first word set, and "invariant object recognition" again as the second.

The similarity does now decrease, with a cosine of only around .114. Thus, we can see that the network's activation dynamics can be influenced to emphasize different senses of a word. Thus, this is potentially a very powerful and flexible form of semantic representation that combines rich, overlapping distributed representations and activation dynamics that can magnify or diminish the similarities of different word combinations.

Question 10.12 *Think of another example of a word that has different senses (that is well represented in this textbook), and perform an experiment similar to the one we just performed to manipulate these different senses. Document and discuss your results.*

A Multiple-Choice Quiz

Finally, we can run an automated multiple-choice quiz on the network. We created ten multiple-choice questions, shown in table 10.13. Note the telegraphic form of the quiz, as it contains only the content words that the network was actually trained on. The best answer is always *A*, and *B* was designed to be a plausible foil, while *C* is obviously unrelated (unlike people, the network can't pick up on these regularities across test items). The quiz is presented to the network by first presenting the "question," recording the resulting hidden activation pattern, and then presenting each possible answer and computing the cosine of the resulting hidden activation with that of the question. The answer that has the closest cosine is chosen as the network's answer.

0.	neural activation function
A	spiking rate code membrane potential point
B	interactive bidirectional feedforward
C	language generalization nonwords
1.	transformation
A	emphasizing distinctions collapsing differences
B	error driven hebbian task model based
C	spiking rate code membrane potential point
2.	bidirectional connectivity
A	amplification pattern completion
B	competition inhibition selection binding
C	language generalization nonwords
3.	cortex learning
A	error driven task based hebbian model
B	error driven task based
C	gradual feature conjunction spatial invariance
4.	object recognition
A	gradual feature conjunction spatial invariance
B	error driven task based hebbian model
C	amplification pattern completion
5.	attention
A	competition inhibition selection binding
B	gradual feature conjunction spatial invariance
C	spiking rate code membrane potential point
6.	weight based priming
A	long term changes learning
B	active maintenance short term residual
C	fast arbitrary details conjunctive
7.	hippocampus learning
A	fast arbitrary details conjunctive
B	slow integration general structure
C	error driven hebbian task model based
8.	dyslexia
A	surface deep phonological reading problem damage
B	speech output hearing language nonwords
C	competition inhibition selection binding
9.	past tense
A	overregularization shaped curve
B	speech output hearing language nonwords
C	fast arbitrary details conjunctive

Table 10.13: Multiple-choice quiz given to the network based on this text. The network compares the activation pattern for each answer with that of the question and selects the closest fitting one.

↪ To run the quiz, first open up a log by doing `View`, `QUIZ_LOG`. Then, open up a process control panel by doing `View`, `QUIZ_PROCESS_CTRL`. The `NEpoch_2` process control panel will appear. Do a `ReInit` and a `Step`.

This presents the first question to the network ("neural activation function").

↪ `Step` 3 more times for each of the possible answers.

After the last step, you should see the `Epoch_2_TextLog` update, with a record of the cosine distances for each of the answers compared to the question, and the answer that the network came up with (*B* in this case, though the correct answer *A* was considerably closer than the clearly wrong answer, *C*). Now let's just run through the rest of the quiz.

↪ Turn off the network `Display` toggle (upper left-hand corner of the NetView), and `Run` the `NEpoch_2` process through the remainder of the quiz.

You should observe that the network does OK, but not exceptionally — 60–80 percent performance is typical. Usually, the network does a pretty good job of rejecting the obviously unrelated answer *C*, but it does not always match our sense of *A* being better than *B*. In question 6, the *B* phrase was often mentioned in the context of the question phrase, but as a *contrast* to it, not a similarity. Because the network does not have the syntactic knowledge to pick up on this kind distinction, it considers them to be closely related because they appear together. This probably reflects at least some of what goes on in humans — we have a strong association between "black" and "white" even though they are opposites. However, we can also use syntactic information to further refine our semantic representations — a skill that is lacking in this network. The next section describes a model that begins to address this skill.

↪ Go to the `PDP++Root` window. To continue on to the next simulation, close this project first by selecting `.projects/Remove/Project_0`. Or, if you wish to stop now, quit by selecting `Object/Quit`.

10.6.3 Summary and Discussion

Perhaps the most important aspects of this semantics model are its ability to represent variations in semantic meaning in terms of rich, overlapping distributed representations, and its ability to develop these representations using Hebbian learning. Because our low-level visual representations model from chapter 8 relies on these same features, this helps to reaffirm our belief that a common set of principles can be used to understand cortical processing across a wide range of different domains, from visual perception to language in this case.

One limitation of this model is that it does not include any task-based learning. The inclusion of this type of learning might help to further refine the distinctions captured by the semantic representations, and improve performance on things like the multiple choice

problems. Indeed, the addition of such task-based learning might serve as a useful model of the beneficial effects of production on comprehension. We have probably all had the experience of feeling as if we understood something, only to find that this feeling was somewhat illusory when it came time to describe the idea orally or in writing. Similarly, the present model has a fairly fuzzy set of representations based on its purely passive, receptive experience with the domain. If we included task-based learning as well, this would be like giving the model practice (and feedback) articulating various ideas, which would presumably clarify and sharpen the representations.

Although the model we explored demonstrates a number of important principles, it falls short of addressing the issue of the topographic organization of different kinds of semantic information across different brain areas. As mentioned in the introduction, this organizational issue has been a major focus of neuropsychological studies, and neural network models such as the one by Farah and McClelland (1991) have played an important, if controversial, role in this field. One could consider extending our model by including recurrent self-connections within the hidden layer, and exploring the topographic organization that develops as a result, much in the same way we explored the topographic organization of visual feature detectors in chapter 8.

However, we are somewhat skeptical of such an approach, because it seems clear that the topographic organization in the human brain depends on all kinds of constraints that might be difficult to capture in such a simple model. Referring back to figure 10.23 and the distributed semantics idea of Allport (1985), it would seem that one would have to build models that include sufficient instantiations of various sensory systems, together with language processing and functional motor-based processing. While not impossible, this is a more formidable challenge that awaits future ambitions.

10.7 Sentence-Level Processing

The semantic representations model we just explored provides one step toward understanding language processing at a level higher than individual words. However, the semantic model was limited in that it com-

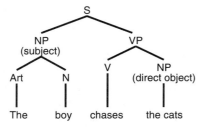

Figure 10.26: Tree diagram of the phrase structure of a simple English sentence. NP = noun phrase, VP = verb phrase, and S is represents the entire sentence.

pletely ignored the issue of syntax. In this section we explore a model developed originally by St. John and McClelland (1990) that combines syntactic and semantic information in the service of sentence-level processing. To begin our discussion of this model, we first introduce some of the main issues in syntactic processing.

The term *syntax* generally refers to the structural regularities of sentences, or in other words, the *grammar* of sentences. We have already seen that neural network models can capture linguistic regularities at the level of the pronunciation and inflection of individual words. Critically, these models demonstrate that principles of neural network learning and processing can be used to understand the kinds of regularities that have traditionally been ascribed to the operation of explicit grammatical rules. Thus, neural network models should provide a similar kind of demonstration in the context of sentence level processing.

The traditional view of syntactic processing involves hierarchically structured tree diagrams of the **phrase structure** of a sentence, like that shown in figure 10.26. This diagram represents the fact that every well-formed English sentence has a **noun phrase** (NP) and a **verb phrase** (VP). These phrases can then be further decomposed into subcomponents until the actual words in the sentence are represented. This same information can be expressed in terms of **rewrite rules** that specify how to rewrite or decompose something into its constituent parts. For example, the top-level structure of figure 10.26 can be written as $S \rightarrow NP\ VP$, meaning that a sentence is composed of a noun phrase and a verb phrase. Traditional computational theories of syntactic

processing involve ways of manipulating these kinds of hierarchical tree structures to produce and comprehend sentences.

For the traditional tree-structured approach to sentence comprehension to work, one must build up the appropriate tree structure by identifying the corresponding role of each of the words in a sentence. Thus, a major aspect of this view of syntax involves using various cues (e.g., word order) to bind words to roles. For the example shown in figure 10.26, one needs to know that "the boy" is the subject of the sentence, and not the direct object. In this case, the fact that "boy" is the first noun in the sentence is a very reliable cue (in English) that it is the subject. However, things can become much more complicated when the sentence structure gets more complex (e.g., with passive constructions, dependent clauses and the like), and when the words have multiple grammatical categories (e.g., "run" can be either a verb or a noun).

In short, the traditional view of sentence processing becomes a combinatorial search problem of large proportions, with the correct tree structure for a given sentence being one out of a huge number of possible such trees. In contrast, a neural network approach to sentence comprehension does not require explicit category labels, or even any kind of explicit representation of the tree structure of a sentence. All that is required is a sufficiently rich distributed representation of the meaning of the sentence, constructed as a result of reading the constituent words.

By way of analogy, consider the difference between the traditional and neural network approaches to object recognition (see chapter 8). The traditional approach posited that an internal object-centered 3-D structural model (e.g., as might be produced in a computer aided design (CAD) program) was constructed from the perceptual input. With such a model, recognizing the object should be simple. However, because the detailed 3-D structure is obscured by the 2-D projection received by the eyes, constructing the 3-D model is a massive underconstrained combinatorial search problem that turned out to be unworkable.

In contrast, the neural network approach only tries to come up with an internal distributed representation that disambiguates different objects, while being roughly invariant to various transformations of the visual input. No detailed structural model needs to be constructed. Instead, the problem becomes one of a massively parallel many-to-few mapping of images to internal object representations that appears to be considerably more practical.

If we apply these ideas to sentence processing, the network can accumulate constraints from the incoming words and produce a distributed representation that best satisfies these constraints. We explored something very much like this in the semantic representation model from the previous section — the network produced a novel semantic representation that reflected the constraints from all the words being presented. This semantics model is also useful for showing that one can get pretty far without processing any syntactic information. Thus, it is possible that the raw collection of words present makes a large contribution to people's interpretations of sentences, with syntactic structure providing additional constraints. This view is consistent with the considerable empirical evidence that semantic properties of individual words can play an important role in sentence comprehension (MacDonald, Pearlmutter, & Seidenberg, 1994).

These kinds of ideas about a constraint-satisfaction approach to sentence comprehension have been developed by Elman (1990, 1991, 1993), and by St. John and McClelland (1990). Elman's models have emphasized purely syntactic processing, while the St. John and McClelland (1990) model combines both semantic and syntactic constraints together into what they referred to as the "Sentence Gestalt" (SG) model. The term *Gestalt* here comes from the holistic notions of the Gestalt psychologists, aptly capturing the multiple constraint satisfaction notion. The Gestalt representation in the SG model is just the kind of powerful distributed representation envisioned above, capturing both semantic and syntactic constraints. We explore a slightly modified version of the SG model in this section (we have also provided a version of the Elman (1991) model as `grammar.proj.gz` in `chapter_10` in case you want to explore that model on your own).

The temporally extended, sequential nature of sentence-level linguistic structure provides perhaps the greatest challenge to using neural network models. In chapter 6, we found that the *context* representation in a simple recurrent network (SRN) is sufficiently powerful to enable a network to learn a simple finite state grammar. The SG model uses this same mechanism for its sentence level processing — indeed, the context representation *is* the sentence gestalt itself. Thus, if you have not yet read section 6.5 (and specifically section 6.6) in chapter 6, we recommend you do so now. Otherwise, you should still be able to follow the main points, but may not have as clear an understanding of the details.

10.7.1 Basic Properties of the Model

The SG model receives input about an environment via sentences. To define the nature of these sentences, we need to specify both the nature of the underlying environment (which provides the *deep structure* of semantics), and the way in which this environment is encoded into the *surface form* of actual sentences (which is a function of both syntax and semantics). We will first discuss the nature of the environmental semantics, followed by a discussion of the syntactic features of the language input. Then, we will discuss the structure of the network, and how it is trained.

Semantics

In contrast with the previous semantics model, where large amounts of actual text served as the semantic database for learning, the SG model is based on a simple "toy world" that captures something like a child's-eye (and stereotypically sex-typed) view of the world. This world is populated with four people (*busdriver* (adult male), *teacher* (adult female), *schoolgirl*, and a boy who is a baseball *pitcher*), who do various different actions (*eat, drink, stir, spread, kiss, give, hit, throw, drive,* and *rise*) in an environment containing various other objects (*spot* (the dog), *steak, soup, ice cream, crackers, jelly, iced tea, kool aid, spoon, knife, finger, rose, bat* (animal), *bat* (baseball), *ball, ball* (party), *bus, pitcher,* and *fur*) and locations (*kitchen, living room, shed,* and *park*).

Eighty underlying events take place in this environment that define the interrelationships among the various entities. Each such event can give rise to a large number of different surface forms. For exam-

```
The busdriver ate steak [with the knife] [with the teacher] [in the kitchen] [with gusto].
The busdriver ate soup [with the spoon] [with the crackers] [in the kitchen] [with gusto].
The busdriver ate ice cream [with the spoon] [with the teacher] [in the park] [with pleasure].
The busdriver ate crackers [with the finger] [with the jelly] [in the kitchen] [with gusto].
The schoolgirl ate soup [with the spoon] [with the crackers] [in the kitchen] [with daintiness].
The schoolgirl ate steak [with the knife] [with the pitcher] [in the kitchen] [with daintiness].
The schoolgirl ate ice cream [with the spoon] [with the pitcher] [in the park] [with pleasure].
The schoolgirl ate crackers [with the finger] [with the jelly] [in the kitchen] [with daintiness].
The busdriver drank iced tea [with the teacher] [in the living room] [with gusto].
The busdriver drank kool aid [with the teacher] [in the kitchen] [with gusto].
The schoolgirl drank iced tea [with the pitcher] [in the living room] [with daintiness].
The schoolgirl drank kool aid [with the pitcher] [in the kitchen] [with daintiness].
The busdriver stirred iced tea [with the spoon] [in the pitcher].
The busdriver stirred kool aid [with the spoon] [in the pitcher].
The schoolgirl stirred iced tea [with the spoon] [in the pitcher].
The schoolgirl stirred kool aid [with the spoon] [in the pitcher].
The busdriver spread jelly [with the knife] [in the kitchen].
The schoolgirl spread jelly [with the knife] [in the kitchen].
The busdriver kissed the teacher [in the park].
The busdriver kissed the schoolgirl [in the park].
The schoolgirl kissed the busdriver [in the park].
The schoolgirl kissed the pitcher [in the shed].
The busdriver gave the rose [to the teacher].
The busdriver gave the ice cream [to the schoolgirl].
The schoolgirl gave the rose [to the busdriver].
The schoolgirl gave the ice cream [to the busdriver].
The busdriver hit the shed [with the bus].
The busdriver hit the ball [with the bat] [in the park].
The busdriver hit the bat [with the bat] [in the shed].
The busdriver hit the pitcher [with the ball] [in the park].
The schoolgirl hit the pitcher [with the spoon] [in the kitchen].
The schoolgirl hit the spot [with the spoon] [in the kitchen].
The schoolgirl hit the teacher [with the spoon] [in the kitchen].
The busdriver threw the ball [in the park] [to the pitcher].
The schoolgirl threw the ball [with the teacher] [in the living room].
The busdriver drove the bus [in the shed] [with gusto].
The busdriver drove the pitcher [in the bus] [with gusto].
The busdriver drove the schoolgirl [in the bus] [with gusto].
The teacher drove the pitcher [with gusto].
The teacher drove the schoolgirl [with gusto].
Spot shed the fur [in the living room].
The busdriver rose [with the teacher] [in the living room].
The schoolgirl rose [with the pitcher] [in the living room].
```

Table 10.14: Examples of the core events that take place in the SG toy world. Only events where the busdriver or school-girl are the agents are shown — similar events apply to the teacher and pitcher (except for the event where spot sheds fur).

ple, *The busdriver ate steak [with the knife] [with the teacher] [in the kitchen] [with gusto]* defines one such event, expressed in sentence form (see table 10.14 for more examples, and the file sg_sents.txt in chapter_10 for a list of all of the events[2]). Each event has an *agent* (here the *busdriver*), an *action* (*ate*), and (usually) a *patient* (*steak*). Then, there are a set of modifying features or *roles* that further qualify the event in terms of any *instrument* used (*knife*), a possible *co-agent* (*teacher*), a possible *co-patient*, the *location* (*kitchen*), a possible *adverb* (*gusto*), and a possible *recipient* (for the *give* action).

The semantics of events are further refined by a set of probabilities associated with the patient selected for each agent/action combination, so that in this somewhat sex-typed toy world, the busdriver is more likely to eat steak than anything else, while the teacher is more likely to eat soup than steak, for example. Refer to sg_frames.txt in chapter_10 for a full specification of the "sentence frames" used to define the environment and its associated probabilities as defined in St. John and McClelland (1990).

Another aspect of the semantics comes in the use of ambiguous words (words with multiple meanings). For example, the word *bat* is used both as a animal and as a piece of baseball equipment. *Pitcher* can also refer to the boy or a vessel for holding beverages. Other ambiguities include: *rose* as in the past tense of rise or the flower, *shed* as in the loosing of hair or a small utility structure, *throw* as in host a party or toss a ball, *ball* as in a party or a baseball, and *drive* as in motivate or to drive a bus. To interpret these words properly, the network must use the semantics of the surrounding context.

Syntax

The underlying semantic event representations are transformed into the surface form sentences that are actually presented to the network. This transformation process involves several syntactic features. The primary syntactic manipulation is in the use of the *active* versus *passive* forms. An example of the active form is "The busdriver ate steak," and the passive form of this sentence is "The steak was eaten by the busdriver." Thus, passive sentences violate the normal syntactic constraint that the first noun is the subject of the sentence. We used an 80 percent rate of the active construction, reflecting the prevalence of this form in normal usage.[3]

Another form of syntactic construction comes in the use of phrases that provide the supplemental information about the event. For example, in "The busdriver ate steak with the teacher," one needs to use syntactic constraints to sort out the different roles of the busdriver

---

[2]Note that the semantics used here represents a best guess reconstruction of the original SG environment, the specifics of which were not fully documented in St. John and McClelland (1990), and are not presently recoverable (St. John, personal communication, 1998).

[3]Note that the original SG model only used the passive form for a subset of events, whereas we use it for all of them here.

(subject) and the teacher (co-agent). This syntactic information is conveyed by the cues of word order and *function words* like *with*.

Importantly, the surface form sentences are always partial and sometimes vague representations of the actual underlying events. The partial nature of the sentences is produced by only specifying at most one (and sometimes none) of the modifying features of the event. The vagueness comes from using vague alternative words such as: *someone, adult, child, something, food, utensil,* and *place*. To continue the busdriver eating example, some sentences might be, "The busdriver ate something," or "Someone ate steak in the kitchen," and so on. As a result of the active/passive variation and the different forms of partiality and vagueness in the sentences, there are a large number of different surface forms corresponding to each event, such that there are 8,668 total different sentences that could be presented to the network.

Finally, we note that the determiners (*the, a,* etc.) were not presented to the network, which simplifies the syntactic processing somewhat.

Network Structure and Training

Having specified the semantics and syntax of the linguistic environment, we now turn to the network (figure 10.27) and how the sentences were presented. Each word in a sentence is presented sequentially across trials in the `Input` layer, which has a localist representation of the words (one unit per word). The `Encode` layer allows the network to develop a distributed encoding of these words, much as in the family trees network discussed in chapter 6. The subsequent `Gestalt` hidden layer serves as the primary gestalt representation, which is maintained and updated over time through the use of the `Gestalt Context` layer. This context layer is a standard SRN context layer that copies the previous activation state from the gestalt hidden layer after each trial.

The network is trained by asking it questions about the information it "reads" in the input sentences. Specifically, the network is required to answer questions of the form "who is the agent?," "who/what is the patient?," "where is the location?," and so on. These

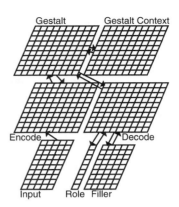

Figure 10.27: The SG model. Localist word inputs are presented in the Input layer, encoded in a learned distributed representation in the Encode layer, and then integrated together over time in the Gestalt and Gestalt Context layers. Questions regarding the sentence are posed by activating a Role unit, and the network answers by Decoding its Gestalt representation to produce the appropriate Filler for that role.

questions are posed to the network by activating one of the 9 different `Role` units (*agent, action, patient, instrument, co-agent, co-patient, location, adverb, and recipient*), and requiring the network to produce the appropriate answer in the `Filler` layer. Importantly, the filler units represent the underlying specific concepts that can sometimes be represented by ambiguous or vague words. Thus, there is a separate filler unit for *bat (animal)* and *bat (baseball)*, and so on for the other ambiguous words. The `Decode` hidden layer facilitates the decoding of this information from the gestalt representation.

The role/filler questions are asked of the network after each input, and only questions that the network could answer based on what it has heard so far are asked. Note that this differs from the original SG model, where all questions were asked after each input, presumably to encourage the network to anticipate future information. However, even though we are not specifically forcing it to do so, the network nevertheless anticipates future information automatically. There are three main reasons for only asking answerable questions during training. First, it just seems more plausible — one could imagine asking oneself questions about the roles of the words one has heard so far. Second, it makes it possible for the network to actually achieve correct performance most of the time, which is not possible with the original method. This enables us to monitor its learning performance over training more easily.

Third, with Leabra, there is no way to present questions about future information during training without effectively exposing the network to that information. Specifically, in Leabra errors are equivalent to activation states, and the entire activation state of the network must be updated for proper error signals to be propagated for each question. Thus, if all of the questions were asked after each input, information about the entire sentence would be propagated into the network (and thus into the gestalt representation) via the plus phases of the questions. To preserve the idea that the gestalt is updated primarily from the inputs, we ask questions only about current or previous inputs. The original SG model instead used a somewhat complicated error propagation mechanism, where all the errors for the questions were accumulated separately in the output end of the network, and then passed back to the encoding portion of the network after the entire sentence has been processed. Thus, there was a dissociation between activation states based on the inputs received so far, and the subsequent error signals based on all the questions, allowing all of the questions to be asked after each input.

Training the network by asking it explicitly about roles is only one of many different possible ways that this information could be learned. For example, visual processing of an event simultaneous with a verbal description of it would provide a means of training the sentence-based encoding to reflect the actual state of affairs in the environment. However, the explicit role-filler training used here is simple and provides a clear picture of how well the gestalt representation has encoded the appropriate information.

The network parameters were fairly standard for a larger sized network, with 25 percent activity in the encoding and decoding hidden layers, and 15 percent activity in the gestalt hidden layer. The proportion of Hebbian learning was .001, and the learning rate was reduced from .01 to .001 after 200 epochs of training. The fm_{hid} and fm_{prv} parameters for updating the context layer were set to the standard values of .7

and .3, which allows for some retention of prior states but mostly copies the current hidden state.

10.7.2 Exploring the Model

↪ Open the project sg.proj.gz in chapter_10 to begin.

As usual, the network is in skeleton form and must be built.

↪ Do BuildNet on the sg_ctrl overall control panel to build it.

↪ Then, you can poke around the network and explore the connectivity using the r.wt button, and then return to viewing act.

Note that the input/output units are all labeled according to the first two letters of the word, role, or concept that they represent.

Training

First, let's see exactly how the network is trained by stepping through some training trials.

↪ Open up a training log by doing View, TRAIN_LOG, and then open up a process control panel for training by doing View, TRAIN_PROCESS_CTRL. Do ReInit. There will be a delay while an entire epoch's worth of sentences (100 sentences) are randomly generated. Then press Step (a similar delay will ensue, due to the need to recreate these sentences at the start of every epoch — because these happen at different levels of processing, the redundancy is difficult to avoid).

You should see the first word of the first sentence presented to the network. Recall that as each word is presented, questions are asked about all current and previous information presented to the network. Because this is the first word, the network has just performed a minus and plus phase update with this word as input, and it tried to answer what the agent of the sentence is.

To understand how the words are presented, let's first look at the training log (Trial_0_TextLog, see figure 10.28 for an example from the trained network). The trial and EventGp columns change with each different word of the sentence, with EventGp showing the word that is currently being processed. Within the presentation of each word, there are one or more events

epoch	trial	EventGp	tick	Event	cnt_se	resp
0	0	busdriver	0	busdriver_busdriver	0	busdriver
0	1	spread	0	spread_spread	0	spread
0	1	spread	1	spread_busdriver	0	busdriver
0	2	jelly	0	jelly_jelly	0	jelly
0	2	jelly	1	jelly_busdriver	0	busdriver
0	2	jelly	2	jelly_spread	0	spread
0	3	with	0	with_jelly	0	jelly
0	3	with	1	with_busdriver	0	busdriver
0	3	with	2	with_spread	0	spread
0	3	with	3	with_jelly	0	jelly
0	4	utensil.	0	utensil_knife	0	knife
0	4	utensil.	1	utensil_busdriver	0	busdriver

Figure 10.28: Output of the `Trial_0_TextLog` for the *trained* network, showing sequence of questions that are asked after each input.

that correspond to the answering of the role/filler questions — these question-level events are counted by the `tick` column, and are labeled in the `Event` column. The first part of the `Event` label is just the input word (same as `EventGp`), and the second part is the correct answer to the current question. The actual output response of the network is shown in the `resp` column, and `cnt_se` is a count of the number of output units with errors (this will be 0 when the network is producing the correct answer).

There is no reason to expect the network to produce the correct answer at the start because the weights are random. Thus, you will probably see that there is a non-zero `cnt_se` value and the `resp` column does not match the second part of the `Event` column. We can now look at the network activations to see what happened in the minus and plus phases.

↪ Press the `act_m` button in the network display to view the minus phase activation states.

You should be able to use the labels on the units to verify that the input word was presented on the `Input` layer, the *agent* (ag) `Role` unit was activated, and the network produced the output shown in the `resp` column in the `Filler` layer.

↪ Now press the `act_p` button to see the plus phase activations.

Here, you should see that the correct answer was provided in the `Filler` layer. Also notice that the `Gestalt Context` layer is zeroed out for this first event — it is automatically reset at the start of each new sentence.

↪ Now press `Step` again on the process control panel to present the next event.

Notice that the question asked about each word when it is first presented is about that word itself, so the network should be asked about the action of the sentence at this point. However, the next question will go back and ask about the agent again.

↪ Press `Step` again.

You should see that the `Role` input asks about the agent while still presenting the second (action) word in the `Input`. Thus, the network has to learn to use the information retained in the gestalt context layer to be able to answer questions about more than just the current input word. You can now step through the remaining words in the sentence, observing that all previous questions are reasked as each new word is presented.

↪ Press `Step` several more times until the `EventGp` word has a period after it, and all the questions have been asked for that last word, as indicated by the period after the word in the `Event` column.

You might have also noticed that the network actually seemed to start remembering things pretty well — this is illusory, and is due to the effects of the small weight updates after each question (it is basically just remembering to say the same thing it just said). As we will see in a moment, the testing that we will perform rules out such weight changes as a source of memory, so that we know the gestalt context representation is responsible. Nevertheless, it is quite possible that people actually take advantage of this kind of priming-like memory (see chapter 9) to encode recently processed information, in addition to the activation-based memory represented by the gestalt context layer. Thus, this model could provide an interesting way of exploring the interactions between weight-based and activation-based memory in sentence processing, but we won't explore this idea here.

After the sentence is over, the gestalt context is cleared, and the next sentence is processed, and so on.

Testing

Now, let's evaluate the trained network's performance, by exploring its performance on a set of specially selected test sentences shown in table 10.15. Because the network takes a considerable amount of time to train,

Task	Sentence
Role assignment	
Active semantic	The schoolgirl stirred the Kool-Aid with a spoon.
Active syntactic	The busdriver gave the rose to the teacher.
Passive semantic	The jelly was spread by the busdriver with the knife.
Passive syntactic	The teacher was kissed by the busdriver.
(control)	The busdriver kissed the teacher.
Word ambiguity	The busdriver threw the ball in the park.
	The teacher threw the ball in the living room.
Concept instantiation	The teacher kissed someone (male).
Role elaboration	The schoolgirl ate crackers (with finger).
	The schoolgirl ate (soup).
Online update	The child ate soup with daintiness.
(control)	The pitcher ate soup with daintiness.
Conflict	The adult drank iced tea in the kitchen (living room).

Table 10.15: Test cases for exploring the behavior of the model, as described in the text.

we will just load in some pretrained weights from a network that was trained for 225 epochs of 100 sentences per epoch.

↪ Do LoadNet on the overall sg_ctrl control panel.

The test sentences are designed to illustrate different aspects of the sentence comprehension task, as noted in the table. First, a set of role assignment tasks provide either semantic or purely syntactic cues to assign the main roles in the sentence. The semantic cues depend on the fact that only animate nouns can be agents, whereas inanimate nouns can only be patients. Although animacy is not explicitly provided in the input, the training environment enforces this constraint. Thus, when a sentence starts off with "The jelly...," we can tell that because jelly is inanimate, it must be the patient of a passive sentence, and not the agent of an active one. However, if the sentence begins with "The busdriver...," we do not know if the busdriver is an agent or a patient, and we thus have to wait to see if the syntactic cue of the word *was* appears next.

↪ To start testing, iconify the training text log and process control panel, and then open a testing log (Trial_1_TextLog) by doing View, TEST_LOG. Then, open a testing process control panel (Epoch_1) using View, TEST_PROCESS_CTRL.

The testing text log has the same columns as the training one (figure 10.28), so the results of testing can be interpreted the same way.

↪ Do ReInit and Step in the process control panel.

Each step here covers all questions for each input

word, to speed things up a bit. The first word of the active semantic role assignment sentence (schoolgirl) is presented, and the network correctly answers that schoolgirl is the agent of the sentence. Note that there is no plus-phase and no training during this testing, so everything depends on the integration of the input words — the small weight changes that we observed during training cannot bias the correct answer.

↪ Continue to Step through to the final word in this sentence (spoon).

You should observe that the network is able to identify correctly the roles of all of the words presented. Because in this sentence the roles of the words are constrained by their semantics, this success demonstrates that the network is sensitive to these semantic constraints and can use them in parsing.

↪ Now Step through the next sentence.

This sentence has two animate nouns (busdriver and teacher), so the network must use the syntactic word order cues to infer that the busdriver is the agent, while using the "gave to" syntactic construction to recognize that the teacher is the recipient. Observe that at the final word in the sentence, the network has correctly identified all the words.

In the next sentence, the passive construction is used, but this should be obvious from the semantic cue that jelly cannot be an agent.

↪ Step through and observe that the network correctly parses this sentence.

In the final role assignment case, the sentence is passive and there are only syntactic constraints available to identify whether the teacher is the agent or the patient. This is the most difficult construction that the network faces, and it does not appear to get it right — it gets confused when busdriver appears at the end of the sentence, and concludes that the busdriver is both the agent and patient of the sentence.

↪ Step through this sentence.

Further testing has shown that the network sometimes gets this sentence right, but often makes errors. This can apparently be attributed to the lower frequency of passive sentences, as you can see from the next sentence, which is a "control condition" of the higher frequency active form of the previous sentence, with which the network has no difficulties.

↪ Step through this next sentence.

The next two sentences test the network's ability to resolve ambiguous words, in this case *throw* and *ball* based on the surrounding semantic context. During training, the network learns that busdrivers throw baseballs, whereas teachers throw parties. Thus, the network should produce the appropriate interpretation of these ambiguous sentences.

↪ Step through these next two sentences to verify that this is the case.

Note that the network makes a mistake here by replacing *teacher* with the other agent that also throws parties, the *schoolgirl*. Thus, the network's context memory is not perfect, but it tends to make semantically appropriate errors, just as people do.

The next test sentence probes the ability of the network to instantiate an ambiguous term (e.g., *someone*) with a more concrete concept. Because the teacher only kisses males (the pitcher or the busdriver), the network should be able to instantiate the ambiguous *someone* with either of these two males.

↪ As you Step through this sentence, observe that *someone* is instantiated with *pitcher*.

A similar phenomenon can be found in the role elaboration test questions. Here, the network is able to answer questions about aspects of an event that were not actually stated in the input. For example, the network can infer that the schoolgirl would eat crackers with her fingers.

↪ Step through the next sentence.

You should see that the very last question regarding the instrument role is answered correctly with fingers, even though fingers was never presented in the input. The next sentence takes this one step further and has the network infer what the schoolgirl tends to eat (soup).

↪ Go ahead and Step through this one.

Question 10.13 *In chapter 9, we discussed a mechanism for using partial cues to retrieve an original stored memory.* **(a)** *Explain the network's role elaboration performance in terms of this mechanism.* **(b)** *Based on what you know about the rates of learning of different brain areas, speculate about differences in where in the brain role elaboration might take place based on how familiar the information in question is.*

The next test sentence evaluates the online updating of information in a case where subsequent information further constrains an initially vague word. In this case, the sentence starts with the word *child*, and the network vacillates back and forth about which child it answers the agent question with. When the network receives the adverb *daintiness*, this uniquely identifies the schoolgirl, which it then reports as the agent of the sentence (even though it does not appear to fully encode the daintiness input, producing *pleasure* instead).

↪ Step through the sentence.

To verify that *daintiness* is having an effect on this result, we can run the next control condition where the pitcher is specified as the agent of the sentence — the network clearly switches from saying *pitcher* to saying *schoolgirl* after receiving the *daintiness* input.

↪ Step through the sentence.

The final test sentence illustrates how the network deals with conflicting information. In this case, the training environment always specifies that iced tea is drunk in the living room, but the input sentence says it was drunk in the kitchen.

↪ Step through this sentence.

Notice that in the middle of the sentence, the network swaps *stirred* for *drank*, only to correct this error (without further input of *drank*) at the end. The main point is that when *kitchen* is input, the network responds with *living room*, as consistent with its prior knowledge. This may provide a useful demonstration of how prior knowledge biases sentence comprehension, as has been shown in the classic "war of the ghosts" experiment (Bartlett, 1932) and many others.

Nature of Representations

Having seen that the network behaves reasonably (if not perfectly), we can explore the nature of its internal representations to get a sense of how it works. First, we can probe the way that the Encode layer encodes the localist input representation of words into more useful distributed representations.

↪ Press WordClust on the overall control panel.

There will be a short delay as all the unambiguous verbs are presented and the corresponding activations over the encoding layer are recorded, followed by a

SG Verb Encodings

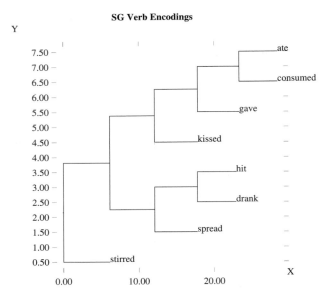

Figure 10.29: Cluster plot of the encoding layer representations of the unambiguous verbs.

SG Noun Encodings

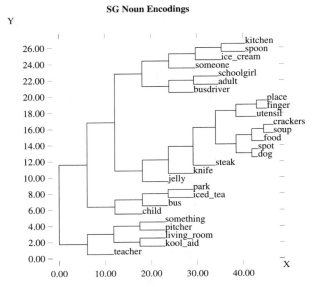

Figure 10.30: Cluster plot of the encoding layer representations of the unambiguous nouns.

cluster plot of the similarity structure for these verbs (which should look like figure 10.29). There is actually not much of interest here, except for the similarity of *ate* and *consumed*, which are the only two verbs that have a close (synonymous) relationship.

After another short delay, the cluster plot for the unambiguous nouns will show up (figure 10.30). Here, there is much greater potential for useful similarity relationships because of the similar roles of some of the nouns, and it is clear that the network has encoded words that appear together in the training sentences as more similar.

Of course, the most important layer in the network is the Gestalt layer. To probe the nature of the gestalt representations, we present the sentences shown in table 10.16, and record the final gestalt layer activation pattern after the last word is presented. These sentences systematically vary the agents, patients, and verbs to reveal how these are represented.

↪ Press SentClust on the overall control panel.

After all the sentences have been processed, a cluster plot will appear (figure 10.31). This plot clearly

Code	Sentence
bu_at_so	The busdriver ate soup.
te_at_so	The teacher ate soup.
pi_at_so	The pitcher ate soup.
sc_at_so	The schoolgirl ate soup.
bu_at_st	The busdriver ate steak.
te_at_st	The teacher ate steak.
pi_at_st	The pitcher ate steak.
sc_at_st	The schoolgirl ate steak.
bu_dr_ic	The busdriver drank iced tea.
te_dr_ic	The teacher drank iced tea.
pi_dr_ic	The pitcher drank iced tea.
sc_dr_ic	The schoolgirl drank iced tea.
bu_st_ko	The busdriver stirred Kool-Aid.
te_st_ko	The teacher stirred Kool-Aid.
pi_st_ko	The pitcher stirred Kool-Aid.
sc_st_ko	The schoolgirl stirred Kool-Aid.

Table 10.16: Probe sentences used to assess the nature of the gestalt representation. The code is used in the corresponding cluster plot (figure 10.31).

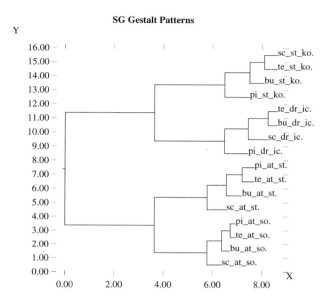

Figure 10.31: Cluster plot of the gestalt layer representations at the end of the probe sentences listed in table 10.16.

shows that the sentences are first clustered together according to verb, and then by patient, and then by agent within that. Furthermore, across the different patients, there appears to be the same similarity structure for the agents. Thus, we can see that the gestalt representation encodes information in a systematic fashion, as we would expect from the network's behavior.

↪ To stop now, quit by selecting `Object/Quit` in the `PDP++Root` window.

10.7.3 Summary and Discussion

The sentence gestalt model has demonstrated that multiple constraints from semantics and syntax can interact in shaping a representation of the meaning of a sentence. Because this meaning is captured in a distributed representation, one would expect it to have all of the advantages of efficiency and generalization we have come to expect from such representations, which it indeed appears to have. This form of sentence representation, and the processing that produces it, differs considerably from the traditional use of phrase structure trees or rewrite rules, which are rigid and difficult to construct.

This model demonstrates how sequential, piecemeal inputs can be integrated together into a coherent summary or gestalt-like distributed representation. This demonstration validates the idea that multiple constraint satisfaction processing can take place across inputs occurring over time, and not just across inputs occurring together at the same time. We will refer to this phenomenon as *temporal integration*.

We think that many important aspects of cognition require temporal integration over piecemeal inputs. For example, in forming a visual representation of all but the most simple scenes, we must integrate over a large number of visual inputs produced by fixating on different aspects of the scene. Clearly, this must be true for representing temporally extended events (e.g., as captured by one scene in a movie). In the domain of language, almost all processing requires temporal integration, from the perception of spoken words to sequences of words (the domain of the present model) to paragraphs and chapters and entire books!

An important unresolved question concerns the role of the context representation in achieving temporal integration. We know that in the present model, the discrete updating and maintenance capabilities of the context representation are essential for its success. In chapter 9, we saw that these properties of the context representation are closely associated with those of the prefrontal cortex. Thus, must we conclude that the frontal cortex is essential for all forms of temporal integration?

People with frontal lesions or schizophrenia (which affects frontal processing) are impaired at some tasks requiring temporal integration (e.g., Shallice, 1988; Cohen & Servan-Schreiber, 1992). However, frontal patients are probably not impaired at integrating over multiple views of a visual scene, or in integrating over the phonemes of a word in speech perception. In the absence of more complete data on this issue, we suggest that temporal integration taking place over fairly short intervals (e.g., up to a few seconds) can be subserved by the natural temporal integration properties of a generic cortical network (e.g., in the posterior cortex), but that integration over longer periods would require the specialized frontal cortex active maintenance capabilities.

Some evidence for the temporal integration of the current input with prior context in the brain comes from a study by Arieli, Sterkin, and Aertsen (1996), who showed that the apparently noisy responses of neurons to discrete inputs can be explained by taking into account the ongoing state of activation in the network. Getting these kinds of temporal integration dynamics right in the model may require that we use units that have a much closer approximation to the true dynamics of cortical neurons. These dynamics are also likely to depend on more detailed parameter settings (e.g., in regulating the balance between hysteresis and accommodation, as discussed in chapter 2). Thus, it may be more practical to continue to use a specialized context representation even when modeling temporal integration phenomena that may not actually depend on such representations.

One important contrast between our model and the original SG model is in the speed of learning. Our model achieved reasonable levels of performance after about 10,000 training sequences, and we stopped training at an apparent asymptote after 25,000 sequences. In contrast, the original SG model required 630,000 total training sequences. We can attribute some of this difference to the benefits of the self-organizing, model learning aspects of Leabra (Hebbian learning and inhibitory competition) in networks having multiple hidden layers, as discussed in chapter 6. Furthermore, temporally extended processing can be viewed as adding more intervening steps in the propagation of error signals, so these model-learning constraints are likely to be even more important in this model.

Finally, we should note that there are a number of limitations of this model. As we saw, its performance is not perfect. Furthermore, the model requires external control mechanisms, like resetting the context after each sentence, that probably should be learned (and more realistically, should be integrated together with paragraph and higher levels of temporal integration). One avenue for further exploration would be to incorporate some of the more powerful frontally mediated context updating and maintenance mechanisms that are discussed in chapters 9 and 11.

Perhaps the biggest limitation of the model is the relatively simplistic form of both the semantic and syntactic features. To demonstrate truly a flexible and powerful form of sentence-level constraint satisfaction processing, one would need to rule out the possibility that the network is doing something akin to "memorization." Although even this relatively simple environment has a combinatorial space of more than 8,000 surface forms (which argues against the memorization idea), one would ideally like to use something approaching the semantic and syntactic complexity managed by an elementary-school child. One optimistic sign that something like this could plausibly be achieved comes from the relatively rapid learning exhibited by the Leabra version of this model, which allows for the possibility that more complex environments could still be learned in reasonable amounts of time.

10.8 Summary

Our explorations of language illustrated some important general principles of computational cognitive neuroscience. For example, a central theme of this chapter is that words are represented in a **distributed lexicon**, and not stored in a single canonical lexicon as in traditional accounts. We explored the distributed lexical components of **orthography** (written word forms), **phonology** (spoken word forms composed of **phonemes**), and **semantics** (representations of word meanings). Various forms of **dyslexia** (reading impairments), including **surface**, **phonological**, and **deep** dyslexia, can be understood in terms of damage to various pathways within an interactive distributed lexicon model.

Another theme is that neural networks can capture both **regularities** and **exceptions** within a unitary system, and that they can **generalize** based on the regularities, for example in producing humanlike pronunciations for **nonwords**. A neural network is ideally suited for modeling the complex continuum of regularities and exceptions in the English orthography to phonology mapping. The tension between regulars and exceptions can be played out over the timecourse of learning, as in the English **past-tense inflectional system**. Here, there is evidence of a **U-shaped curve** over development, where irregulars are initially produced correctly, and are then sporadically **overregularized**, followed by eventual mastery. Both Hebbian learning and inhibitory competition contribute to a reasonable account of the U-shaped curve in our model.

We explored one of many possible shaping influences on the development of distributed semantic representations, **word co-occurrence**. CPCA Hebbian learning produced useful representations of the semantic meanings of a large number of words by "reading" this textbook. The resulting network can dynamically construct representations of conjunctions of words, and can perform multiple choice tests with reasonable accuracy.

Moving beyond the single word level, we explored the **sentence gestalt** model of sentence comprehension, which performs multiple constraint satisfaction on both **syntax** and semantics to produce a distributed overall representation of sentence meaning. This model also provides a paradigm example for the **temporal integration** of information encountered sequentially into a common underlying representation.

10.9 Further Reading

Almost any textbook on language will contain more detailed information about phonology if you are interested in learning more (e.g., Fromkin & Rodman, 1993).

Shallice (1988) is the classic neuropsychological treatment of language and other cognitive phenomena.

Kintsch (1998) provides a wealth of information about higher levels of discourse comprehension using neural-network like spreading-activation mechanisms (combined with latent-semantic analysis mechanisms like those used in the semantics model).

The following are generally useful papers on the neural basis of language and computational models thereof: Saffran (1997); Plaut (1999); Saffran and Schwartz (1994); Damasio et al. (1996); Hodges, Patterson, and Tyler (1994).

One topic that has not received the attention it deserves in this text is language production. Dell, Burger, and Svec (1997) provide a neural network model of this phenomenon.

Chapter 11

Higher-Level Cognition

Contents

11.1	**Overview**	**379**
11.2	**Biology of the Frontal Cortex**	**384**
11.3	**Controlled Processing and the Stroop Task**	**385**
	11.3.1 Basic Properties of the Model	*387*
	11.3.2 Exploring the Model	*388*
	11.3.3 Summary and Discussion	*391*
11.4	**Dynamic Categorization/Sorting Tasks**	**392**
	11.4.1 Basic Properties of the Model	*395*
	11.4.2 Exploring the Model	*397*
	11.4.3 Summary and Discussion	*402*
11.5	**General Role of Frontal Cortex in Higher-Level Cognition**	**403**
	11.5.1 Functions Commonly Attributed to Frontal Cortex	*403*
	11.5.2 Other Models and Theoretical Frameworks .	*407*
11.6	**Interacting Specialized Systems and Cognitive Control**	**408**
11.7	**Summary**	**409**
11.8	**Further Reading**	**410**

11.1 Overview

Higher-level cognition includes important and complex phenomena such as planning, problem solving, abstract and formal reasoning, and complex decision-making. These phenomena are distinguished in part from those discussed in previous chapters by involving the coordinated action of multiple more basic cognitive mechanisms over longer periods of time. Therefore, they are intrinsically more difficult to model — one can imagine combining several of the models from previous chapters to get a sense of the complexity involved. For these and other reasons (e.g., the lack of suitable animal models, differences in learned strategies between individuals), progress in understanding the neural basis of higher-level cognition has been slower than for the more basic mechanisms covered in previous chapters. Thus, much of our treatment of this topic will be based on ideas within one particular framework (Cohen et al., 1996; O'Reilly et al., 1999a; Braver & Cohen, 2000) that has been developed relatively recently. These ideas should be regarded as relatively speculative and not necessarily widespread. We present them to give some sense of modeling at this level, and also in the hope that they may provide a solid basis for future research in this area. This overview section is a bit longer than in previous chapters to allow us to sketch the overall framework.

Framing the Challenge of Higher-Level Cognition

Although neural network models of higher-level cognition are in their relative infancy, the more traditional symbolic approach to this domain has a long history of successful models (e.g., Newell & Simon, 1972; Anderson, 1983). One of our objectives in this chapter is to sketch the relationship between these symbolic models and the biologically based models discussed here. In symbolic models, the relative ease of chaining together sequences of operations and performing arbitrary symbol binding makes it much more straightforward to simulate higher-level cognition than in a neural network.

However, this relative ease can also lead symbolic models to *over*estimate the power and flexibility of human symbolic reasoning.

For example, many symbolic models have no difficulty with simple abstract logic problems that confound people. In the neural network framework, higher-level cognition instead emerges from interactions among the kinds of more basic neural mechanisms covered in previous chapters, and it remains strongly constrained by them. This framework clearly predicts that people should have difficulty with abstract logic problems, and that they should have less difficulty with more concrete, familiar versions of such problems, which would engage the rich semantic representations built up over experience in a neural network. Indeed, people are much better at solving logic problems when they are stated in more concrete and familiar terms (e.g., Cheng & Holyoak, 1985; Johnson-Laird, Legrenzi, & Legrenzi, 1972).

Thus, we view the challenge of this chapter as one of building a more flexible, dynamic cognitive system out of neural mechanisms that use dedicated, content-specific representations, without relying on implausible symbolic machinery (even as implemented in neural hardware; see chapter 7). The resulting cognitive system should be capable of appropriate levels of deliberate, explicit processing involving relatively abstract constructs, and it should be able to chain together a series of cognitive operations over a relatively long period of time, all focused on achieving a specific goal or series of goals.

The Importance of Activation-Based Processing

The core idea behind our approach to this challenge involves a distinction between activation- and weight-based processing, which builds on the distinction between activation- versus weight-based memory as discussed in chapter 9. Activation-based processing is based on the activation, maintenance, and updating of active representations to influence cognitive processing, whereas weight-based processing is based on the adaptation of weight values to alter input/output mappings. An appropriately configured and dynamically controlled activation-based memory system, like the

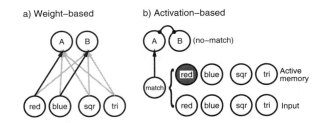

Figure 11.1: Weight- versus activation-based processing in the context of a categorization task. (a) weight-based solution involves associating discriminating feature ("red") with category A, other features (or just "not red") with category B. (b) activation-based solution maintains critical feature in active memory, and does a match comparison with the current input, such that if input matches this feature, the response is A, otherwise it is B. The match unit could detect enhanced activation from mutual support between input and maintained feature. The activation-based solution is much more rapidly updatable (i.e., flexible), and the categorization rule is easily accessible to other parts of the system.

prefrontal working memory system developed in chapter 9, is likely to be essential for achieving the flexible, dynamic style of processing that lies at the heart of higher-level cognitive processes such as explicit, abstract reasoning, planning, and problem solving.

To make the activation- versus weight-based processing distinction more concrete, consider the example (which we model later) of performing a simple categorization task (figure 11.1). The task is to categorize stimuli as either As or Bs based on their distinguishing features (e.g., respond A for red stimuli, B for any other color). A weight-based solution to this problem would involve learning associations (weights) between the critical input feature units and the category response units. An alternative activation-based solution involves maintaining in active memory a representation of the discriminating feature(s) (e.g., "red"), and then performing a matching operation that compares the similarity of the maintained features with those of the current input, and responds appropriately (e.g., if the input matches the maintained feature "red," respond A, else B).

The activation-based solution, though more complex, has a distinct advantage in the speed with which the categorization rules can be switched. By simply activating a different active memory representation and applying the same generic matching operation, an entirely different categorization rule can be applied. This speed produces flexibility, for example enabling one to rapidly adapt to changing situations (e.g., different categorization rules), or rapidly search through a number of different possible rules. In contrast, the weight-based solution requires slow, constant learning and unlearning to switch categorization rules. The categorization simulation later in the chapter explores this flexibility property of activation-based processing.

Activation-based processing also has important advantages in terms of the accessibility and impact of the representations. When information is actively maintained, it is immediately accessible to other parts of the system and constantly influences the activation of other representations. In contrast, encoding information by changing weights requires that those weights be reused for the information to influence behavior, and the effects tend to be more specific and less accessible to other parts of the system (Munakata, 1998, in press). One important consequence of accessibility is that activation-based processing representations are likely to be more easily verbalized (i.e., accessed by verbal output pathways) than weight-based processing representations. Going in the other direction, it is also likely that verbal inputs (e.g., task instructions) can more easily affect activation-based representations than weight-based ones.

In short, accessibility may play a defining role in the distinction between explicit, consciously driven ("declarative") cognitive processing and more implicit, automatic processing. In the categorization example, the activation-based strategy would make it easy to state what the defining feature is ("red"), whereas the weight changes underlying the weight-based strategy are not directly accessible. Furthermore, the categorization rule in the activation-based case can be easily influenced by verbal or other inputs, which need only activate a different feature (e.g., "blue") to impose a different rule.

The ability of actively maintained information to constantly influence processing elsewhere in the system is important for focusing and coordinating processing around a specified goal, as opposed to simply reacting

based on learned input/output associations. This distinction is typically characterized as one of *controlled* versus *automatic* processing (Schneider & Shiffrin, 1977; Shiffrin & Schneider, 1977). A paradigmatic example requiring controlled processing is the Stroop task. In this task, color words (e.g., "red") are presented in different colors, and people are instructed to either read the word or name the color of ink that the word is written in. Because we have so much experience reading, we naturally tend to read the word, even if instructed to name the color — effortful controlled processing is needed to overcome the prepotent bias toward word reading. As demonstrated by Cohen et al. (1990) (and explored later in this chapter), the ability to override the prepotent word-reading response in favor of color naming can be explained in terms of sustained goallike activation that favors the color-naming process. This account is consistent with the finding that frontal patients, who are thought to be impaired in activation-based processing, make disproportionately many errors in the Stroop conflict conditions.

In addition to the activation- versus weight-based processing distinction, one particularly interesting source of intuition into the nature of the distinction between frontal and posterior cortex comes from considering the nature of dreams. Recent data suggests that the frontal cortex (and other areas including the thalamus) is inactivated during REM sleep (Braun, Balkin, & Herscovitch, 1998). Thus, the spreading activation of associations and generally fuzzy, graded nature of dream-state cognition is just what we would expect from a system operating mostly on the basis of the posterior cortex. The absence of long-term continuity and focus is also what one would expect without the frontal involvement in controlled processing. Although there are many other things going on during REM sleep besides frontal inactivation, it may nonetheless provide a useful and universally accessible source of intuitions.

Before the kind of activation-based processing sketched here can produce anything approaching human-like higher-level cognition, two central issues must be solved: (a) the control of activation-based processing, and (b) the nature of activation-based processing representations. We consider each of these problems in turn.

The Control of Activation-Based Processing

The first issue is one that we began to address in chapter 9: How can the updating and maintenance of active representations be controlled in a systematic, task-relevant fashion? As explored in chapter 9, an active-memory-based working memory system requires a dynamic control system. In this chapter, we continue to explore the use of the dopamine-based gating system developed in chapter 9. We see that this mechanism can be used to drive a kind of trial-and-error search through activation space, which can provide greater flexibility than weight-based learning. As discussed in chapter 9, it is likely that more complex models will require additional control mechanisms, including a mechanism based speculatively on the basal ganglia for dynamically restricting the set of working memory representations subject to updating.

We emphasize the following important features of these control mechanisms: (a) control is an emergent phenomenon resulting from the interaction of basic neural mechanisms (e.g., multiple constraint satisfaction) with more specialized control mechanisms like the dopaminergic gating system; (b) strategic, task-based control develops through experience-based learning; (c) control typically involves a hierarchical set of goallike structures that decompose problems into a number of simpler steps (e.g., the high-level goal is to make a sandwich, which constrains the lower-level goal of applying peanut butter and jelly, which constrains the actions of finding these ingredients) — goals can thus both control lower-level goals and be controlled by higher-level goals.

In short, even though it can be useful to distinguish control mechanisms from other parts of the system, this distinction is often not a clear-cut one, and care should be taken to treat the system as an interactive whole and not as a master-slave kind of system; this later view inevitably leads to conceptions of controlling mechanisms having homunculus-like powers. The reliance on learning mechanisms is also important for avoiding the need to posit these homunculus-like powers — there is no need for a homunculus if "intelligent" control can be shown to emerge through experience.

The Nature of Activation-Based Processing Representations

The second issue for activation-based processing concerns the development of the necessary representations. How does a network like the activation-based categorization one (figure 11.1b) get set up in the first place? The general problem is that when the burden of processing depends mainly on the strategic activation of appropriate representations (e.g., goals, discriminating features, etc.), then there must be an existing vocabulary of such representations available for immediate use. Furthermore, one must be able to activate novel combinations of such representations to solve novel tasks, which is an essential aspect of many higher-level cognitive phenomena.

To understand better the existing vocabulary constraint, consider the categorization task example — to be able to switch rapidly among different categorization rules by simply activating different representations (e.g., "red," "blue," etc.), these representations have to already exist and have appropriate associations with corresponding posterior representations. It is not reasonable to imagine that the necessary associations could be developed dynamically on the fly — how could only a few trials of learning develop appropriately rich and systematic associations? Consider the analogy of trying to have a reasonable conversation with someone in an unfamiliar language — it is impossible to both learn a large number of new vocabulary words and dynamically use them for communicating. Even with a good, quick dictionary, extensive experience is required to learn the appropriate uses of words.

Therefore, the kind of slow, interleaved learning hypothesized to be the specialty of the cortex (chapters 7, 9) may build up a rich vocabulary of frontal activation-based processing representations, with appropriate associations to corresponding posterior-cortical representations. An activation-based control mechanism could then rapidly select among an existing vocabulary. Nevertheless, this general principle does not provide much substantial insight into what kinds of things are actually represented in frontal cortex. Are they like "goals" or "productions" or would simple copies of posterior stimulus-based representations work just as well?

In this section, we discuss a number of different ideas about the general nature of frontal activation-based processing representations. Unlike representations in the visual system, for example, where it is likely that humans are similar to monkeys and relatively much is known (chapter 8), human frontal representations may be qualitatively different than those in monkeys, because our capacities for higher-level activation-based processing are qualitatively different. Therefore, we have no solid empirical data about what kinds of things neurons in human frontal cortex actually encode, so we must draw on a diverse set of more functionally driven ideas, including inspiration from symbolically based production systems, performance on Stroop and categorization tasks, and language-based representations.

Because traditional symbolically based *production systems* have been successful at modeling higher-level cognitive tasks such as problem solving (e.g., Anderson, 1983; Newell, 1990), it is useful to consider the idea that frontal representations may resemble the kinds of *productions* used in these systems. A production is an elemental cognitive action that is activated when a specific set of conditions is met. The effect of production activation is ultimately to activate subsequent productions, typically by manipulating the contents of active memory to trigger the enabling conditions of other productions. Thus, productions control the flow of processing in a goal-driven manner via these enabling conditions — one could imagine a similar weight-based mechanism for detecting the enabling conditions of a production. However, symbolic production systems take liberal advantage of arbitrary symbol binding operations, whereas the goallike active memory representations in the neural system may have a more content-specific, dedicated nature. Thus, we are not advocating the use of neural mechanisms that simply reimplement existing symbolic processing frameworks (see chapter 7 for discussion). Nevertheless, the general notion of a production might be a useful way of conceptualizing the nature of the representations used in activation-based processing.

Another relatively simple idea is that some of the activation-based processing representations encode stimulus-level information. In the categorization example, correct task performance can be achieved by simply maintaining active representations of the discriminating features (e.g., "red"). At a somewhat more abstract level, the Stroop task can be solved by maintaining an active representation that specifically favors processing in the color-naming pathway — this could be a representation corresponding to the sensory perception of color, for example.

Language-based representations also provide a potential source of insight into the nature of frontal representations, in two different senses. In a strictly metaphorical sense, frontal representations may constitute a "vocabulary" that can be systematically combined to produce an effectively infinite combinatorial space of context, goal and task representations. In a more literal sense, the considerable time and effort spent developing the ability to combine flexibly verbal representations into complex, meaningful structures is undoubtedly directly leveraged by the frontal cortex.

Thus, the frontal cortex may have a strong tendency to rely on linguistic representations in the service of complex task performance. Support for this idea is the nearly ubiquitous finding of activation localized around Broca's area during working memory or other frontal tasks (e.g., Awh, Jonides, Smith, Schumacher, Koeppe, & Katz, 1996; Braver, Cohen, Nystrom, Jonides, Smith, & Noll, 1997; Paulesu, Frith, & Frackowiak, 1993; Fiez, Raife, Balota, Schwarz, Raichle, & Petersen, 1986). This area is commonly thought to subserve the *phonological loop* function engaged in verbal rehearsal (Baddeley, 1986). Thus, a simple, intuitively appealing idea is that people engage in verbal rehearsal of task-relevant information during the performance of complex tasks.

One overarching characterization of frontal representations, which is consistent with the above ideas, is that they are more *discrete* in nature, whereas posterior cortical representations encode information in a more continuous fashion (O'Reilly, Mozer, Munakata, & Miyake, 1999b; O'Reilly et al., 1999a). For example, productions are discrete because they either fire or not, and language is based on discrete symbols (words). Interestingly, discreteness can confer increased noise tolerance for working memory representations, as we explored in chapter 9, suggesting a synergy between a number of constraints.

Chapter Organization

After a brief discussion of the biological organization
of the frontal cortex, we begin with the first exploration, which covers a model of the Stroop task and illustrates how the prefrontal cortex can exhibit strategic,
goal-directed control over cognitive processing by simply maintaining appropriate goallike representations in
active memory. Then, we explore a version of the categorization task described previously that is based on the
widely-studied Wisconsin Card Sorting Task. We simulate performance of intact and frontally-lesioned monkeys on this task.

Having explored two important principles of frontal
function, we then consider a broader range of data regarding the role of frontal cortex in humans and monkeys (e.g., lesion data, electrophysiology, neuroimaging). These data provide a more general sense of frontal
contributions to cognitive functioning, which we can
then account for using the mechanisms developed in the
explorations. We also discuss other major theoretical
frameworks for understanding frontal function.

Having focused primarily on the role of the frontal
cortex in higher-level cognition, we conclude with a
broader perspective on the interactions among different
brain areas as they contribute to controlled processing.

11.2 Biology of the Frontal Cortex

From a biological perspective, the emphasis we place
on activation-based processing in higher-level cognition
clearly points to an important role for the prefrontal
cortex, with its ability to sustain robust yet rapidly
updatable activation-based memories (see chapter 9).
Thus, we focus primarily on the properties of this system. However, it is important to keep in mind that the
true complexity and power of human higher-level cognition is undoubtedly an emergent property involving
important contributions from posterior cortical systems
as well as other brain areas such as the hippocampus.
Unfortunately, the complexity of developing models of
these emergent phenomena is prohibitive at this time.
We focus on the prefrontal cortex to develop the central
theme of activation-based processing and to introduce
an important set of principles.

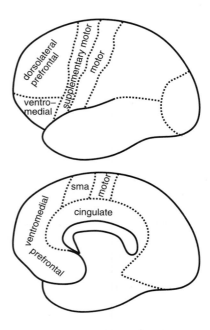

Figure 11.2: Primary subdivisions of the frontal cortex,
shown for both a lateral (top panel) and medial (bottom panel)
perspective.

The frontal cortex can be subdivided into a number of
different regions, and lesions of these different regions
can have different effects on behavior, as we discuss
later. Figure 11.2 shows the primary subdivisions of
frontal cortex, including the more posterior motor and
supplementary motor areas, and the dorsolateral (top
and side) and ventromedial (bottom and middle) prefrontal areas. The cingulate cortex, located in the medial wall, is typically included in discussions of frontal
cortex.

In general, one can think of the frontal representations as becoming progressively more abstract in the direction from the posterior (primary motor) to the more
anterior (prefrontal) areas. The supplementary (also
called premotor) areas constitute an intermediate level
of abstraction, consisting of larger-scale motor plan representations that integrate a number of more basic motor movements. By extension, one can think of the prefrontal areas as having yet more abstract action plans.

There also appear to be some functional differences associated with the dorsolateral and ventromedial regions of prefrontal cortex, but the precise characterization of these differences is controversial. For example, some theories hold that dorsolateral areas are important for active/working memory, while ventromedial areas perform behavioral inhibition and other kinds of more affective processing (e.g., Fuster, 1989; Diamond, 1990). Others hold that the dorsolateral region is important for more complex processing, while the ventromedial region performs simpler memory functions (e.g., Petrides, 1996). In the context of the dynamic categorization model explored below, we posit a dorsolateral/ventromedial distinction between more abstract and more concrete representations, respectively. However, we regard all of these ideas as speculative and incomplete at this point, because there is simply insufficient evidence.

At a finer grain of organization, we reviewed in chapter 9 that there is evidence that the prefrontal cortex may have more isolated patterns of connectivity — neurons there appear to be interconnected within self-contained "stripe" patterns (Levitt et al., 1993), and iso-coding microcolumns of neurons have been recorded (Rao et al., 1999). This biological data can influence ideas about the nature of frontal representations — isolated stripes may facilitate the development of representations that are more easily and flexibly combined with each other for novel task performance (O'Reilly et al., 1999a; O'Reilly et al., 1999b).

One other important aspect of frontal biology has to do with its extensive interconnectivity with the basal ganglia. The frontal cortex provides one of the primary inputs to the striatum of the basal ganglia, and the basal ganglia project via the thalamus back up to the frontal cortex, creating a series of "loops" (Alexander, De-Long, & Strick, 1986). As discussed in chapters 7 and 9, these loops through the basal ganglia may provide a fine-grained gating/motor initiation mechanism. This intimate association of the basal ganglia and the frontal cortex can help to explain why basal ganglia lesions (e.g., in Parkinson's disease) often produce frontal-like behavioral deficits (which are reviewed in a later section).

11.3 Controlled Processing and the Stroop Task

Our first exploration focuses on the distinction between controlled and automatic processing using a model of the Stroop task (Stroop, 1935). As mentioned in the introduction, the controlled-processing aspect of the Stroop task involves naming the ink color of a conflicting color word (e.g., saying "red" to the word "green" printed in red ink). Our model is based on that developed by Cohen and colleagues (Cohen et al., 1990; Cohen & Servan-Schreiber, 1992; Cohen & Huston, 1994), and demonstrates how top-down activation-based biasing from the frontal cortex can enable controlled processing by overriding prepotent associations encoded in the posterior cortex. That is, the frontal activation supports the weaker process of color naming over the prepotent response of word reading. Frontal cortex is uniquely important for this biasing function because it can robustly maintain the appropriate task-relevant representations in an active state over time without being overcome by the activity from the stronger processing pathway.

At a mechanistic level, the model is very simple, involving only a handful of units and relying on the simple idea that additional activation (from the frontal cortical units) can support processing in a weaker pathway. Nevertheless, these simple principles are sufficient to replicate important aspects of the behavioral data. Furthermore, we think that these same simple principles can be applied to understanding the role of frontal cortex in much more complex tasks (e.g., problem solving). These more complex tasks would require more sophisticated control mechanisms for activation-based processing, and a richer vocabulary of representations that can be combined in complex ways — you should recognize these as the two central problems outlined in the introduction. We begin to address the control problem in the subsequent simulation, which is followed by a more detailed discussion of the representation issue. Thus, the Stroop model establishes the basic principles of top-down control that are elaborated in the subsequent sections.

The standard pattern of reaction time performance in the Stroop task is shown in figure 11.3 (data from

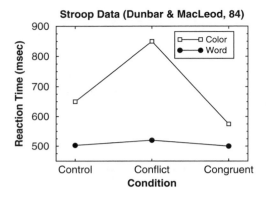

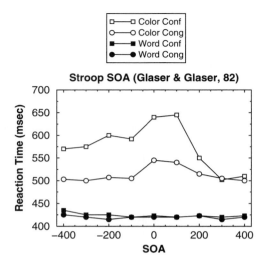

Figure 11.3: Reaction times for standard Stroop task, showing strong interference effect in the color naming conflict condition, and little effect of color on word reading. The control conditions have no influence from the other process (i.e., just reading a color word written in black ink, or naming a patch of color or colored X's). In the conflict condition, color and word conflict (e.g., "red" written in green ink), and in the congruent condition they agree. Data from Dunbar & MacLeod, 1984.

Figure 11.4: Reaction time data from a Stroop task where colors and words were presented at different times relative to each other (stimulus onset asynchrony, SOA). For word reading negative SOA means the color preceded the word. For color naming, negative SOA means the word preceded the color. Even when presented 400 msec before the word, color fails to significantly affect word reading, invalidating the processing speed model. Data from Glaser & Glaser, 1982.

Dunbar & MacLeod, 1984). There are several important features of these data: (a) the relative weakness of the color naming process is revealed by slower overall reaction times; (b) the color naming conflict condition is particularly slowed, because the conflicting prepotent word reading response must be overcome; (c) there is a slight facilitation effect for congruent stimuli in the color naming condition (color and word the same) compared to the control condition where no other information is present (e.g., naming a color patch or colored X's); (d) the relative automaticity of word reading is evident by virtue of its imperviousness to the color condition — reaction times are essentially flat across conditions (though there are small effects that are consistent with the conditions).

One standard account of the Stroop effect is in terms of processing speed — word reading is faster, and thus drives the response before the color information is processed, explaining the lack of effect of color on word reading. Color naming, being slower, must overcome the word reading response which is already influencing the response. To test this processing speed account,

Glaser and Glaser (1982) independently varied the onset of color and word information (i.e., the stimulus onset asynchrony, or SOA). If the processing speed account is correct, presenting the color prior to the word should result in color interfering with word reading. However, as shown in figure 11.4, this was not the observed result — color still had virtually no effect on word reading even when presented 400 msec prior to the word.

Thus, as argued by Cohen et al. (1990), a strength-based account, where the word-reading pathway is stronger than the color-naming one and thus dominates it in the context of competitive activation dynamics, provides a better model of the Stroop effect. In the model, the strength differences are due to learning, which is sensitive to the differential frequencies of word reading and color naming. Thus, the word reading pathway has stronger, better-trained weights than the color naming pathway. These differences result both in faster reaction times for word reading and in a strength-based competition between color naming and word reading that results in the conflict slowing effect.

Another illuminating piece of behavioral data comes from a training study in which subjects learned to label novel shapes with color names (e.g., to respond "blue" to a squiggle shape) (MacLeod & Dunbar, 1988). Subjects with different amounts of this shape-naming training were tested on naming the shapes (the trained task) and the ink colors (the Stroop task), under congruent and conflicting conditions. For relatively brief amounts of shape-naming training (one day), conflicting color interfered with shape naming, just like word reading usually interferes with color naming in the standard Stroop task. Meanwhile, color naming was essentially unaffected by the shapes (again, like word reading normally is). After more extensive training (20 days), the shape naming task acted like word reading in the standard Stroop task — it interfered with color naming, and was itself relatively insensitive to color. Thus, automatic versus controlled processing is a relative distinction, depending on where the competing stimuli lie along a continuum of strength. All of these aspects of Stroop behavior are important for understanding the nature of the phenomenon in normals, and they provide important constraints for the model.

Additional evidence from frontal patients and schizophrenics speaks directly to the role of frontal cortex in the Stroop task (e.g., Cohen & Servan-Schreiber, 1992; Vendrell, Junque, & Grafman, 1995). Both of these populations exhibit differentially impaired performance on the color naming conflict condition, indicating an impairment in overriding the prepotent response of word reading based on task instructions to name the color. The frontal patient data clearly support the idea that frontal cortex is important for this controlled-processing function. The schizophrenic data are also supportive, because schizophrenia apparently involves an impairment of frontal dopamine function (among other things).

Cohen and Servan-Schreiber (1992) showed that the schizophrenic data could be modeled by assuming that dopamine affects the gain of the activity of frontal neurons (e.g., γ in equation 2.19 from chapter 2). A reduction of gain in the frontal task units in the Stroop

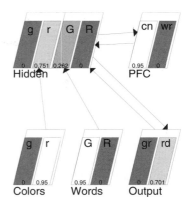

Figure 11.5: The Stroop model, where the PFC (prefrontal cortex) represents the task context (cn = color naming, wr = word reading). Activity pattern corresponds to color naming conflict condition, where the color input is red (r), the word input is green (G), and the task context activated in the PFC is color naming (cn), which biases the color naming hidden units (the left two units in the hidden layer) and enables the network to respond "red" (rd) in the output.

model, corresponding to lower dopaminergic gain in schizophrenics, produces a differential impairment in the color naming conflict condition. The net effect of the gain reduction is to lower the amount of top-down support to the color naming pathway, supporting the general idea that the critical contribution of frontal cortex in this task is to provide this top-down support.

11.3.1 Basic Properties of the Model

Figure 11.5 shows the Stroop model. Two different colors and color words are represented, red and green. The color and word inputs feed into a hidden layer with separate hidden units for processing color and word information. These hidden units, which are intended to represent posterior-cortical processing pathways, are combined into a single layer to enable them to compete amongst each other under a kWTA constraint — it is this competition that produces the slowed reaction times in the color naming conflict condition. The kWTA constraint is set so that there is more stringent competition within each processing pathway than between pathways (achieved by setting the k parameter to 1 within subgroups representing the pathways, and a k value of 2 for the entire layer — the resulting inhibition is the maximum of these two).

The top-down prefrontal cortex (PFC) task units are each connected to the corresponding group of 2 hidden units (i.e., color naming PFC (cn) connects to g and r color hidden units, and word reading PFC (wr) connects to G and R word hidden units). This connectivity assumes that the PFC has a set of representations that differentially project to color naming versus word reading pathways — we discuss this representation issue in a subsequent section. We also simulate the robust maintenance of these PFC units by simply clamping them with external input — we explore the mechanisms of activating and maintaining these representations in the next simulation.

The prepotent nature of word reading is produced by training with a frequency ratio of 3:2 for word reading compared to color naming. Although this ratio likely underestimates the actual frequency difference for reading color words versus naming colors, the inhibitory competition and other parameters of the model cause it to be very sensitive to differences in pathway strength, so that this frequency difference is sufficient to simulate typical human behavior. If the actual frequencies were known, one could easily adjust the sensitivity of the model to use these frequencies. As it is, we opted for default network parameters and adjusted the frequencies.

Because of its simplified nature, training in this model does not actually shape the representations — it only adapts the weight strengths. The 2 word reading training events simply present a color word input (G or R) and clamp the word reading PFC unit (wr), and train the network to produce the corresponding output (gr or rd). Similarly, the color naming training has the color naming PFC unit active (cn) and trains the output to the color inputs. Thus, the network never experiences either a conflict or a congruent condition in its training — its behavior in these conditions emerges from the frequency effects.

To record a "reaction time" out of the model, we simply measure the number of cycles of settling, with the stopping criterion being whenever an output unit exceeds an activation value of .7. As is typical when the

units in the model represent entire pathways of neurons (i.e., when using a highly scaled down model), we lower the unit gain (to 50). Otherwise, default parameters are used.

11.3.2 Exploring the Model

↪   Open the project `stroop.proj.gz` in `chapter_11` to begin.

You should see the network just as pictured in figure 11.5.

↪ Begin by exploring the connectivity using `r.wt`.

You will notice that all of the units for red versus green are connected in the way you would expect, with the exception of the connections between the hidden and output units. Although we assume that people enter the Stroop task with more meaningful connections than the random ones we start with here (e.g., they are able to say "Red" and not "Green" when they represent red in the environment), we did not bother to preset these connections here because they become meaningful during the course of training on the task.

Next, let's look at the training environment patterns.

↪ Press `View`, `TRAIN_EVENTS` on the `stroop_ctrl` control panel.

You will see 4 events, 2 for training the word reading pathway, and 2 for color naming (one event for each color). The frequency of these events is controlled by a parameter associated with each event.

↪ Locate the `Evt Label` menu in the upper left-hand corner of the environment window, which controls what is displayed as the label for each event in the window. Change the selection from `Event::name` (the name of the event) to `FreqEvent::freq` (the frequency of the event).

Now you can see that the word reading events have a frequency of .3, while the color naming events are at .2 (note that the sum of all frequencies equals 1). This frequency difference causes word reading to be stronger than color naming. Note that by using training to establish the strength of the different pathways, the model very naturally accounts for the MacLeod and Dunbar (1988) training experiments.

↪ Iconify the environment window.

Now, let's train the network.

↪ Open a training log using View, TRAIN_LOG, and the press Train on the control panel. You might also want to turn off the Display on the network to speed things up.

We next explore the differential weight strengths for the two pathways that develop as a result of training. Although the observed weight differences are not huge, they are enough to produce the behavioral effects of word reading being dominant over color naming.

↪ Use r.wt, and click on the output units — note that the word reading pathway is stronger. Similarly, press on the g and G hidden units in sequence, and note that the G (word reading) hidden unit has stronger weights overall.

Question 11.1 (a) *Report the weights for the* g *and* G *hidden units from their respective input, PFC, and output units (you need only report the* gr *output weight).* **(b)** *At which layers in the network are the differences greatest?* **(c)** *Can you explain this in terms of the error signals as they propagate through the network?*

Basic Stroop Task

Now, let's test the network on the Stroop task. First, we will view the testing events.

↪ Press View, WORDREAD_EVENTS.

You should see the control, conflict, and congruent conditions for word reading, all of which have the word reading PFC task unit clamped (wr). All patterns have the R word unit active. Control does not have any active color units, conflict adds the g (green) color unit active, and congruent adds the r (red) color unit.

↪ Iconify the word reading environment, and then press View, COLORNAME_EVENTS to observe a similar pattern of inputs for color naming. Iconify that environment before continuing.

Now, we can actually test the network.

↪ Iconify the training log, and then open a testing log using View, TEST_LOG. Then press TEST.

You will see the reaction times (cycles of settling) plotted in the upper graph log, which should resemble figure 11.6. The data points are plotted at X-axis values of 0, 1, and 2, corresponding to the Control, Conflict, and Congruent conditions, respectively.

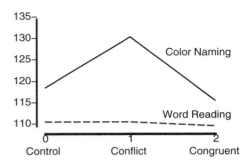

Figure 11.6: GraphLog results for the Stroop task in the model. Compare this pattern of results with those for people as shown in figure 11.3.

↪ You may need to press the Init button on the graph log to rescale it to better fit the display.

If you compare this with the human data shown in figure 11.3, you will see that the model reproduces all of the important characteristics of the human data as described previously: interference in the conflict condition of color naming, the imperviousness of word reading to different conditions, and the overall slowing of color naming.

Now, we can single-step through the testing events to get a better sense of what is going on.

↪ First, be sure your Display is on for the network, and that you are viewing act (activations). Then, do StepTest.

Each StepTest of the process will advance one step through the three conditions of word reading in order (control, conflict, congruent) followed by the same for color naming. For the word reading conditions, you should observe that the corresponding word reading hidden unit is rapidly activated, and that this then activates the corresponding output unit, with little effect of the color pathway inputs. The critical condition of interest is the conflict color naming condition.

Question 11.2 (a) *Describe what happens in the network during the conflict color naming condition, paying particular attention to the activations of the hidden units.* **(b)** *Explain how this leads to the observed slowing of reaction time (settling).*

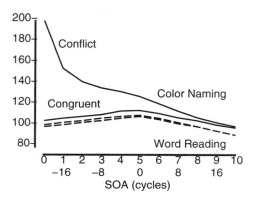

Figure 11.7: GraphLog results of the SOA test in the model. Compare this pattern of results with those for people as shown in figure 11.4. See text for a discussion of the comparison.

SOA Timing Data

Another important set of data for the model to account for are the effects of differential stimulus onset times Glaser and Glaser (1982) discussed previously. To implement this test in the model, we simply present one stimulus for a specified number of cycles, and then add the other stimulus and measure the final reaction time (relative to the onset of the second stimulus). We use five different SOA (stimulus onset asynchrony) values covering a range of 20 cycles on either side of the simultaneous condition. For word reading, color starts out preceding the word by 20 cycles, then 16, 12, 8, and 4 cycles (all indicated by negative SOA), then color and word are presented simultaneously as in standard Stroop (0 SOA), and finally word precedes color by 4, 8, 12, 16, and 20 cycles (positive SOA). Similarly, for color naming, word initially precedes color (negative SOA), then word and color are presented simultaneously (0 SOA), and finally color precedes word (positive SOA). To simplify the simulation, we run only the most important conditions – conflict and congruent.

↪ To run the SOA test, first View SOATEST_LOG, and then press the SOA_Test button. You may want to turn the network Display off.

You will see that the lower graphlog has been replaced with a new one, which displays the reaction time as a function of SOA on the X axis. You should see

something like figure 11.7 when the test is complete — because it is not possible to label the lines in the simulation, you should rely on the figure to decode what is going on. The two solid lines represent the color naming conflict and congruent conditions. The two dotted lines represent the word reading conflict and congruent conditions – these lines basically fall on top of one another and so are not labeled separately, but the conflict condition line is slightly higher at the earliest SOA's.

By comparing the simulation data with the human data shown in figure 11.4, you can see that the model's performance shows both commonalities and contrasts with the behavioral data. We first consider the commonalities. The model simulates several important features of the behavioral data. Most importantly, the model shows that word reading is relatively impervious to color conditions (conflict vs. congruent), even when the colors precede the word inputs, as indicated by the similarity of the two dotted lines in the graph. Thus, the dominant effect in the model is a strength-based competition — the word reading pathway is sufficiently strong that even when it comes on later, it is relatively unaffected by competition from the weaker color naming pathway. Note that there is some evidence of an interference effect (congruent vs. conflict difference) in the model for the earliest color SOA's — there is also a hint of this in the behavioral data.

Another important feature of the human data captured by the model is the elimination of the interference effect of words on color naming when the color precedes the word by a relatively long time (right hand side of the graph). Thus, if the color pathway is given enough time to build up activation, it can drive the response without being affected by the word.

There are two important differences between the model and the human data, however. One difference is that processing is relatively slowed across all conditions as the two inputs get closer to being presented simultaneously. This is particularly evident in the two word reading conditions and in the congruent color naming condition, in the upward slope from -20 to 0 SOA, followed by a downward slope from 0 to 20. This effect can be attributed to the effects of competition — when inputs are presented together, they compete with one another and thus slow processing. This may be an artifact of the kWTA form of competition, as it was not found in the original Cohen et al. (1990) model.

Another difference, which was present in that model, is the increasingly large interference effect for earlier word SOA's on color naming in the model, but not in people. It appears that people are somehow able to reduce the word activation if it appears sufficiently early, thereby minimizing its interfering effects. Cohen et al. (1990) suggested that people might be habituating to the word when it is presented early, reducing its influence. However, this explanation appears unlikely given that the effects of the early word presentation are minimal even when the word is presented only 100 msec early, allowing little time for habituation. Further, this model and other models still fail to replicate the minimal effects of early word presentation even when habituation (accommodation) is added to the models.

An alternative possibility is that the minimal effects of early word presentation reflect a strategic use of perceptual (spatially mediated?) attentional mechanisms (like those explored in chapter 8) that can be engaged after identifying the stimulus as a word. According to this account, once the word has been identified as such, it can be actively ignored, reducing its impact. Such mechanisms would not work when both stimuli are presented together because there would not be enough time to isolate the word without also processing its color.

Effects of Frontal Damage

Now that we have seen that the model accounts for several important aspects of the normal data, we can assess the importance of the prefrontal (PFC) task units in the model by weakening their contribution to biasing the posterior processing pathways (i.e., the hidden layer units in the model). The strength of this contribution can be manipulated using a weight scaling (wt_scale) parameter for the connections from the PFC to the Hidden layer. This parameter is shown as pfc_gain in the control panel, with a default value of .8. Because the model is relatively sensitive, we only need to reduce this value to .75 to see an effect. Note that this reduction in the impact of the PFC units is functionally equivalent to the gain manipulation performed by Cohen and Servan-Schreiber (1992).

↪ Reduce the pfc_gain parameter from .8 to .75, and do a Test.

You should see that the model is now much slower for the conflict color naming condition, but not for any of the other conditions. This is exactly the same pattern of data observed in frontal and schizophrenic patient populations (Cohen & Servan-Schreiber, 1992). Thus, we can see that the top-down activation coming from the PFC task units is specifically important for the controlled-processing necessary to overcome the prepotent word reading response. Note that to fit the model to the actual patient reaction times, one must adjust for overall slowing effects that are not present in the model (see chapter 8 for a discussion of how to compare model and patient data).

Although we have shown that reducing the PFC gain can produce the characteristic behavior of frontal patients and schizophrenics, it is still possible that other manipulations could cause this same pattern of behavior without specifically affecting the PFC. In other words, the observed behavior may not be particularly *diagnostic* of PFC deficits. For example, one typical side effect of neurological damage is that overall processing is slower — what if this overall slowing had a differential impact on the color naming conflict condition? To test this possibility in the model, let's reduce the dt_vm parameter in the control panel, which determines the overall rate of settling in the model.

↪ Restore pfc_gain to the default value of .8, and then reduce dt_vm from .01 to .008, and do a Test.

Question 11.3 *Compare the results of this overall slowing manipulation to the PFC gain manipulation performed previously. Does slowing also produce the characteristic behavior seen in frontal and schizophrenic patients?*

↪ Go to the PDP++Root window. To continue on to the next simulation, close this project first by selecting .projects/Remove/Project_0. Or, if you wish to stop now, quit by selecting Object/Quit.

11.3.3   Summary and Discussion

The Stroop model demonstrates how the frontal cortex might contribute to controlled processing by providing a top-down source of activation that can support weak forms of processing (e.g., color naming). The model simulated several important features of the behavioral data, and, importantly, simulated the effects of frontal damage, thereby more directly supporting frontal involvement in this kind of controlled processing.

There have been a number of follow-ups to the original Cohen et al. (1990) Stroop model. The Cohen and Huston (1994) model improved on the original by using an interactive (bidirectionally connected) network instead of a feedforward one. Other papers have addressed other variations of the task, and other aspects of the fit to behavioral data (Schooler, Neumann, & Roberts, 1997; Kanne, Balota, & Faust, 1998; Cohen, Usher, & McClelland, 1998). However, the somewhat strange effects of early word SOA's on color naming reported by Glaser and Glaser (1982) have yet to be successfully accounted for by a model. Thus, many details remain to be resolved, but the general principles behind the model remain sound.

11.4 Dynamic Categorization/Sorting Tasks

In the Stroop model, we simulated the robust maintenance abilities of the prefrontal cortex by simply clamping the units with appropriate external input. In the present model, based on O'Reilly, Noelle, Braver, and Cohen (submitted), we retain the principle of top-down biasing, and turn our focus to the mechanisms of maintenance and updating of prefrontal representations. The task we explore is a version of the Wisconsin card sorting task, which can also be regarded as a dynamic categorization task where the rules change periodically. As discussed in the introduction, categorization tasks can be solved in two qualitatively different ways — either by using weight-based associations between distinctive features and responses, or by using activation-based maintenance of the distinctive features that can be compared with the inputs to generate a response. The activation-based approach has the distinct advantage of flexibility — a new categorization rule can be adopted simply by activating a new set of critical features.

There is actually another way that activation-based processing can contribute to a categorization task that involves a combination of activation-based and weight-based processing, instead of just pure activation-based processing. This third alternative is also more consistent with the role of the prefrontal cortex in the Stroop model, as it involves a top-down biasing of the relevant features in the posterior cortex, so that it is easier for weight-based learning to associate these features with the relevant response.

This top-down biasing is specifically relevant if a new categorization rule must be learned that conflicts with a prior rule. Here, the top-down biasing can facilitate the activation of representations appropriate for the new rule and enable them to better compete against the strengthened representations from the prior rule, just as top-down biasing from the prefrontal cortex enabled the weaker color-naming pathway to compete with the stronger word-reading pathway in the Stroop model. However, if there is no existing imbalance in the posterior representations (e.g., when learning an entirely new categorization rule), then this top-down biasing would not make that much of a difference, and learning would proceed according to the rate of weight-based learning. The A-not-B model from chapter 9 also has this general characteristic — the frontal cortex is specifically important for overcoming prior biases in where to reach.

As we will see in a moment, the pattern of data we will be modeling shows this characteristic that new categorization learning is unaffected by prefrontal lesions, while *reversals* of existing categorization rules (which involve conflict from prior learning) are affected. In contrast, if we were to adopt the kind of more purely activation-based categorization solution discussed in the introduction (involving a comparison between maintained information and the sensory input), we would expect that both initial acquisition of rules and reversal learning would be faster because no weight-based learning at all would be involved. Interestingly, this pattern of data has been found in humans for easily verbalizable categorization rules (i.e., those that can be easily maintained in activation-based memory), which were found to be more rapidly learned than other nonverbalizable (but equally reliable and salient) categorization rules (Ashby, Alfonso-Reese, & Waldron, 1998).

Thus, we suggest that the purely activation-based approach may be something that only humans have devel-

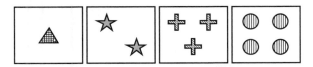

Figure 11.8: Example stimuli used in the Wisconsin Card Sorting Test. Cards vary in three dimensions: shape, color, and number, with four values along each dimension, as shown (different hatching patterns indicate different colors). When matching according to shape, for example, all cards containing a triangle should be placed under the first card shown in the figure, regardless of the number or color of the triangles. Similarly, when matching according to number, all cards having two stimuli, regardless of their color or shape, should be placed under the second card.

oped the strategies for, whereas the top-down biasing approach is something that all animals with a frontal cortex could readily apply. Given that the present model focuses on data from monkeys, it is appropriate that the top-down biasing approach is used here. Nevertheless, we expect that if similar tasks were run with people, the purely activation-based approach would be employed, resulting for example in more rapid overall learning with frontally intact people.

The Dynamic Categorization Task

The task we explore is similar to the Wisconsin card sorting test (WCST). In the WCST, participants sort sequentially presented cards according to one of three different stimulus dimensions (shape, color, and number; see figure 11.8). They must induce the correct sorting dimension based on feedback from the experimenter, and the experimenter periodically switches the categorization rule without notifying the subject. Normal subjects will pick up on this switch relatively quickly, and adopt the appropriate rule. In contrast, frontal patients tend to perseverate and retain the current sorting rule even in the face of mounting errors on the task.

In the top-down biasing model, frontal cortex contributes to the WCST by maintaining a representation of the currently relevant dimension in frontal active memory, which focuses top-down activation on the corresponding perceptual processing pathway, thereby facilitating sorting along this dimension. As we have ar-

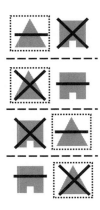

Figure 11.9: Example stimuli from the feature & dimension switching categorization task studied by Dias et al. (1997). Each row represents one trial. Subjects were rewarded for choosing the target (indicated by the surrounding box, which was not presented to the subjects). The stimuli were created by combining one of two possible line-shapes and one of two possible filled-shapes (all four possible test combinations are shown for these line-shape and filled-shape dimensions). The target was determined by one feature from one dimension, in this case, the triangle feature from the filled-shape dimension.

gued, the active representation can be relatively rapidly switched when the sorting rules changes, whereas a weight-based solution must unlearn the previous weights and learn the new ones. The perseveration observed in frontal patients on the WCST can be accounted for by the loss of the more flexible, frontally mediated activation-based facilitation to a less flexible weight-based one.

The actual task that our model implements, called the ID/ED task, has been explored in monkeys, neurologically intact humans, frontal patients, and Parkinson's patients (Dias, Robbins, & Roberts, 1997; Roberts, Robbins, & Everitt, 1988; Owen, Roberts, Hodges, Summers, Polkey, & Robbins, 1993). Instead of sorting, the task involves a two-alternative choice decision, which simplifies things somewhat. Also, as we will see in a moment, Dias et al. (1997) found an intriguing pattern of behavioral deficits associated with lesions of different frontal areas — this may shed some light on the topographic organization of frontal representations.

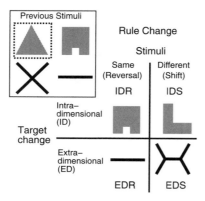

Figure 11.10: Types of changes in categorization rule following criterion performance on the original rule (figure 11.9), organized by same versus different stimuli across the rule change, and intradimensional or extradimensional target change. The target stimulus is again indicated by the surrounding box.

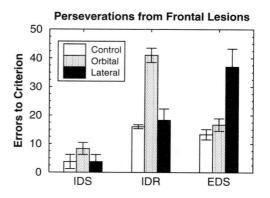

Figure 11.11: Perseverations from different types of frontal lesions in the WCST-like task studied by Dias et al. (1997). Orbital lesions (ventromedial) selectively impair intradimensional (IDR) reversals, whereas lateral lesions selectively impair extradimensional shifts (EDS, which are actually reversals to a previously ignored dimension). Intradimensional shifts (IDS) are never impaired. Data from Dias et al. (1997).

In this task, two stimuli are presented on each trial (figure 11.9), and the subject is rewarded for choosing the target stimulus. Each stimulus varies among two dimensions (e.g., filled-shape and line-shape), with each dimension having two different possible features (e.g., within line-shapes, either a bar or an X). The target is determined by one feature from one dimension (e.g., the triangle feature from the filled-shape dimension). Thus, reward is initially ambiguous between the two features of the stimulus on the rewarded side. Then, the pattern of reward across trials specifies the single target feature.

After the subject has achieved criterion level performance (e.g., 90% correct), the target feature is changed, and the stimuli either change or remain the same (figure 11.10). The target feature is changed either to a feature within the same dimension (*intradimensional*, or ID), or to a feature in the other dimension (*extradimensional*, or ED). The stimuli either stay the same, or they are changed such that each dimension (filled-shape or line-shape) now has two new possible features.

When the stimuli remain the same, the rule change results in a *reversal*, because the selection of a previously rewarded feature must be reversed to become a nonselection, and the nonselection of a previously unrewarded feature must be reversed to become a selec-

tion. When the stimuli change, the rule change results in a *shift*, because the selection of a previously rewarded feature must be shifted onto a novel feature. Thus, there are four different types of changes to the categorization rule: intradimensional reversal (IDR), intradimensional shift (IDS), extradimensional reversal (EDR), and extradimensional shift (EDS). The EDS case involves a reversal at the dimensional level, because a previously irrelevant dimension must be reversed to become relevant, and a previously relevant dimension must be reversed to become irrelevant.

Dias et al. (1997) tested marmosets (a type of Old World monkey) with lesions in different regions of frontal cortex on three of these changes: IDR, IDS, and EDS. They found selective impairment of intradimensional reversals with orbital (ventromedial) lesions, selective impairment of extradimensional shift with dorsolateral lesions, and no significant impairments on intradimensional shifts with either frontal lesion (figure 11.11).

Dias et al. (1997) interpreted their data in terms of the inhibitory roles of both orbital and dorsolateral areas, because frontal effects are only seen when the target change is a reversal (either IDR or EDS). Presumably, only reversals require the inhibition of learned associations between the target feature or target dimension and the response. They specifically dismissed the notion that an active-memory ("on-line" processing) account of frontal function could explain the data. However, as we saw in the Stroop model, the top-down biasing of correct information from active memory can in fact serve to inhibit incorrect (previous, prepotent) information.

Dias et al. (1997) further argued that the orbital area is important for "affective" inhibitory processing, whereas the dorsolateral area is important for "attentional selection." Under their logic, the intradimensional reversal requires a reversal of affective associations, whereas the extradimensional shift requires higher-order shifting of attentional focus to another dimension. This way of characterizing these different frontal areas is partially consistent with other notions in the literature, but also inconsistent with several others.

Our alternative interpretation of these findings consists of two parts. First, the effects of these frontal areas are seen only in reversal conditions because of the prepotent responses that must be overcome, through top-down biasing from active memory. As discussed above, this is essentially the same idea that we explored in the Stroop task, except that here we must establish how the frontal cortex can switch categorization rules more rapidly than the posterior system to provide an appropriate bias in the reversal conditions.

Second, we posit that different frontal areas represent information at different levels of abstraction. Specifically, orbital areas contain more detailed representations of the featural information within a dimension, and thus facilitate the intradimensional switching of targets, whereas the dorsolateral areas contain more abstract representations of dimensions per se, and thus facilitate switching to another dimension. There is some empirical evidence consistent with such a distinction between orbital and lateral areas. For example, a number of neural recording studies in monkeys suggest that ventral (orbital) areas encode object or pattern information (e.g. Mishkin & Manning, 1978; Wilson, Scalaidhe, & Goldman-Rakic, 1993). Other researchers have hypothesized based on a variety of data that the dorsolateral areas are involved in more complex, ab-

stract processing, whereas the ventral (e.g., orbital) areas are used for simpler memory processes that require maintaining specific information (e.g., Petrides, 1996).

The model we explore here implements this posited distinction between detailed and abstract representations in different frontal areas, combined with activation-based memory control mechanisms that enable the simulated prefrontal cortex to switch categorization rules more rapidly than the posterior cortex.

We use the same dopamine-based gating principles developed in chapter 9 to control the updating and maintenance of prefrontal representations. Recall that the dopamine-based system is based on the temporal differences (TD) reinforcement learning mechanism, which we explored in chapter 6. We can think of this mechanism as producing a form of *trial-and-error search*. Specifically, prefrontal representations are initially randomly activated, and persist until errors are made, at which time they are deactivated by the negative TD error signal, allowing other representations to be activated. Thus, in contrast with weight-based learning, the prefrontal representations can be rapidly deactivated, and new ones activated very quickly. This speed in discarding a previous categorization rule and switching to a new one produces the frontal advantage in our model.

11.4.1 Basic Properties of the Model

Figure 11.12 shows the structure of the model. The input layer represents the stimuli in a simple format, with separate units for the 2 different dimensions in each of the 2 different locations (left and right). There are 4 units within each dimension, and features are encoded using simple distributed representations having 2 out of the 4 units active. The hidden layer is organized in the same way as the input, but critically it is limited so that it can only have 2 units active at the same time, so that once a given target feature has been learned, the hidden representations of the other features are naturally suppressed. The output response is then produced via connections directly from the hidden layer, which is consistent with the top-down biasing model of frontal contribution — all of the actual learning is performed via weight-based associations between hidden and output units.

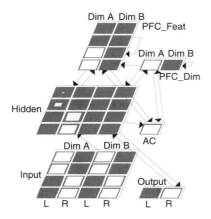

Figure 11.12: Dynamic categorization network: The input display contains two stimuli – one on the left and one on the right – and the network must choose one. The two stimuli differ along two dimensions (Dim A and B). Individual features within a dimension are composed of 2 active units within a column. The Input and Hidden layers encode these features separately for the left (L) and right (R) side display. Response (Output) is generated by learned associations from the Hidden layer. Because there are a large number of features in the input, the hidden layer cannot represent all of them at the same time. Learning in the hidden layer ensures that relevant features are active, and irrelevant ones are therefore suppressed. This suppression impairs learning when the irrelevant features become relevant. The prefrontal cortex (PFC) layers (representing feature-level and dimension-level information) help by more rapidly focusing hidden layer processing on previously irrelevant features.

The prefrontal cortex (PFC) areas are `PFC_Feat`, corresponding to orbital areas that represent featural information, and `PFC_Dim`, which corresponds to the dorsolateral areas that represent more abstract dimension-level information. These areas are reciprocally interconnected with the hidden units, and their activity thus biases the hidden units. The featural nature of the `PFC_Feat` representations is accomplished by having the individual PFC units connect in a one-to-one fashion with the featural units within the 2 dimensions. We only included one set of 4 such featural units per dimension because this area does not encode the location of the features, only their identity. The dimensional nature of the `PFC_Dim` representations comes from the

fact that there are only two such units, one for each dimension, with each unit fully connected with the feature units in the hidden layer from the corresponding dimension.

During initial learning, the network has no difficulty activating the target item representation, because all hidden units are roughly equally likely to get activated, and the correct item will get reinforced through learning. However, if the target is then switched to one that was previously irrelevant (i.e., a reversal), then the irrelevant item will not tend to be activated in the hidden layer, making it difficult to learn the new association. The top-down PFC biasing can overcome this problem by supporting the activation of the new target item, giving it an edge in the kWTA competition.

The AC layer is the adaptive critic for the temporal differences reward-based learning mechanism, which controls the dopamine-based gating of PFC representations and is thus critical for the trial-and-error search process. In this model, there is no temporal gap between the stimulus, response, and subsequent reward or lack thereof, but the AC still plays a critical role by learning to expect reward when the network is performing correctly, and having these expectations disconfirmed when the rule changes and the network starts performing incorrectly. By learning to expect rewards during correct behavior, the AC ends up stabilizing the PFC representations by not delivering an updating gating signal. When these expectations are violated, the AC destabilizes the PFC and facilitates the switching to a new representation.

More specifically, three patterns of AC unit activation – increasing, constant, and decreasing – affect the PFC units in different ways. If the network has been making errors and then makes a correct response, the AC unit transitions from near-zero to near-1 level activation, resulting in a positive TD δ value (computed as the difference in minus and plus phase AC activation, and indicating a change in expected reward), and thus in a transient strengthening of the gain on the weights from the hidden units to the PFC. This causes the PFC to encode the current pattern of hidden activity. If the network is consistently making errors or consistently performing correctly (and expecting this performance), then there is no change in the AC activation, and the

δ value is zero. This keeps the hidden to PFC weights at their low tonic value, so the PFC tends to maintain its current values. However, there is some noise added to the gating function, so it is possible for transitions to occur even with no AC change, especially if there is nothing presently active in the PFC. Finally, if an error is made after correct performance, then there is a negative δ value, which causes the PFC weight gain to decrease significantly in strength, including the gain on the recurrent self-maintenance weights. This effectively resets the PFC activations.

Note that although we generally describe this process of AC-mediated activation and deactivation of the frontal representations in terms of trial-and-error search, the search process is not actually completely random. The PFC units that are likely to get activated are those that receive the strongest input from the hidden layer. Thus, the search process is guided by the activations of the hidden units, which has the advantage of restricting the search to only relevant aspects of the input (i.e., it doesn't randomly search through the entire space of possible PFC representations).

We test the model on the three types of rule changes tested by Dias et al. (1997): IDR, IDS, and EDS. For each of these rule changes, we test an intact network first and then networks with lesions to the feature-level (orbital) prefrontal cortex or to the dimension-level (lateral) prefrontal cortex.

Before each rule change, each network receives 2 blocks of training (as did Dias et al.'s (1997) monkeys). In the first block, features from only one dimension are presented, where one feature is rewarded and the other is not. In the second block (described earlier in our initial presentation of the task), the two features from the other dimension are added, but the categorization rule remains the same as before. The network receives multiple trials within each of the 2 training blocks and proceeds from each block after completing two epochs without error. After the 2 training blocks are completed, the categorization rule changes so that the target: (1) shifts to be a newly presented feature within the dimension (IDS), (2) reverses to be the other (previously seen) feature within the dimension (IDR), or (3) shifts to a newly presented feature within the other dimension (EDS), thereby reversing at the dimensional level.

11.4.2 Exploring the Model

↪ Open the project `id_ed.proj.gz` in `chapter_11` to begin.

The network is as pictured in figure 11.12.

↪ Begin by exploring the network connectivity using `r.wt` and clicking on units in each of the different layers.

You should notice that the hidden units receive directly from their corresponding input unit, and from the appropriate units in both the PFC layers. Note also that the PFC units do not encode the location information, only the object properties. The PFC units each receive a single self-connection, which provides their maintenance ability (using isolated representations). The output units have random initial weights from the hidden layer units — it is these weights that are adapted during learning to solve the task.

Training

Now, let's step through the categorization learning. As described earlier, the first block of training trials presents features from only one dimension.

↪ First, make sure that you are viewing `act` (activations). Then, open up two logs to monitor training by doing `View`, `EPOCH_LOG`, and `View`, `NEPOCH_LOG`. Then, do `ReInit` and `StepSettle` on the overall `id_ed` control panel.

You will see the minus phase of the first categorization trial, which has the first 2 units within dimension A representing one feature on the left, and the second 2 units representing the other feature on the right. The location of these features (which is on the left and which is on the right) varies randomly. In this simulation, the target feature is represented by the activation of the first 2 units in dimension A. The hidden layer cannot initially decide which of the two features to represent, so it has weak activation for both of them.

↪ Press `StepSettle` again to get to the plus phase.

You should now see that the output unit corresponding to the location of the first feature is activated, providing the correct response. Because the network did not get this answer correct, the AC unit is provided with the absence of reward. (For purely technical implementation reasons, this is actually encoded by a very small positive value, 1.0e-12, which you should see as the value for that unit. Values of exactly 0 indicate no reward information at all, not the absence of reward.)

↪ Press StepSettle again to get to the second plus phase. Note that the network window displays all the counter information, so you can more easily keep track of where you are — phase_no should be 2 now.

Recall from chapter 9 that this second plus phase is viewed as part of one overall plus phase, but gets separated out for ease of determining first the change in the AC unit activation over the initial minus-plus phase set, and then the consequences for the PFC. You should see that in this case the PFC units are not updated, because the temporal differences TD signal across the AC unit minus and plus phases was zero, meaning that the hidden-to-PFC weights were not transiently strengthened. Note that there is noise added on top of this basic TD signal, but, because we are using the same set of random numbers (via the ReInit function), we know that this noise was negative and did not activate the PFC.

You can see the actual TD values used for gating the PFC units in the PFC_td values displayed near the respective PFC layers (both should be negative). Although random noise in the gating signal can activate the PFC units by chance, it turns out that on this run, the units will only get activated when the network produces the correct output.

↪ Press StepTrial (which steps through all three phases of one event) a few times, until you see the PFC units get activated.

When the network produces the correct output, the AC unit then receives a positive reward value in the first plus phase. To see that the network did produce the correct output in the minus phase, we can look at the minus phase activations.

↪ Press act_m in the network window to view the minus phase activations.

You should see that the right output unit is active above .5. The reward for producing the correct output that is provided to the AC unit produces a positive TD signal, which modulates the strength of the hidden-to-PFC weights by a large amount as shown in the PFC_td values, which should both be around 1. This large input strength causes the PFC units to now represent the most strongly active hidden units.

↪ Press act in the network window to view the plus phase activations, where you can see the active PFC units. Press StepSettle several times, observing the AC unit activation in the minus and plus phases. Stop when you see the other dimension getting activated in the input — the network is moving on to the second training block at this point.

You should notice for the next several trials that the network continues to perform correctly, so that the AC unit is activated in the plus phase, but it is not activated in the minus phase because that depends on learning to predict or expect the reward. This learning is taking place, and early in the next block it will come to expect this reward in the minus phase.

At this point, the network is responding correctly to the location of the first feature, and so has completed the first training block. However, you may have noticed that there is not necessarily a clear correspondence in the feature-level PFC to this target stimulus for the initial training block. This is because the second stimulus is actually perfectly anticorrelated with the first one in location, so the network could just as easily learn "press in the opposite direction of the second stimulus." Monkeys (and people) probably have biases to learn the more direct "press in the same direction as the first stimulus," but this bias is not captured in the model. Nevertheless, this bias turns out not to be critical, as we shall see.

To monitor the performance of the network on this task, it is useful to check the Epoch_0_GraphLog, which contains a plot of the error over epochs. You can see that the network error has descended to zero during this first training block, and completed one additional epoch with zero error, indicating that it is time to move on to the next block.

We next present the second training block, where the features from the other dimension (B) are included, but the target remains the same (the first feature in dimension A). The network has no difficulty with this problem. It should complete the block to criterion after the minimum of 2 epochs. During this time, the AC unit will come to strongly expect the reward signal in the minus phase.

↪ StepTrial through the second training block, stopping when the patterns in the input change (you can

batch	batch	env	epc_ctr	Epoch	cur_task
0	0	0	4	4	intact_ids
0	0	1	2	6	intact_ids
0	0	2	2	8	intact_ids
1	0	0	4	4	fetles_ids
1	0	1	2	6	fetles_ids
1	0	2	2	8	fetles_ids
2	0	0	6	6	dimles_ids
2	0	1	2	8	dimles_ids
2	0	2	4	12	dimles_ids

Figure 11.13: Output of `NEpoch_0_TextLog` for all lesion conditions of the IDS task.

cur_task	onedim	twodim	rule_change
intact_ids	4	2	2
fetles_ids	4	2	2
dimles_ids	6	2	4
intact_idr	4	2	9
fetles_idr	4	2	17
dimles_idr	4	2	9
intact_eds	3	2	8
fetles_eds	4	2	5
dimles_eds	7	2	13

Figure 11.14: Output of `RepiBatch_0_TextLog` for the entire set of lesions and categorization rule conditions. The first line of output discussed in the text is at the top row.

#	Task	Network	Log Label
1	IDS	Intact	intact_ids
2		Feat lesion	fetles_ids
3		Dim lesion	dimles_ids
4	IDR	Intact	intact_idr
5		Feat lesion	fetles_idr
6		Dim lesion	dimles_idr
7	EDS	Intact	intact_eds
8		Feat lesion	fetles_eds
9		Dim lesion	dimles_eds

Table 11.1: Schedule of categorization tasks and network lesion conditions that the simulation automatically steps through, and the label used in the text log `cur_task` column.

also monitor the `env:` counter in the network — stop just when it gets to 2.

Intradimensional Shift

Now, we are ready to change the categorization rule and test the network's ability to react appropriately. We begin with the intradimensional shift rule change: the network is presented with two new features within each of the two previous dimensions, and the new target is one of the new features from the same dimension previously rewarded.

↪ `StepSettle` through the phases for the first few trials in this sequence.

You should see that the network is still getting this problem correct — it just happened to learn weights that work for both problems. Now, let's accelerate the rate of stepping as the network comes to acquire the new categorization rule.

↪ First, open one more log that will record the summary of this sequence of training by doing `View`, `BATCH_LOG`. Then, press `StepEpoch` (which steps over epochs, not settling phases) until the input patterns switch back to the single-dimension (A) patterns, which indicates the start of the first training block for the next sequence of blocks.

To evaluate the overall performance of the intact network on the IDS task, let's examine the other two logs (you should have noticed that the `Epoch_0_GraphLog` was automatically cleared at the start of the next block). First, look at the `NEpoch_0_TextLog` (figure 11.13), specifically the `epc_ctr` column, which shows the number of epochs required to reach criterion on each of the 2 training blocks (4 and 2 epochs) and on the rule change block (2 epochs). Also shown in this log is the `cur_task` column, which reads `intact_ids` indicating that the network is intact and that the task was IDS.

Next, look at the `RepiBatch_0_TextLog` (figure 11.14), which summarizes the `epc_ctr` values across a single line, with the three blocks labeled `onedim`, `twodim`, and `rule_change`. The `rule_change` column is the key one for comparison with the Dias et al. (1997) results.

Next we will test the importance of the PFC areas for performance on this IDS task. We first test the network with a lesioned (deactivated) `PFC_Feat` layer (orbital prefrontal cortex), and then with a lesioned `PFC_Dim` layer (dorsolateral prefrontal cortex). The simulation will automatically cycle through the appropriate lesions and task conditions as you step the process, according to the schedule shown in table 11.1.

↪ `StepEpoch`, monitoring the `NEpoch_0_TextLog`. Stop just after the network has completed all three blocks (two training and one rule change) with both lesions — there are no interesting lesion effects for the IDS task so we can just skip over these two lesions.

The `cur_task` column in both logs shows `fetles_ids` and `dimles_ids` to indicate the two different lesion conditions — the first with lesioned `PFC_Feat` layer and the second with lesioned `PFC_Dim` layer — tested on IDS. In `RepiBatch_0_TextLog`, the `rule_change` column reports a 2 and a 4 for both the lesioned networks. Thus, the network, like Dias et al.'s (1997) monkeys, does not seem to rely on prefrontal cortex for the IDS task.

Question 11.4 *Explain why PFC lesions do not affect learning in the IDS task in the network (focus on the advantages of the PFC, and why the demands of the task do not require these advantages).*

Intradimensional Reversal

Now, we will change the categorization rule in a different way, with an intradimensional reversal. The network is presented with the same stimuli during training and after the rule change, but the target reverses to be the other feature within the previously rewarded dimension. As with the previous exercise, we will test an intact network first and then two lesioned networks, providing each network with 2 blocks of training before the rule change.

↪ `StepEpoch`, monitoring the `NEpoch_0_TextLog`, and stopping just after the first 2 training blocks have been completed. Note the two `PFC_Feat` units that are active.

Now, we are in the position to watch what happens during an intradimensional reversal trial. We will switch back to stepping at the level of a single phase of settling, and watch the network's response to the errors that are produced.

↪ `StepSettle` through a few trials observing what happens to the PFC units as errors are made.

You should observe that the PFC units are deactivated as a result of the network's errors, because the network produces exactly the opposite of the correct responses (due to the reversal of the target stimuli). This rapid deactivation of the PFC units facilitates switching to another categorization rule. Next, we will observe as the deactivated PFC units are reactivated.

↪ Continue to `StepSettle` until the PFC units are reactivated (even though they are in the wrong dimension). Monitor the `PFC_td` values associated with each PFC layer.

Question 11.5 **(a)** *Report the* `PFC_td` *values that led to the PFC units being reactivated.* **(b)** *Explain these values in terms of what happened on the trial — did the network produce a correct response, or was the activation due to random noise?*

↪ Continue to `StepSettle` for several more trials, until PFC units in the *A* dimension units get activated again.

Over this next set of trials, a combination of random gating noise and initial correct responses caused the PFC units to get deactivated and then reactivated again in a new configuration, which facilitates producing a different response.

Because of the redundancy in the way the problem can be solved, either by responding to the same side as the target stimulus or to the side opposite of the nontarget, it is not always clear that the network has reversed its focus from the previous target to the current target. Thus, the critical property to observe is that *different* `PFC_Feat` units get activated, and thereby support the activation of different hidden units, which facilitates the learning of a different response mapping. You should see that this is indeed what has happened.

↪ `StepEpoch` through the remaining trials in the IDR block with the intact network.

You should see that the logs have recorded the `intact_idr rule_change` value, which should be 9 epochs.

Next we will test the importance of the PFC areas for performance on this intradimensional reversal task. The automatic schedule calls for the network with a lesioned `PFC_Feat` layer (orbital prefrontal cortex) to be run next, and then with a lesioned `PFC_Dim` layer (dorsolateral prefrontal cortex).

We can step through the orbital lesion at the level of epochs, observing the general patterns of activation of the hidden units.

↪ StepEpoch through the training and rule change blocks, focusing on the patterns of activity in the hidden layer.

You should have observed that the hidden unit activations never get very sharply differentiated from each other (because of the absence of top-town differentiating support from the PFC), but that there is a noticeable change in the hidden activation patterns as a result of the IDR task. Without the feature-level PFC top-down influence, the slower weight-based learning takes longer to master this task, resulting in a rule_change epc_ctr value of 17 instead of 9 with the intact network.

We next test the network with a dorsolateral lesion on the intradimensional reversal.

↪ StepEpoch through the training and rule change blocks.

You should see that there is no effect of this dorsolateral lesion compared to the intact network.

Question 11.6 *Explain why the dorsolateral (dimensional) lesion has no effect on the intradimensional reversal.*

Extradimensional Shift

Finally, we will change the categorization rule according to an extradimensional shift (which includes a reversal at the level of dimensions). The network is presented with two new features within each of the two previous dimensions, and the new target is one of the new features from the previously nonrewarded dimension. Again, we will test an intact network first and then two lesioned networks, providing each network with 2 blocks of training before the rule change.

↪ StepEpoch through the first 2 training blocks for the intact network.

Now we are in a position to watch what happens during an extradimensional shift. Let's do phase-wise stepping as the network comes to activate the other, previously ignored dimension.

↪ StepSettle through the remainder of the sequence, observing the PFC units.

Question 11.7 *Provide a narrative account of what happens during this EDS trial and explain this in general terms with respect to the AC-mediated trial-and-error search mechanism.*

Again, we see that the ability of the PFC to more rapidly switch to a new representation plays an important role in this reversal task.

Now, let's see how the lesioned networks perform. We first test the network with a lesioned PFC_Feat layer (orbital prefrontal cortex).

↪ StepEpoch through the training and rule change blocks for the orbital lesioned network (fetles_eds).

You should see from the rule_change column in the batch text log that the orbital lesion actually enabled the network to learn more rapidly than the intact network (5 epochs for the lesioned case compared to 8 for the intact — this appears to be a somewhat reliable trend for the network).

We next test the network with a lesioned PFC_Dim layer (dorsolateral prefrontal cortex).

↪ First, StepEpoch through the 2 training blocks for the orbital lesioned network (dimles_eds).

Now, we can step more carefully, though still at the epoch level, through the EDS task, and observe what happens without the benefit of the dimension-level PFC units.

↪ StepEpoch through the epochs, observing the activation of the remaining PFC_Feat units and the hidden units, specifically with respect to when the dimension B units become activated.

You should observe that there is no coordinated switch of the PFC units to the other dimension, resulting in a protracted period of incorrect performance before the PFC_Feat units switch over to dimension B. This switch took 13 epochs to work itself out, compared to 8 for the intact and feature-PFC lesioned network.

Question 11.8 *Explain why the absence of the dimension-level (dorsolateral) PFC units impairs extradimensional shift performance in this way.*

Because of the important role of noise in determining the network's performance, multiple runs through the tasks need to be averaged to provide a more complete

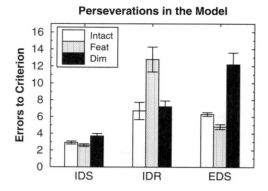

Perseverations in the Model

Figure 11.15: Perseverations from different types of simulated frontal lesions in the model. *Feat* is lesions of the feature-level PFC representations, which correspond to the orbital lesions (ventromedial) in the Dias et al. (1997) monkeys — intradimensional reversals (IDR) are selectively impaired. *Dim* is lesions of the dimension-level PFC representations, which correspond to the lateral lesions in monkeys — extradimensional shift/reversals (EDS) are selectively impaired. Intradimensional shifts (IDS) are never impaired.

picture. Figure 11.15 shows a graph of the averages for 10 runs on each task, plotted in a manner comparable with figure 11.11 showing the empirical data from Dias et al. (1997). The qualitative patterns of effects of PFC damage are comparable in the simulation and the monkeys. Feature (orbital) lesions selectively impair intradimensional reversal, dimensional (lateral) lesions selectively impair extradimensional reversal, and neither lesion affects intradimensional shift. These effects demonstrate that the model captures the essential contribution of the PFC in facilitating more flexible (less perseverative) processing via activation-based processing.

One interesting difference between the model and monkey data is that the featural (orbital) lesions appear to *improve* extradimensional shift performance (EDS). This effect can be attributed to the fact that top-down activation organized *not* along the direction of the reversal can actually *impair* performance (i.e., the featural level organization impairs reversal across dimensions), such that a lesion of this area can actually improve performance slightly. Although this effect makes sense in the model, it is likely that other collateral effects of dam-

age, or a less perfect division of dimensional and featural representations, could obscure such an effect in the monkeys.

↪ To stop now, quit by selecting `Object/Quit` in the `PDP++Root` window.

11.4.3   Summary and Discussion

This simulation provides a first step toward characterizing the kinds of control mechanisms that enable activation-based processing to be more flexible and dynamic than weight-based processing. The model extends the simpler working-memory model from chapter 9 by accounting for empirical data that implicates the frontal cortex in more flexible, less perseverative processing.

More specifically, we found that by simulating the role of dopamine in regulating the frontal cortex in terms of an adaptive-critic mechanism, a rapid trial-and-error searching process emerged. This searching process deactivated the prefrontal cortex when errors were made, and activated it either through noise or when performance was successful. The model matched at a qualitative level the effects of orbital and lateral prefrontal cortex damage on the dynamic categorization task by encoding more detailed feature-level information in orbital areas, while encoding more abstract dimension-level information in lateral areas. These different levels of representation, when combined with the trial-and-error control mechanism, provided a quick way of reconfiguring the categorization rule used by the network via top-down biasing (as in the Stroop model) of different representations. This biasing was specifically beneficial when the rules were reversed, in which case the cortical system had a difficult time overcoming the prior (dominant) pattern of responding without the help of top-down activity.

Although the model is successful at a qualitative, demonstration-of-principles level, its detailed patterns of behavior do not precisely match those of the monkeys in the Dias et al. (1997) studies. The monkeys experienced two different training sequences across two different experiments that involved a sequence of intradimensional shifts and reversals, and an extradimensional shift/reversal. To implement these sequences in the model would require a more complex network capable of representing 16 different stimuli, whereas our simplified model can only represent 4. One of the most interesting phenomena that could be addressed by such a model is the finding that a second reversal does not produce the same patterns of frontal deficits as observed with the first reversal. We suspect that this may emerge as a result of the posterior system establishing a more equal balance among the representations involved, but this may not entirely account for the effect.

Another aspect of the model worth noting is the way in which object and location information has been represented in the hidden layer. Although we know that object ("what") and location ("where") information are represented in separate pathways in the brain (chapter 8), we have used combined what/where representations in the hidden layer, so that each hidden unit represents an object feature in a particular location. This avoids having to deal with the what-where binding problem that is likely resolved by more complex sequential attention mechanisms in the real system (again see chapter 8 for models of this). The basic principles of the frontal involvement in this task are not likely to be affected by these implementational factors.

11.5 General Role of Frontal Cortex in Higher-Level Cognition

We have now explored two primary ways in which frontal cortex contributes to higher-level cognitive function. In the Stroop model, robust active maintenance provides top-down activation to facilitate weaker processing in the posterior cortex, and in the dynamic categorization model frontal cortex contributes to flexible behavior by virtue of dynamic activation-based processing control mechanisms.

11.5.1 Functions Commonly Attributed to Frontal Cortex

In this section, we more broadly review several functions, not necessarily mutually exclusive, that have been attributed to the frontal cortex based on cognitive neuroscience data. We show that these functions can be understood within the activation-based processing frame-

work, which we then discuss in relation to other major theoretical frameworks for understanding frontal function. The following functions have generally been attributed to the frontal cortex:

Activation-based working memory This attribution is based largely on monkey electrophysiology data in simple delayed response tasks that require information to be maintained during the delay (e.g., Fuster, 1989; Goldman-Rakic, 1987; Miller et al., 1996; see chapter 9 for a more detailed discussion of these data).

Inhibition The frontal cortex appears to be important for inhibiting prepotent responses, (e.g., word reading in the Stroop task) or "reflexive" or "instinctual" behaviors.

Flexibility Frontal patients tend to lack flexibility, for example by perseverating in producing old responses even after the task has changed (e.g., in the reversal conditions of the dynamic categorization task).

Fluency Frontal patients have difficulty generating a variety of responses to a given stimulus, for example in coming up with novel uses for a familiar object.

Executive control Frontal cortex is important for goal-directed behavior like planning, coordinating, and the like.

Monitoring/evaluation To control behavior, an executive also needs to monitor and evaluate the status of ongoing behavior — some frontal areas seem to be specialized for these functions.

After discussing the data in support of these attributions, we will see how each of them can be understood within the common framework of an activation-based processing model of frontal function. Because chapter 9 covers the working memory data, we focus on the other themes here.

Inhibition

Failures of inhibition are sometimes the most salient effect of frontal damage. A classic example is the case of Phineas Gage, who had a metal spike penetrate his ventromedial prefrontal cortex in a railroad construction accident. After the accident, the previously mild-mannered man began to engage in inappropriate behaviors and say rude and inappropriate things, often in outbursts of rage. One interpretation is that he could no longer inhibit these inappropriate urges.

In the laboratory, inhibition has been studied primarily using simple motor response tasks, for example the anti-saccade task (Roberts, Hager, & Heron, 1994) where subjects have to saccade (move their eyes) in the opposite direction of a visual stimulus. Here, the prepotent response is to saccade toward the stimulus, so this must be inhibited. Frontal lesions produce deficits in this task (e.g., Guitton, Buchtel, & Douglas, 1985). Inhibition also can be invoked to explain aspects of several of the other attributions to frontal cortex, as described in subsequent sections.

Although some researchers have proposed that frontal areas, specifically ventromedial, are specialized for inhibitory processing per se (e.g., Fuster, 1989; Diamond & Goldman-Rakic, 1989), other researchers have characterized the inhibitory functions of frontal cortex as a consequence of activation-based processing (Cohen et al., 1990; Kimberg & Farah, 1993; Munakata, 1998; O'Reilly et al., 1999a). For example, as we saw in the Stroop model, top-down support for color naming can inhibit the word-reading process as a consequence of direct competition among these processes. Our framework is more consistent with this activation-based characterization. With widespread inhibitory competition throughout our networks (and presumably the cortex), any differential support for one set of representations or processes will automatically result in inhibition of other competing ones.

In many ways, the inhibition versus competition distinction is similar to the case of the disengage mechanism for attention discussed in chapter 8. Recall that Posner and colleagues had proposed that to switch attention to a new location, one first needed to disengage (i.e., inhibit) the previously attended location. We saw that instead of requiring a specialized disengaging mechanism, competition from the engaging of attention elsewhere could produce the necessary disengagement. This competition model seems to be more consistent with the attentional data from patients and normals, and

arises quite naturally within the modeling framework developed here.

Further evidence against the notion of a specialized inhibitory system comes from the nature of the connections from prefrontal cortex to other areas. Long-range intracortical connections (e.g., from the prefrontal cortex to other posterior cortical areas) are all excitatory rather than inhibitory. These excitatory connections also synapse on inhibitory interneurons, but they do not do so exclusively. Further, the inhibitory interneurons have very diffuse patterns of connectivity that would not facilitate the precise inhibition of only selected types of information.

Flexibility

The contribution of frontal cortex to flexibility is revealed by the perseverations of frontal patients. Recall that perseveration is the tendency to persist in making a previously valid response even when task conditions have changed. Probably the most well-known paradigm where perseveration is observed is the Wisconsin card sorting task as we explored previously, but it is also found across a range of other paradigms, including the A-not-B task as discussed in chapter 9.

One standard interpretation of these perseverative effects is that they reflect a failure of inhibition, where the frontal patient fails to properly inhibit the previous response or categorization rule (e.g., Diamond & Goldman-Rakic, 1989; Dias et al., 1997). However, as we saw in the dynamic categorization exploration and the A-not-B model in chapter 9, perseveration can be explained in terms of a weak active memory system that cannot overcome the effects of prior learning.

In short, perseveration in frontal patients may reveal the flexibility benefits in normals of an activation-based solution over a weight-based one. When the activation-based solution is eliminated or impaired (via a frontal lesion), the system resorts to a weight-based solution, which is slower to react to changes (i.e., exhibits perseveration) and is generally less flexible. The apparent need to inhibit prior responses to avoid perseveration falls naturally out of the competitive model described earlier — one does not need to hypothesize a specific inhibitory system.

Fluency

Another important angle on the issue of flexibility comes from the study of fluency tasks with frontal patients. These tasks typically require the subject to generate as many different responses to a given stimulus as possible, for example by naming as many different animals that they can think of in a limited amount of time, or by generating as many different words that begin with a given letter. Interestingly, frontal patients do not show deficits on the animal-naming version of the fluency task (Newcombe, 1969), but do show deficits on the word initial-letter version (Milner, 1964). These findings show that the deficit is not necessarily associated with the control aspects of the generation task, but rather with the arbitrary nature of the initial-letter version. Thus, when the responses are all very familiar and fit within a well-established category (e.g., animals), posterior areas appear to be capable of generating the responses. In contrast, one is not often required to generate words based on initial letters, so this requires a kind of flexibility in adapting to the novel demands of the task.

Another fluency task, the Alternative Uses test, appears to place even greater demands on the frontal cortex because it is more sensitive to frontal damage (Butler, Rorsman, Hill, & Tuma, 1993). This test requires the subject to generate as many atypical uses for a common object as possible (e.g., using newspaper to make a hat, wrap fish, start a fire). In addition to requiring novel responses, these responses must overcome the prepotent responses of the typical uses for an object.

The continuum of frontal involvement in these fluency tasks is consistent with the activation-based model of frontal function. In short, top-down support from the frontal cortex is needed to support the unfamiliar processing involved in the initial-letter word fluency task, but not in the familiar animal-naming task. The Alternative Uses test is even more demanding of frontal function because strong prepotent responses must be overcome, presumably via strong top-down activation from the frontal cortex.

Executive Control

Deficits in executive control associated with frontal lesions are commonly observed, but can be difficult to characterize due to the complex nature of these processes. One important aspect of executive control is goal-directed behavior. As early as Bianchi (1922), frontal lesions have been characterized as impairing the ability to organize a series of actions around a common goal. For example, Bianchi described a frontally lesioned monkey that grabbed a door handle but then failed to open the door because it became engaged in looking at the handle; then it just sat on the handle. It appears that actions under frontal damage are more often reactions to environmental cues rather than deliberate and goal-directed. Lhermitte (1986) has described an *environmental dependency syndrome* accompanying frontal damage. For example, a patient visiting a physician's home reacted to seeing a hammer, nail, and picture by hanging the picture on the wall, and another saw a set of dirty dishes and immediately began washing them!

In addition to not seeming to be able to generate goal-driven behavior themselves, frontal patients have difficulty following explicit task instructions, even for relatively simple everyday tasks. For example, Shallice and Burgess (1991) described frontal trauma patients who were given explicit instructions for a sequence of everyday tasks (shopping for a small set of items, keeping an appointment, and collecting information). These patients, who scored *above* average on an IQ test, nevertheless failed to remain focused on the tasks, and became distracted by various intervening events. A simple lack of memory for the goals can be ruled out as an explanation for their failure because they were given a written list of the tasks.

Laboratory problem solving tasks can provide somewhat more controlled tests of frontal executive functions. One such task that has been studied with frontal patients is the Tower of London task (Shallice, 1982). In this task, a variant of the Tower of Hanoi, colored balls placed on a set of three sticks must be moved one at a time to achieve a specified goal state where the balls are in a specific arrangement on the sticks. Because the sticks are of varying heights so that they can only support a limited number of balls, there are constraints as to which balls can be moved at any given point to achieve the goal state. To achieve the goal state in a minimal number of moves, the sequence of moves must be planned to take into account the constraints. Frontal patients are significantly impaired on this task, requiring many more moves than controls to achieve the goal state, and generally making moves in a rather aimless fashion (Shallice, 1982). Further, neurologically intact individuals show activation of the frontal pole as they solve this task (Baker, Rogers, Owen, Frith, Dolan, Frackowiak, & Robbins, 1996).

As should be clear from our activation-based processing framework, we view activation-based memory and controlled processing as two sides of the same coin (e.g., O'Reilly et al., 1999a; Cohen et al., 1997), but this view is certainly not universally accepted (e.g., Baddeley, 1986; Grafman, 1989; Petrides, 1996). Although an abstract problem solving task like the Tower of London may require different sets of goallike control representations as compared to a more stimulus-based categorization task, the basic mechanisms of rapid updating and robust maintenance of information are clearly important for formulating executing a plan. Planning in particular requires that activations be updated not based on current stimuli, but rather on internally activated representations of future situations. This requires that the representations involved be protected from interference from ongoing perceptual processing. Also, once a plan has been activated, goal states must be maintained and updated as processing proceeds.

Monitoring/Evaluation

For controlled processing to be effective, the current state of processing in the cognitive system must be monitored and evaluated. There is growing evidence that areas of the frontal cortex are important for these monitoring and evaluation tasks. One area that has received considerable attention is the cingulate, specifically the anterior portion (see figure 11.2). Gehring, Goss, Coles, Meyer, and Donchin (1993) observed that the anterior cingulate appeared to be the source of an error-related activation signal that arises when people detect that they have made an erroneous response. Carter,

Braver, and Cohen (1998) showed that this area could alternatively be interpreted as representing the level of response conflict (i.e., the extent to which two different responses are strongly competing with each other, as opposed to there being one dominant response), which is correlated with the probability of making an error.

Processes like error monitoring are clearly important for controlling goal-driven kinds of behaviors. Indeed, we showed in chapter 9 that the adaptive critic mechanism from the temporal-differences learning procedure, which computes differences between expected and actual reward, could regulate the updating and maintenance of active memories in a simple working memory task. We think this kind of monitoring process is an essential aspect of the activation-based processing in frontal cortex. In addition to the anterior cingulate, neighboring regions of ventromedial prefrontal cortex are likely to be important for this function (e.g., Bechara et al., 1996).

Summary

To summarize, the frontal cortex appears to be important for a range of different behavioral manifestations of what we have characterized as activation-based processing. Beyond the basic function of actively maintaining information, this type of processing can provide flexibility and fluency, and serves to inhibit task-irrelevant information via intrinsic competition while reducing perseveration by being more rapidly updatable than weight-based systems. Executive-like controlled processing can emerge out of the effects of this system, combined with an effective monitoring and evaluation system and other nonfrontal areas, as elaborated later.

Although we think that the common mechanism of activation-based processing underlies the full spectrum of frontal functions, this has not yet been conclusively demonstrated, and must be regarded as a speculative hypothesis — one that, as we have pointed out, is not necessarily widely held.

Finally, it is important to note that despite the wide variety of effects of frontal damage, frontal patients often have completely normal IQ scores. Indeed, as emphasized by Shallice (1988), the frontal cortex was regarded as largely unimportant for several decades (roughly from the 1940s to the '60s) because the effects of frontal damage did not show up on standardized tests. It turns out that these tests largely tap routine knowledge and cognitive procedures, and not the kinds of temporally-extended, novel tasks where the frontal cortex plays its largest role. Thus, despite the temptation to associate intelligence with frontal processing and higher-level cognition, the standard IQ measure appears to tap more posterior, well-learned cognitive processes. This fact should serve as an important reminder against the temptation to attribute too much power and importance to the frontal cortex — intelligence is truly distributed and the posterior cortex plays a very important role in "intelligent" processing.

11.5.2 Other Models and Theoretical Frameworks

There are a number of other models and theoretical frameworks for understanding frontal function in the literature. Perhaps the most relevant for the dynamic categorization model is the framework of Ashby et al. (1998), who focus on the different brain areas involved in category learning. They discuss the role of the prefrontal cortex in terms of verbalizable, rule-based categorization processes, whereas the posterior cortex is involved in more holistic, similarity-based processes. This is very compatible with the ideas that we have presented here. One contribution our model makes is in providing a self-sufficient, learning-based searching mechanism — the Ashby et al. (1998) leaves these mechanisms biologically underspecified.

Dehaene and Changeux (1991) developed a model of the Wisconsin card-sorting task (WCST), which is closely related to the dynamic categorization task we explored previously. They proposed that the frontal deficit impaired the ability to use feedback to select alternative responses, which is also similar to the idea proposed by Levine and Prueitt (1989). Both of these models share basic principles in common with the model we developed.

Using a model based on a production-system framework, Kimberg and Farah (1993) accounted for a range of frontal deficits, including perseveration on the WCST. The essence of the model is that frontal damage reduces the influence of specific information on production firing, such that the productions end up falling back on perseverative and noisy firing biases that operate in the absence of other specific information. Thus, they build in perseveration as the behavior that the model resorts to after a frontal lesion. In contrast, we see perseveration as a result of learning in the weight-based processing of the posterior cortex. Nonetheless, this paper makes a number of more general points that resonate well with the framework presented here. For example, Kimberg and Farah (1993) emphasize the idea that frontal cortex can be understood as performing a single function, that, when damaged, produces a range of different behavioral manifestations. Furthermore, this common frontal function has something generally to do with working memory, which is consistent with our emphasis on activation-based processing.

In addition, there are many points of overlap between the framework outlined above and theoretical frameworks in the literature that have not yet been specified at the level of explicit neural network models.

Perhaps the most commonly cited theoretical framework for frontal function is the supervisory attentional system (SAS) of Shallice (1982; Shallice & Burgess, 1991). The SAS is a *central-executive* mechanism (Gathercole, 1994; Shiffrin & Schneider, 1977) that is deployed for nonroutine behavior, and it has been characterized in the context of a production system architecture, in which the SAS is responsible for maintaining goal states in working memory to coordinate the firing of productions involved in complex behaviors. These notions of frontal involvement in attentional and nonroutine processing are similar to the top-down biasing we discussed above, and we have discussed the maintenance of goal states as a likely role of the specialized frontal activation-based memory system. Thus, many aspects of the SAS are consistent with our approach, but its rather underspecified framing in terms of a production system hinder any attempt to provide a more detailed mapping between the two frameworks.

There are several more biologically based theoretical frameworks, which lack specific computational mechanisms but do provide important general themes. For example, Fuster (1989) suggests that frontal cortex plays an important role in mediating sensory-motor mappings at the highest levels of a hierarchy of many such mapping systems. The lower-level mappings can subserve more reflexive and well-learned mappings, while the frontal cortex is important for more novel and temporally-extended, complex mappings. This is clearly very consistent with our activation-based processing framework. Another important example is the framework of Goldman-Rakic (1987), which is based on the idea of actively maintained representations in frontal cortex. Although her research has focused on relatively simple maintenance tasks that do not place significant demands on either dynamic control mechanisms or representational complexity (e.g., more abstract goallike representations), her basic ideas can be extended to cover these issues, as we have done within our framework.

Finally, there are a range of other theoretical perspectives that we do not have the space to cover, but which also share aspects in common with our framework, and offer a variety of different ideas as well (e.g., Baddeley, 1986; Grafman, 1989; Petrides, 1996).

11.6 Interacting Specialized Systems and Cognitive Control

Although we have focused our discussion to this point on the role of the frontal cortex in higher-level cognition and controlled processing, it is clear that these phenomena depend on the interaction of multiple brain areas. In this section we elaborate some specific ideas regarding the nature of these interactions as they contribute to controlled (versus automatic) processing. These ideas are based on the *cognitive architecture* comprised of three interacting specialized systems: the posterior cortex, the hippocampus, and the frontal cortex as sketched in chapter 7 and explored in the context of memory function in chapter 9.

We focus on the interactions between frontal cortex and hippocampus here, because a relatively simple story can be told. This should not be taken to exclude other interactions. The goal is to understand the nature of the continuum between controlled and automatic processing in terms of the differential involvement of the frontal cortex and hippocampus (figure 11.16). As we've seen, the frontal cortical contribution can be characterized in terms of top-down *biasing*. The hippocampal contribu-

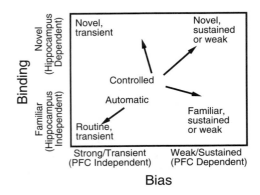

Figure 11.16: Ways in which the hippocampus and frontal cortex contribute to the automatic versus controlled-processing distinction. **Bias** is provided by the frontal cortex, and can be used to perform sustained processing, can facilitate the processing of weakly-learned (i.e., relatively infrequent) tasks, and can serve to coordinate processing across different areas. **Binding** is provided by the hippocampus, and can be used to rapidly learn and store the information necessary to perform novel tasks or processing. Controlled processing can involve either or both of these contributions, whereas automatic processing can be performed independent of them.

tion can be characterized in terms of a *binding* function for rapidly encoding and binding together information (Cohen & O'Reilly, 1996). This binding can be useful in the context of controlled processing for encoding the different components of a task as given by verbal instructions, or encoding intermediate states of processing for later retrieval. Thus, we hypothesize that the extent of controlled processing in a task is defined by the extent to which the following conditions exist:

• Sustained, weakly learned (i.e., relatively infrequent), or coordinated processing is required (engaging the frontal cortex biasing function).

• Novel information must be rapidly stored and accessed (engaging the hippocampus binding function).

The extent of automatic processing is defined by the relative absence of these factors.

We can apply this framework to the case of text comprehension to obtain a fuller picture of the kinds of interactions that are possible. As one is reading, the limited capacity of the frontal active memory system will necessitate the offloading of information to the hippocampal system. Thus, the comprehension of prior paragraphs is encoded only within the hippocampus, and must be recalled as necessary during later processing (e.g., when encountering a reference like, "this would be impossible, given Ms. Smith's condition," which refers to previously introduced information that may not have remained active in the frontal cortex). This later reference can be used to trigger recall of the previous information from the hippocampus, perhaps with the addition of some strategic activation of other relevant information that has persisted in the frontal cortex (e.g., the fact that Ms. Smith lives in Kansas). A successful recall of this information will result in the activation of appropriate representations within the both the frontal and posterior cortex, which combined with the current text results in comprehension (e.g., Ms. Smith was hit by a tornado, and can't come into work for an important meeting).

Although we can visualize these kinds of interactions in terms of the hippocampal and frontal models we have explored, models that incorporate both of these components, together with a distributed posterior cortical system, are just beginning to be developed. Such models are very complex, and represent the frontier of current computational capacity. Therefore, it is too early to say how well our account of controlled processing works in practice, but as a conceptual model, it clearly captures important aspects of the controlled-versus-automatic processing distinction.

11.7 Summary

We have presented a speculative but hopefully intriguing framework for approaching the issue of higher-level cognition. This framework is centered around the notion of **activation-based processing** as distinct from **weight-based processing**, with the idea that the frontal cortex is specialized for activation-based processing. Two key issues for activation-based processing are the nature of the **control mechanisms** for updating and maintenance, and the nature of the **activation-based representations**, which need to exist prior to their use and be flexibly recombined to solve novel tasks.

We first explored this framework by modeling several patterns of human performance on the **Stroop** task, the critical condition of which involves a **conflict** between a more dominant word-reading pathway and a weaker color-naming pathway when subjects are asked to name the color of a color word written in another color (e.g., "red" written in blue ink). The Stroop model is based on the principle of **top-down biasing** from the prefrontal cortex, which can support the weaker color-naming pathway and help it compete against the stronger word-reading pathway. In the absence of this top-down support (e.g., in frontal patients and in schizophrenics, or in the lesioned model), the word-reading pathway dominates, resulting in slower and more error-prone performance in the conflict condition.

Building on the basic principles of top-down biasing from the Stroop task, we explored a **dynamic categorization task** based on the **Wisconsin Card Sorting Test**, which is widely known to be sensitive to frontal function. The model demonstrates that the frontal cortex can more rapidly switch categorization rules by using activation-based processing, whereas the posterior cortex depends on less flexible weight-based processing. Thus, frontal lesions result in *perseverations* when the system resorts to the weight-based processing, and the model can account for two different kinds of perseverations that result from lesions in two different frontal areas. The model uses the same **dynamic control mechanism** based on the neuromodulator **dopamine** as was explored in chapter 9 for controlling updating and maintenance in active memory. This mechanism results in **trial-and-error search** in activation-space, which is what produces more flexible behavior.

Having explored two important manifestations of the activation- versus weight-based framework, we then reviewed a range of phenomena from monkey electrophysiology, the behavior of frontally damaged patients, and functional neuroimaging, which can all be accounted for within the activation-based processing framework. These phenomena include **inhibition**, **perseveration**, **fluency/flexibility**, **executive control**, and **monitoring/evaluation**. We concluded with a discussion of the ways in which other brain areas, including the **hippocampus**, can interact with the frontal cortex in higher-level cognitive phenomena.

As a final comment, the work in this chapter was more speculative than in previous chapters. Although we had to rely on intuition and analogy instead of implemented computational models for many critical arguments in developing the framework, we hope that future modeling work will address these issues in a more satisfying manner.

11.8   Further Reading

Shallice (1988) contains a nice historical summary of the course of thinking about frontal function over this century, as well as covering his supervisory attentional system (SAS) model, which has been very influential.

Miyake and Shah (1999) provides a collection of very recent, high-quality articles from leading researchers on the topic of working memory, which is intimately intertwined with higher-level cognition.

Newell and Simon (1972) and Anderson (1983) provide classic treatments of human problem solving from the traditional symbolic perspective.

Fuster (1989) provides an excellent treatment of the biological perspective on frontal function, as well as his theoretical ideas.

Ashby et al. (1998) review a range of behavioral and biological data on the involvement of the frontal cortex and other related brain areas (cingulate, basal ganglia) in categorization tasks.

Chapter 12

Conclusions

Contents

12.1 Overview 411
12.2 Fundamentals 411
12.3 General Challenges for Computational Modeling 413
    12.3.1 Models Are Too Simple 414
    12.3.2 Models Are Too Complex 417
    12.3.3 Models Can Do Anything 418
    12.3.4 Models Are Reductionistic 418
    12.3.5 Modeling Lacks Cumulative Research . . . 419
12.4 Specific Challenges 419
    12.4.1 Analytical Treatments of Learning 419
    12.4.2 Error Signals 420
    12.4.3 Regularities and Generalization 420
    12.4.4 Capturing Higher-Level Cognition 421
12.5 Contributions of Computation to Cognitive Neuroscience 421
    12.5.1 Models Help Us to Understand Phenomena 421
    12.5.2 Models Deal with Complexity 422
    12.5.3 Models Are Explicit 423
    12.5.4 Models Allow Control 423
    12.5.5 Models Provide a Unified Framework 423
12.6 Exploring on Your Own 424

12.1 Overview

In this chapter we revisit some of the fundamental issues in computational cognitive neuroscience covered in previous chapters, with an eye toward integration across chapters. Then we explore remaining challenges for the field at both the general level of the computational modeling endeavor and in terms of more specific issues, and speculate about how these might be addressed and what the next generation of models will bring. We conclude by highlighting the ways in which computational models have contributed toward the development of cognitive neuroscience.

12.2 Fundamentals

We covered quite a broad range of topics in this text, from the movements of ions at the individual neuron level up through learning in the service of complex cognitive functions such as planning. Our goal has been to understand findings across these different levels through an interactive, balanced approach that emphasizes connections between neurobiological, cognitive, and computational considerations.

In chapter 2, we saw that individual neurons act like detectors, constantly monitoring their inputs and responding when something matches their pattern of weights (synaptic efficacies). The ion channels of the neuron compute a balance of excitatory, inhibitory, and leak currents reflected in the membrane potential. When this potential exceeds a threshold, the neuron fires and sends inputs to other neurons in the network. The rate of firing can be encoded as a continuous variable, activation.

Chapter 3 showed how individual detectors, when wired together in a network, can exhibit useful collective properties that provide the building blocks of cognition. These network properties build on the ability of individual detectors to compute a balance of excitatory and inhibitory inputs, and include: transforming input patterns into patterns that emphasize some distinctions and collapse across others; bidirectional top-down and bottom-up processing, pattern completion, amplification, and bootstrapping; attractor dynamics; inhibitory competition and activity regulation, leading to sparse distributed representations; and multiple constraint satisfaction, where the network's activation updates attempt to satisfy as many constraints as possible.

Chapters 4–6 built on the basic network properties by showing how neurons within a network can learn by adapting their weights according to activation values of the sending and receiving units. Such learning uses local variables, yet results in coherent and beneficial effects for the entire network. We analyzed two main learning objectives: model learning and task learning. Model learning causes the network to capture important aspects of the correlational structure of the environment. Task learning enables the network to learn specific tasks. These learning objectives are complementary and synergistic, and can both be achieved using known properties of synaptic modification mechanisms. Extra mechanisms, including an internal context representation and a mechanism for predicting future rewards, can also be used to learn temporally extended or sequential tasks.

In chapter 7, we sketched an overall cognitive architecture that builds on the mechanisms just described. Three different brain areas can be defined on the basis of fundamental tradeoffs that arise from basic neural network mechanisms. One tradeoff captures the distinction between the hippocampal system and the rest of cortex in terms of learning rate — one system cannot both learn arbitrary things rapidly and also extract the underlying regularities of the environment. Another tradeoff captures the difference between the prefrontal cortex and the posterior cortex in terms of the ability to perform rapidly updatable yet robust active maintenance. Active maintenance suffers when representations are richly interconnected, because spreading activation bleeds away memory. But these interconnections are useful for many kinds of processing (e.g., pattern completion, constraint-satisfaction, and *inference* more generally). The posterior cortex can thus be understood in terms of its relationship to these other specialized brain areas. More generally, the posterior cortex can be seen as a set of specialized but interacting, hierarchically organized pathways of transformations building upon each other.

Chapter 8 provided a good example of a hierarchically organized sequence of transformations that lead to the ability to recognize objects in a spatially invariant fashion. At each level, units transformed the input by both combining features and integrating over different locations and sizes. At the lowest level of cortical visual processing, neurons encode the correlational structure present in visual images. Although the object recognition model could recognize individual objects quite well, it got confused when multiple objects were present. Adding spatial representations that interacted with this object processing pathway enabled the system to sequentially process multiple objects, and also accounted for effects of lesions in the spatial processing pathway on performance in the Posner spatial cuing task.

Chapter 9 explored two different ways that neural networks can implement memories — in weights and activations. We saw how priming tasks might tap cortical memories taking the form of small weight changes produced by gradual learning, or residual activation in the network. However, we saw that the basic cortical model fell short of capturing other human memory abilities, consistent with our discussion of fundamental computational tradeoffs in chapter 7. First, a basic cortical model like those used for learning regularities in the perceptual domain performs badly when required to rapidly learn and retain novel information — it suffers from catastrophic interference. The hippocampus, using very sparse, pattern separated representations, can avoid this interference while learning rapidly. Second, the basic cortical model cannot both be rapidly updated and robustly maintain activation, and spreading activation via overlapping distributed representations limit its maintenance abilities. The prefrontal cortex overcomes these limitations by having an adaptive, dynamic gating mechanism and relatively isolated representations. Finally, the interaction between activation and weight-based memory can be complex, as we saw in a model of the A-not-B task.

Language, explored in chapter 10, requires a number of specialized processing pathways and representations, that interact with (and build from) perceptual and other pathways and representations. These specialized pathways operate according to the same principles as any other pathway. We saw that a distributed, multipathway model of word representations can account for various patterns of dyslexia when damaged. Focusing on the direct pathway from orthographic input to phonological output, we saw how a network captured regularities that enabled it to generalize pronunciation to nonwords in much the same way humans do. Focusing on the pathway from semantics to phonology, we saw how a network could learn the regularities and exceptions of inflectional morphology, and that it produced a U-shaped overregularization curve as it learned, much as children do. We also explored a model of semantic representation learning based on co-occurrence statistics of words over large samples of text. The resulting semantic representations capture many relevant aspects of word similarity. Finally, we saw that a network can perform multiple constraint satisfaction across both semantic and syntactic constraints in sentence processing, producing a distributed representation that captures the overall meaning or gestalt of the sentence. This model provides a good example of how sequential information can be integrated over time.

Chapter 11 took on the challenge of applying the biologically realistic neural network mechanisms explored in previous chapters to modeling higher-level cognition. We saw that activation-based processing, as implemented in the frontal cortex, is a critical factor in enabling the kind of dynamic, flexible, and verbally accessible processing that is characteristic of higher-level cognitive function. Focusing on the role of the prefrontal cortex, we saw that a very simple model can account for normal and patient performance on the Stroop task. An important next step was to see how dynamic control over maintained prefrontal activations via gating (implemented by the neuromodulator dopamine) leads to more flexible task performance compared to simple weight-based task learning. We explored this in the context of a simple dynamic categorization task based on the Wisconsin Card Sorting task. One major outstanding challenge in the domain of higher-level cognition

is to understand how appropriate prefrontal representations can be learned over experience to enable this flexible task performance without invoking something like a homunculus.

12.3 General Challenges for Computational Modeling

From the brief summary above, it is clear that computational models have a lot to say about many different aspects of cognitive neuroscience, and that the current framework can address an exciting range of phenomena. However, a number of important challenges remain for future work. In this section, we revisit the general problems that computational models face that we outlined in the introductory chapter, and see how the models we have explored have addressed these challenges, and where future work needs to continue to make progress. In the subsequent section, we address more specific issues that are faced by neural network models and the framework adopted here.

First, we note that the history of neural network modeling has been dominated by periods of either extreme hype or extreme skepticism. In the past, the entire approach has been rejected based on limitations that were subsequently overcome (e.g., the limitations of delta-rule learning). Readers taking a similarly skeptical approach may find this list of future challenges so long, or some of the issues here (or others we don't cover) so damaging, that they question the validity of the entire enterprise. On the other hand, other readers may be so enamored with existing successes that they ignore important limitations.

We encourage all readers to strike a balance between rejecting the approach outright, and simply ignoring remaining challenges. Indeed, we feel that in recent years, the hype that resurged in the '80s has leveled off into a productive balance of skepticism and optimism (although not usually within the same researcher). Hopefully, this balance will continue along with the progress in future years.

12.3.1 Models Are Too Simple

The need for and use of simplification is at once one of
the greatest strengths and weaknesses of neural network
modeling. It is a strength because it allows one to extract, for example, the essential kernel of insight about
which biological properties are important for a particular behavior, and why. It is a weakness because behind
each simplification lies a largely uncharted sea of details, any one of which could render the simplification a
blatant misconstrual of the facts.

An example of the importance of simplification
comes from chapter 2, where the neuron was intention-
ally presented as simpler than its biological complexity
might otherwise suggest. To summarize, detailed complexity in the integration of neural inputs, or a complex
encoding of information in the detailed timing of the
spiking output, is inconsistent with several prominent
properties of the brain. For example, the brain is noisy
and needs to be robust, but these complex mechanisms
are brittle and would be too easily disturbed. Neurons
have only one output signal, yet receive thousands of inputs — there isn't enough bandwidth for complex processing over thousands of inputs to be conveyed in any
useful form through a single output. Furthermore, neurons act collectively and each individual one makes only
a minor, incremental contribution.

This example provides a cautionary statement against
becoming swept away with bottom-up detail — these
details must always be considered within a larger (and
often simplified) functional framework. In this example, although certain biological details might suggest
that the neuron is a very complex computational device, these details must be evaluated in the context of
the overall nature of neural computation, which strongly
supports a simpler, graded conception of the neuron.

Furthermore, simpler things often just work better.
We are reminded of the currently popular technique of
making mosaic images out of a large number of smaller
images that serve as pixels in the larger image. If you
get too close to one of these images, it just looks like
a random ensemble of little images. However, if you
step back and squint your eyes, the larger overall picture emerges. Thus, it is simpler to describe the overall
image as "A picture of Princess Diana" instead of de-

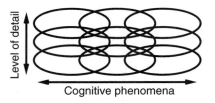

Figure 12.1: Ideal relationship between different levels of
modeling, varying in level of detail and in the range of cognitive phenomena covered. If each modeling effort overlaps
to some extent with others at different levels of detail or addressing other phenomena, then there are beneficial mutual
constraints between models.

scribing the properties and configurations of all the individual component images. Similarly, it may be that
squinting our eyes and ignoring some of the biological
details produces a simpler, more relevant picture of neural computation. Obviously as scientists we cannot take
it on faith that this is so — instead we must also laboriously assemble the mosaic from its pieces and confirm
that when you put it together right, it really does look
like something simple.

Although individual researchers must face tradeoffs
in deciding what is most important to study at any given
point in time, the larger plurality of the field allows for,
and benefits from, multiple parallel approaches. We see
this as the key to ultimately solving the simplification
problem — many different models at distinct but overlapping levels of analysis and detail (figure 12.1). Thus,
where one model makes a simplification, another delves
into further detail. To the extent that the two models
can be compared in their area of overlap, the simplified
model can be either validated or improved by taking
into account the behavior of the more detailed model
(or at least the limitations of the simplified model will
be known). Likewise, the simplified model can point
to the *functionally relevant* details, and focus the more
detailed model on them.

Examples of the effective use of multiple overlapping models exist throughout this book. For example, in
chapter 2, we compared the performance of a unit that
fires discrete spikes with one that computes a rate code.
In chapter 3, we compared inhibition using detailed
inhibitory interneurons with the kWTA simplification.

These examples showed that the simplifications are reasonable approximations to the more detailed case, but it was also clear that there were differences. However, these simplifications made it possible to explore models that otherwise would have been impractical.

The language chapter (10) provided additional examples of overlapping models. There, we explored a number of phenomena using a simplified model with all three main representations involved in reading, and then used larger, more realistic models to explore detailed aspects of performance specific pathways. The simplified model made it possible to explore certain broader aspects of behavior and effects of damage in a manageable and more comprehensible manner, and provided a general framework for situating the more detailed models. These examples provide a sample of the kinds of benefits of multiple overlapping levels of analysis.

In the sections that follow we discuss various areas where simplifications have been made and more detailed models might be revealing.

Details of Neurobiology

Reading through *The Journal of Neuroscience, Brain Research,* and other neuroscience journals, one can be overwhelmed with biological details. How is it that many of these biological properties can be largely ignored in our models? One general answer to this question is that we have used powerful simplifications that require lots of biological machinery to actually implement — our simplifications undoubtedly fail to capture all the subtlety of these mechanisms, but perhaps they capture enough of the main effect. Thus, generally speaking, it will be useful to relate the functional properties of these more detailed mechanisms to the simpler abstractions to find out exactly what the differences are and how much they matter. The following may be particularly relevant.

First, the kWTA function is a powerful simplification for activity regulation — a lot of biological machinery is likely necessary to keep neurons firing in the right zone of activation (not too much, not too little). In addition to the basic feedforward and feedback inhibition, the relevant biological machinery probably includes lots of channels along the lines of those discussed in the sec-

tion on self-regulation in chapter 2, but also factors like cellular metabolism, gene expression, and glia.

Second, most neural network models make dramatic simplifications in the initial wiring of the networks, often simply starting with random connectivity (with or without additional topographic constraints) within a network already constrained to receive particular types of inputs. A huge and largely unsolved problem in biology, not to mention cognitive neuroscience, is to understand how biological structure emerges through a complex sequence of interactions between genetic switches, chemical gradients, surface protein markers, and so on. Probably a significant portion of the initial wiring of the brain derives from this kind of process. The development of the brain, to a much greater degree than other organs, is also subject to influences of experience. We know specific examples in some detail — in the early visual system, for example, random noise coming from the retina plays an important role in configuring the wiring of neurons in V1 (e.g., Shatz, 1996; Miller et al., 1989). Thus, the line between when the setup of the initial configuration ends and learning begins is undoubtedly a fuzzy one, so understanding how the brain gets to its "initial configuration" may be critical to understanding later effects of learning.

Third, we have typically vastly simplified the control of processing and learning. Inputs are presented in a carefully controlled fashion, with the network's activations reset between each input and between phases of input (plus and minus), and learning is neatly constrained to operate on the appropriate information. The real system is obviously not that simple — boundaries between events are not predefined, and activation resetting (if it occurs at all) must be endogenously controlled. Although tests with various simulations show that activation resetting is important for rapid and successful learning with rate-code units, this needs to be explored in the context of spiking models, which generally exhibit less persistence of prior states (hysteresis) than rate-code models. The constant output of activation among interconnected rate-code units reinforces existing activation patterns more strongly than sporadic spiking. If activation resetting proves to be important even for discrete spiking models, then its biological reality and potential implementation should be explored.

We will take up the issue of phases of learning and co-ordination of learning more generally in a later section.

Missing Brain Areas

The models in this text have focused on the cortex (including the hippocampus), with the exception of a few that dealt in a very superficial way with the thalamus and the basal ganglia. There are a number of good reasons for this focus on cortical networks, including: (1) Much of cognition depends most critically on the cortex; (2) a cortical model can usually be initialized rather simply, because learning apparently plays a very strong role in structuring the cortical network; (3) the cortical pyramidal neuron, with supporting inhibitory interneurons, provides a common structural basis for neural computation throughout the cortex, so a common algorithm can be used for modeling many different cognitive phenomena.

In reality of course, the cortex operates in the context of a large number of other brain areas. There are several difficulties in including these other areas in computational models, including the fact that they are generally evolutionarily older and correspondingly more determined by genetics. This usually means that they have more complex, specialized neuron types that cannot be easily parameterized in terms of just patterns of weight values in an otherwise generic unit model. At a more practical level, adding other brain areas to a model can substantially increase computational complexity of the model.

Many of the missing brain areas serve as extensions of the sensory input or motor output pathways, and are often not particularly relevant for cognitive-level models. However, others have more profound effects on the nature of processing in the cortex because they secrete neuromodulatory substances. We explored the role of the neuromodulator dopamine in the context of reinforcement learning (chapter 6) and prefrontal active maintenance and learning (chapters 9 and 11). A number of other neuromodulators probably have similarly important roles. For example, norepinephrine, secreted by the locus ceruleus (LC), may regulate the ability of cortical neurons to remain focused on a particular task as a function of task performance or other variables.

Serotonin is another important neurotransmitter that has been linked to the regulation of states of arousal (i.e., sleeping versus waking), and also to mood.

It is possible to ignore these neuromodulators to the extent that we assume an awake cortex that is completely focused on the task at hand. However, a richer and more complete model of cognition will require the inclusion of such neuromodulatory factors, which play a critical role in human and animal performance both in the "wild" and in psychological task situations.

Aside from the basal ganglia and thalamus, probably the most cognitively relevant brain area, which has received scant attention in this book, is the cerebellum. Long known to be important for motor control, the cerebellum has been recently implicated as also playing a more cognitive role (e.g., Gao et al., 1996; Doyon, Gaudreau, & Bouchard, 1997). One useful focus of future research would be to understand the exact contributions of the cerebellum at a mechanistic level. Another area that is likely to be important is the amygdala, which is important for assigning emotional salience to stimuli, and has been the subject of some recent modeling efforts (Armony et al., 1997).

Scaling

We have argued that the brain possesses a kind of self-similar, fractal structure, so that coarse-grained models of multiple brain areas using relatively few units should employ the same principles as more fine-grained models of individual columns using a large number of units. Although a number of factors support this fractal assumption, the multiple models approach is an ideal one to test the validity of these scaling assumptions. That is, one could literally test how well a very detailed, fine-grained model can be approximated by a coarse-grained one. Clearly, the coarse-grained model can only represent a small fraction of the information compared to the fine-grained one, but its overall dynamics and some relevant behavioral characteristics should be comparable.

Ultimately, the limitation is one of computational power — it is nearly impossible to use fine-grained models of multiple brain areas on today's computers. However, the computational horizons are rapidly expanding (for example, computer power more than doubled during the period this book was written). Thus, it should be increasingly possible to implement large fine-grained models to test whether the simplified, scaled-down models provide a reasonable approximation to more realistic implementations.

12.3.2 Models Are Too Complex

A common criticism of neural network models is that they are not useful theoretical tools, because they are much more complicated than a simple verbal theory (McCloskey, 1991). A nice reply to this criticism has been given by Seidenberg (1993), where he emphasizes the distinction between *descriptive* and *explanatory* theories. McCloskey's arguments depend on a descriptive theoretical framework, where the goal is to describe a set of phenomena with theoretical constructs that can be relatively transparently mapped onto the phenomena — these kinds of theories essentially provide a concise and systematic description of a set of data.

The complexity of neural network models can sometimes make them unsuitable as purely descriptive theories, which is the thrust of McCloskey's argument. However, as we hope this book has demonstrated, neural network models are very well suited for developing explanatory theories, which explain a set of phenomena in terms of a small set of deeper, *independently motivated* principles. The implemented model serves as a test of the sufficiency of these principles to account for data, and is thus an essential tool in the development and refinement of the theory.

For example, McClelland et al. (1995), leveraging work on statistical learning by White (1989b), provided a theoretical account of the tradeoff between rapid arbitrary and slow integrative learning, and related this tradeoff to the complementary roles of the hippocampus and neocortex in learning and memory. The arguments in this work are based on general principles, not particular implementations, and therefore are truly theoretical. Instantiations of these principles were then made to demonstrate their applicability.

These instantiations required all the concomitant assumptions, simplifications, and the like that McCloskey (1991) argued irrevocably cloud the theoretical importance of network models. However, because the issues were analyzed in terms of more general principles that apply to virtually any kind of statistical learning mechanism (which includes all commonly used neural network learning algorithms) the models could be understood in terms of these principles.

Another good example comes from Plaut et al. (1996), who provided both an analytical and implemented model of the effects of regularity and frequency on learning and reaction time in reading.

Another major aspect of model complexity is the issue of *interpretability* — a traditional complaint about neural network models (typically backpropagation networks) is that they cannot be inspected after learning to discover anything about what they have learned. That is, network performance is uninterpretable (e.g., Young & Burton, 1999). This issue has also been emphasized by people who use neural networks for solving practical problems.

However, we must accept that the brain is a complex dynamic system and is not likely to be easy to reverse-engineer. Thus, restricting oneself to overly simplistic models that are easy to understand is not likely to be a good approach (O'Reilly & Farah, 1999).

Further, as discussed in chapter 6, the standard backpropagation algorithm is likely to be aberrantly opaque to interpretation; interpretability may become less of an issue with the development of additional algorithms and constraints on learning. Backpropagation is typically highly underconstrained in its learning, so the weights do not tend to strongly align themselves with the relevant aspects of the task. Hebbian model learning provides a generally useful bias that produces much more constrained, easily interpretable weights. This advantage of Hebbian constraints was exploited throughout the text, for example, in the object recognition model (chapter 8) and the reading and past-tense language models (chapter 10).

The resulting models provide a nice balance between computational power and interpretability. Hopefully, such models will appeal to those who currently advocate computationally weak localist models just because they are more interpretable.

Thus, although a number of published models constitute relatively unanalyzed and/or uninterpreted implementations that show effects without a clear principled understanding of why, this is becoming increasingly rare as the field matures and standards improve. Nevertheless, it is important to maintain a concerted focus on understanding models' performance in terms of a set of principles that transcend particular implementations.

12.3.3   Models Can Do Anything

A number of challenges focus on the free parameters in neural network models. For example, critics have argued that with so many parameters, one can get these models to learn anything, so it is uninteresting to show that they do. And it is hard to know which parameters were crucial for the learning. Further, multiple models that differ greatly from one another may all successfully simulate a particular phenomenon, making it even more difficult to identify the critical mechanisms underlying behavior (the *indeterminacy* problem).

One might be able to train a network to do anything, perhaps even using multiple, very different models. However, many models are subjected to further tests of *untrained* aspects of performance, such as generalization to new problems or response to damage. A network's behavior when damaged, for example, is not due to it being trained to behave this way. Instead, the network was trained to perform correctly, and the performance following damage emerged from the basic computational properties of the model (O'Reilly & Farah, 1999). Many of the most psychologically interesting aspects of neural network models are based on such untrained aspects of performance.

Moreover, such tests, beyond what networks were trained to do, may provide important constraints on resolving indeterminacy issues. Two very different networks may be equally good at modeling what they were trained to do, but one may provide a better match to untrained aspects of performance. Similarly, two very different networks may appear to be equally faithful to known properties of neurobiology, but one may provide a better match to a more detailed model, or to subsequent discoveries. Thus, with the vast and growing collection of top-down (behavioral) and bottom-up (biological) constraints on neural network models, it seems increasingly unlikely that we will face the indetermi-

nacy problem of multiple, very different models that are completely equally good, and thus, impossible to choose between.

Further, learning, which shapes the weight parameters in the model, is not ad hoc and under the researcher's precise control. Instead, learning is governed by a well-understood set of principles that shape the network's weights in interaction with the environment. Thus, by understanding the principles by which a network learns, the apparent complexity of the model is reduced to the relatively simple application of a small set of principles.

Importantly, the majority of the models in this book use the same set of standard parameters. The few exceptions are generally based on principled consideration, not ad-hoc parameter fitting. For example, we varied the parameter for the activity level of the hidden layers between models. As we saw in chapter 9, this manipulation maps onto known properties of different brain regions, and has important implications for the trade-off between learning specific information about individual patterns (sparse activations) versus integrating over many patterns (more distributed activations).

Novice modelers often ask how to determine how many units, layers, and the like should be used in a model. We have emphasized with the Leabra algorithm that performance does not depend very much on these parameters, as long as there are enough units and layers (chapter 4). The network will generally behave very much the same with excess units, though it may have more redundancy. Adding excess layers usually slows learning, but not nearly as much as in a backpropagation network. We think this robustness to excess degrees of freedom is essential for any plausible model of the brain, which is clearly overparameterized relative to the constraints of any given task. Thus, one basic approach is to include as many units and layers as the network appears to need to learn the task; and it really should not matter (except in computational time) if you have too many.

12.3.4   Models Are Reductionistic

How can a computational model tell us anything about love, hate, free will, consciousness and everything else that goes along with being a human being? There are two extreme positions to this issue that are typically staked out, but we think the truth, as usual, lies somewhere in between. At one extreme are essentially dualistic beliefs that amount to the idea that there is something ineffable about the human brain/mind that can never be captured in a purely mechanistic system. Even if people do not explicitly think of themselves as dualists, they view the standard notions of mechanistic systems, inspired by present day computers and machines, as so far removed from the sublime complexity of human experience that a mechanistic reduction seems impossible, even repulsive. At the other extreme is the reductionistic notion that someday psychology will disappear as a field of study and human cognition will be discussed in terms of neurons, or neurochemicals, or...where does it end?

As emphasized in the introductory chapter, it is essential to pursue the complementary process of *reconstructionism* while engaging in the reductionist enterprise. We think that computational models are uniquely well suited for developing reconstructionist understanding, and we hope that this has become clear in the course of this text. For example, we spent much of chapter 2 discussing ion channels and their effects on electrical conductances within individual neurons, but we quickly found in chapter 3 that a whole new terminology was necessary to understand the emergent properties of networks of interacting neurons. The introduction of learning mechanisms then led to another whole new set of emergent phenomena. In subsequent chapters, we then relied on these emergent network phenomena to explain complex cognitive phenomena like attention, object recognition, processing of regularities and exceptions in language, and so on.

Getting more to the heart of the matter is the issue of consciousness. Although we have not focused much on this issue, it has received a considerable amount of attention lately from computational modelers and other theoreticians. One interesting theme emerging from this work is that one can usefully characterize the properties of things that are within the scope of conscious awareness in terms of the duration, persistence, stability, and level of influence of representations (e.g., Kinsbourne, 1997; Mathis & Mozer, 1995). These are emergent

properties that are within the purview of a reconstructionist modeling endeavor, and we anticipate that future models will inevitably continue to make progress in understanding the "ineffable."

12.3.5 Modeling Lacks Cumulative Research

Neural network models are often criticized for their lack of cumulative research, even very recently (e.g., Gazzaniga, Ivry, & Mangun, 1998). As we noted in the introduction, this criticism might be applied to any new field where there is a lot of territory to be covered — indeed, it would be easy to level this same charge at the current explosion of neuroimaging studies. We hope that this book helps to allay this criticism in the domain of computational cognitive neuroscience. We have revisited, integrated, and consolidated a wide range of ideas from many years of computational modeling research. It should be very clear that the field as a whole has developed a set of largely consistent ideas that provides a solid basis for further refinement and exploration, as in any maturing scientific discipline.

12.4 Specific Challenges

Having discussed challenges that apply generally to the computational modeling endeavor, we now turn to a set of more specific challenges faced by neural network models and the specific modeling framework adopted in this book. As with the more general challenges, some of these have been met by existing models but are listed here because they continue to be leveled at neural network models, while others remain for future models to resolve.

12.4.1 Analytical Treatments of Learning

Mathematically based analyses of neural networks are an important part of the overall endeavor. These provide in-general proofs that our algorithms are likely to achieve something useful, and they also provide insights into the behavior of these algorithms. In developing the Leabra algorithm, we included such analyses wherever we could.

One outstanding problem for mathematical analysis is caused by the nature of the inhibitory competition between units within a layer. The two easily analyzed extremes for this type of competition either produce a single winner-take-all localist representation, or employ a noncompetitive constraint that enters into each unit's activation function or learning rule completely independent from the other units. In contrast, the kWTA function produces complex competitive and cooperative dynamics in the resulting sparse distributed representation, which we regard as essential aspects of cortical cognition. However, these complex interactions among units renders the algorithm analytically intractable, because of the combinatorial explosion involved in treating these interactions (analogous to the n body problem in physics).

Future research will hopefully make advances in developing useful approximations or other methods that can enable such analyses to go forward, without sacrificing the unique and essential virtues of the kWTA function.

12.4.2 Error Signals

Chapter 5 presented biological mechanisms that could implement error-driven task learning, and showed how models could learn on the basis of such mechanisms. However, these models simply imposed the necessary minus and plus phase structure required for learning, and provided target (outcome) patterns in the output layer. An open challenge is to demonstrate how expectation *and* outcome representations actually arise naturally in a simple perceptual-motor system operating within a simulated environment, particularly when the perception of the outcome happens through the same layers that represented the expectation. A second challenge is to address how the system knows when it is in the plus-phase so that it can perform learning then. Although the resolution of these challenges awaits further modeling and empirical work, there is evidence in the brain for the kind of phase-switching proposed to underlie error-driven learning, as well as for signals that might signal when to learn.

The issue of when to learn is probably related to dopamine. We examined its role in driving learning

based on differences between expected and obtained *reward* in chapters 6 and 11. Relating these findings back to basic error-driven learning requires that the dopamine signal occur for any difference in expected versus obtained *outcome*, not only reward. Electrophysiological recording studies should be able to test these ideas.

Finally, a growing body of evidence suggests that the anterior cingulate cortex is involved in detecting "errors" (e.g., Gehring et al., 1993) — it thus seems likely that this brain area plays an important role in error-driven learning, but its exact role remains to be specified (Carter et al., 1998).

12.4.3 Regularities and Generalization

An early and enduring criticism of neural networks is that they are just rote memorizers in the tradition of associationism or behaviorism, and are thus incapable of the kind of rule-like systematic behavior sometimes characteristic of human cognition (e.g., Pinker & Prince, 1988; Marcus, 1998).

Some of these critiques fail to appreciate the basic points addressed in chapter 7: networks generalize by systematic recombination of *existing* representations (cf. Marcus, 1998), and by forming such representations at an appropriate level of abstraction that naturally accommodates subsequent novel instances. These processes allow neural networks to capture many aspects of human generalization. Some particularly relevant examples include the demonstration by Hinton (1986) (see also chapter 6) that networks can form systematic internal re-representations that go beyond the surface structure of a problem. Two of the models in the language chapter (10) specifically demonstrate that a neural network can simulate human generalization performance in pronouncing nonwords, and in overregularizing irregular past tense inflections.

Some of the generalization critiques stem from the present limitations of neural network models for dealing with higher-level cognitive function. The applicability of such critiques may be somewhat narrow — many cases of systematic, rulelike processing are not the result of higher-level, deliberate, explicit rules, but can instead be readily explained in terms of basic neural network principles, and so generalization abilities can be captured as in the models mentioned earlier. Nevertheless, the explicit forms of cognition are obviously real and are largely unaccounted for by present neural network models. We revisit this issue next.

12.4.4 Capturing Higher-Level Cognition

Initial forays into the challenging task of capturing higher-level cognition (temporally extended tasks, planning, task-switching, "executive function," etc.) were described in chapter 11, but this is clearly a frontier area where much more work needs to be done. We are nevertheless optimistic that the distinction between activation- and weight-based processing captures an essential aspect of what differentiates explicit/declarative from implicit/procedural processes. It is clear that neural network models are just beginning to make progress in the activation-based processing domain, but we think that such models will soon provide an important alternative to traditional symbolic models for understanding higher-level cognitive phenomena.

An important question that must be faced is whether higher-level cognition necessarily requires large-scale models, or whether important aspects of it can be captured in smaller more manageable models. In other words, does higher-level cognition happen only when a large critical mass of cortex gets going, or can more basic principles be instantiated in scaled-down models? We clearly believe the latter to be at least partially true, suggesting that continued progress can be made with models of the scale of those presented in chapter 11.

12.5 Contributions of Computation to Cognitive Neuroscience

In this section, we highlight some of the main contributions of the computational approach to the broader field of cognitive neuroscience. In other areas of science, computational and formal models are used by the theoretical branch of the discipline (e.g., theoretical physics, computational chemistry), and their advantages are clear to all involved. This general appreciation of computational modeling is not as widespread in cognitive neuroscience. One possible reason for this lack of appreciation is that computational models have

been viewed as relatively removed from empirical approaches, for example because of the biological implausibility of the backpropagation algorithm. Furthermore, any empirical researchers have felt they can get by with "common sense" theoretical approaches (e.g., simple box-and-arrow process models and introspection).

Throughout this book, we have demonstrated how the computational/theoretical approach can play an essential role in cognitive neuroscience, because of the complexity and subtlety of the brain, behavior, and their interactions. We have shown how this approach can actually speak to the practical concerns facing empiricists. Here we highlight some of the main contributions using the same categories as in the introductory chapter.

12.5.1 Models Help Us to Understand Phenomena

In general, theories are important for making sense of behavior. It is one thing to observe patterns of neural responding in various cortical areas, or to observe different patterns of spared and impaired performance with brain damage, but quite another to actually make sense of these findings within a coherent overall framework. The computational approach can relate cognitive neuroscience data to a set of functional principles that help us understand *why* the brain subserves the behaviors that it does.

One example is in the explanation of why oriented bars of light constitute our basic representations of the visual world. The model in chapter 8 (based on the work of Olshausen & Field, 1996) shows that these bars of light constitute the basic statistical structure of the visual environment, and thus provide a principled basis for visual representations.

In memory, constructs like *repetition priming* and *semantic priming* have traditionally been considered separate entities. Repetition priming is typically identified with long-term effects, whereas semantic priming is typically identified with transient effects. From a computational/mechanistic basis, the space of priming effects can be accommodated with three dimensions (weight versus activation based, content, and similarity, see chapter 9). Within this framework, one can have both activation-based and weight-based semantic and repetition priming. Researchers working from the neural network perspective have recently confirmed this possibility in the case of semantic priming (Joordens & Becker, 1997).

Also in the domain of memory, we can now understand in terms of computational principles why the brain *should* separate out the rapid learning of arbitrary information from the slow incremental learning of semantic and procedural information (i.e., to avoid a tradeoff). This perspective can considerably deepen our understanding of the nature of memory in the brain in ways that purely verbal labels simply cannot.

In addition, we have seen in our explorations how the neural network approach can have significant implications for neuropsychological interpretation, for making inferences about normal function from people with brain damage (see also Farah, 1994). For example, Posner et al. (1984) used a simple box-and-arrow process model and the effects of parietal lobe damage in attentional cuing tasks to argue that the parietal cortex was responsible for "disengaging" attention. In contrast, we explored a model (based on that of Cohen et al., 1994) that showed how these effects (and other data on parietal lobe function) can be more plausibly explained within the basic principles of computational cognitive neuroscience, without any specific "disengage" mechanism (chapter 8).

In chapter 10, we saw that reading deficits following brain damage (dyslexia) can have complex and somewhat counterintuitive properties based on the premorbid division of labor over different processing pathways. This division of labor can be explained based on principles of learning in neural networks, and the resulting model provides a good fit to available data. Accounting for these data within a standard modular framework would require complex and improbable patterns of damage.

12.5.2 Models Deal with Complexity

Although it is convenient when we can explain nature using simple constructs, this is not always possible, especially in a system as complex as the brain. One major contribution of the computational approach is to provide a means of implementing and validating complex explanatory constructs.

For example, one of the basic principles emphasized in this text is multiple constraint satisfaction. Although this principle can be expressed relatively simply in mathematical and verbal terms, the way that this process actually plays out in an implemented model can be very complex, capturing the corresponding complexity of processing in the interactive brain. Without a firm mechanistic basis, the principle of multiple constraint satisfaction might come across as vague handwaving.

The sentence gestalt model from chapter 10 provides an instantiation of the complex idea that rich, overlapping distributed representations can capture sentence meaning and syntactic structure. When relatively simple representational structures (e.g., hierarchical trees) have been used to try to achieve insight into the nature of sentence-level representations, they always seem to fall short of capturing the rich interdependencies between semantics and syntax, among other things. Furthermore, if one were to simply postulate verbally that some kind of magical distributed representation should have all the right properties, this would likely come off as mere optimistic hand-waving. Thus, one needs to actually have an implemented model that demonstrates the powerful complexity of distributed representations. These complex representations also require the use of sophisticated learning procedures, because they would be nearly impossible to hand-code.

Another example of the benefits of harnessing the complexity of distributed representations comes from the language models that can represent both regular and exception mappings using the same set of distributed representations. Previously, researchers were unable to conceive of a single system capable of performing both kinds of mappings. Similarly, the object recognition model from chapter 8 exhibits powerful and generalizable invariant recognition abilities by chaining together several layers of transformations — the invariance transformation is not a simple, one step process, and this was difficult to imagine before the advent of network models such as that of Fukushima (1988).

The semantic representations model from chapter 10 (based on the work of Landauer & Dumais, 1997) showed that word co-occurrence statistics contain a surprising amount of semantic information. In this example, the complexity is in the environment, because extracting the relevant semantic information requires sampling over very large bodies of text. It is very difficult to imagine anyone making a convincing verbal or otherwise purely intuitive argument that this complex and subtle information could be as useful as it appears to be. Thus computational models can be essential for appreciating and taking advantage of the complexity of environments, as well as behaviors.

12.5.3   Models Are Explicit

A major consequence of the fact that models force one to be explicit is that they can help to replace vague, functionally defined constructs with more explicit, mechanistically based ones. Cognitive neuroscience has adopted a number of psychological constructs — such as attention, memory, working memory, and consciousness — that are vague and unlikely to be the product of single mechanisms. Neural network models can help the field progress beyond these somewhat simplistic constructs by "deconstructing" them, and introducing in their stead more mechanistically based constructs that fit better with the underlying biology.

For example, we saw that attention can emerge through the interaction of brain areas with inhibitory competition mechanisms. The overall process of multiple constraint satisfaction operating within these inhibitory constraints dictates which representations will dominate in a given situation. Something close to this view of attention has been proposed from a non neural-network perspective (e.g., Allport, 1989; Desimone & Duncan, 1995). The naturalness of this idea from the neural network perspective both lends considerable support, and provides an explicit mechanistic basis for it.

Another deconstruction example addressed the variety of verbal characterizations of distinct memory types (declarative, explicit, episodic, procedural, semantic, etc.). We saw that principles of neural computation provided a more precise and fundamental characterization of the properties of cortical and hippocampal memory (O'Reilly & Rudy, 1999; McClelland et al., 1995).

Another example of a deconstructed box is the "disengage" mechanism described in the previous section. A similar example is the notion of a specific "inhibitor"

system in the brain, for example in explaining the function of the prefrontal cortex. Instead, inhibitory effects can emerge due to competing activation elsewhere. The A-not-B model in chapter 9 (Munakata, 1998) and the Stroop model in chapter 11 (Cohen et al., 1990) both make this point.

Another important benefit of the explicitness of models is that they can directly generate predictions. We have discussed a number of such predictions throughout the text. Although we think these predictions are important, we caution against an apparent tendency to overemphasize them, as if they were the only real test of a model's value. It should be clear from all of the important contributions discussed in this section that this is far from the truth — predictions are one of many different contributions that models can make.

12.5.4   Models Allow Control

In virtually every exploration in this text, we have poked and prodded the networks in ways that experimentalists can only dream about. With a few simple clicks we can directly visualize the synaptic connectivities that underlie neural firing patterns in the models, while at the same time presenting these models with stimuli and observing the entire state of activation in response. Having this kind of access to the mechanics of the models leads to levels of understanding that would be impossible to achieve in the intact system. We can leverage this understanding to establish better and better correspondences between the models and reality, so that our detailed and sophisticated understanding of the artificial system can further inform our understanding of the real one.

12.5.5   Models Provide a Unified Framework

We have stressed the importance of developing and using a coherent, integrated set of principles for computational cognitive neuroscience. The broader field of cognitive neuroscience should also benefit from such a coherent framework, for a number of reasons, some of which were alluded to in previous sections (e.g., in making sense of the data). Another benefit is the ability to relate two seemingly disparate phenomena by understanding them in light of a common set of basic principles. For example, our models of the learning of semantic representations of word meanings and the encoding of basic features of visual structure exploited virtually identical principles and network structures. This link opens up the possibility for empirical data in these two very different domains to be related and provide mutual understanding.

The coherent set of principles that we have exploited in this book and incorporated into the Leabra algorithm have been around for a while, and have each been validated a number of times in different implementations. However, in using a single algorithm for this entire book we are not implying that everyone in computational cognitive neuroscience should use one particular algorithm, or that this algorithm has some privileged connection with the truth. Nevertheless, we do believe that this collection of principles is important, and, when combined together in an appropriate fashion, can help us to understand a wide range of phenomena, from ion channels to language processing to higher-level cognitive skills like planning.

Undoubtedly, better performance in one way or another could be obtained in specific cases by using a different implementation or a different set of principles. However, we do not at this time know of any obvious alternative algorithm or set of principles that could provide as good a fit to such a wide range of performance criteria as the ones used in this book. As such alternatives emerge, we will gladly adopt them for subsequent editions of this book!

12.6   Exploring on Your Own

We hope that you are now filled with a sense of balanced optimism and general excitement for the endeavor of computational cognitive neuroscience! We close by encouraging you to continue in the exploration of computational cognitive neuroscience by constructing your own models. The following appendixes provide a starting tutorial, and the many models in the various chapters can be used as points of departure for exploring other related phenomena. Enjoy!

Part III

Simulator Details

Appendix A

Introduction to the PDP++ Simulation Environment

Contents

A.1 Overview 427
A.2 Downloading and Installing the Software 427
A.3 Overall Structure of PDP++ 427
A.4 Buttons and Menu Commands 429
A.5 Edit Dialogs 429
A.6 Control Panels 430
A.7 Specs 430
A.8 Networks and NetViews 431
    A.8.1 NetView 431
A.9 Environments and EnviroViews 431
A.10 Processes 432
    A.10.1 Process Control Panels 432
    A.10.2 Statistics 432
A.11 Logs 433
    A.11.1 TextLog 433
    A.11.2 GraphLog 433
    A.11.3 GridLog 433
A.12 Scripts 433

A.1 Overview

This chapter provides a brief introduction and reference for the basic aspects of the PDP++ simulation environment used for the exercises in this text. There is also a full PDP++ manual freely available on the web at www.cnbc.cmu.edu/PDP++/PDP++.html, and a print-format version that can be downloaded from that site. The user is encouraged to take advantage of this more detailed documentation to supplement the brief introduction given here and the step-by-step instructions contained in the exercises within each chapter. The next chapter contains a tutorial for constructing a basic simulation from scratch, which can be useful for students (and researchers) doing their own simulation projects.

This chapter should be read over once before attempting any of the exercises, and later, as your knowledge of the underlying computation increases, you can reread those sections that are particularly relevant to a given exercise. Eventually, we hope this all will make sense!

A.2 Downloading and Installing the Software

The PDP++ software (specifically leabra++) and simulation projects for this text are available for downloading from the internet. Go to the MIT Press website, http://mitpress.mit.edu, and then locate the website for this book by searching for it using the title. This page will lead you to detailed, platform-specific instructions for downloading and installing the software.

A.3 Overall Structure of PDP++

PDP++ is organized into a collection of hierarchically arranged **objects**. Each object generally contains all the data and functionality that applies to a given type

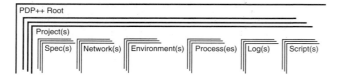

Figure A.1: Hierarchical structure of main objects in PDP++ software.

of thing in the simulation (e.g., the `Unit` object contains the data and functionality for computing unit (neural) activations). Many objects contain other objects, which leads to the hierarchical organization shown in figure A.1, starting with the most basic of all objects, the **Root** object (so named because it is the *root* or base of the tree of objects). The root object has a corresponding window, which is the only thing on the screen when you start the simulator without any arguments. This window is always around when the simulator is running, and provides the highest level of control over the basic loading, saving, and exiting operations. The root contains **Projects**, which group together all of the other objects that pertain to a particular simulation project. Each project object has a corresponding project window (typically this is iconified in the explorations), which simply contains a menu with entries for each of the objects that live within the project. These objects are of the following types (there are others, but they are less commonly used):

Spec(s) These are **Spec**ifications or *parameters* for how other objects should behave. For example, much of the behavior of a **Unit** object is specified by a corresponding **UnitSpec**, leaving the unit itself to primarily just represent the *variables* particular to each unit (e.g., activation value). This separation of data (variables) and specifications (parameters) is critical for enabling the user to change the behavior of a large number of units (or other objects) by acting on a single object (the Spec), instead of acting on each individual object (e.g., each unit in the network).

Network(s) All of the layers, units, connections and related objects that define a particular network are contained within the **Network** object. In addition, the network object contains an object called the

NetView, which implements a graphical display of the network within a separate window (a NetView window) on your computer screen. There can be multiple such views of the underlying network object, each of which can display different aspects of it.

Environment(s) The *environment* in which the network exists and with which it interacts is defined by the **Environment** object. Each environment contains a number of **Event** objects, which contain the discrete, individual **Pattern**s that a network encounters within the environment. Like the network, environments have an **EnviroView** object that provides a graphical display. Unlike most other objects, the *Specs* that define the nature and behavior of the events (called **EventSpec**s) are contained within each environment, instead of being at the level of the entire project. This makes environments more self-contained, so they can more easily be exchanged between different projects, and so on.

Process(es) This is perhaps the most difficult of the object types to understand, because it is a bit more abstract. A **Process** object instantiates a procedure or process, which is just a set of steps that are taken at a particular point to make the simulation *Run*. Typically, there are a number of such process objects, organized hierarchically (as usual), with each process instantiating a particular *grain* of processing. Take an example simulation where we train a network on a particular environment for 100 **epochs** (presentations of the entire environment). The outermost (highest) level of processing is at the level of orchestrating the overall training, which is handled by the **TrainProcess**. This process loops 100 times, and within each loop, it delegates the details of the individual epoch processing to the **EpochProcess**. This epoch process then loops through all the events in the environment, and delegates the processing of each event to the **TrialProcess** (a **trial** happens when a single event is presented to the network). As you will see in the book, the processing of a single trial itself contains further levels of sub-processing, which are handled by yet more processes. Finally, each grain or level of processing can have associated with it a number of **Statistics** which compute values that help you to understand how the processing is going, how the network is responding, etc. (In addition, miscellaneous other processes can be attached to a given grain of overall processing). Now you know why it can be confusing! Do not panic — you will not have to fully understand these processes to follow the examples in the text. However, you will need to know some of the important buttons that make a given process work, which are covered in section A.10.

Log(s) The results (i.e., *statistics*) from processing are displayed in *Logs*, which can also be configured to send data to a file for later examination. Because the word *Log* is also the name of a mathematical function, the Log object in PDP++ is called the **PDPLog**. There is basically just one type of PDPLog, but it can have several different types of *View* objects which display the underlying data in different ways. The **TextLogView** just displays the data as rows of text organized in columns, while the **GraphLogView** displays data as line graphs, and the **GridLogView** displays data as matrixes (grids) of colored (or shaded) squares. To simplify things, there are trivial subtypes of the PDPLog object which set the default view type to one of the above, giving us **TextLog**'s, **GraphLog**'s, and **GridLog**'s. Each type of log view has its own set of controls, which are briefly explained in section A.11, and in more depth where relevant in the exercises in the text. A given log is typically associated with a particular level (grain) of *process* object (see above), so that it is updated and displays information relevant to that level of processing.

Script(s) are somewhat like Processes, in that they automate routine tasks. However, a script is different from a process in several ways. Most importantly, it is designed to be executed on an ad hoc basis, and not as part of the elaborate sequence of processing orchestrated by the Process objects. In addition, a **Script** object doesn't know how to do much of anything until it is associated with a **script file**, which is just a standard text file containing C++-like code (actually **CSS** code, which is the scripting language that is built into PDP++). The script object just makes it easier to manage these script files within the project, and provides a simple graphical interface for running them. The most important category of script objects are the **Control Scripts** with their associated **Control Panel**s, that are used for every exercise project to simplify and automate the execution of the exercise. Please read section A.6 for more information on these control scripts.

A.4 Buttons and Menu Commands

The exercises will typically ask you to select certain actions by pressing a button on the overall control panel. Just press the named button with the left mouse button to perform that action. Often, the button will bring up another window where you can fill in more details about the action you want to perform (e.g., the `View` button on the control panel will bring up a window asking which window you want to view). After specifying this further information, pressing the `Ok` button will actually carry out the action, while `Cancel` will cancel the action.

Less frequently, you will be instructed to perform a menu command in a specific window (not the control panel window). Each window in PDP++ will typically have a number of different menu options at the top of the window. The window in question will either be specified by description (i.e., "the project window"), or as part of the menu specification. Assuming the latter, let's examine the following example: `Project/.specs/Edit/UnitSpec_0`. Each element or item in the menu specification is separated by a slash (`/`), and the first term (in this case) specifies the type of window. Once you have located the Project window, then look for the menu labeled with the next term (`.specs`), and click on it. Then a submenu will appear, and you should be able to locate the next item (`Edit`) in that menu, and so on.

A.5 Edit Dialogs

Every object in PDP++ can be *edited*, which means that a window containing all of the modifiable values and functions associated with that object can be called up, manipulated, changes made to the underlying object (or not), and then closed. Most menus in the system contain an `Edit` menu item, which lists the objects available for editing as submenus of that item. After selecting one of these objects, the **edit dialog** window will appear. Every edit dialog has the following four buttons on the bottom, which control the editing process:

Ok This *applies* any changes made to the object in the edit dialog, and closes the edit dialog window. Note that this button is not available on the overall exercise control panels, because they should never be closed (except of course when the project itself is closed, which happens automatically).

Apply This *applies* any changes made to the object in the edit dialog, and keeps the window around for subsequent use. **Always press** `Apply` **after changing something in the edit dialog!**.

Revert This effectively *undoes* any changes made by the user in the edit dialog, and *reverts* the object to its unedited state. It is also possible that something else other than the edit dialog could have changed the value(s) of the object (e.g., if the network is being changed, an edit dialog displaying a Unit or a Connection will have different values after processing than those shown in the edit dialog). If this has happened, then the revert button will also update the display to show those changes.

Cancel Aborts any changes made in the edit dialog, and closes the window. Again, this button does not appear on the overall control panels.

In addition to these standard buttons, different edit dialogs and control panels can have other buttons that appear just above the standard ones. These have descriptive names, and are described in more detail in the explorations.

Edit dialogs also can have menus on the top of the window. These menus contain less frequently executed functions that apply to the object in question.

Finally, the main guts of the edit dialog are the values, which are arranged vertically with *name — value* fields on each line. The name field identifies the nature of the value, while the value field provides the necessary interface for editing the field. Note that you can

click on the name field to view a more detailed (but still somewhat brief) description of the value.

A.6   Control Panels

A control panel is an edit dialog associated with a Script object that contains parameters and functions (buttons, menus) that are specifically relevant to a particular exercise. These windows can be identified in several ways. They typically have a title that appears in the top border surrounding the window that ends with `_ctrl` (and typically starts with something like the name of the project that was loaded). These windows typically float to the top after a project is loaded, and they are positioned under the mouse pointer. These edit dialogs are also identifiable because they do not have `Ok` or `Cancel` buttons.

All control panels have a `View` button on the left, which opens other windows to view. Selecting the `NOTHING` option under `View` will close all windows (except the Root and the control panel itself) — this is useful for cleaning things up if you get lost in a sea of windows. Also, `View` will always raise the window in question to the top if it is already open somewhere. Control panels almost always have a `Defaults` button, which restores the original default parameters. This is useful to restore standard settings after playing around with various parameters.

It is a good idea to move the control panel to a location where it will not get covered up by other windows, because it is your lifeline for controlling the simulation!

A.7   Specs

The details of the specs for the Leabra algorithm are presented in appendix C. You will not need to use the actual spec objects themselves for any of the provided simulations, but they will be essential should you try to develop a model on your own. The tutorial in appendix B provides more details on how to use these specs when building a network.

A.8 Networks and NetViews

A network consists of **Layer** objects containing **Unit** objects, which are connected with **Connection** objects. One possibly confusing aspect of the network is the **Projection** object, which specifies connectivity on a layer-to-layer basis (e.g., the projection specifies that the hidden layer receives from the input layer). It is the responsibility of the Projection object to actually create all the individual connections between units in the respective layers. The patterns of connectivity are determined by the **ProjectionSpec**, which is the spec object associated with the Projection.

There are also Spec objects associated with Layers, Units, and Connections. These are where you should look for all the controlling parameters for the network.

A.8.1 NetView

The **NetView** displays a graphical representation of the network, showing the individual units as colored squares organized within layers, with projections represented by arrows. The units in the display obtain their color as a function of the currently selected variable (other modes of display are available through the `Disp Md` menu on the right-hand side of the window. The available variables are represented by buttons arranged in the lower left hand side of the display. Note that there may be more buttons than space to display them, in which case the scroll bar may be used to view them all. Clicking with the left mouse button on one of these variables will select it for display over the units in the network. In this way, one can alternately view all of the important state variables associated with the units.

Viewing weights and other values associated with connections is also possible, but it requires one extra step. Buttons associated with connection variables are at the bottom of the list of variables, and begin with either an `r.` (for *receiving* connection values) or an `s.` (for *sending* connection values). For example, to view the weights coming into a particular unit, you would select the `r.wt` button. Then, however, you must also select the unit for which you wish to view the weights. You can only view the weights for one unit at a time,

since the weight values are displayed over the other unit squares in the display. After selecting a connection variable, simply click with the left mouse button any unit in the display, and this will show the connection values on the corresponding units that are on the other side of connection. Thus, somewhat confusingly, when you select to view the receiving weights, the units that are lit up in the display are the sending units, since these are the ones that the selected unit receives from.

It is also possible to view *multiple* variables at the same time, by using an extended selection procedure. Select the first variable to view as before with the left mouse button. To view an additional variable, simply select it with the *middle* mouse button (or hold down the shift key while pressing the left mouse button). The units will now be split, showing both variables in each unit. Any number of additional variables may be selected (though it is typically quite difficult to actually interpret such displays).

A.9 Environments and EnviroViews

The **EnviroView** provides a display of the environment object, showing the events listed in buttons down the left hand side of the display. When one of these event buttons is clicked, the pattern values for that event are displayed over on the right. Multiple such events can be selected by using the middle button, or shift and left-click. To turn a selected event off, also use middle button or shift and left-click.

The various buttons at the top left of the window control the display of the events. `Evt Label` allows one to select what information is displayed at the top (header) of each event display. This is normally the event name, but could be its frequency or other such information. `Pat Label` controls what is displayed as the header for each Pattern within the event (a pattern typically corresponds to one layer's worth of event information — the pattern of activity that is presented to a layer). The `Pat Block` field controls what is displayed in the values (blocks) for each pattern. Normally this is just the activation value for the event, but there are also special flags that could be displayed.

The configuration and behavior of events is controlled by corresponding event specs — these can be edited by pressing the `Edit Specs` button, which switches the display to spec editing mode. Pressing `Edit Events` switches back to editing the events.

A.10   Processes

The main action of most processes is simply to loop over its subordinate processes. Almost all processes have a *loop counter*, which reflects the number of times the process has looped over its subordinate processes (e.g., the number of epochs that have been processed in a TrainProcess, or the number of events that have been processed in an EpochProcess). Processes also act as placeholders for actions that take place at a given grain size (epochs, trials, phases, etc.), so that, for example, the network display can be updated at different grain sizes by linking its updating to a given process. Similarly, logs are associated with a given process to record information summarized at that grain size.

As we mentioned, statistics, processes and scripts can be hung off of any level of process to provide very flexible control mechanisms. There are three levels within each process where such things can be attached: init, loop, and final, which correspond to the start of a given grain size, within each loop, or at the end.

A.10.1   Process Control Panels

Somewhat confusingly, processes also have control panels, but unlike the overall project-wide control panels described in section A.6, these control panels just apply to the individual process in question. The following special buttons are available on a process object:

New Init, Re Init initialize the process (cause it to start over), with the only difference between the two being that `Re Init` reuses the previous random seed, so that the next run will precisely replicate the prior one, even if random numbers (e.g., noise, random event presentation order) are involved, while `New Init` gets a new random seed and will do different things if randomness is involved.[1]

Run will run the process, starting from wherever it was last stopped or initialized, and continuing until it is done — in the case of the epoch process, running means presenting all the different events in the environment to the network.

Step will do one step of running at a time, with the granularity of processing and the number of steps determined by the `step` parameters in the window.

Stop will stop a running process (and is otherwise unavailable — "ghosted").

Go To will skip to a given value of the loop counter (e.g., event number in the EpochProcess).

A.10.2   Statistics

As we have mentioned, statistics are attached to processes, and compute useful information about the state of the network so that it can be reported in a log. An example is the SE (squared error) statistic, which computes the squared error of the network's output relative to the training target values. This SE statistic must be computed at the trial level, because that is where the actual and target activation states are available. However, we often want to see how the network is performing at a higher grain size, for example at the epoch level. To do this, each statistic is capable of **aggregating** information from another statistic of the same type at a lower grain level. These aggregators can perform different operations such as sum, average, and so on. All statistics associated with a given grain of processing are automatically logged when that process is logged, unless specifically told not to log (using the `log_stat` toggle on the statistic object).

A particularly important type of statistic is the **MonitorStat**, which records (monitors) state information from the network for display in the log. These monitor stats can be configured from within the NetView display, by clicking on a set of units to monitor, and then creating a new monitor stat from the `Monitor Values` menu.

---

[1]Note that random numbers on a computer are really pseudorandom — the sequence can be replicated given the starting *seed* number, but there is no systematic relationship between one number and the next, which makes the sequence effectively random.

A.11 Logs

There are three main types of log displays, the TextLog, the GraphLog, and the GridLog. Each displays the same information, but using a different output format. The specific content displayed in the log is determined entirely by the process that is updating the log — the job of the log is to then take this information and display it in a specified manner.

All of the logs have VCR-like buttons at the top that perform full rewind, fast rewind, slow rewind, slow forward, fast forward, and full forward. These buttons move the (small) window of currently-displayed information across the (larger) set of total information recorded by the log. The logs will not automatically update unless they are at the end of this total set of data (to allow you to view prior information even as new data is being recorded).

If for some reason the log does not appear to be updating when the simulation is being run, press the full forward button to make sure it is at the end of the data (where the latest information is).

A.11.1 TextLog

The text log simply displays the information as columns of numbers. Each row corresponds to a different iteration of processing of the updating process object. This type of log is most useful for summary levels of processing, such as training or batch level information.

A.11.2 GraphLog

The variables being plotted in the GraphLog are represented by buttons along the lower left hand side of the window. The display state of the variable is indicated by the little "led" in the button. To toggle the display state on or off, just click with the *left* mouse button. One of the variables must serve as the X (horizontal) axis of the graph. This is indicated by the presence of the X to the right of the button. To select a different variable as the X axis, use the *middle* mouse button.

Some variables will share a common Y (vertical) axis scale. The Y axes are color coded, with the color of the line to the right of the variable button indicating which axis the variable is using. *Note that the first variable (from the top) which has this color Y axis must be displayed, or else all the other variables will create their own Y axis.*

Various display attributes of the variables can be edited by clicking with the *right* mouse button on the variable button. This will bring up an edit dialog. This should not be necessary for any of the provided projects, and further documentation is available in the full PDP++ manual.

Finally, the user can click with the left mouse button on any line in the graph to view the precise numerical value at a given point. Pressing the Init button in the upper right hand side of the window will remove any numerical values being displayed. Further, this button will generally fix any display problems that might occur with the graph. The Update button can also be used if for some reason the graph does not display the most current information.

A.11.3 GridLog

The grid log displays information as grids of colored blocks, which is very useful for monitoring network state over time (i.e., from a MonitorStat). The display is organized like a text log in columns of variables with each row representing a new iteration of the updating process. The layout and display properties (i.e., whether to display text or as a colored block) of the items within the log can be manipulated by clicking with the right mouse button on the label at the top of the column, though this should not be necessary for any of the existing simulations.

A.12 Scripts

The final type of objects within the project are the scripts. Scripts can be accessed through their edit dialogs, which provide the ability to Run and Compile (turn the textual script code into an executable form). It will not be necessary to understand the details of scripts for any of the exercises, but they are used in the next chapter, which provides more information.

Appendix B

Tutorial for Constructing Simulations in PDP++

Contents

B.1 Overview **435**
B.2 Constructing a Basic Simulation **436**
    B.2.1 Creating a Project *436*
    B.2.2 Recording a Script *436*
    B.2.3 Creating a Network and Layers *437*
    B.2.4 Creating Projections and Connections . . . *438*
    B.2.5 Specifying Layer Activity Levels *439*
    B.2.6 Creating an Environment *440*
    B.2.7 Creating Training Process *441*
    B.2.8 Creating a Training Log and Running the
           Model *442*
B.3 Examining the Script **442**
    B.3.1 Object Paths *443*
    B.3.2 Object-Oriented Function Calls *443*
    B.3.3 Assigning Member Values *444*
    B.3.4 Scoped Variables *444*
    B.3.5 Running Processes from the Script *444*
    B.3.6 Saving Files from the Script *445*
    B.3.7 Compiling and Running the Script *445*
B.4 Creating a Testing Process **446**
    B.4.1 Monitoring Unit Activities *446*
    B.4.2 Creating a New Statistic for Testing *447*
    B.4.3 Automatically Testing during Training . . . *448*
B.5 Writing Script Code to Create an Environment . **448**
    B.5.1 Setting a Stopping Criterion for Training . . *450*
B.6 Creating an Overall Control Panel **450**
B.7 Creating SRN Context Layers **452**

B.1 Overview

Constructing a simulation from scratch in PDP++ (leabra++) is relatively easy, at least until you have to do something out of the ordinary (which ends up being quite often, unfortunately). However, even when you have to do something more complex, it is often the case that an elegant, or at least fairly straightforward solution, exists within the simulator. The problem is finding it. This tutorial will give you an introduction to the easy stuff, and some pointers as to how to solve harder problems. Beyond that, the exercises contain a wide range of solved examples of different simulation tasks, some of them quite complex. You will, we hope, be able to find something similar to what you want to accomplish in one or more of these exercises, and can then figure out how it was solved there and apply this to your own project. It is assumed here that you have read the previous chapter and explored a range of the exercises and are familiar with the Leabra algorithm and can successfully navigate the prepared simulations.

We will initially be creating a simulation that learns to perform an arbitrary input-output mapping between sets of randomly generated patterns. Then, we will create a script that automatically generates input/output patterns according to a simple rule. Finally, we will embellish the network with a testing process, some additional statistics, and a custom control panel. We will also keep a record of all the actions we take in the interface, producing corresponding script code that, if run, would recreate the simulation just as we had made it. However, we will not rely on this script to actually save our project (we can just save the final product as a project file), so you need not be concerned about making mistakes during project construction. Instead, we will use this script code to learn how to program in PDP++, by examining the script versions of the actions that you took. Many complex tasks can be efficiently automated by a little bit of appropriate script code, so it can really pay off to invest a little bit of effort learning the script language.

B.2   Constructing a Basic Simulation

B.2.1   Creating a Project

↪ Let's start by going to the `tutorial` directory.

This directory should be empty, but it provides a place to save the files you create during this tutorial for later reference.

↪ Now, start `leabra++` with no additional arguments.

You will see the `PDP++ Root` window. The `.projects` menu within this window allows you to manipulate projects — we want to create a new one.

↪ Select `.projects/New/Project`.

This will bring up the **new object dialog**, which shows up whenever you create any new object in PDP++. It allows you to select how many objects to create (often just 1), and which **type** of object to create — this should correspond to the type of object you selected in the menu just before the dialog came up (i.e., `Project` in this case), but you might want to change it (in this case there is only one type of project, so don't).

If you do click on the `Of Type:` button (i.e., `Project` in this case), you will see that there is always some type of `Group` type at the bottom of the list. This reflects a powerful feature of PDP++, which enables you to create arbitrary groupings of objects to organize them in ways that make sense to you as a user. In this case, if you were going to be having multiple projects open at the same time, you could create groups to keep more related projects together. Because we typically just have one project at a time, this is not so useful here, but it will be later. Most of the time, the simu-

lator just ignores this group structure, so it is just for your convenience. However, sometimes it is important, as we will see below. For technical reasons, sometimes these groups are called `_MGroup` and sometimes just `_Group` — they are both essentially the same thing, except that the `_MGroup` has the ability to produce a graphical menu of the objects in the group. Thus, whenever you are creating things from a menu, the relevant group type will be `_MGroup`.

↪ Just press `Ok` to create the project.

You should see a project window appear. Like the `PDP++ Root` window, the project window is basically just a set of menus, which allow you to create and manage all the objects that belong in a project. Every major window has an `Object` menu at the very left, which has actions that apply to the particular object that the window corresponds to (i.e., the project in this case). This allows you to `Save`, `Load`, and `Close` the object, among other things.

The menus in the project window are arranged in the order you should typically use them, from left to right, when creating a new project. Many times (including this one), you can skip right to the `.network` window, since the `.defaults` are usually appropriate, and the objects you create in the network (units, etc.) will automatically create their corresponding initial `.specs`.

B.2.2   Recording a Script

Because we want to record all of our actions in a script, we will violate this general rule (already!) and start with the `.scripts` menu at the far right side of the project window.

↪ Do `.scripts/New/Script`.

You will get a new object dialog. The initial values in the dialog are fine. However, there is an important time-saving trick that we will use now, because we want to edit this new Script object that we will be creating. Instead of clicking on the `Ok` button with the usual left mouse button and then going back to the `.scripts/Edit/Script_0` menu, we can just use the **right mouse button** to click on the `Ok` button, which will create the object and immediately pull up an edit window on that object.

↪ Right-click on the `Ok` button.

The script edit window has a `script_file` field that we need to set to the name of the script file that we want to record our actions into.

↪ Click on the `----No File----` button, and select `Open` from the menu you get, and then type in a new file name (e.g., `constr`) in the file dialog that comes up, and press the `Open` button.

You will now see that `script_file` has `constr.css` next to it, telling you the file name.

↪ The `Apply` button is highlighted, so go ahead and press it to apply this change.

You may notice that the original xterm window reports an error that it can't open the file — this makes sense because this file doesn't exist yet!

↪ Now, hit the `Record` button.

This will record all subsequent actions to this script file.

↪ Use your window manager to iconify this script window.

We will return to this window later. You should notice that the pointer now has a `rec` under it, indicating that recording is active.

B.2.3 Creating a Network and Layers

↪ Now, let's go to the `.network` menu, and select `New/Network`. Again you will see the new object dialog, which you can just press `Ok` to.

An empty network window will now appear. The buttons at the left of the window give you the tools for constructing and configuring your network. Notice that the `New Layer(s)` button is highlighted for you. These highlighted buttons often (but not always) are the right ones to press.

↪ Press `New Layer(s)` now. Again, you see the new object dialog. This time, let's create 3 objects (`LeabraLayer`s). Note that you can use those little up/down arrows to change the `Number` field without having to type in a number.

You will see 3 layers in the network, but they are of zero dimension so they look like lines. The `ReShape` tool is activated, indicating that you can reshape the layers to the size that they should be. Let's make all 3 layers $5x5$ in size.

↪ Just click on the line, and drag to the upper right.

You will see a grid representing the units as you drag, and the size of the layer will be displayed in the upper left hand side of the network window. After each layer is reshaped the display will automatically resize and re-center to fit the current layer sizes.

After reshaping all the layers, you will notice that the `Build All` button is highlighted.

↪ Press `Build All`.

This will create the actual units to fill in the layers to the size they were shaped. Before continuing, let's consider what would happen if you wanted to later change the size of one of these layers. Let's say you wanted to reduce the hidden layer to $4x4$ in size.

↪ Try clicking on the `ReShape` button again, and then reshaping the layer to a smaller size — you should see that it does not work.

You should notice that you can alter the geometry of the layer (e.g., making it $4x7$), but you can't shrink it. This is because `ReShape` works differently on layers that already have units in them as opposed to those that are empty. When empty, `ReShape` sets the geometry (and number of units) to whatever shape you want. When units are present, it simply rearranges the shape, but does not affect the number of units. Thus, to change the number of units, you need to remove the existing ones, reshape it, and then build it again. You can do this in one of two ways — we will do the procedure that should be used if you only want to reshape one layer.

↪ Press the `Select` button, and then click twice on the hidden layer, so that the `Rmv UnitGp(s)` button shows up as one of the options on the left hand side of the window. Then, you just click on this, and it will remove the entire group of units that were selected (i.e., all the units in the layer).

Alternatively, you could have selected `Actions/Remove Units` from the network window menu, and this would have removed all units in the network, enabling you to reshape any layer.

↪ Now, `ReShape` the layer to be $4x4$, and then hit `Build All` again.

It is also possible to set the number of units in a layer to be different than the full geometry of the layer (e.g., if you wanted 7 units in a $4x2$ layer shape). To do this, you must select an empty layer that has been shaped to the desired geometry, and then hit the `New Unit(s)` button, where you can enter the specific number of units you want within the layer. We will not do this here, though.

Now let's give the layers names.

↪ Click on the Select tool, and then click twice on the layer name (i.e., until there is a box around this name, and the Edit Name(s) button shows up on the left).

Note that you have to click twice because the first time you click you select the entire layer, the second time you select the lower-level object within the layer that the pointer is over (i.e., the name in this case, but the group of units in the previous case), and the next time you get the next level down, if applicable (i.e., an individual unit, if you were over a unit). After the first layer name is selected, you can **extend** the selection to include the second and third layer's names.

↪ Either use the middle mouse button or hold down shift and use the left mouse button, and click twice on the second and third layer's names. Then, click on Edit Name(s).

You should get an edit dialog with all three names in it.

↪ Click into the first name, and press Ctrl-u (the control (ctrl) key plus u), which highlights the entire name. Then, just type in Input, which will overwrite the highlighted text. Then, press the Tab key, which will go to the next field, and use Ctrl-u again and type Hidden, and then label the last layer Output. Press Ok when done.

B.2.4 Creating Projections and Connections

The connectivity between layers is specified in terms of a **Projection**, which must be created first before individual units get connected to each other.

↪ To create a projection, select the *receiving layer* first (i.e., the Hidden layer), using the left mouse button. Then extend the selection as before to the *sending layer* (i.e., the Input layer) using either the middle button or shift plus the left button.

You should see the New Prjn(s) button get highlighted.

↪ Press the New Prjn(s) button.

You will see that an arrow going from the input to the hidden was created. This arrow has an empty ar-

rowhead, indicating that the actual connections between individual units have not yet been created — we have merely specified how to create such connections, without actually doing it yet. This is similar to the way we first reshaped the layer to a desired size, and then used the build command to fill in the actual units. As you can see, the Connect All button is highlighted, which would create the actual connections for all projections. Let's create some more projections before we do this, though.

↪ Select the output layer, and then extend the selection to the hidden layer. This time, we will press the New BiPrjns button (to the left of New Prjn(s)), which will create bidirectional connectivity between the two selected layers.

This bidirectional connectivity is essential for the GeneRec error driven learning to work (only the input layer can get by with only feedforward projections).

↪ Now you can press Connect All, and see that the arrowheads have been filled in.

Now, you can do the usual inspection of the weights.

↪ Select r.wt and click on various units.

Notice that the layers are fully interconnected — this is the default type of connectivity pattern. We could change this by creating a new ProjectionSpec object in the .specs menu of the project, and then setting a given projection to use this new spec. Let's do this.

↪ Go to .specs and first just click on Edit.

Notice that several Spec objects have automatically been created. The LeabraUnitSpec_0 provides the default specifications for the all the units in the network, LeabraBiasSpec_0 specifies the parameters for the bias weights on the units, LeabraLayerSpec_0 specifies applies to all the layers, LeabraConSpec_0 provides the specifications for all the connections within the network, and FullPrjnSpec_0 specifies that the projections have full connectivity.

↪ Go down to New in the .specs menu, then select ProjectionSpec/TesselPrjnSpec.

This is one of the most useful forms of projection specs, which allows you to specify repeated "tilings" or receptive fields.

↪ Be sure to press Ok using the right mouse button, so you can edit this new spec.

There are many parameters that can be set in this object. We will just leave these all at their defaults, and create a rectangular receptive field for each unit.

↪ Go to the `Actions` menu at the top of this edit dialog, and select `Make Rectangle`.

The parameters for this function are shown in the next window that comes up.

↪ Enter a width and height of 2, and x and y center values (`ctr_x` and `ctr_y`) of 1. Then press `Ok`, and then `Ok` again on the `TesselPrjnSpec` dialog itself.

We have now created a connectivity pattern, but we have not yet specified which projection will use this new connectivity pattern.

↪ To do this, go to the network window and first click on the `Select` button at the top (`View` was active because we were viewing network weights), and then click on the projection arrow going from the input to the hidden layer. Then, use the far right `Selections` menu in the network window and choose `Set Prjn Spec`. You then need to select which projection spec to use in the window that comes up — choose the `TesselPrjnSpec_0`, which we just created.

↪ Now, you can just press `Connect All` again.

The network is now reconnected using the newly specified connectivity pattern.

↪ Use `r.wt` to view the connectivity into the hidden units — you need to click back on `View` at the top of the display to pick the different units for viewing.

Notice how they only receive from a $2x2$ square from the input units. This is what the tessel prjn spec does! Its many options allow you to determine how much the input square moves in relation to the position of the output units (here the input is directly proportional to the output), and lots of other things. Tessel prjn specs were used extensively in the object recognition simulations in chapter 8 — use these simulations for further examples of what they can do.

B.2.5 Specifying Layer Activity Levels

The default parameters contained in the automatically created unit, connection, and layer specs are probably reasonable for most simulations. However, one thing that usually must be specified on a layer-by-layer basis is the kWTA activity level for each layer. We can do this using the same technique as we did for the tessel prjn

spec, by creating a new spec object and then using the `Selections` menu to apply that spec to the different layers.

Usually, the only thing that differs about the different layers is their activity level — all other parameters in the layer spec should apply to all the layers. Fortunately, PDP++ has a special mechanism for dealing with just this kind of situation. The idea is that you can create **children** of a **parent** spec, where the children **inherit** parameters from the parent (except for specific parameters that are marked as special to a given child). First, let's edit the default layer spec.

↪ Do `.specs/Edit/LeabraLayerSpec_0`.

We can use this layer spec to control the hidden layer, so let's set the name appropriately.

↪ Do `Ctrl-u` and type in `HiddenLayer` in the `name` field.

Then, we can set the `kwta` field to a specific number of active units for the hidden layer.

↪ First, change `USE PCT` to `USE K`, and then set the k value to 4.

The default inhibitory function is `KWTA INHIB` (because it is more dependable), but `KWTA AVG INHIB` often works better for hidden layers.

↪ Set `compute i` to `KWTA AVG INHIB`. When this parameter is changed, you should also change `i kwta pt` to .6 instead of .25. Go ahead and `Apply` these changes.

Now, we can create two new children of this layer spec, one for the input layer one for the output layer.

↪ Use the `New Child` menu item in the `.specs` menu of the project window, and select `HiddenLayer` as the parent to create a child from.

You will then get a new object dialog. We will just create one new spec at a time, so leave the parameters as they are.

↪ Use the right mouse button on the `Ok` button to edit the new child layer spec.

Let's make this one for the output layer.

↪ Do `Ctrl-u` and type in `OutputLayer`. Then, click on the button right next to the `kwta` field label.

This will mark this as **unique** to this child, and not inherited from the parent.

↪ Then, change the `kwta k` parameter to 6, and `Ok` the edit dialog.

Next, we can create the input layer spec.

↪   Repeat the above process to create an `InputLayer` **spec, with a** `k` **value of 5.**

We're not done yet — we have to apply these new specs to the appropriate layers (this step is often forgotten!).

↪ **Select the** `Input` **layer, and then do** `Selections/ Set Layer Spec`**, and select** `InputLayer`**. Then do the same for the output layer.**

One optional step in configuring a network that is sometimes a good idea is to move the bias spec to be a child of the basic con spec, so that changes in the learning rate will automatically propagate to the bias spec.

↪ **Do this by editing the** `LeabraConSpec_0` **object, and then selecting** `Transfer` **from the menu under the** `children` **field, and select** `LeabraBiasSpec_0`**.**

Now when you look in the specs menu, you can see that the bias spec is under the con spec. Now you are done configuring the network!

B.2.6   Creating an Environment

The next menu down the line in the project window is the `.environments` menu.

↪   **Do** `.environments/New/Environment`**, and press** `Ok` **(using the left mouse button).**

(notice that there are several other types of environments that one could create, but we will just make the generic one.) An environment window will appear. Note that the `New Event` button is highlighted.

↪ **Press** `New Event`**, and create 5 events.**

These new events appear in the list on the left side of the window. We could select and extend-select these events to view them in this window, or we could use the following shortcut.

↪   **Use the** `View:Actions/SelectEvents` **menu (on the right side of the event window), and just press** `Ok`**.**

This will select all the events. We could manually click into the events to enter different activation patterns, as we did in some of the explorations. However, we can also use various automatic event generation techniques.

↪   **Select** `Permuted Binary Min Dist` **in the** `Generate` **menu, which will bring up a dialog window.**

This function will create random patterns that all have the same number of active values, and ensure that these patterns do not overlap too much (this is the min dist part). The `pat_no` field specifies which pattern in the event to generate patterns for (0 is the input layer, and 1 is for the output layer). Keep this at 0.

↪ **Set the** `n_on` **parameter to 5.**

This will cause each pattern to have 5 active units (1's), and the rest inactive (0's).

↪ **Set** `dist` **to 8, and the** `metric` **to** HAMMING.

This ensures that all the patterns will overlap by no more than 1 active unit (a hamming distance of 8 means there are 4 units that are different between the 2 patterns, meaning that there is 1 out of the 5 in common). Don't worry about the remaining two parameters, which just affect the way that the distance is computed, and aren't relevant for hamming distance.

↪ **Press** `Ok`**.**

You should now see that the input patterns for all the events contain random activity patterns.

Let's repeat this process for the output layer.

↪ **Select** `Permuted Binary Min Dist` **again, and set** `pat_no` **to 1,** `n_on` **to 6, and** `dist` **to 10 (again ensuring only 1 bit of overlap).**

This will provide a simple input-output mapping task for the network to learn.

As you can see, configuring the environment for a simple input-output learning task is relatively simple. To see how to configure a more complex example, we can create a second output layer in the network, and then configure the environment to provide a target for this new layer.

↪ **In the network window, do** `New Layer(s)` **and create one new layer. Reshape this layer to be** $5x1$ **units, and do** `Build All`**.**

Then, we can move this new layer down to the same level as the Output layer, and to its right.

↪ **Do** `Move` **and drag the layer into that position.**

Note that because the network geometry is three-dimensional, and the screen is only two-dimensional, we can only move layers in two dimensions at one time. By default, movement is in the X (horizontal) and Z (vertical) dimensions. Using the right mouse button moves within the Y (depth, into the screen) dimension. We can rename this layer as before.

↪ Select and edit the label and call it "Output2". Then, bidirectionally connect this layer to the hidden layer (New BiPrjns), and do Connect All.

Now, we return to the environment window to create a pattern corresponding to this new layer.

↪ Press the Edit Specs button.

This switches the environment to editing the EventSpec and associated PatternSpec objects. Pressing Edit Events would take you back to the previous mode of editing the events. The event specs control the layout and action of the events that they are associated with — each event points to its associated event spec and obtains its configuration and the way it interacts with the network from this spec. The event spec that was automatically created when we created events is shown as EventSpec_0 on the lower left side of the window.

↪ Select EventSpec_0 to edit.

You should see the PatternSpecs that define the input and output patterns of the events. The lower left hand corner of each pattern spec shows some of the critical parameters associated with each pattern. One thing you should notice is that the to_layer of the Output pattern spec is set to LAST — because we created a new layer in the network, this means that this pattern will automatically go to this new last layer, which is no longer appropriate.

↪ To fix this, click with the right mouse button on the to_layer text until an edit dialog appears (three times — the first click selects the event spec and the second the pattern spec), and then set the to_layer for this pattern to LAY_NAME (and hit OK).

This will ensure that the pattern is presented to the layer specified in the layer_name field, which should be Output.

Now, we need to create the new pattern spec for the new output layer.

↪ Select the event spec by clicking once on a grid in the display, and then hit the New Pattern button. Then, select this new pattern (at the top of the display) by clicking twice on it, and then hit the Set To Layer button, and select the Output2 layer (ignore the error message about not being able to find the PatternSpec_2 layer in the network).

This will automatically configure the pattern to fit the Output2 layer, including placing it in the same location as the corresponding layer in the network. If this automatic positioning is not appropriate, the Move button can be used to move patterns around (you must double-click on the pattern and hold down the button after the second click to select and move the pattern). Return to Select if you did move.

Finally, we need to specify that this pattern will be a TARGET, providing a plus-phase training signal to this output layer.

↪ Do this by editing the type field for this pattern (which shows an initial value of INACTIVE), using the right mouse button clicking trick.

Another way of editing these values is to select the field using the left button, and then click the Edit Val(s) button. Once the specs are configured, we can go back to view the events.

↪ Press Edit Events to see the events.

You will see that the events now have the new output layer. We can set some activation values for this new pattern.

↪ Click on one of the Output2 units for each event to provide some activation target for this layer (don't forget to Apply).

We will return to the environment in a later section when we take up the issue of programming in the PDP++ script language, which can enable you to create more sophisticated environments in a relatively efficient manner. You can iconify the window now.

B.2.7 Creating Training Process

Having created a network and an environment to train it on, we just need to create a set of processes which will systematically control the presentation of the events to the network, and generally orchestrate the processing and learning of the network. As you should recall from the previous appendix, processes are organized into a hierarchy, with each process responsible for a different temporal scale of processing. Thus, the TrainProcess simply calls the EpochProcess a number of times, which in turn iterates over the events in the environment, calling the TrialProcess on each one. Each event is processed by one or more

`SettleProcess` iterations, one for each phase of settling (minus then plus, or just minus during testing), and finally each settling phase consists of multiple iterations over the `CycleProcess`, which performs one cycle of activation updating in the network. Fortunately, we can usually just create the top-level process, and all the others will be created automatically.

Creating processes happens in the `.processes` menu in the project window (the next one down the line).

↪ Do `New/TrainProcess` (note that there are many different types of processes shown here that one could create).

Note that the new object dialog that comes up has a `Create Sub Procs` option — if this is clicked (as it is by default), then appropriate subprocesses under this one will be automatically created (which you want to do).

In addition to the subprocesses that are automatically created (the `EpochProcess`, `TrialProcess`, `SettleProcess`, and `CycleProcess` as described above), two commonly used statistics are also automatically created, these are a sum-squared error statistic, and a cycles-to-settle statistic. Thus, there is nothing else necessary to do for a basic set of training processes. We can now just create a process control panel for the train process.

↪ Do `.processes/Control Panel/Train_0`.

This brings up a small window that allows you to initialize, run and step the process using the buttons along the bottom of the window (many of these functions were performed in the explorations by similarly-named buttons on the overall control panel).

B.2.8   Creating a Training Log and Running the Model

Moving down to the next menu in the project window, we will create a graph log to monitor the progress of training.

↪ Do `.logs/New/Graph Log`.

Notice that there is an option on this new object dialog as well (`AddUpdater`), which if checked will automatically prompt you to specify which process should update this new log.

↪ Keep `AddUpdater` checked, and just hit `Ok`.

Then, the `AddUpdater` window will come up.

↪ Select the `Epoch_0` epoch process to update this log, so that we can see the error after every epoch of training.

Now you are ready to run the network!

↪ Do `ReInit` to reinitialize the network (using the previous random seed — to get a new random seed do `NewInit`) and `Run`.

The network should rapidly learn the task, as evidenced by the red line in the graph log. Depending on how your random event patterns turned out, the network may or may not learn the task completely (due to the small receptive fields for the hidden units).

↪ Go ahead and press `Stop` when it looks like training has plateaued.

You can enter in a smaller upper limit value (e.g., 50 epochs) in the `max` field if you want, so that training will stop then. We will see how to stop training based on the training error level later.

Next, we will add various refinements to this basic simulation. However, it might be useful to save this new project in its current state, and stop recording the script at this point.

↪ Do `Object/Save As` in the project window, and give it any name you wish. Then, locate the iconified script window, deiconify it, and press the `StopRec` button to stop recording.

B.3   Examining the Script

We can now examine the script that recorded all of your actions.

↪ Do `Edit` in the `script file` field of the script edit dialog (on some platforms, you may need to edit the script file using a simple text editor that you start separately).

An editor window should appear, showing the script. Let's step through some of this script (for those with programming experience the script language (css) is essentially C++, with some minor extensions and limitations). Note that the script code generated often contains some problems (which will be pointed out below), and should not be run without first looking at it and correcting these problems.

The first line of the script should be:

```
.projects[0].networks->New(1, Network);
```

This corresponds to the first action you took after starting the script recording, which was to create a new network. There are two key principles at work in this corresponding script code.

B.3.1 Object Paths

The first principle is that objects are specified with a **path**, where each element in the path is separated by a period (.). All paths start with the **root** object, which is represented graphically with the PDP++ Root window. This root is represented in the script code by the initial period (.) before `.projects...`. If you want to be very explicit, you can also write this as `root.projects...`. The subsequent elements of the path are specified in terms of particular **members** (aka fields, data items, sub objects) of a given object. Thus, the root object has as one of its members the `projects` group, where projects are located. Since almost everything is contained within a project, all of the script lines start with `.project`.

Because you could have multiple projects, you need to specify which one you want. This is done using the bracket syntax `[0]` after `.projects`. The `0` indicates that you want the first project (which is the only one in this case). Thus, we can understand `.projects[0].networks` in the script as specifying the `networks` member of the first project. There is a shortcut mechanism built into the script, which allows you to only specify the distinctive parts of the path. Thus, it will automatically look into the first element of every group and search for the member name you give it in the path. So, this first line could have been written `.networks->New(1, Network);`, because the networks member is assumed to be the one in the first element of the `.projects` group, which is correct in this case. In general, it is safe to skip the initial `.projects[0]`, and often the `.networks[0]` too, but beyond that you might end up not giving enough distinctive information, or pointing to the wrong place, so it is safer just to be explicit.

B.3.2 Object-Oriented Function Calls

The second principle is that the script language is **object oriented**, which means that the **function** that is being performed (i.e., New, which creates new objects) is called from the relevant object, and not as a global function. Thus, this function is called by first specifying the path to the object that owns the function (and will be responsible for making the new object, which it will subsequently "own' as one of its elements), and then specifying the function and its arguments. The alternative, more traditional way of doing this would be to have a global function called New, which would be called with the path to the object that will own the new object as its first argument:

```
New(.projects[0].networks, 1, Network);
```

The advantage of the object oriented approach is that it allows each object to have its own custom set of functions, and to do different things with standard functions if necessary. Instead of having a big if-then statement in the global New function to handle each different type of object that could be created, the object-specific New function just implements the code relevant to that particular object.

To complete our analysis of this one line of script code, note that the arguments to the function (1, Network) correspond to the values in the new object dialog box. In this case, and in general, there is a close homology between the structure of things and actions taken in the interface, and the corresponding script code. Finally, observe that there is a semicolon (;) at the end of the entire line — this is necessary to indicate that this is one complete **statement** or program action.

The next line of code in the script is similar to the first, except that it is creating layers in the newly created network:

```
.projects[0].networks[0].layers->New(3, \
    LeabraLayer);
```

Note that the backslash (\) in the above code and in subsequent examples indicates that the following line should continue at the end of the current line — these lines are too long to be typeset as one line in the book, but should appear as one line in the program, without the \.

B.3.3 Assigning Member Values

The next line after that is somewhat different, in that it does not involve a function (e.g., New), but instead involves setting (assigning) the value of a given member (field) in an object:

```
.projects[0].networks[0].layers[0].geom \
   = "{x=5: y=5: z=1: }";
```

Here, we are setting the geom member of the first layer (layers[0]) to have an x value of 5, a y value of 5, and a z value of 1. This was generated after we resized the layer using the ReSize tool. This line could have been written more laboriously as the three following lines:

```
.projects[0].networks[0].layers[0].geom.x=5;
.projects[0].networks[0].layers[0].geom.y=5;
.projects[0].networks[0].layers[0].geom.z=1;
```

where it is clear that x, y, and z are just members of the geom object. The shortcut that was actually used obviously makes for a more compact script.

The next line after this one is a function call to the UpdateAfterEdit() function, which performs any updating necessary to take into account any "edit" changes made by setting new member values. In this case, it multiplies x times y in the geom, and computes the total number of units that will fit within that geometry, making this the default number of units to create when the Build() function is later called. You should see that the script proceeds to set the geometries for the other layers in the network, and then calls this Build() function, which is the equivalent of hitting the Build All button in the network window. After that, you will see various attempts to resize the hidden layer (layers[1]), and at some point a

```
.projects[0].networks[0].layers[1].units.\
   RemoveAll();
```

function call which removed all the units in the layer, enabling you to subsequently resize it as desired.

B.3.4 Scoped Variables

After the network is built again, you will notice a set of three lines of the following general form:

```
{ taNBase* ths = .projects[0].networks[0].?.[0];
  ths->name = "Input";
}
```

This is a somewhat complicated construction that you will see occasionally in recorded script code. The surrounding curly brackets ("{" and "}") are there to **scope** the enclosed script code, so that any new **variables** that get created only apply within the scope enclosed by the brackets. This allows you to reuse the same variable name without worrying about where else it is used in the script. The variable that gets created is called ths (short for "this"), and it is just a shortcut way of referring to an object. The motivation for doing this is to allow multiple members of the ths object to be set without having to repeat the long path name each time. However, in this case, there is only one member being set, so it was unnecessary (but the script code generator was too dumb to figure this out in this case).

There is also a *bug* in this line of script code (which is difficult to fix for technical reasons, but can be easily corrected by editing the script code) — the path name contains a question mark (?), indicating that it couldn't quite figure out this part of the path. You might be able to guess that this should say layers, since we want to set the layer names here. Thus, you should change these paths to fit the following example:

```
{ taNBase* ths = .projects[0].networks[0].\
   layers[0];
  ths->name = "Input";
}
```

The next chunk of code deals with the creation of the projections between the layers, ending with the calling of the Connect() function. Then you can see where you created the different layer specifications (which provides a better example of the use of the scoped ths variable). Then you can see where the environment was created, and the PermutedBinary_MinDist function called (with the same arguments you gave it in the dialog).

B.3.5 Running Processes from the Script

Finally we see where the .processes[0] object is ReInit() and then run. Only the ReInit() function call shows up, because the others don't make sense to run in the script. If you were to do:

```
.projects[0].processes[0].Run();
```

then the function call would be processed to completion before going on to the next line in the script, meaning that the process would complete running all the way! You can do this with a script call, but since you can't `Stop()` from within the script, it doesn't get recorded by default.

B.3.6 Saving Files from the Script

There is one final (and difficult to correct) bug on what should be the last line of your script:

```
.projects[0].SaveAs(ostream_ref);
```

The problem is that it has this `ostream_ref` argument instead of the actual file name that we want to save into. This happens because by the time the `SaveAs` function is called, it has lost any record of the actual file name, and so cannot record it here in the script. Thus, you have to edit this line, providing the entire name of the project you want to save (including the extension, which is added automatically for you in the graphical interface, but not here):

```
.projects[0].SaveAs("constr.proj.gz");
```

Be sure to save the resulting script file with your bug fixes before proceeding.

B.3.7 Compiling and Running the Script

Now that we have made it all the way through the script, and you have edited out any mistakes that you might have made along the way, we can actually compile and run it, which should result in the reproduction of the same project we just finished setting up. To do this, we have to start out with an empty project.

↪ Go to the project window and do `Object/Close` and click on `Ok` to get rid of the current project. Then, do `.projects/New/Project` in the remaining `PDP++ Root` window, to create a new project. As before, create a new script object in the `.scripts` menu, and this time, `Open` the recorded script file.

When you hit the `Apply` button in the script window, this script will automatically be **compiled**. Compiling the script turns the text file into something that the computer can actually run. If you were to make changes to the script file at this point in the editor, then you should hit the `Compile` button in the script window to re-compile the script and incorporate your changes into the thing that actually gets run. You might notice that you get a couple of warning messages about not finding the `SetUnique` function — ignore these. If you made a mistake in editing the file, you might notice other errors or warnings — it is always a good idea to look at these (especially errors) when you hit `Compile`, and see if you can figure out what is wrong.

Now, you are ready to run the script.

↪ Hit the `Run` button.

You should see several windows coming up as the objects were created (network, environment, etc.). However, these windows are blank initially — don't panic. Just hit the `Init` buttons to initialize these displays. You can poke around the network, environment, and so on, and `ReInit` and `Run` the process to see that everything is the same as when you first created it!

One thing you might have noticed is that the original window positions were not saved in the script. We can remedy this in the following way.

↪ First, position the windows in the way that you want them. Then, start `Record` again in the script window.

This will *append* newly recorded script code to the end of your existing program.

↪ Then, do `Object/Edit` in the process window. In the resulting edit dialog, select `Script All Win Pos` from the `Object` menu in the edit dialog (this is an expanded version of the `Object` menu that appears in the project window). Then, hit `Stop Rec` in the script window, and `Edit` the script file again (or just revert your editor if you still have it there).

You should notice some additional lines at the end of the script that call `SetWinPos` functions on the various objects (and `Place` on the control panel). Then close this project, and repeat the steps for creating a new project and running the script again. You should find that the windows appear in their saved locations this time around.

While this exercise of using the script to create the project is useful for learning how to program in the script language, it is not the most useful way to save and load projects. It is much easier just to use `SaveAs` on the project object, and then do `Open In` to load it back in, as we have done with all of the projects for the explorations in the book. The following sections will provide more useful applications of the script technology.

B.4   Creating a Testing Process

The set of processes that we created above is configured for training the network. Although it is possible to modify these processes to make them suitable for testing the network after it has been trained, it is usually a much better idea just to create a new set of processes for each different task you want to perform on the network (i.e., one for training, another for testing). We will go one step further here and link in the testing process to the training process, so that testing is performed automatically during the course of training. This technique was used in a number of the exercises.

To keep the different sets (hierarchies) of processes organized, we will put each set into a different **group**. Since this is commonly done, it has been automated.

↪   Edit the highest-level process in the hierarchy (the `Train_0` process in this case) (i.e., do `.processes/Edit/Train_0` in the project window), and then do `Actions/Move To Sub Gp` in the menu of the resulting edit dialog for `Train_0`. It will then prompt you for the name of the group, to which you should enter `Train`, to indicate that this is the training group of processes.

If you now do `.processes/Edit`, you will see that all of the processes are now grouped together in the `Train` subgroup.

↪ Go ahead and `Ok` the `Train_0` edit dialog.

Now, let's create a testing process hierarchy. The typical way that testing is done is to present a single epoch of events while measuring the network's responses to these events. Thus, we will create an `EpochProcess`.

↪ Do `.processes/New/EpochProcess`. When the new object dialog comes up, press `Ok` with the right mouse button, so that we can edit it.

Notice that this object is called `Epoch_1` — all objects are created with sequentially increasing numbers as a function of the number of other objects of that type that have been created. This is useful, since all of these testing objects will have the same number, and can thus be identified as belonging to the same hierarchy. In cases when this isn't true (i.e., a testing process has a new type of process object), then it is useful to change the names to all have the same number.

There are two parameters that are typically changed on the epoch process to make it more appropriate for testing rather than training.

↪   The first is the `order` field, which should be changed from `PERMUTED` to `SEQUENTIAL`.

The order of event presentation is usually permuted (random, without replacement) so that there aren't any unusual learning effects that arise from the events being presented in the same order every time. During testing, it is more useful to have the events in a predictable, sequential order.

↪   The other parameter is the `wt_update` field, which should be set to `TEST` instead of `ON_LINE` so that no weight changes (learning) takes place during testing. `Apply` these changes, and then do `Actions/Move To Sub Gp` for this set of testing processes, calling the group `Test`.

Now, we can get a control panel for this new testing epoch process, and step through some testing events.

↪   Do `.processes/Control Panel/Test /Epoch_1`. Set the `step` process in this control panel to be `Trial_1` instead of `Epoch_1`, so that when we hit the `Step` button, it will go one event (trial) at a time. Then, hit `ReInit` and then the `Step` button. You should see the first event presented to the network. Continue to `Step` through the entire epoch.

B.4.1   Monitoring Unit Activities

Let's imagine that we were interested in the hidden unit activity patterns in response to these different events. As we have seen in a number of the exercises, it is useful to use a grid log to view activity patterns over time. There are two steps that we need to do, (a) create the log, and then (b) **monitor** the hidden unit activities so that they end up in the log.

↳ Do `.logs/New/GridLog`, and set the `updt_proc` (updating process) to `Trial_1`. Then, `Run` the test epoch process, just to see what shows up in the log by default.

One thing you will notice is that the `sum_se` and `1st_cycles` statistics (only `su` and `ls` are visible as the header labels for these columns) are displayed as colored squares instead of as textual values. This is fine, but it will do strange things to the color scale when we also display activity values in the $0 - 1$ range, so we will switch the display to a textual output.

↳ Click with the right mouse button on the header buttons for these columns. When you do this, an edit dialog will appear, where you can switch the `display_style` from `BLOCK` to `TEXT`. Then, if you `Run` again, you will see the errors and cycles as text.

Now we are ready to monitor the hidden layer.

↳ Click on the hidden layer in the network window (make sure that the `Select` tool is active first). Then, make sure you are viewing the `act` variable. Then, do `Monitor Values/New`, which is just below the tool and action buttons on the left side of the network window.

When we monitor network variables, we are actually creating a `MonitorStat` object, which is reflected in the first field of the resulting dialog that comes up. The second field, `In Process`, is critical.

↳ Set `In Process` to `Trial_1`, so that the monitored values show up in our testing process instead of in the training one.

You can leave the remaining fields as they are, but be aware that you have an option here to not just `COPY` the values, but alternatively you could perform simple computations like `AVG` or `SUM` over them.

↳ Then press `Ok`.

Although you could just `Run` the testing process, it is a good idea to `Clear` the log first, because the new data will have a different format. Now, when you `Run` your testing process again, you will see that the hidden unit activations appear on the right hand side. If you didn't hit clear first, you may need to hit the `Init` button. Also, you will probably want to resize the window to fit all the events at once.

B.4.2 Creating a New Statistic for Testing

In addition to monitoring unit activations, you can create a wide range of different statistics. We will create a closest-event statistic, that compares the output produced by the network to the target events in the environment, and reports on the closest such event. This statistic was used in the weight-based priming simulation in section 9.2.1.

The simplest way to create a new statistic is to use the `New Stat` menu item in the `.processes` menu.

↳ Select `.processes/New Stat/Closest Event Stat`.

The dialog that comes up contains three important parameters. The `In Process` field specifies in which process to create the statistic, the `Loop/Final` field specifies at which point in the processing this statistic should be computed, and the `CreateAggregates` toggle determines if higher-level aggregations of the statistic are created.

↳ Select `Trial_1` for the process, to compute as each testing event is presented.

Each statistic usually has a reasonable `DEFAULT` value for the `Loop/Final` field, but you may need to change it sometimes. `LOOP` means that the statistic will be computed during each iteration of the process (e.g., after every event if created in the loop of an epoch process), and `FINAL` means that it will be computed when the process is done (e.g., at the end of the epoch in the above example). Let's just leave it at `DEFAULT` for now.

The `CreateAggregates` flag is set by default, since it is often useful to have higher-level aggregation of a given statistic. For example, the `sum_se` statistic, which is computed during each trial, has to be aggregated by summing over the trials to get a total error for the entire epoch. We can leave this flag set here, even though we don't have any immediate need for the aggregated values of this statistic.

↳ Press the `Ok` button using the right mouse button, so that you can edit the resulting statistic object.

You will then get another dialog window asking for the type of aggregation to perform.

↳ Select `SUM` here.

When the edit window comes up, you will notice that the `layer` field has been set to `Input` by default.

↪ You actually want to set `layer` to the `Output` layer. Also, to replicate the tolerance typically used in the squared error statistic, you should set `dst_tol` to .5. Then `Ok` this edit dialog.

↪ Now you should `Clear` the grid log again, and then `Run` the testing process.

You will probably get a little dialog warning of overlap in the grid log, to which you should press the `ResetLayout` button to fix this situation. You probably want to switch the one column (`min_dst`) that shows up as a `BLOCK` over to `TEXT`. Also, you will probably have to stretch the window wider to fit all the information.

B.4.3 Automatically Testing during Training

So far, this setup is sufficient for testing the network after training — what if you want to run a test after each epoch of training? We will **link** the testing process into the training process hierarchy. Each level of processing has three different places (groups) where other processes can be attached: `init_procs`, `loop_procs`, and `final_procs`. As you might guess, the difference is whether the attached processes are run at the start (init), during the iteration (loop), or at the end (final) of the given process's running. Further a given process can either be created and "live" entirely within one of these groups, or in the current case, it can live elsewhere and just be linked into the group. The difference between being owned versus linked is important — if the owning process is removed, then you lose all the other processes that it owns. If it is linked, then it persists independently (and must have been already created, just like our testing process).

Given the above considerations, we want to link the testing process into the `final_procs` of the training `EpochProcess`. Thus, at the end of an epoch of training, we will run an epoch of testing.

↪ To do this, edit the training epoch process (`.processes/Edit/Train/Epoch_0`). Then, go to the `final_procs` field, select `Link`, and select `EpochProcess/Epoch_1` as the `item` to link. Leave the `idx` field at -1, so that it will be put at the end of the

list (since it is the 1st item, this is irrelevant). Press `Ok`, and then `Ok` again on the `Epoch_0` edit dialog.

↪ Now, `ReInit` the `Train_0` train process, and then `Run` it.

You should see that testing is run after every epoch of training. Often, you want to run testing only every n (e.g., 5 or 10) epochs of training. We can do this by setting the `mod` parameters of the testing epoch process, so that it will be run **modulo** the training epoch count (where modulo gives the remainder after dividing by n, which cycles between 0 and n-1).

↪ Edit the `Epoch_1` process, and set the `mod` m value to 5 (for example). `Run` the training process again, and observe that testing only occurs every 5 training epochs.

B.5 Writing Script Code to Create an Environment

One of the most useful applications of the script language is for creating environments, often saving considerable time and effort over manually clicking in the events. We will do a simple example here, which will contain all the basic elements necessary for doing more elaborate things. Our objective will be to create events that have sequentially overlapping patterns (i.e., the first event has the first 5 units active, the second has 5 units active starting at unit 3, etc.).

The first thing we need to do is create a home for the script code that we will write. If the environment were something that changed dynamically every epoch, then one would want to associate the script code with the environment itself (i.e., in a `ScriptEnv` object), which has provisions for automatically calling the script every epoch (or whenever new events are needed). In the present case, we will just create the environment once, so that we can do the same thing we did when we recorded a script — create a `Script` object in the `.scripts` menu.

↪ Do `.scripts/New/Script` in the project window. Use the right mouse button on the new object `Ok` button, and then `Open` a new `script_file` called `make_env.css`. Then `Apply` on the script edit window, and then do `Edit` on the `script_file` to bring up a text editor, which we will use to enter the script code.

To write this script, we will create a new *object type* in the script language, which will provide a way of organizing and interacting with the script. We will later edit an instance of this object type, and obtain an edit dialog like those you are accustomed to using, with all the necessary parameters and functions visible. The script should begin with the following lines:

```
class MakeEnv {
  // makes environment
public:
```

This declares the object (class) type name (MakeEnv), gives it a little descriptive comment, and then makes all of what follows publicly accessible (as opposed to private to the class object itself — this is not really necessary in the script language, but is needed if you were to later compile this using a C++ compiler).

Next, we will define a number of variables which will parameterize the algorithm for creating the environment, including first a pointer to which environment object to operate on. The backslashes (\) in the following code indicate that the subsequent line should continue at the end of the current line — these lines are too long to be typeset as one line in the book, but should appear as one line in the program (without the \).

```
Environment*  env;              \
  // environment to operate on
int           n_events;         \
  // number of events to create
int           in_active;        \
  // number active in the input layer
int           out_active;       \
  // number active in the output layer
int           in_skip;          \
  // number to skip per event in input
int           out_skip;         \
  // and in output layer
```

Notice that these are defined in three parts, first a *type* name (e.g., int for integer), then the name of the parameter, and finally a descriptive comment.

Now, we define a set of functions that will accomplish the creation of the environment:

```
void  Make();                 \
  // #BUTTON make the full environment
void  MakeEvent(Event* ev, int idx); \
```

```
  // make one event (number idx)
void  MakePattern(Pattern* pat, int idx, \
  int active, int skip);
```

Note that these also have the same basic parts, a return type (which is void because these functions do not return anything), a function name (including arguments, which are defined as a comma-separated list of type-name pairs), and a descriptive comment. The #BUTTON after the Make function means that this function will have a button associated with it in the edit dialog. We will define the actual code that goes with each of these functions later, but we need to **declare** them here first (so that, for example, other functions can call them).

Finally, we need to declare the class **constructor**, which initializes an instance of this class type whenever one is created. Thus, we will use this to set the default values for all the parameters.

```
  MakeEnv(); // constructor to set defaults
};
```

Note that the constructor is just a function (with no return type and no arguments) that has the same name as the class type. Also, we have terminated the class type definition by including the }; at the end.

Now, it is time to define the functions themselves. Let's start with the constructor:

```
MakeEnv::MakeEnv() {
  env = .environments[0];
  n_events = 5;
  in_active = 5;
  out_active = 6;
  in_skip = 4;
  out_skip = 4;
}
```

Notice that the function definition starts with a **scoping** operator MakeEnv:: which identifies this as applying to a function of this particular class type.

Next, we will define the Make function, and its helpers. Note that in these functions, we are directly manipulating the Event objects and their constituent Patterns, instead of for example writing a text file of patterns and then reading that in — manipulating these structures often makes for easier programming.

```
void MakeEnv::Make() {
  env.events.Reset();            \
    // get rid of any existing events
  int i;
  for(i=0;i<n_events;i++) {      \
    // iterate over events
    Event* ev = env.events.New(1, Event); \
    // create new event
    MakeEvent(ev, i);            \
    // hand off to subroutine
  }
  env.UpdateAllViews();          \
    // update display to reflect changes
}

void MakeEnv::MakeEvent(Event* ev, int idx) {
  ev->name = "seq_ev_" + idx; \
    // name the event according to index
  // first make the input pattern
  MakePattern(ev->patterns[0], idx, \
    in_active, in_skip);
  // then the output pattern
  MakePattern(ev->patterns[1], idx, \
    out_active, out_skip);
}
```

Note that we are ignoring the second output layer in the above code.

```
void MakeEnv::MakePattern(Pattern* pat, \
    int idx, int active, int skip) {
  int i;
  for(i=0;i<active;i++) {
    pat.value[skip*idx + i] = 1.0;
  }
}
```

Finally, we just need to create an instance of the MakeEnv type, and then edit it, and we're done:

```
MakeEnv make_env;
EditObj(make_env);
```

Be sure to save the file after you have entered the above lines of code.

↪ Then just hit `Compile` in the script object window.

You should not get any error messages — if you do, then compare the line(s) in question with those here and correct any discrepancies (and then hit `Compile` again to make the changes take effect). Now, you are ready to run your new script.

↪ Press the `Run` button.

You should see an edit dialog appear, with the appropriate parameter fields and the `Make` button across the

bottom. You can click on the field labels, and see the descriptive comment you entered (and the overall comment at the top of the file appears at the top of the edit window). This is the same basic technology that is used throughout the PDP++ system for providing a graphical interface to the underlying class objects.

↪ Hit the `Make` button on your new edit dialog, and then click on a few of the new events in the environment window.

The events should have patterns as you would expect from the algorithm. You can play with the parameters and hit `Make` again to see the effects of the parameters. When you are done, you can go ahead and `Run` the training process again with this new environment.

B.5.1 Setting a Stopping Criterion for Training

One thing you might notice with this new environment is that the network learns all the way to completion (since the patterns now work better with the limited receptive fields of the hidden units). Thus, it would be convenient to arrange it so that the training process stops when the error goes to zero. Any statistic can provide a means for stopping the process it is attached to, by simply setting a flag and establishing the conditions under which stopping should occur. For training, we will edit the squared error statistic object in the training process.

↪ Do `.processes/Edit/Train/Train_0/loop_stats/..SE_Stat`.

Notice that the `se` field has some `stopcrit` parameters, which specify the stopping criteria parameters.

↪ Click the toggle button on, to indicate that there is a stopping criterion associated with this statistic value, and just leave the `<=` and `0` parameters as is.

Thus, when the `se` value gets less than or equal to zero, this statistic will signal the training process to stop running. Now, when you `Run` the training process again, you should see that it stops just as the red error line goes to zero.

B.6 Creating an Overall Control Panel

The last thing we will do with the simulation is to create one of those overall control panels that have been so handy in the exercises. We will put some important spec parameters in this control panel, and include some buttons for switching between training and testing windows and logs, and running the training and testing processes. A control panel is really just a script object that is edited to create an edit dialog, just like we did with the environment creation script above.

↪ Go through the same steps of creating a new script object, set the file name to `constr_ctrl.css`, and edit this file.

We start the script just like we did before, creating a new type of object:

```
class ConstrCtrl {
  // control panel for the tutorial \
    on constructing simulations
public:
```

Again, we start with some parameters. We will just put in the learning rate and the activity level of the hidden layer.

```
  c_float*       lrate;            \
    // learning rate
  c_int*         hid_kwta;         \
    // activity of the hidden layer
```

The types of these variables start with a `c_`, which indicates that they are really just **pointers** to internal, hard-coded C/C++ variables that were created when PDP++ itself was compiled. Thus, there is an important distinction between variables defined within the script, and hard coded variables. Script variables can point to these hard coded variables, but they must be treated differently since the script does not actually own the underlying variables (it just points to them). We will establish this pointing relationship in the constructor.

Next, let's define some functions:

```
  void  Run();                     \
    // #BUTTON run training
  void  RunTest();                 \
    // #BUTTON run testing
  void  Train();                   \
    // #BUTTON display training windows
  void  Test();                    \
    // #BUTTON display testing windows
```

and we also need one helper function that iconifies all the windows before turning on other windows, and of course the constructor for initializing things, and the closing bracket:

```
  void  EverythingOff();           \
    // iconify all windows
  ConstrCtrl();                    \
    // constructor
};
```

Now, we define the constructor:

```
ConstrCtrl::ConstrCtrl() {
  // point lrate to the actual lrate parameter
  lrate = .specs.ConSpec.lrate;
  // point hid_kwta to actual parameter
  hid_kwta = .specs.HiddenLayer.kwta.k;
}
```

where we just specify the path to the actual parameter to point the `c_` variables to these actual hard coded parameters.

Then, we define the functions for running the training and testing processes, which simply call the appropriate functions:

```
void ConstrCtrl::Run() {
  // note that we need to specify subgroup
  // for the training process (.gp.Train)
  .processes.gp.Train[0].ReInit();
  .processes.gp.Train[0].Run();
}
```

```
void ConstrCtrl::RunTest() {
  .processes.gp.Test[0].ReInit();
  .processes.gp.Test[0].Run();
}
```

Next, we define the window manipulation routines:

```
void ConstrCtrl::Train() {
  EverythingOff();                 \
    // turn everything off first
  .processes.gp.Train[0].ControlPanel();
  .logs.Epoch_0_GraphLog.DeIconify();
}
```

```
void ConstrCtrl::Test() {
  EverythingOff();                 \
    // turn everything off first
  .processes.gp.Test[0].ControlPanel();
  .logs.Trial_1_GridLog.DeIconify();
}
```

which just turn everything off, and then deiconify the appropriate windows (you might want to deiconify the testing grid log too, since it is updated during training, but we will leave that out for the time being just to make these functions seem more useful).

The `EverythingOff` function is somewhat complicated, but essentially it just iconifies things (or gets rid of control panels), and then makes sure all of the resulting windowing actions actually get processed before continuing:

```
void ConstrCtrl::EverythingOff() {
  if(!taMisc::iv_active)        return;
  int i;
  for(i=0; i<.logs.size; i++)
    .logs[i].Iconify();

  // don't actually iconify network - only one
//   for(i=0; i<.networks.size; i++)
//     .networks[i].Iconify();

  for(i=0; i<.environments.size; i++)
    .environments[i].Iconify();

  for(i=0; i<.processes.leaves; i++)
    taivMisc::CloseEdits(.processes.Leaf(i),\
    .processes.Leaf(i));

  // this is necessary to make sure all the
  // processing for closing the windows
  // happens before we continue
  taivMisc::FlushIVPending();
}
```

Finally, we again need to create a instance of this new type, and then edit it:

```
ConstrCtrl constr_ctrl;
EditObj(constr_ctrl);
```

↪ Then, just `Compile` and `Run` the new script.

You should see the control panel window, and can press the buttons and alter the parameters as you want.

You now have performed all the basic tasks that go into creating a simulation! While there are many other things you can do, you should now at least have some idea as to where to start to accomplish the things you want.

Finally, we would strongly recommend reading one of the many good C++ books available to learn how to use the script language better. Also, the PDP++ users manual, available at

`www.cnbc.cmu.edu/PDP++/PDP++.html`, contains a wealth of detailed information on all of the general PDP++ objects, and is an essential reference guide for constructing more complex simulations.

B.7   Creating SRN Context Layers

This section describes the specific steps that need to be taken to construct an SRN context layer. First, the `LayerSpec` needs to be set to be a `LeabraContextLayerSpec`, which has the `fm_hid` and `fm_prv` parameters on it, and controls the updating of the units. Do this by going to `.specs/New/` and selecting `LeabraContextLayerSpec` as the type of object. Then, select the layer that is to be the context layer, and do `Selections` in the network window, and set the layer spec to be this new layer spec you created.

Second, a projection with a `OneToOnePrjnSpec` projection spec from the hidden layer to the context layer needs to be created, which tells each context unit which hidden unit to get the activation from. Again, create the spec in `.specs`, then use the `Selections` menu to set this for the appropriate projection in the network. A standard full projection can be made going the opposite direction (from context to hidden).

Finally, the `LeabraTrialProcess` needs to be told to not completely initialize the network at the start of each trial, so that the context layer can grab the previous hidden and context layer activations. This is done by editing this trial processes (from the `.processes` menu in the project), and setting the `trial_init` parameter to `DECAY_STATE` instead of `INIT_STATE`. The `decay.event` decay parameter on the layer specs, which is 1 by default, will still ensure that the network starts settling with an initialized state (the context uses the `act_p` state variables, which are not used in processing, and which are preserved by decay state but not by init state).

Then, you probably also need to use an environment with grouped events, and a `Sequence` process, to control the presentation of the events. The example networks can be consulted for how these are set up. There are defaults that can be loaded into the `.defaults` menu that make constructing the sequence-based processes easier. These default files are located in the `defaults` file included with the software. The `leabra_seq.def` sets up the sequence defaults.

Appendix C

Leabra Implementation Reference

Contents

C.1 Overview 455
C.2 Pseudocode 456
C.3 Connection-Level Variables 456
C.4 Unit-Level Variables 459
C.5 Layer-Level Variables 463
C.6 Process-Level Variables 465

C.1 Overview

This appendix provides a summary of the Leabra implementation in PDP++. This should be useful for reference, for exploring the existing simulations more in depth on your own, and for creating your own simulations using the simulator. First, we provide the pseudocode listing of the steps in computing Leabra, and then we describe all the parameters and their roles, organized as they are within the Spec objects of the simulator (see appendix A for more general information about these).

C.2   Pseudocode

Outer loop: Iterate over events (trials) within an epoch. For each event:

1. Iterate over minus and plus phases of settling for each event.

   (a) At start of settling, for all units:

      i. Initialize all state variables (activation, v_m, etc).

      ii. Apply external patterns (clamp input in minus, input & output in plus).

      iii. Compute net input scaling terms (constants, computed here so network can be dynamically altered).

      iv. Optimization: compute net input once from all static activations (e.g., hard-clamped external inputs).

   (b) During each cycle of settling, for all non-clamped units:

      i. Compute net input (net or η_j, and g_i if unit-based inhib) – sender-based optimization by ignoring inactives.

      ii. Unless doing unit-based inhibition, compute kWTA inhibition, based on g_i^Θ (equation 3.2):

         A. Sort units into two groups based on g_i^Θ: top k and remaining $k+1$ to n.

         B. If basic kWTA, find k and $k+1th$ highest, if average-based, compute average of 1 to k and $k+1$ to n.

         C. Set inhib conductance g_i between k and $k+1$ for basic kWTA, or between averages for average-based.

      iii. Compute point-neuron activation (incorporating netinput and inhibition).

   (c) After settling, for all units:

      i. Record final settling activations as either minus or plus phase (act_m or act_p).

2. After both phases, for all units & connections:

   (a) Compute weight changes from plus-minus activations (error-driven) and plus-phase activations (Hebbian).

   (b) Increment the weights according to computed changes.

C.3   Connection-Level Variables

We first describe the connection object, and then the specifications that control that object. Most object variables are computed by the software, and should not be changed manually (they will just get overwritten) — only the specifications should be changed.

LeabraCon connection object:

Variable	Description
wt	The weight value (shows up in NetView as r.wt for receiving, s.wt for sending
dwt	Accumulated change in weight value computed for current trial: this is usually zero by the time NetView is updated
pdw	Previous dwt weight change value: this is what is visible in NetView.

LeabraConSpec connection-level specifications:

Variable	Default	Description
rnd		Controls the random initialization of the weights:
.type		Select type of random distribution to use (e.g., UNIFORM (default), NORMAL (Gaussian)).
.mean	.5	Mean of the random distribution (mean rnd weight val).
.var	.25	Variance of the distribution (range for UNIFORM).
.par	0	2nd parameter for distributions like BINOMIAL and GAMMA that require it (not typically used).
wt_limits		Sets limits on the weight values — Leabra weights are constrained between 0 and 1 and are initialized to be symmetric:
.type		Type of constraint (GT_MIN = greater than min, LT_MAX = less than max, MIN_MAX (default) within both min and max)
.min	0	Minimum weight value (if GT_MIN or MIN_MAX).
.max	1	Maximum weight value (if LT_MAX or MIN_MAX).
.sym	true	Symmetrizes the weights (only done at initialization).
inhib	false	Makes the connection inhibitory (net input goes to g_i instead of net).
wt_scale		Controls relative and absolute scaling of weights from different projections (see equation 2.17):
.abs	1	Absolute scaling (s_k): directly multiplies weight value.
.rel	1	Relative scaling (r_k): effect is normalized by sum of rel values for all incoming projections.
wt_sig		Parameters for the sigmoidal weight contrast enhancement function:
.gain	6	Gain parameter: how sharp is the contrast enhancement. 1=linear function.
.off	1.25	Offset parameter: for values > 1, how far above .5 is neutral point on contrast enhancement curve (1=neutral is at .5, values < 1 not used, 2 is probably the maximum usable value).
lrate	.01	Learning rate (ϵ).
cur_lrate	.01	Current learning rate as affected by lrate_sched: note that this is only updated when the network is actually run (and only for ConSpecs that are actually used in network).
lrate_sched		Schedule of learning rate over training epochs: to use, create elements in the list, assign start_ctr's to epoch vals when lrate's (given by start_val's) take effect. These start_val lrates *multiply* the basic lrate, so use .1 for a cur_lrate of .001 if basic lrate = .01.
lmix		Sets mixture of Hebbian and err-driven learning:
.hebb	.01	Amount of Hebbian learning: unless using pure Hebb (1), values greater than .05 are usually to big. For large networks trained on many patterns, values as low as .00005 are still useful.
.err	.99	Amount of error-driven: automatically set to be 1-hebb, so you can't set this independently.

Variable	Default	Description
fix_savg		Sets fixed sending avg activity value for normalizing netin: i.e., α_k in equation 2.15: $g_{e_k} = \frac{1}{\alpha_k}\langle x_i w_{ij}\rangle_k$. This is useful when expected activity of sending region that projection actually receives is different from that of sending layer as a whole.
.fix	false	Toggle for actually fixing the sending avg activation to value set in savg.
.savg	.25	The fixed sending average activation value — should be between 0 and 1.
.div_gp_n	false	Divide by group n, not layer n, where group n is the number of actual connections in the connection group that this unit receives from (corresponds to a given projection). Usually, the netinput is averaged by dividing by layer n, so it is the same even with partial connectivity — use this flag to override where projection n is more meaningful.
savg_cor		Correction for sending average activation levels in hebbian learning — renormalizes weights to use full dynamic range even with sparse sending activity levels that would otherwise result in generally very small weight values (equations 4.18, 4.19, 4.20).
.cor	1	Amount of correction to apply (0=none, 1=all, .5=half, etc): q_m in equation 4.20: $\alpha_m = .5 - q_m(.5 - \alpha)$, where $m = \frac{.5}{\alpha_m}$ (equation 4.19), and $\Delta w_{ij} = \epsilon[y_j x_i(m - w_{ij}) + y_j(1 - x_i)(0 - w_{ij})]$ (equation 4.18).
.src		Source of the sending average act for use in correction. SLAYER_AVG_ACT (default) = use actual sending layer average activation. SLAYER_TRG_PCT = use sending layer target activation level. FIXED_SAVG = use value specified in fix_savg.savg. COMPUTED_SAVG = use actual computed average sending activation *for each specific projection* — this is very computationally expensive and almost never used.
.thresh	.01	Threshold of sending average activation below which Hebbian learning does not occur — if the sending layer is essentially inactive, it is much faster to simply ignore it. Note that this also has the effect of preserving weight values for projections coming from inactive layers, whereas they would otherwise uniformly decrease.

LeabraBiasSpec connection specification for bias weight (bias weights do not have the normal weight bounding and wt_limits settings, are initialized to zero with zero variance, and do not have a Hebbian learning component):

Variable	Default	Description
dwt_thresh	.1	Don't change weights if dwt (weight change) is below this value — this prevents bias weights from slowly creeping up or down and growing ad-infinitum even when the network is basically performing correctly — essentially a tolerance factor for how accurate the actual activation has to be relative to the target.

C.4 Unit-Level Variables

LeabraUnit unit object:

Variable	Description
spec	Determines the spec that controls this unit (not in NetView).
pos	Determines location of unit within layer (not in NetView).
ext_flag	Reflects type of external input to unit (not in NetView).
targ	Target activity value (provided by external input from event).
ext	External activation value when clamped (provided by external input from event).
act	Activation value (what is sent to other units, y_j).
net	Net input value (η_j) computed as normalized weights times activations — excitation only (equation 2.16), inhibition is computed separately as g_i (gc.i) either by kWTA or directly by unit inhib.
bias	The bias weight is a LeabraCon object hanging off of the unit — it is managed by its own LeabraBiasSpec in the LeabraUnitSpec.
act_eq	Rate-code equivalent activity value (time-averaged spikes when using discrete spiking activation, or just a copy of act when already using rate code activation).
act_avg	Average activation over long time intervals, as integrated by time constant in adapt_thr (see UnitSpec). Useful to see which units are dominating, and to adapt their thresholds if that is enabled.
act_m	Minus phase activation value, set after settling in minus phase and used for learning.
act_p	Plus phase activation value, set after settling in plus phase and used for learning.
act_dif	Difference between plus and minus phase activations — equivalent to the error contribution for unit (δ_j).
da	Delta activation: change in activation from one cycle to the next, used for determining when to stop settling.
vcb	Voltage-gated channel basis variables that integrate activation over time to determine if channels should be open or closed (channels are not active by default):
.hyst	Hysteresis channel (excitatory) basis variable — typically hysteresis is triggered after unit achieves brief sustained level of excitation as reflected in this basis variable.
.acc	Accommodation channel (inhibitory) basis variable — typically accommodation (fatigue) is triggered after unit is active for a relatively long time period as reflected in this more slowly-integrating basis variable.
gc	Channel conductances for the different input channel types except excitatory input (which is in net).
.l	Leak channel conductance (a constant, not visible in NetView).
.i	Inhibition channel conductance, computed by kWTA or direct unit inhibition.
.h	Hysteresis (voltage-gated excitation) channel conductance.
.a	Accommodation (voltage-gated inhibition) channel conductance.
I_net	Net current produced by all channels: what drives the changes in membrane potential.
v_m	The membrane potential, integrates over time weighted-average inputs across different channels, provides basis for activation output via thresholded, saturating nonlinear function.

Variable	Description
thr	Threshold for firing as used in computing activation from v_m, as a state variable so that it can be adapted as a function of activation over time (not done by default, done if `adapt_thr.t_dt > 0` in UnitSpec — if adapting, treated like a weight and only initialized with weights).

LeabraUnitSpec unit-level specifications:

Variable	Default	Description
act_range	0, 1	Range of activation for units: Leabra units are bounded between 0 (min) and 1 (max).
bias_con_type		Type of bias connection to make: almost always LeabraCon.
bias_spec		The LeabraBiasSpec that controls the bias connection on the unit.
act_fun		The activation function to use: NOISY_XX1 (default), XX1 (not convolved with noise), LINEAR (act is linear function of v_m above threshold (0 below threshold)), SPIKE (discrete spiking).
act		Specifications for the activation function:
.thr	.25	The threshold value Θ in equation 2.19: $y_j = \frac{\gamma[V_m - \Theta]_+}{\gamma[V_m - \Theta]_+ + 1}$. Note that the units have their own adjustable thr parameter used if `adapt_thr.t_dt > 0`.
.gain	600	Gain of the activation function (γ in equation 2.19: $y_j = \frac{\gamma[V_m - \Theta]_+}{\gamma[V_m - \Theta]_+ + 1}$).
.nvar	.005	Variance of the Gaussian noise kernel for convolving with XX1 function in NOISY_XX1.
spike		Specifications for the discrete spiking activation function (SPIKE):
.dur	3	Spike duration in cycles — models extended duration of effect on postsynaptic neuron via opened channels, etc.
.v_m_r	0	Post-spiking membrane potential to reset to, produces a refractory effect and controls overall rate of firing (0 std).
.eq_gain	10	Gain for computing act_eq relative to actual time-average spiking rate (γ_{eq} in equation 2.18: $y_j^{eq} = \gamma_{eq} \frac{N_{spikes}}{N_{cycles}}$).
.ext_gain	.4	Gain for clamped external inputs, multiplies the ext value before clamping, needed because constant external inputs otherwise have too much influence compared to spiking ones.
adapt_thr		Adapting threshold specifications (not used by default):
.a_dt	.005	Time constant for integrating activation average act_avg: $y_j^{avg}(t) = y_j^{avg}(t - 1) + a\_dt(y_j(t) - y_j^{avg}(t - 1))$.
.min	.01	Minimum avg act, above which no adaptation occurs.
.max	.35	Maximum avg act, below which no adaptation occurs.
.t_dt	0	Time constant for integrating threshold changes when avg act is outside of min,max bounds. When set to 0, adaptive threshold mechanism is turned off. To use, set to .1.
.mx_d	.04	Maximum amount to change threshold — even if avg act is not restored to min,max bounds by changing threshold, don't keep changing beyond this deviation from orig threshold.

Variable	Default	Description
`opt_thresh`		Optimization thresholds for speeding up computation:
`.send`	.1	Don't send activation when act $<=$ send.
`.learn`	0	Don't learn on recv unit weights when both phase acts $<=$ learn.
`.updt_wts`	true	Whether to apply `learn` threshold to updating weights (otherwise always update).
`.phase_dif`	0	Don't learn when +/- phase difference ratio (- / +) < phase_dif. This is off (0) by default, but can be useful if network is failing to activate output (e.g., in a deep network) on minus phase of some trials — learning in this case is just massive increase in all weights, and tends to produce "hog" units for all the active units. To use, set to .8 as a good initial value.
`clamp_range`	0, .95	Range of clamped (external) activation values (`min`, `max`) — Don't clamp to 1 because NOISY_XX1 activations can't reach that value, so use .95 as max.
`vm_range`	0, 1	Membrane potential range (`min`, `max`), 0-1 for normalized, -90-50 for bio-based.
`v_m_init`		Random distribution for initializing the membrane potential (constant by default):
`.type`		Select type of random distribution to use (e.g., UNIFORM (default), NORMAL (Gaussian)).
`.mean`	.15	Mean of the random distribution, .15 is default resting potential (a.k.a. `v_rest` or V_{rest}).
`.var`	0	Variance of the distribution (range for UNIFORM), no var by default.
`.par`	0	2nd parameter for distributions like BINOMIAL and GAMMA that require it (not typically used).
`dt`		Time constants for integrating values over time:
`.vm`	.2	Membrane potential `v_m` time constant: dt_{vm} in equation 2.8: $V_m(t+1) = V_m(t) + dt_{vm}I_{net-}$.
`.net`	.7	Net input `net` time constant: dt_{net} in equation 2.16: $g_e(t) = (1 - dt_{net})g_e(t-1) + dt_{net}\left(\frac{1}{n_p}\sum_k g_{e_k} + \frac{\beta}{N}\right)$.
`g_bar`		Maximal conductances for channels:
`.e`	1	Excitatory (glutamatergic synaptic sodium (Na) channel).
`.l`	.1	Constant leak (potassium, K+) channel.
`.i`	1	Inhibitory GABA-ergic channel (computed by kWTA or directly).
`.h`	.1	Hysteresis (excitation) voltage-gated channel (Ca++).
`.a`	.5	Accommodation (fatigue, inhibition) voltage-gated channel (K+).
`e_rev`		Reversal potentials for each channel (see above, defaults: 1, .15, .15, 1, 0).
`hyst`		Hysteresis (excitation) voltage-gated channel specs, see accommodation (`acc`) for details, defaults are: false, .05, .8, .7, .1 and true).
`acc`		Accommodation (fatigue, inhibition) voltage-gated channel:
`.on`	false	Activate use of channel if true.
`.b_dt`	.01	Time constant for integrating basis variable, dt_{b_a} in equation 2.41: $b_a(t) = b_a(t-1) + dt_{b_a}(y_j(t) - b_a(t-1))$.
`.a_thr`	.5	Activation threshold for basis variable, when exceeded opens the channel, Θ_a in equation 2.39.
`.d_thr`	.1	Deactivation threshold for basis variable, when less than closes channel (after having been opened), Θ_d in equation 2.39.
`.g_dt`	.1	Time constant for changing conductance when activating or deactivating, dt_{g_a} in equation 2.39.

Variable	Default	Description
`.init`	true	If true, initialize basis variables when state is initialized (else with weights).
`noise_type`		Where to add noise in the processing (if at all): NO_NOISE (default) = no noise, VM_NOISE = add to `v_m` (most commonly used), NETIN_NOISE = add to `net`, ACT_NOISE = add to activation `act`.
`noise`		Distribution parameters for random added noise, default = GAUSSIAN, mean = 0, var = .001.
`noise_sched`		Schedule of noise variance over settling cycles, can be used to make an *annealing* schedule (rarely needed), use same logic as `lrate_sched` described in Leabra-ConSpec.

C.5   Layer-Level Variables

LeabraLayer layer object:

Variable	Description
n_units	Number of units to create with Build command (0=use geometry).
geom	Geometry (size) of units in layer (or of each subgroup if geom.z $>$ 1).
pos	Position of layer within network.
gp_geom	Geometry of subgroups (if geom.z $>$ 1).
projections	Group of receiving projections for this layer.
units	Units or groups of units in the layer.
unit_spec	Default unit specification for units in this layer: only applied during Build or explicit SetUnitSpec command.
lesion	Inactivate this layer from processing (reversible).
ext_flag	Indicates which kind of external input layer received.
netin	Average and maximum net input (net) values for layer (avg, max). These values kept for information purposes only.
acts	Avg and max activation values for the layer — avg is used for sending average activation computation in savg_cor in the ConSpec.
acts_p	Plus-phase activation stats for the layer.
acts_m	Minus-phase activation stats for the layer.
acts_dif	Difference between plus and minus phase vals above.
phase_dif_ratio	Phase-difference ratio (acts_p.avg / acts_m.avg) that can be used with phase_dif in UnitSpec to prevent learning when network is inactive in minus phase but active in plus phase.
kwta	values for kwta – activity levels, etc:
.k	Actual target number of active units for layer.
.pct	Actual target percent activity in layer.
.k_ithr	Inhib threshold for kth most active unit (top k for avg-based).
.k1_ithr	Inhib threshold for k+1th unit (other units for avg-based).
.ithr_r	Log of ratio of ithr values, indicates sharpness of differentiation between active and inactive units.
i_val	Computed inhibition values: kwta = kWTA inhibition, g_i = overall inhibition (usually same as kwta, but not for UNIT_INHIB).
un_g_i	Average and stdev (not max) values for unit inhib.
adapt_pt	Adapting kwta point values (if adapting, not by default).
spec	Determines the spec that controls this layer.
layer_links	List of layers to link inhibition with (not commonly used).
stm_gain	Actual stim gain for soft clamping, can be incremented to ensure clamped units active.
hard_clamped	If true, this layer is actually hard clamped.

LeabraLayerSpec layer-level specifications:

Variable	Default	Description
kwta		How to calculate desired activity level:
.k_from		How is the actual k determined: USE_K = directly by given k, USE_PCT = by pct times number of units in layer (default), USE_PAT_K = by number of units where external input ext > .5 (pat_q).
.k	12	Desired number of active units in the layer (default is meaningless — change as appropriate).
.pct	.25	Desired proportion of activity (used to compute a k value based on layer size).
gp_kwta		Desired activity level for the unit groups (not applicable if no unit subgroups in layer, or if not in inhib_group). See kwta for values.
inhib_group		What to consider the inhibitory group. ENTIRE_LAYER = layer (default), UNIT_GROUPS = unit subgroups within layer each compute kwta separately, LAY_AND_GPS = do both layer and subgroup, inhib is max of each value.
compute_i		How to compute inhibition (g_i): KWTA_INHIB = basic kWTA between k and k+1 (default), KWTA_AVG_INHIB = average based, between avg of k and avg of k+1-n, UNIT_INHIB = units with inhib flag send g_i directly.
i_kwta_pt	.25	Point to place inhibition between k and k+1 for kwta (.25 std), between avg of k and avg of k+1-n for avg-based (.6 std).
adapt_pt		Adapt the i_kwta_pt point based on difference between actual and target pct activity level (for avg-based only, and rarely used).
.a_dt	.005	Time constant for integrating average average activation.
.tol	.05	Tolerance around target avg act before changing i_kwta_pt.
.pt_dt	0	Time constant for integrating i_kwta_pt changes (0 = no adapt, .1 when used).
.mx_d	.2	Maximum deviation from initial i_kwta_pt allowed (.2 std).
clamp		How to clamp external inputs.
.hard	true	Whether to hard clamp external inputs to this layer (directly set activation, resulting in much faster processing), or provide external inputs as extra net input (soft clamping, if false).
.gain	.5	Starting soft clamp gain factor (net = gain * ext).
.d_gain	0	For soft clamp, delta to increase gain when target units not > .5 (0 = off, .1 std when used).
decay		Proportion of decay of activity state vars between various levels of processing:
.event	1	Decay between different events.
.phase	1	Decay between different phases.
.phase2	0	Decay between 2nd set of phases (if applicable).
layer_link		Link inhibition between layers (with specified gain), rarely used. Linked layers are in layer objects.
.link	false	Whether to link the inhibition.
.gain	.5	Strength of the linked inhibition.

C.6   Process-Level Variables

In addition to having parameters in the specification objects listed above, which are associated with state variable objects in the network, the process objects contain some important variables, as described here.

EpochProcess epoch process-level specifications:

Variable	Description
order	Order to present events within the epoch in: SEQUENTIAL, PERMUTED (default), and RANDOM.
wt_update	Determines weight update mode. Leabra always uses either ON_LINE (default) for learning, or TEST for just presenting events but not learning.

LeabraTrialProcess trial process-level specifications:

Variable	Description
phase_order	Number and order of phases to present.
phase_no	Current phase number.
phase	Type of phase, minus or plus.
trial_init	How to initialize network state at start of trial. INIT_STATE (default) initializes activation state, but you must use DECAY_STATE to retain context information across trials for networks with context layers.
no_plus_stats	Don't do stats or logging in the plus phase — true by default.
no_plus_test	Don't run the plus phase when testing — true by default.

LeabraSettleProcess settle process-level specifications:

Variable	Default	Description
min_cycles	60	Minimum number of cycles to settle for — this may need to be set larger for larger networks that take longer to settle. Also, settling is typically cut off sooner by the LeabraMaxDa statistic described below.

LeabraMaxDa Maximum delta-activation statistic, used to cut off settling after network has reached a stable state:

Variable	Default	Description
da_type		Type of activation change measure to use: can either use da (DA_ONLY) or I_Net (INET_ONLY) or both (INET_DA — the default), where I_Net is used while there is no activity in the layer, and after that point da is used.
inet_scale	1	How to scale the inet measure to be like da.
lay_avg_thr	.01	For INET_DA, threshold for layer average activation to switch to da from Inet.
da		The absolute value of activation change (either da or Inet) — use this to set a stopping criterion.

References

Abbott, L., & Sejnowski, T. J. (Eds.). (1999). *Neural codes and distributed representations.* Cambridge, MA: MIT Press.

Abbott, L. F. (1999). Lapicque's introduction of the integrate-and-fire model neuron (1907). *Brain Research Bulletin, 50,* 303.

Abbott, L. F., & LeMasson, G. (1993). Analysis of neuron models with dynamically regulated conductances. *Neural Computation, 5*(6), 823–842.

Abbott, L. F., Varela, J. A., Sen, K., & Nelson, S. B. (1997). Synaptic depression and cortical gain control. *Science, 275,* 220.

Ackley, D. H., Hinton, G. E., & Sejnowski, T. J. (1985). A learning algorithm for Boltzmann machines. *Cognitive Science, 9,* 147–169.

Aggleton, J. P., & Brown, M. W. (1999). Episodic memory, amnesia, and the hippocampal-anterior thalamic axis. *Behavioral and Brain Sciences, 22,* 425–490.

Ahmed, A., & Ruffman, T. (1998). Why do infants make A not B errors in a search task, yet show memory for the location of hidden objects in a non-search task? *Developmental Psychology, 34,* 441–453.

Alexander, G. E., DeLong, M. R., & Strick, P. L. (1986). Parallel organization of functionally segregated circuits linking basal ganglia and cortex. *Annual Review of Neuroscience, 9,* 357–381.

Alexander, M. P. (1997). Aphasia: Clinical and anatomic aspects. In T. E. Feinberg, & M. J. Farah (Eds.), *Behavioral neurology and neuropsychology* (pp. 133–150). New York: McGraw-Hill.

Allport, A. (1989). Visual attention. In M. I. Posner (Ed.), *Foundations of cognitive science* (pp. 631–682). Cambridge, MA: MIT Press.

Allport, D. A. (1985). Distributed memory, modular systems and dysphasia. In S. K. Newman, & R. Epstein (Eds.), *Current perspectives in dysphasia.* Edinburgh: Churchill Livingstone.

Alvarez, P., & Squire, L. R. (1994). Memory consolidation and the medial temporal lobe: A simple network model. *Proceedings of the National Academy of Sciences, USA, 91,* 7041–7045.

Amari, S., & Maginu, K. (1988). Statistical neurodynamics of associative memory. *Neural Networks, 1,* 63–73.

Amit, D. J., Gutfreund, H., & Sompolinsky, H. (1987). Information storage in neural networks with low levels of activity. *Physical Review A, 35,* 2293–2303.

Amitai, Y., Friedman, A., Connors, B., & Gutnick, M. (1993). Regenerative activity in apical dendrites of pyramidal cell in neocortex. *Cerebral Cortex, 3,* 26–38.

Andersen, R. A., Essick, G. K., & Siegel, R. M. (1985). Encoding of spatial location by posterior parietal neurons. *Science, 230,* 456–458.

Anderson, J. A. (1995). *An introduction to neural networks.* Cambridge, MA: MIT Press.

Anderson, J. A., & Rosenfeld, E. (1988). *Neurocomputing: Foundations of research.* Cambridge, MA: MIT Press.

Anderson, J. R. (1983). *The architecture of cognition.* Cambridge, MA: Harvard University Press.

Anderson, J. R. (1990). *The adaptive character of thought.* Hillsdale, NJ: Lawrence Erlbaum Associates.

Arbib, M. A. (Ed.). (1995). *The handbook of brain theory and neural networks.* Cambridge, MA: MIT Press.

Arieli, A., Sterkin, A., & Aertsen, A. (1996). Dynamics of ongoing activity: Explanation of the large variability in evoked cortical responses. *Science, 273,* 1868.

Armony, J. L., Servan-Schreiber, D., Cohen, J. D., & LeDoux, J. E. (1997). Computational modeling of emotion: explorations through the anatomy and physiology of fear conditioning. *Trends in Cognitive Sciences, 1,* 28–34.

Artola, A., Brocher, S., & Singer, W. (1990). Different voltage-dependent thresholds for inducing long-term depression and long-term potentiation in slices of rat visual cortex. *Nature, 347,* 69–72.

Ashby, F. G., Alfonso-Reese, L. A., & Waldron, E. M. (1998).

a neuropsychological theory of multiple systems in category learning. *Psychological Review*, *105*, 442.

Atick, J. J., & Redlich, A. N. (1990). Towards a theory of early visual processing. *Neural Computation*, *2*(3), 308–320.

Awh, E., Jonides, J., Smith, E. E., Schumacher, E. H., Koeppe, R. A., & Katz, S. (1996). Dissociation of storage and rehearsal in verbal working memory: Evidence from positron emission tomography. *Psychological Science*, *7*, 25–31.

Baddeley, A. D. (1986). *Working memory*. New York: Oxford University Press.

Baillargeon, R., DeVos, J., & Graber, M. (1989). Location memory in 8-month-old infants in a non-search AB task: Further evidence. *Cognitive Development*, *4*, 345–367.

Baillargeon, R., & Graber, M. (1988). Evidence of location memory in 8-month-old infants in a non-search AB task. *Developmental Psychology*, *24*, 502–511.

Baker, S. C., Rogers, R. D., Owen, A. M., Frith, C. D., Dolan, R. J., Frackowiak, R. S. J., & Robbins, T. W. (1996). Neural systems engaged by planning: A PET study of the Tower of London task. *Neuropsychologia*, *34*, 515.

Ballard, D. H. (1997). *An introduction to natural computation*. Cambridge, MA: MIT Press.

Banich, M. T. (1997). *Neuropsychology: The neural bases of mental function*. Boston: Houghton Mifflin.

Barch, D. M., Braver, T. S., Nystrom, L. E., Forman, S. D., Noll, D. C., & Cohen, J. D. (1997). Dissociating working memory from task difficulty in human prefrontal cortex. *Neuropsychologia*, *35*, 1373.

Barlow, H. B. (1989). Unsupervised learning. *Neural Computation*, *1*, 295–311.

Barnes, C. A., McNaughton, B. L., Mizumori, S. J. Y., Leonard, B. W., & Lin, L.-H. (1990). Comparison of spatial and temporal characteristics of neuronal activity in sequential stages of hippocampal processing. *Progress in Brain Research*, *83*, 287–300.

Barnes, J. M., & Underwood, B. J. (1959). Fate of first-list associations in transfer theory. *Journal of Experimental Psychology*, *58*, 97–105.

Barone, P., & Joseph, J. P. (1989). Prefrontal cortex and spatial sequencing in macaque monkey. *Experimental Brain Research*, *78*, 447–464.

Bartlett, F. C. (1932). *Remembering: A study in experimental and social psychology*. Cambridge: Cambridge University Press.

Bashir, Z., Bortolotto, Z. A., & Davies, C. H. (1993). Induction of LTP in the hippocampus needs synaptic activation

of glutamate metabotropic receptors. *Nature*, *363*, 347–350.

Bear, M. F. (1996). A synaptic basis for memory storage in the cerebral cortex. *Proceedings of the National Academy of Sciences*, *93*, 3453.

Bear, M. F., Conners, B. W., & Paradiso, M. A. (1996). *Neuroscience: Exploring the brain*. Baltimore: Williams & Wilkins.

Bear, M. F., & Malenka, R. C. (1994). Synaptic plasticity: LTP and LTD. *Current Opinion in Neurobiology*, *4*, 389–399.

Bechara, A., Tranel, D., Damasio, H., & Damasio, A. R. (1996). Failure to respond autonomically to anticipated future outcomes following damage to prefrontal cortex. *Cerebral Cortex*, *6*, 215–225.

Becker, S. (1996). Mutual information maximization: Models of cortical self-organization. *Network : Computation in Neural Systems*, *7*, 7–31.

Becker, S., Moscovitch, M., Behrmann, M., & Joordens, S. (1997). Long-term semantic priming: A computational account and empirical evidence. *Journal of Experimental Psychology: Learning, Memory, and Cognition*, *23*, 1059–1082.

Behrmann, M., & Tipper, S. P. (1994). Object-based attentional mechanisms: Evidence from patients with unilateral neglect. In C. Umilta, & M. Moscovitch (Eds.), *Attention and performance XV: Conscious and nonconscious information processing* (pp. 351–375). Cambridge, MA: MIT Press.

Beiser, D. G., Hua, S. E., & Houk, J. C. (1997). Network models of the basal ganglia. *Current Opinion in Neurobiology*, *7*, 185.

Bell, A. J., & Sejnowski, T. J. (1995). An information maximization approach to blind separation and blind deconvolution. *Neural Computation*, *7*, 1129–1159.

Berndt, R. S. (1998). Sentence processing in aphasia, 3rd ed. In M. T. Sarno (Ed.), *Acquired aphasia* (pp. 229–267). San Diego, CA: Academic Press.

Berndt, R. S., & Caramazza, A. (1980). A redefinition of the syndrome of Broca's aphasia: Implications for a neuropsychological model of language. *Applied Psycholinguistics*, *1*, 225–278.

Bianchi, L. (1922). *The mechanism of the brain and the function of the frontal lobes*. Edinburgh: Livingstone.

Biederman, I. (1987). Recognition-by-components: A theory of human image understanding. *Psychological Review*, *94*(2), 115–147.

Biederman, I., & Cooper, E. E. (1991). Priming contour-deleted images: Evidence for intermediate representations in visual object recognition. *Cognitive Psychology*, *23*, 393–419.

Biederman, I., & Cooper, E. E. (1992). Size invariance in visual object priming. *Journal of Experimental Psychology: Human Perception and Performance*, *18*, 121–133.

Biederman, I., & Gerhardstein, P. C. (1995). Viewpoint-dependent mechanisms in visual object recognition: Reply to Tarr and Bülthoff (1995). *Journal of Experimental Psychology: Human Perception and Performance*, *21*, 1506–1514.

Bienenstock, E. L., Cooper, L. N., & Munro, P. W. (1982). Theory for the development of neuron selectivity: Orientation specificity and binocular interaction in visual cortex. *Journal of Neuroscience*, *2*(2), 32–48.

Bishop, C. M. (1995). *Neural networks for pattern recognition.* Oxford: Oxford University Press.

Blasdel, G. G., & Salama, G. (1986). Voltage-sensitive dyes reveal a modular organization in monkey striate cortex. *Nature*, *321*, 579–585.

Bliss, T. V. P., & Lomo, T. (1973). Long-lasting potentiation of synaptic transmission in the dentate area of the anaesthetized rabbit following stimulation of the perforant path. *Journal of Physiology (London)*, *232*, 331–356.

Bolton, J. S. (1910). A contribution to the localization of cerebral function, based on the clinicopathological study of mental disease. *Brain*, *26-147*, 33.

Boss, B. D., Peterson, G. M., & Cowan, W. M. (1985). On the numbers of neurons in the dentate gyrus of the rat. *Brain Research*, *338*, 144–150.

Boss, B. D., Turlejski, K., Stanfield, B. B., & Cowan, W. M. (1987). On the numbers of neurons in fields CA1 and CA3 of the hippocampus of Sprague-Dawley and Wistar rats. *Brain Research*, *406*, 280–287.

Bower, J. M. (1992). Modeling the nervous system. *Trends in Neurosciences*, *15*, 411–412.

Bower, J. M., & Beeman, D. (1994). *The book of GENESIS: Exploring realistic neural models with the GEneral NEural SImulation System.* New York: TELOS/Springer Verlag.

Braun, A. R., Balkin, T. J., & Herscovitch, P. (1998). Dissociated pattern of activity in visual cortices and their projections during human rapid eye movement sleep. *Science*, *279*, 91.

Braver, T. S., & Cohen, J. D. (2000). On the control of control: The role of dopamine in regulating prefrontal function and working memory. In S. Monsell, & J. Driver (Eds.), *Attention and performance XVII*. Cambridge, MA: MIT Press.

Braver, T. S., Cohen, J. D., Nystrom, L. E., Jonides, J., Smith, E. E., & Noll, D. C. (1997). A parametric study of frontal cortex involvement in human working memory. *NeuroImage*, *5*, 49–62.

Braver, T. S., Cohen, J. D., & Servan-Schreiber, D. (1995). A computational model of prefrontal cortex function. In D. S. Touretzky, G. Tesauro, & T. K. Leen (Eds.), *Advances in neural information processing systems* (pp. 141–148). Cambridge, MA: MIT Press.

Brown, L. L., Schneider, J. S., & Lidsky, T. I. (1997). Sensory and cognitive functions of the basal ganglia. *Current Opinion in Neurobiology*, *7*, 157.

Brown, R. G., & Marsden, C. D. (1990). Cognitive function in parkinson's disease: From description to theory. *Trends in Neurosciences*, *13*, 21–29.

Brown, T. H., Kairiss, E. W., & Keenan, C. L. (1990). Hebbian synapses: Biophysical mechanisms and algorithms. *Annual Review of Neuroscience*, 475–511.

Bryson, A. E., & Ho, Y. C. (1969). *Applied optimal control.* New York: Blaisdell.

Burgess, N. (1995). A solvable connectionist model of immediate recall of ordered lists. In D. S. Touretzky, G. Tesauro, & T. K. Leen (Eds.), *Advances in neural information processing systems* (pp. 51–58). Cambridge, MA: MIT Press.

Burgess, N., Recce, M., & O'Keefe, J. (1994). A model of hippocampal function. *Neural networks*, *7*, 1065–1083.

Burgund, E. D., & Marsolek, C. J. (in press). Viewpoint-invariant and viewpoint-dependent object recognition in dissociable neural subsystems. *Psychonomic Bulletin and Review*.

Butler, R. W., Rorsman, I., Hill, J. M., & Tuma, R. (1993). The effects of frontal brain impairment on fluency: Simple and complex paradigms. *Neuropsychology*, *7*, 519–529.

Camperi, M., & Wang, X. J. (1997). Modeling delay-period activity in the prefrontal cortex during working memory tasks. In J. Bower (Ed.), *Computational neuroscience* (Chap. 44, pp. 273–279). New York: Plenum Press.

Carpenter, G., & Grossberg, S. (1987). A massively parallel architecture for a self-organizing neural pattern recognition machine. *Computer Vision, Graphics, and Image Processing*, *37*, 54–115.

Carter, C. S., Braver, T. S., & Cohen, J. D. (1998). Anterior cingulate cortex, error detection, and the online monitoring of performance. *Science*, *280*, 747.

Cauller, L., & Connors, B. (1994). Synaptic physiology of horizontal afferents to layer I in slices of rat SI neocortex. *Journal of Neuroscience*, *14*, 751–762.

Chauvin, Y., & Rumelhart, D. E. (1995). *Backpropagation: Theory, architectures, and applications.* Hillsdale, NJ: Erlbaum.

Cheng, P., & Holyoak, K. J. (1985). Pragmatic reasoning schemas. *Cognitive Psychology, 17*, 391–416.

Chiodo, L., & Berger, T. (1986). Interactions between dopamine and amino-acid induced excitation and inhibition in the striatum. *Brain Research, 375*, 198–203.

Chomsky, N. (1965). *Aspects of the theory of syntax.* Cambridge, MA: MIT Press.

Churchland, P. S. (1986). *Neurophilosophy: Toward a unified science of the mind-brain.* Cambridge, MA: MIT Press.

Cleeremans, A., & McClelland, J. L. (1991). Learning the structure of event sequences. *Journal of Experimental Psychology: General, 120*, 235–253.

Cleeremans, A., Servan-Schreiber, D., & McClelland, J. L. (1989). Finite state automata and simple recurrent networks. *Neural Computation, 1*, 372–381.

Cohen, J. D., Braver, T. S., & O'Reilly, R. C. (1996). A computational approach to prefrontal cortex, cognitive control, and schizophrenia: Recent developments and current challenges. *Philosophical Transactions of the Royal Society (London) B, 351*, 1515–1527.

Cohen, J. D., Dunbar, K., & McClelland, J. L. (1990). On the control of automatic processes: A parallel distributed processing model of the Stroop effect. *Psychological Review, 97*(3), 332–361.

Cohen, J. D., & Huston, T. A. (1994). Progress in the use of interactive models for understanding attention and performance. In C. Umilta, & M. Moscovitch (Eds.), *Attention and performance XV* (pp. 1–19). Cambridge, MA: MIT Press.

Cohen, J. D., & O'Reilly, R. C. (1996). A preliminary theory of the interactions between prefrontal cortex and hippocampus that contribute to planning and prospective memory. In M. Brandimonte, G. O. Einstein, & M. A. McDaniel (Eds.), *Prospective memory: Theory and applications.* Mahwah, New Jersey: Lawrence Earlbaum Associates.

Cohen, J. D., Perlstein, W. M., Braver, T. S., Nystrom, L. E., Noll, D. C., Jonides, J., & Smith, E. E. (1997). Temporal dynamics of brain activity during a working memory task. *Nature, 386*, 604–608.

Cohen, J. D., Romero, R. D., Farah, M. J., & Servan-Schreiber, D. (1994). Mechanisms of spatial attention: The relation of macrostructure to microstructure in parietal neglect. *Journal of Cognitive Neuroscience, 6*, 377.

Cohen, J. D., & Servan-Schreiber, D. (1992). Context, cortex, and dopamine: A connectionist approach to behavior and biology in schizophrenia. *Psychological Review, 99*, 45–77.

Cohen, J. D., Usher, M., & McClelland, J. L. (1998). A PDP approach to set size effects within the Stroop task: Reply to Kanne, Balota, Spieler, and Faust (1998). *Psychological Review, 105*, 188.

Cohen, N. J., & Eichenbaum, H. (1993). *Memory, amnesia, and the hippocampal system.* Cambridge, MA: MIT Press.

Colby, C. L., Duhamel, J. R., & Goldberg, M. E. (1996). Visual, presaccadic, and cognitive activation of single neurons in monkey lateral intraparietal area. *Journal of Neurophysiology, 76*, 2841.

Collingridge, G. L., & Bliss, T. V. P. (1987). NMDA receptors - their role in long-term potentiation. *Trends in Neurosciences, 10*, 288–293.

Coltheart, M., Curtis, B., Atkins, P., & Haller, M. (1993). Models of reading aloud: Dual route and parallel-distributed-processing approaches. *Psychological Review, 100*, 589–608.

Coltheart, M., Patterson, K., & Marshall, J. C. (Eds.). (1980). *Deep dyslexia, 2nd ed.* London: Routledge & Kegan Paul.

Coltheart, M., & Rastle, K. (1994). Serial processing in reading aloud: Evidence for dual-route models of reading. *Journal of Experimental Psychology: Human Perception and Performance, 20*, 1197–11211.

Contreras-Vidal, J. L., Grossberg, S., & Bullock, D. (1997). A neural model of cerebellar learning for arm movement control: Cortico-spino-cerebellar dynamics. *Learning and Memory, 3*, 475–502.

Coslett, H. B., & Saffran, E. (1991). Simultanagnosia. To see but not two see. *Brain, 114*, 1523–1545.

Crick, F. (1984). Function of the thalamic reticular complex: The searchlight hypothesis. *Proceedings of the National Academy of Sciences, 81*, 4586–90.

Crick, F. H. C. (1989). The recent excitement about neural networks. *Nature, 337*, 129–132.

Crick, F. H. C., & Asanuma, C. (1986). Certain aspects of the anatomy and physiology of the cerebral cortex. In J. L. McClelland, & D. E. Rumelhart (Eds.), *Parallel distributed processing: Explorations in the microstructure of cognition*, Vol. 2 (Chap. 20, pp. 333–371). Cambridge, MA: MIT Press.

Damasio, H., Grabowski, T. J., & Damasio, A. R. (1996). A neural basis for lexical retrieval. *Nature, 380*, 499.

Daneman, M., & Carpenter, P. A. (1980). Individual differences in working memory and reading. *Journal of Verbal Learning and Verbal Behavior, 19*, 450–466.

Das, A., & Gilbert, C. D. (1995). Receptive field expansion in adult visual cortex is linked to dynamic changes in strength of cortical connections. *Journal of Neurophysiology, 74*, 779.

Daugherty, K., & Seidenberg, M. S. (1992). Rules or connections? The past tense revisited. *Proceedings of the 14th Annual Conference of the Cognitive Science Society* (pp. 259–264). Hillsdale, NJ: Lawrence Erlbaum Associates.

Dayan, P. (1992). The convergenece of TD(λ) for general λ. *Machine Learning, 8*, 341.

Dayan, P., Hinton, G. E., Neal, R. N., & Zemel, R. S. (1995). The Helmholtz machine. *Neural Computation, 7*, 889–904.

Dayan, P., & Zemel, R. S. (1995). Competition and multiple cause models. *Neural Computation, 7*, 565–579.

de Sa, V. R., & Ballard, D. H. (1998). Category learning through multimodality sensing. *Neural Computation, 10*, 1097–1118.

Dehaene, S., & Changeux, J. P. (1989). A simple model of prefrontal cortex function in delayed-response tasks. *Journal of Cognitive Neuroscience, 1*, 244–261.

Dehaene, S., & Changeux, J. P. (1991). The Wisconsin Card Sorting Test: Theoretical analysis and modeling in a neuronal network. *Cerebral Cortex, 1*, 62–79.

Dell, G. S., Burger, L. K., & Svec, W. R. (1997). Language production and serial order: A functional analysis and a model. *Psychological Review, 104*(1), 123–147.

Desai, N. S., Rutherford, L. C., & Turrigiano, G. G. (1999). Plasticity in the intrinsic excitability of cortical pyramidal neurons. *Nature Neuroscience, 2*, 515–520.

Desimone, R., & Duncan, J. (1995). Neural mechanisms of selective visual attention. *Annual Review of Neuroscience, 18*, 193.

Desimone, R., & Ungerleider, L. G. (1989). Neural mechanisms of visual processing in monkeys. In F. Boller, & J. Grafman (Eds.), *Handbook of neurophysiology, vol. 2* (Chap. 14, pp. 267–299). Amsterdam: Elsevier.

Diamond, A. (1990). The development and neural bases of memory functions as indexed by the A-not-B task: Evidence for dependence on dorsolateral prefrontal cortex. In A. Diamond (Ed.), *The development and neural bases of higher cognitive functions* (pp. 267–317). New York: New York Academy of Science Press.

Diamond, A., & Goldman-Rakic, P. S. (1986). Comparative development in human infants and infant rhesus monkeys of cognitive functions that depend on prefrontal cortex. *Society for Neuroscience Abstracts, 12*, 742.

Diamond, A., & Goldman-Rakic, P. S. (1989). Comparison of human infants and rhesus monkeys on Piaget's A$\overline{B}$ task: Evidence for dependence on dorsolateral prefrontal cortex. *Experimental Brain Research, 74*, 24–40.

Dias, R., Robbins, T. W., & Roberts, A. C. (1997). Dissociable forms of inhibitory control within prefrontal cortex with an analog of the Wisconsin Card Sort Test: Restriction to novel situations and independence from "on-line" processing. *Journal of Neuroscience, 17*, 9285–9297.

Dilmore, J. G., Gutkin, B. G., & Ermentrout, G. B. (1999). Effects of dopaminergic modulation of persistent sodium currents on the excitability of prefrontal cortical neurons: A computational study. *Neurocomputing, 26*, 104–116.

Douglas, R. J., & Martin, K. A. C. (1990). Neocortex. In G. M. Shepherd (Ed.), *The synaptic organization of the brain* (Chap. 12, pp. 389–438). Oxford: Oxford University Press.

Doyon, J., Gaudreau, D., & Bouchard, J. P. (1997). Roles of the striatum, cerebellum, and frontal lobes in the learning of a visumotor sequence. *Brain and Cognition, 34*, 218.

Duda, R. O., & Hart, P. E. (1973). *Pattern classification and scene analysis.* New York: John Wiley.

Dunbar, K., & MacLeod, C. M. (1984). A horse race of a different color: Stroop interference patterns with transformed words. *Journal of Experimental Psychology: Human Perception and Performance, 10*, 622–639.

Duncan, J. (1984). Selective attention and the organization of visual information. *Journal of Experimental Psychology: General, 113*, 501–517.

Duncan, J., & Humphreys, G. W. (1989). Visual search and stimulus similarity. *Psychological Review, 96*(3).

Edelman, G. (1987). *Neural Darwinism.* New York: Basic Books.

Elman, J. L. (1990). Finding structure in time. *Cognitive Science, 14*, 179–211.

Elman, J. L. (1991). Distributed representations, simple recurrent networks, and grammatical structure. *Machine Learning, 7*, 195–225.

Elman, J. L. (1993). Learning and development in neural networks: The importance of starting small. *Cognition, 48*(1), 71–99.

Elman, J. L., Bates, E. A., Johnson, M. H., Karmiloff-Smith, A., Parisi, D., & Plunkett, K. (1996). *Rethinking innate-*

ness: A connectionist perspective on development. Cambridge, MA: MIT Press.

Engel, A. K., Konig, P., Kreiter, A. K., Schillen, T. B., & Singer, W. (1992). Temporal coding in the visual cortex: New vistas on integration in the nervous system. *Trends in Neurosciences, 15*(6), 218–226.

Ermentrout, G. B. (1994). Reduction of conductance-based models with slow synapses to neural nets. *Neural Computation, 6,* 679–695.

Erwin, E., Obermayer, K., & Schulten, K. (1995). Models of orientation and ocular dominance columns in the visual cortex: A critical comparison. *Neural Computation, 7,* 425–468.

Farah, M. J. (1990). *Visual agnosia.* Cambridge, MA: MIT Press.

Farah, M. J. (1992). Is an object an object an object? *Current Directions in Psychological Science, 1,* 164–169.

Farah, M. J. (1994). Neuropsychological inference with an interactive brain: A critique of the "locality" assumption. *Behavioral and Brain Sciences, 17,* 43–104.

Farah, M. J. (1999). *The cognitive neuroscience of vision.* Oxford: Blackwell.

Farah, M. J., & McClelland, J. L. (1991). A computational model of semantic memory impairment: Modality-specificity and emergent category-specificity. *Journal of Experimental Psychology: General, 120*(4), 339–357.

Farah, M. J., O'Reilly, R. C., & Vecera, S. P. (1993). Dissociated overt and covert recognition as an emergent property of a lesioned neural network. *Psychological Review, 100,* 571–588.

Felleman, D. J., & Van Essen, D. C. (1991). Distributed hierarchical processing in the primate cerebral cortex. *Cerebral Cortex, 1,* 1–47.

Fellous, J. M., Wang, X. J., & Lisman, J. E. (1998). A role for NMDA-receptor channels in working memory. *Nature Neuroscience, 1,* 273–275.

Field, D. J. (1994). What is the goal of sensory coding? *Neural Computation, 6*(4), 559–601.

Fiez, J. A., Raife, E. A., Balota, D. A., Schwarz, J. P., Raichle, M. E., & Petersen, S. E. (1986). A positron emission tomography study of the short-term maintenance of verbal information. *Journal of Neuroscience, 16,* 808–822.

Fodor, J. (1983). *The modularity of mind.* Cambridge, MA: MIT/Bradford Press.

Francis, W. N., & Kučera, H. (1982). *Frequency analysis of English usage.* Boston: Houghton Mifflin.

French, R. M. (1992). Semi-distributed representations and catastrophic forgetting in connectionist networks. *Connection Science, 4,* 365–377.

Friedman, R. B. (1996). Recovery from deep alexia to phonological alexia. *Brain and Language, 52,* 114–128.

Fromkin, V., & Rodman, R. (1993). *An introduction to language, 5th ed.* Fort Worth, TX: Harcourt Brace College Publishers.

Fukushima, K. (1988). Neocognitron: A hierarchical neural network capable of visual pattern recognition. *Neural Networks, 1,* 119–130.

Fuster, J. M. (1989). *The prefrontal cortex: Anatomy, physiology and neuropsychology of the frontal lobe.* New York: Raven Press.

Fuster, J. M., & Alexander, G. E. (1971). Neuron activity related to short-term memory. *Science, 173,* 652–654.

Galland, C. C. (1993). The limitations of deterministic Boltzmann machine learning. *Network: Computation in Neural Systems, 4,* 355–379.

Galland, C. C., & Hinton, G. E. (1990). Discovering high order features with mean field modules. In D. S. Touretzky (Ed.), *Advances in Neural Information Processing Systems, 2.* San Mateo, CA: Morgan Kaufmann.

Galland, C. C., & Hinton, G. E. (1991). Deterministic Boltzmann learning in networks with asymmetric connectivity. In D. S. Touretzky, J. L. Elman, T. J. Sejnowski, & G. E. Hinton (Eds.), *Connectionist Models: Proceedings of the 1990 Summer School* (pp. 3–9). San Mateo, CA: Morgan Kaufmann.

Gao, J. H., Parsons, L. M., & Fox, P. T. (1996). Cerebellum implicated in sensory acquisition and discrimination rather than motor control. *Science, 272,* 545.

Gathercole, S. E. (1994). Neuropsychology and working memory: A review. *Neuropsychology, 8*(4), 494–505.

Gazzaniga, M. S., Ivry, R. B., & Mangun, G. R. (1998). *Cognitive neuroscience: The biology of the mind.* New York: W. W. Norton.

Gehring, W. J., Goss, B., Coles, M. G. H., Meyer, D. E., & Donchin, E. (1993). A neural system for error detection and compensation. *Psychological Science, 4*(6), 385–390.

Geman, S., Bienenstock, E. L., & Doursat, R. (1992). Neural networks and the bias/variance dilemma. *Neural Computation, 4,* 1–58.

Gerfen, C. R. (1985). The neostriatal mosaic. I. Compartmental organization of projections of the striatonigral system in the rat. *Journal of Comparative Neurology, 236,* 454–476.

Gershberg, F. B., & Shimamura, A. P. (1995). Impaired use of organizational strategies in free recall following frontal lobe damage. *Neuropsychologia, 33*, 1305–1333.

Gillund, G., & Shiffrin, R. M. (1984). A retrieval model for both recognition and recall. *Psychological Review, 91*, 1–67.

Glaser, M. O., & Glaser, W. R. (1982). Time course analysis of the Stroop phenomenon. *Journal of Experimental Psychology: Human Perception and Performance, 8*, 875–894.

Gluck, M. A., & Myers, C. E. (1993). Hippocampal mediation of stimulus representation: A computational theory. *Hippocampus, 3*, 491–516.

Glushko, R. J. (1979). The organization and activation of orthographic knowledge in reading aloud. *Journal of Experimental Psychology: Human Perception and Performance, 5*, 674–691.

Goldman-Rakic, P. S. (1987). Circuitry of primate prefrontal cortex and regulation of behavior by representational memory. *Handbook of Physiology — The Nervous System, 5*, 373–417.

Goodale, M. A., & Milner, A. D. (1992). Separate visual pathways for perception and action. *Trends in Neurosciences, 15*(1), 20–25.

Graf, P., Squire, L. R., & Mandler, G. (1984). The information that amnesic patients do not forget. *Journal of Experimental Psychology: Learning, Memory, and Cognition, 10*, 164–178.

Grafman, J. (1989). Plans, actions, and mental sets: Managerial knowledge units in the frontal lobes. In E. Perecman (Ed.), *Integrating theory and practice in clinical neuropsychology* (pp. 93–138). Hillsdale, NJ: Erlbaum.

Gray, C. M., Engel, A. K., Konig, P., & Singer, W. (1992). Synchronization of oscillatory neuronal responses in cat striate cortex — temporal properties. *Visual Neuroscience, 8*, 337–347.

Graybiel, A. M., Ragsdale, C. W., & Mood Edley, S. (1979). Compartments in the striatum of the cat observed by retrograde cell labeling. *Experimental Brain Research, 34*, 189–195.

Grossberg, S. (1976). Adaptive pattern classification and universal recoding I: Parallel development and coding of neural feature detectors. *Biological Cybernetics, 23*, 121–134.

Grossberg, S. (1978). A theory of visual coding, memory, and development. In E. L. J. Leeuwenberg, & H. F. J. M. Buffart (Eds.), *Formal theories of visual perception* (Chap. 1, pp. 7–26). New York: Wiley.

Guitton, D., Buchtel, H. A., & Douglas, R. M. (1985). Frontal lobe lesions in man cause difficulties in suppressing reflexive glances and in generating goal-directed saccades. *Experimental Brain Research, 58*, 455–472.

Hare, M., & Elman, J. L. (1992). A connectionist account of English inflectional morphology: Evidence from language change. *Proceedings of the 14th Annual Conference of the Cognitive Science Society* (pp. 265–270). Hillsdale, NJ: Lawrence Erlbaum Associates.

Hasselmo, M. E., & Wyble, B. (1997). Free recall and recognition in a network model of the hippocampus: Simulating effects of scopolamine on human memory function. *Behavioural Brain Research, 67*, 1–27.

Hebb, D. O. (1949). *The organization of behavior*. New York: Wiley.

Hertz, J., Krogh, A., & Palmer, R. G. (1991). *Introduction to the theory of neural computation*. Redwood City, CA: Addison-Wesley.

Hillis, A. E., & Caramazza, A. (1991). Category-specific naming and comprehension impairment: A double dissociation. *Brain, 114*, 2081–2094.

Hillyard, S. A., & Picton, T. W. (1987). Electrophysiology of cognition. In F. Plum (Ed.), *Handbook of physiology, section I: Neurophysiology, volume V: Higher functions of the brain* (pp. 519–584). American Physiological Society.

Hines, M. L., & Carnevale, N. T. (1997). The NEURON simulation environment. *Neural Computation, 9*, 1179–1209.

Hinton, G. E. (1981). A parallel computation that assigns canonical object-based frames of reference. *Proceedings of the 7th IJCAI* (pp. 683–685). Vancouver.

Hinton, G. E. (1986). Learning distributed representations of concepts. *Proceedings of the 8th Conference of the Cognitive Science Society* (pp. 1–12). Hillsdale, NJ: Lawrence Erlbaum Associates.

Hinton, G. E. (1989a). Connectionist learning procedures. *Artificial Intelligence, 40*, 185–234.

Hinton, G. E. (1989b). Deterministic Boltzmann learning performs steepest descent in weight-space. *Neural Computation, 1*, 143–150.

Hinton, G. E., & Ghahramani, Z. (1997). Generative models for discovering sparse distributed representations. *Philosophical Transactions of the Royal Society (London) B, 352*, 1177–1190.

Hinton, G. E., & McClelland, J. L. (1988). Learning representations by recirculation. In D. Z. Anderson (Ed.), *Neural Information Processing Systems, 1987* (pp. 358–366). New York: American Institute of Physics.

Hinton, G. E., McClelland, J. L., & Rumelhart, D. E. (1986). Distributed representations. In D. E. Rumelhart, J. L. McClelland, & PDP Research Group (Eds.), *Parallel distributed processing. Volume 1: Foundations* (Chap. 3, pp. 77–109). Cambridge, MA: MIT Press.

Hinton, G. E., & Sejnowski, T. J. (1983). Optimal perceptual inference. *Proceedings of the IEEE Conference on Computer Vision and Pattern Recognition*. Washington, DC.

Hinton, G. E., & Sejnowski, T. J. (Eds.). (1999). *Unsupervised learning*. Cambridge, MA: MIT Press.

Hinton, G. E., & Shallice, T. (1991). Lesioning an attractor network: Investigations of acquired dyslexia. *Psychological Review*, 98(1), 74–95.

Hintzman, D. L. (1988). Judgments of frequency and recognition memory in a multiple-trace memory model. *Psychological Review*, 95, 528–551.

Hochreiter, S., & Schmidhuber, J. (1995). *Long short term memory* (Technical Report FKI-207-95). Technische Universität München.

Hochreiter, S., & Schmidhuber, J. (1997). Long short term memory. *Neural Computation*, 9, 1735–1780.

Hodges, J. R., Patterson, K., & Tyler, L. K. (1994). Loss of semantic memory: Implications for the modularity of mind. *Cognitive Neuropsychology*, 11, 505.

Hodgkin, A. L., & Huxley, A. F. (1952). A quantitative description of membrane current and its application to conduction and excitation in nerve. *Journal of Neurophysiology (London)*, 117, 500–544.

Hoeffner, J. H. (1992). Are rules a thing of the past? The acquisition of verbal morphology by an attractor network. *Proceedings of the 14th Annual Conference of the Cognitive Science Society* (pp. 861–866). Hillsdale, NJ: Lawrence Erlbaum Associates.

Hoeffner, J. H. (1997). *Are rules a thing of the past? A single mechanism account of English past tense acquistion and processing*. PhD thesis, Department of Psychology, Carnegie Mellon University, Pittsburgh, PA.

Hofstadter, M. C., & Reznick, J. S. (1996). Response modality affects human infant delayed-response performance. *Child Development*, 67, 646–658.

Hopfield, J. J. (1982). Neural networks and physical systems with emergent collective computational abilities. *Proceedings of the National Academy of Sciences*, 79, 2554–2558.

Hopfield, J. J. (1984). Neurons with graded response have collective computational properties like those of two-state neurons. *Proceedings of the National Academy of Sciences*, 81, 3088–3092.

Hubel, D., & Wiesel, T. N. (1962). Receptive fields, binocular interaction, and functional architecture in the cat's visual cortex. *Journal of Physiology*, 160, 106–154.

Hummel, J. E., & Biederman, I. (1992). Dynamic binding in a neural network for shape recognition. *Psychological Review*, 99(3), 480–517.

Hummel, J. E., & Holyoak, K. J. (1997). Distributed representations of structure: A theory of analogical access and mapping. *Psychological Review*, 104(3), 427–466.

Husain, M., & Stein, J. (1988). Rezso Bálint and his most celebrated case. *Archives of Neurology*, 45, 89–93.

Ikeda, J., Mori, K., Oka, S., & Watanabe, Y. (1989). A columnar arrangement of dendritic processes of entorhinal cortex neurons revealed by a monoclonal antibody. *Brain Research*, 505, 176–179.

Jacobs, R. A., Jordan, M. I., Nowlan, S. J., & Hinton, G. E. (1991). Adaptive mixtures of local experts. *Neural Computation*, 3, 79–87.

Jacoby, L. L., & Witherspoon, D. (1982). Remembering without awareness. *Canadian Journal of Psychology*, 32, 300–324.

Jacoby, L. L., Yonelinas, A. P., & Jennings, J. M. (1997). The relation between conscious and unconscious (automatic) influences: A declaration of independence. In J. D. Cohen, & J. W. Schooler (Eds.), *Scientific approaches to consciousness* (pp. 13–47). Mahway, NJ: Lawrence Erlbaum Associates.

Jaffe, D. B., & Carnevale, N. T. (1999). Passive normalization of synaptic integration influenced by dendritic architecture. *Journal of Neurophysiology*, 82, 3268–3285.

Joanisse, M. F., & Seidenberg, M. S. (1999). Impairments in verb morphology after brain injury: A connectionist model. *Proceedings of the National Academy of Sciences*, 96, 7592.

Johnson-Laird, P., Legrenzi, P., & Legrenzi, M. S. (1972). Reasoning and a sense of reality. *British Journal of Psychology*, 63, 395–400.

Johnston, D., & Wu, S. M. (1995). *Foundations of cellular neurophysiology*. Cambridge, MA: MIT Press.

Joordens, S., & Becker, S. (1997). The long and short of semantic priming effects in lexical decision. *Journal of Experimental Psychology: Learning, Memory, and Cognition*, 23, 1083.

Jordan, M. I. (1986). Attractor dynamics and parallelism in a connectionist sequential machine. *Proceedings of the 8th Confererence of the Cognitive Science Society* (pp. 531–546). Hillsdale, NJ: Lawrence Erlbaum Associates.

Kalat, J. W. (1995). *Biological psychology, 5th ed.* Pacific Grove, CA: Brooks Cole.

Kandel, E. R., Schwartz, J. H., & Jessell, T. M. (1991). *Principles of neural science, 3rd ed.* Norwalk, CT: Appleton & Lange.

Kanne, S. M., Balota, D. A., & Faust, M. E. (1998). Explorations of Cohen, Dunbar, and McClelland's (1990) connectionist model of Stroop performance. *Psychological Review, 105,* 174.

Kay, J., Floreano, D., & Phillips, W. (1998). Contextually guided unsupervised learning using local multivariate binary processors. *Neural Networks, 11,* 117–140.

Keith, J. R., & Rudy, J. W. (1990). Why NMDA-receptor-dependent long-term potentiation may not be a mechanism of learning and memory: Reappraisal of the NMDA-receptor blockade strategy. *Psychobiology, 18,* 251–257.

Kimberg, D. Y., & Farah, M. J. (1993). A unified account of cognitive impairments following frontal lobe damage: The role of working memory in complex, organized behavior. *Journal of Experimental Psychology: General, 122,* 411–428.

Kinsbourne, M. (1997). What qualifies a representation for a role in consciousness? In J. D. Cohen, & J. W. Schooler (Eds.), *Scientific approaches to consciousness* (pp. 335–355). Mahway, NJ: Lawrence Erlbaum Associates.

Kintsch, W. (1998). *Comprehension: A paradigm for cognition.* Cambridge: Cambridge University Press.

Kirkpatrick, S., Gelatt, C. D., & Vecchi, M. P. (1983). Optimization by simulated annealing. *Science, 220,* 671–680.

Koch, C., & Segev, I. (Eds.). (1998). *Methods in neuronal modeling, 2d ed.* Cambridge, MA: MIT Press.

Koechlin, E., Basso, G., & Grafman, J. (1999). The role of the anterior prefrontal cortex in human cognition. *Nature, 399,* 148.

Kohonen, T. (1984). *Self-organization and associative memory.* Berlin: Springer Verlag.

Kortge, C. A. (1993). Episodic memory in connectionist networks. *Proceedings of the Twelfth Annual Conference of the Cognitive Science Society* (pp. 764–771). Hillsdale, NJ: Erlbaum.

Kosslyn, S. M. (1994). *Image and brain: The resolution of the imagery debate.* Cambridge, MA: MIT Press.

Kubota, K., & Niki, H. (1971). Prefrontal cortical unit activity and delayed alternation performance in monkeys. *Journal of Neurophysiology, 34,* 337–347.

LaBerge, D. (1990). Thalamic and cortical mechanisms of attention suggested by recent positron emission tomographic experiments. *Journal of Cognitive Neuroscience, 2,* 358–372.

Landauer, T. K., & Dumais, S. T. (1997). A solution to Plato's problem: The latent semantic analysis theory of acquisition, induction, and representation of knowledge. *Psychological Review, 104,* 211–240.

LeCun, Y., Boser, B., Denker, J. S., Henderson, D., Howard, R. E., Hubbard, W., & Jackel, L. D. (1989). Backpropagation applied to handwritten zip code recognition. *Neural Computation, 1,* 541–551.

Lecuyer, R., Abgueguen, I., & Lemarie, C. (1992). 9- and 5-month-olds do not make the AB error if not required to manipulate objects. In C. Rovee-Collier (Ed.), *Abstracts of papers presented at the 8th International Conference on Infants Studies.* Norwood, NJ: Ablex.

Lenat, D. B. (1995). CYC: A large-scale investment in knowledge infrastructure. *Communications of the ACM, 38,* 32–38.

Levine, D. S., & Prueitt, P. S. (1989). Modeling some effects of frontal lobe damage-novelty and perseveration. *Neural Networks, 2,* 103–116.

Levitt, J. B., Lewis, D. A., Yoshioka, T., & Lund, J. S. (1993). Topography of pyramidal neuron intrinsic connections in macaque monkey prefrontal cortex (areas 9 & 46). *Journal of Comparative Neurology, 338,* 360–376.

Levy, W. B. (1989). A computational approach to hippocampal function. In R. D. Hawkins, & G. H. Bower (Eds.), *Computational models of learning in simple neural systems* (pp. 243–304). San Diego, CA: Academic Press.

Lewis, D. A., Hayes, T. L., Lund, J. S., & Oeth, K. M. (1992). Dopamine and the neural circuitry of primate prefrontal cortex: Implications for schizophrenia research. *Neuropsychopharmacology, 6,* 127–134.

Lhermitte, F. (1986). Human autonomy and the frontal lobes: Part II. Patient behavior in complex and social situations: The "environmental dependency syndrome". *Annals of Neurology, 19,* 335–343.

Linsker, R. (1986). From basic network principles to neural architecture (a three-part series). *Proceedings of the National Academy of Sciences, 83,* 7508–7512, 8390–8394, 8779–8783.

Linsker, R. (1988). Self-organization in a perceptual network. *Computer, 21*(3), 105–117.

Lisman, J. (1994). The CaM Kinase II hypothesis for the storage of synaptic memory. *Trends in Neurosciences, 17,* 406.

Lisman, J. E. (1989). A mechanism for the Hebb and the anti-Hebb processes underlying learning and memory. *Proceedings of the National Academy of Sciences, 86,* 9574–9578.

Livingstone, M., & Hubel, D. (1988). Segregation of form, color, movement, and depth: Anatomy, physiology, and perception. *Science*, *240*, 740–749.

Logothetis, N. K., & Sheinberg, D. L. (1996). Visual object recognition. *Annual Review of Neuroscience*, *19*, 577–621.

Lowe, D. G. (1987). The viewpoint consistency constraint. *International Journal of Computer Vision*, *1*, 57–72.

Luciana, M., Depue, R. A., Arbisi, P., & Leon, A. (1992). Facilitation of working memory in humans by a D2 dopamine receptor agonist. *Journal of Cognitive Neuroscience*, *4*, 58–68.

MacDonald, M. C., Pearlmutter, N. J., & Seidenberg, M. S. (1994). The lexical nature of syntactic ambiguity resolution. *Psychological Review*, *101*(4), 676–703.

MacLeod, C. M., & Dunbar, K. (1988). Training and Stroop-like interference: Evidence for a continuum of automaticity. *Journal of Experimental Psychology*, *14*, 126–135.

MacWhinney, B., & Leinbach, J. (1991). Implementations are not conceptualizations: Revising the verb learning model. *Cognition*, *40*, 121–153.

MacWhinney, B., & Snow, C. (1990). The child language data exchange system: An update. *Journal of Child Language*, *17*, 457–472.

Majani, E., Erlarson, R., & Abu-Mostafa, Y. (1989). The induction of multiscale temporal structure. In D. S. Touretzky (Ed.), *Advances in Neural Information Processing Systems, 1* (pp. 634–642). San Mateo, CA: Morgan Kaufmann.

Malenka, R. C., & Nicoll, R. A. (1993). NMDA receptor-dependent synaptic plasticity: Multiple forms and mechanisms. *Trends in Neurosciences*, *16*, 521–527.

Marcus, G. F. (1998). Rethinking eliminative connectionism. *Cognitive Psychology*, *37*, 243.

Marcus, G. F., Pinker, S., Ullman, M., Hollander, M., Rosen, J. T., & Xu, F. (1992). Overregularization in language acquisition. *Monographs of the Society for Research in Child Development*, *57*(4), 1–165.

Marr, D. (1969). A theory of cerebellar cortex. *Journal of Physiology (London)*, *202*, 437–470.

Marr, D. (1970). A theory for cerebral neocortex. *Proceedings of the Royal Society (London) B*, *176*, 161–234.

Marr, D. (1971). Simple memory: A theory for archicortex. *Philosophical Transactions of the Royal Society (London) B*, *262*, 23–81.

Marr, D. (1982). *Vision*. New York: Freeman.

Mathis, D. A., & Mozer, M. C. (1995). On the computational utility of consciousness. In G. Tesauro, D. S. Touretzky, & T. K. Leen (Eds.), *Advances in Neural Information Processing Systems, 7* (pp. 10–18). Cambridge, MA: MIT Press.

Matthews, A. (1992). Infants' performance on two versions of AB: Is recall memory a critical factor? In C. Rovee-Collier (Ed.), *Abstracts of papers presented at the 8th International Conference on Infants Studies*. Norwood, NJ: Ablex.

Maunsell, J. H. R., & Newsome, W. T. (1987). Visual processing in monkey extrastriate cortex. *Annual Review of Neuroscience*, *10*, 363–401.

Maylor, E. (1985). Facilitatory and inhibitory components of orienting in visual space. In M. I. Posner, & O. S. M. Marin (Eds.), *Attention and performance XI*. Hillsdale, NJ: Lawrence Erlbaum Associates.

Mazzoni, P., Andersen, R. A., & Jordan, M. I. (1991). A more biologically plausible learning rule for neural networks. *Proceedings of the National Academy of Sciences*, *88*, 4433–4437.

McCann, R. S., & Besner, D. (1987). Reading pseudohomophones: Implications for models of pronunciation and the locus of the word-frequency effects in word naming. *Journal of Experimental Psychology: Human Perception and Performance*, *13*, 14–24.

McClelland, J. L. (1993). The GRAIN model: A framework for modeling the dynamics of information processing. In D. E. Meyer, & S. Kornblum (Eds.), *Attention and performance XIV: Synergies in experimental psychology, artificial intelligence, and cognitive neuroscience* (pp. 655–688). Hillsdale, NJ: Lawrence Erlbaum Associates.

McClelland, J. L. (1994). The interaction of nature and nurture in development: A parallel distributed processing perspective. In P. Bertelson, P. Eelen, & G. D'Ydewalle (Eds.), *Current advances in psychological science: Ongoing research* (pp. 57–88). Hillsdale, NJ: Erlbaum.

McClelland, J. L. (1998). Connectionist models and Bayesian inference. In N. Chater, & M. Oaksford (Eds.), *Rational models of cognitive processes*. Oxford: Oxford University Press.

McClelland, J. L., & Chappell, M. (1998). Familiarity breeds differentiation: a subjective-likelihood approach to the effects of experience in recognition memory. *Psychological Review*, *105*, 724.

McClelland, J. L., & Goddard, N. H. (1996). Considerations arising from a complementary learning systems perspective on hippocampus and neocortex. *Hippocampus*, *6*, 654–665.

McClelland, J. L., McNaughton, B. L., & O'Reilly, R. C. (1995). Why there are complementary learning systems in the hippocampus and neocortex: Insights from the successes and failures of connectionst models of learning and memory. *Psychological Review, 102*, 419–457.

McClelland, J. L., & Rumelhart, D. E. (1981). An interactive activation model of context effects in letter perception: Part 1. An account of basic findings. *Psychological Review, 88*(5), 375–407.

McClelland, J. L., & Rumelhart, D. E. (1986). A distributed model of human learning and memory. In J. L. McClelland, D. E. Rumelhart, & PDP Research Group (Eds.), *Parallel distributed processing. Volume 2: Psychological and biological models* (pp. 170–215). Cambridge, MA: MIT Press.

McClelland, J. L., & Rumelhart, D. E. (Eds.). (1988). *Explorations in parallel distributed processing: A handbook of models, programs, and exercises*. Cambridge, MA: MIT Press.

McClelland, J. L., Rumelhart, D. E., & PDP Research Group (Eds.). (1986). *Parallel distributed processing. Volume 2: Psychological and biological models*. Cambridge, MA: MIT Press.

McCleod, P., Plunkett, K., & Rolls, E. T. (1998). *Introduction to connectionist modelling of cognitive processes*. Oxford: Oxford University Press.

McCloskey, M. (1991). Networks and theories: The place of connectionism in cognitive science. *Psychological Science, 2*, 387–395.

McCloskey, M., & Cohen, N. J. (1989). Catastrophic interference in connectionist networks: The sequential learning problem. In G. H. Bower (Ed.), *The psychology of learning and motivation, vol. 24* (pp. 109–164). San Diego, CA: Academic Press, Inc.

McCulloch, W. S., & Pitts, W. (1943). A logical calculus of the ideas immanent in nervous activity. *Bulletin of Mathematical Biophysics, 5*, 115–133.

McNaughton, B. L., & Morris, R. G. M. (1987). Hippocampal synaptic enhancement and information storage within a distributed memory system. *Trends in Neurosciences, 10*(10), 408–415.

McNaughton, B. L., & Nadel, L. (1990). Hebb-marr networks and the neurobiological representation of action in space. In M. A. Gluck, & D. E. Rumelhart (Eds.), *Neuroscience and connectionist theory* (Chap. 1, pp. 1–63). Hillsdale, NJ: Lawrence Erlbaum Associates.

McRae, K., & Hetherington, P. A. (1993). Catastrophic interference is eliminated in pretrained networks. *Proceedings of the Fifteenth Annual Conference of the Cognitive Science Society* (pp. 723–728). Hillsdale, NJ: Erlbaum.

Mel, B. A., & Fiser, J. (2000). Minimizing binding errors using learned conjunctive features. *Neural Computation, 12*, 731–762.

Miller, E. K., & Desimone, R. (1994). Parallel neuronal mechanisms for short-term memory. *Science, 263*, 520–522.

Miller, E. K., Erickson, C. A., & Desimone, R. (1996). Neural mechanisms of visual working memory in prefontal cortex of the macaque. *Journal of Neuroscience, 16*, 5154.

Miller, G. A. (1956). The magical number seven, plus or minus two: Some limits on our capacity for processing information. *Psychological Review, 63*, 81–97.

Miller, K. D. (1994). A model for the development of simple cell receptive fields and the ordered arrangement of orientation columns through activity-dependent competition between ON- and OFF-center inputs. *Journal of Neuroscience, 14*, 409–441.

Miller, K. D., Keller, J. B., & Stryker, M. P. (1989). Ocular dominance column development: Analysis and simulation. *Science, 245*, 605–615.

Milner, B. (1964). Some effects of frontal lobectomy in man. In J. M. Warren, & K. Akert (Eds.), *The frontal granual cortex and behavior* (pp. 313–331). New York: McGraw-Hill.

Minsky, M. L., & Papert, S. A. (1969). *Perceptrons*. Cambridge, MA: MIT Press.

Mishkin, M., & Manning, F. J. (1978). Nonspatial memory after selective prefrontal lesions in monkeys. *Brain Research, 143*, 313–323.

Miyake, A., & Shah, P. (Eds.). (1999). *Models of working memory: Mechanisms of active maintenance and executive control*. New York: Cambridge University Press.

Moll, M., & Miikkulainen, R. (1997). Convergence-zone episodic memory: Analysis and simulations. *Neural Networks, 10*, 1017.

Montague, P. R., Dayan, P., & Sejnowski, T. J. (1996). A framework for mesencephalic dopamine systems based on predictive Hebbian learning. *Journal of Neuroscience, 16*, 1936–1947.

Moran, J., & Desimone, R. (1985). Selective attention gates visual processing in the extrastriate cortex. *Science, 229*, 782–784.

Motter, B. C. (1993). Focal attention produces spatially selective processing in areas V1, V2 and V4 in the presence of competing stimuli. *Journal of Neurophysiology, 70*, 909–919.

Movellan, J. R. (1990). Contrastive Hebbian learning in the continuous Hopfield model. In D. S. Touretzky, G. E. Hinton, & T. J. Sejnowski (Eds.), *Proceedings of the 1989 Connectionist Models Summer School* (pp. 10–17). San Mateo, CA: Morgan Kaufman.

Movellan, J. R., & McClelland, J. L. (1993). Learning continuous probability distributions with symmetric diffusion networks. *Cognitive Science, 17*, 463–496.

Mozer, M. C. (1987). Early parallel processing in reading: A connectionist approach. In M. Colthheart (Ed.), *Attention and Performance XII: The Psychology of Reading.* (pp. 83–104). Hillsdale, NJ: Lawrence Erlbaum Associates.

Mozer, M. C. (1991). *The perception of multiple objects: A connectionist approach.* Cambridge, MA: MIT Press.

Mozer, M. C. (1993). Neural net architectures for temporal sequence processing. In A. Weigend, & N. Gershenfeld (Eds.), *Predicting the future and understanding the past.* Redwood City, CA: Addison-Wesley.

Mozer, M. C., & Sitton, M. (1998). Computational modeling of spatial attention. In H. Pashler (Ed.), *Attention* (pp. 341–393). London: UCL Press.

Mozer, M. C., Zemel, R. S., Behrmann, M., & Williams, C. K. I. (1992). Learning to segment images using dynamic feature binding. *Neural Computation, 4*, 650–665.

Munakata, Y. (1998). Infant perseveration and implications for object permanence theories: A PDP model of the $A\overline{B}$ task. *Developmental Science, 1*, 161–184.

Munakata, Y. (in press). Task-dependency in infant behavior: Toward an understanding of the processes underlying cognitive development. In F. Lacerda, C. v. Hofsten, & M. Heimann (Eds.), *Emerging cognitive abilities in early infancy.* Mahwah, NJ: Lawrence Erlbaum.

Munakata, Y., McClelland, J. L., Johnson, M. J., & Siegler, R. S. (1997). Rethinking infant knowledge: Toward an adaptive process account of successes and failures in object permanence tasks. *Psychological Review, 104*, 686–713.

Newcombe, F. (1969). *Missile wounds of the brain: A study of psychological deficits.* Oxford: Oxford University Press.

Newell, A. (1990). *Unified theories of cognition.* Cambridge, MA: Harvard University Press.

Newell, A., & Simon, H. A. (1972). *Human problem solving.* Englewood Cliffs, NJ: Prentice-Hall.

Noelle, D. C., & Cottrell, G. W. (1996). In search of articulated attractors. In G. W. Cottrell (Ed.), *Proceedings of the 18th Annual Conference of the Cognitive Science Society* (pp. 329–334). Mahwah, NJ: Lawrence Erlbaum.

Norman, K. A., & Schacter, D. (submitted). List strength affects recollection but not familiarity.

Nowlan, S. J. (1990). Maximum likelihood competitive learning. In D. S. Touretzky (Ed.), *Advances in neural information processing systems, 2* (pp. 574–582). San Mateo, CA: Morgan Kaufmann.

Oja, E. (1982). A simplified neuron model as a principal component analyzer. *Journal of Mathematical Biology, 15*, 267–273.

Oja, E. (1989). Neural networks, principal components, and subspaces. *International Journal of Neural Systems, 1*, 61–68.

O'Keefe, J., & Nadel, L. (1978). *The hippocampus as a cognitive map.* Oxford: Oxford University Press.

Olshausen, B. A., & Field, D. J. (1996). Emergence of simple-cell receptive field properties by learning a sparse code for natural images. *Nature, 381*, 607.

O'Reilly, R. C. (1996a). Biologically plausible error-driven learning using local activation differences: The generalized recirculation algorithm. *Neural Computation, 8*(5), 895–938.

O'Reilly, R. C. (1996b). *The Leabra model of neural interactions and learning in the neocortex.* PhD thesis, Carnegie Mellon University, Pittsburgh, PA, USA.

O'Reilly, R. C. (1998). Six principles for biologically-based computational models of cortical cognition. *Trends in Cognitive Sciences, 2*(11), 455–462.

O'Reilly, R. C. (in press). Generalization in interactive networks: The benefits of inhibitory competition and Hebbian learning. *Neural Computation.*

O'Reilly, R. C., Braver, T. S., & Cohen, J. D. (1999a). A biologically based computational model of working memory. In A. Miyake, & P. Shah (Eds.), *Models of working memory: Mechanisms of active maintenance and executive control.* (pp. 375–411). New York: Cambridge University Press.

O'Reilly, R. C., & Farah, M. J. (1999). Simulation and explanation in neuropsychology and beyond. *Cognitive Neuropsychology, 16*, 49–72.

O'Reilly, R. C., & Hoeffner, J. H. (in preparation). Competition, priming, and the past tense U-shaped developmental curve.

O'Reilly, R. C., & McClelland, J. L. (1994). Hippocampal conjunctive encoding, storage, and recall: Avoiding a tradeoff. *Hippocampus, 4*(6), 661–682.

O'Reilly, R. C., Mozer, M., Munakata, Y., & Miyake, A. (1999b). Discrete representations in working memory: A hypothesis and computational investigations. *The Second International Conference on Cognitive Science* (pp. 183–188). Tokyo: Japanese Cognitive Science Society.

O'Reilly, R. C., Noelle, D., Braver, T. S., & Cohen, J. D. (submitted). Prefrontal cortex and dynamic categorization tasks: Representational organization and neuromodulatory control.

O'Reilly, R. C., Norman, K. A., & McClelland, J. L. (1998). A hippocampal model of recognition memory. In M. I. Jordan, M. J. Kearns, & S. A. Solla (Eds.), *Advances in neural information processing systems 10* (pp. 73–79). Cambridge, MA: MIT Press.

O'Reilly, R. C., & Rudy, J. W. (1999). *Conjunctive representations in learning and memory: Principles of cortical and hippocampal function* (Institute of Cognitive Science TR 99-01). Boulder: University of Colorado Boulder.

O'Reilly, R. C., & Rudy, J. W. (in press). Conjunctive representations in learning and memory: Principles of cortical and hippocampal function. *Psychological Review*.

Owen, A. M., Roberts, A. C., Hodges, J. R., Summers, B. A., Polkey, C. E., & Robbins, T. W. (1993). Contrasting mechanisms of impaired attentional set-shifting in patients with frontal lobe damage or Parkinson's disease. *Brain, 116*, 1159–1175.

Parker, D. B. (1985). *Learning logic* (Technical Report TR-47). Cambridge, MA: Center for Computational Research in Economics and Management Science, Massachusetts Institute of Technology.

Paulesu, E., Frith, C. D., & Frackowiak, R. S. J. (1993). The neural correlates of the verbal component of working memory. *Nature, 362*, 342–345.

Pearlmutter, B. A. (1989). Learning state space trajectories in recurrent neural networks. *Neural Computation, 1*(2), 263–269.

Penit-Soria, J., Audinat, E., & Crepel, F. (1987). Excitation of rat prefrontal cortical neurons by dopamine: An in vitro electrophysiological study. *Brain Research, 425*, 263–274.

Peterson, C., & Anderson, J. R. (1987). A mean field theory learning algorithm for neural networks. *Complex Systems, 1*, 995–1019.

Peterson, M., & Zemel, R. S. (1998). Location-specificity in memories of novel objects. *The 39th Annual Meeting of the Psychonomic Society*. The Psychonomic Society.

Petrides, M. E. (1996). Specialized systems for the processing of mnemonic information within the primate frontal cortex. *Philosophical Transactions of the Royal Society (London) B, 351*, 1455–1462.

Piaget, J. (1954). *The construction of reality in the child*. New York: Basic Books.

Pinker, S. (1991). Rules of language. *Science, 253*, 530–535.

Pinker, S., & Prince, A. (1988). On language and connectionism: Analysis of a parallel distributed processing model of language acquisition. *Cognition, 28*, 73–193.

Plaut, D. C. (1995). Double dissociation without modularity: Evidence from connectionist neuropsychology. *Journal of Clinical and Experimental Neuropsychology, 17*(2), 291–321.

Plaut, D. C. (1997). Structure and function in the lexical system: Insights from distributed models of word reading and lexical decision. *Language and Cognitive Processes, 12*, 767–808.

Plaut, D. C. (1999). Computational modeling of word reading, acquired dyslexia, and remediation. In R. M. Klein, & P. A. McMullen (Eds.), *Converging methods in reading and dyslexia* (pp. 339–372). Cambridge, MA: MIT Press.

Plaut, D. C., & McClelland, J. L. (1993). Generalization with componential attractors: Word and nonword reading in an attractor network. *Proceedings of the 15th Annual Conference of the Cognitive Science Society* (pp. 824–829). Hillsdale, NJ: Lawrence Erlbaum Associates.

Plaut, D. C., McClelland, J. L., Seidenberg, M. S., & Patterson, K. E. (1996). Understanding normal and impaired word reading: Computational principles in quasi-regular domains. *Psychological Review, 103*, 56–115.

Plaut, D. C., & Shallice, T. (1993). Deep dyslexia: A case study of connectionist neuropsychology. *Cognitive Neuropsychology, 10*(5), 377–500.

Plunkett, K., & Elman, J. L. (1997). *Exercises in rethinking innateness: A handbook for connectionist simulations*. Cambridge, MA: MIT Press.

Plunkett, K., & Marchman, V. A. (1991). U-shaped learning and frequency effects in a multi-layered perceptron: Implications for child language acquisition. *Cognition, 38*, 43–102.

Plunkett, K., & Marchman, V. A. (1993). From rote learning to system building: Acquiring verb morphology in children and connectionist nets. *Cognition, 48*(1), 21–69.

Posner, M. I. (1980). Orienting of attention. *Quarterly Journal of Experimental Psychology, 32*, 3–25.

Posner, M. I., Inhoff, A. W., Friedrich, F. J., & Cohen, A. (1987). Isolating attentional system: A cognitive-anatomical analysis. *Psychobiology, 15*, 107–121.

Posner, M. I., Walker, J. A., Friedrich, F. J., & Rafal, R. D. (1984). Effects of parietal lobe injury on covert orienting of visual attention. *Journal of Neuroscience, 4*, 1863–1874.

Rakic, P. (1994). Corticogenesis in human and nonhuman primates. In M. S. Gazzaniga (Ed.), *The cognitive neurosciences* (pp. 127–145). Cambridge, MA: MIT Press.

Rao, S. G., Williams, G. V., & Goldman-Rakic, P. S. (1999). Isodirectional tuning of adjacent interneurons and pyramidal cells during working memory: Evidence for microcolumnar organization in PFC. *Journal of Neurophysiology*, *81*, 1903.

Reber, A. S. (1967). Implicit learning of artificial grammars. *Journal of Verbal Learning and Verbal Behavior*, *6*, 855–863.

Reid, R. C., & Alonso, J. M. (1995). Specificity of monosynaptic connections from thalamus to visual cortex. *Nature*, *378*, 281–284.

Reike, F., Warland, D., van Steveninck, R., & Bialek, W. (1996). *Spikes: Exploring the neural code*. Cambridge, MA: MIT Press.

Rescorla, R. A., & Wagner, A. R. (1972). A theory of Pavlovian conditioning: Variation in the effectiveness of reinforcement and non-reinforcement. In A. H. Black, & W. F. Prokasy (Eds.), *Classical conditioning II: Theory and research* (pp. 64–99). New York: Appleton-Century-Crofts.

Rissanen, J. (1986). Stochastic complexity. *Annals of Statistics*, *14*, 1080–1100.

Roberts, A. C., Robbins, T. W., & Everitt, B. J. (1988). The effects of intradimensional and extradimensional shifts on visual discrimination learning in humans and non-human primates. *Quarterly Journal of Experimental Psychology*, *40*, 321–341.

Roberts, R. J., Hager, L. D., & Heron, C. (1994). Prefrontal cognitive processes: Working memory and inhibition in the antisaccade task. *Journal of Experimental Psychology: General*, *123*, 374.

Rosch, E. (1975). Cognitive representations of semantic categories. *Journal of Experimental Psychology: General*, *104*, 192–223.

Rosenblatt, F. (1958). The perceptron: A probabilistic model for information storage and organization in the brain. *Psychological Review*, *65*, 386–408.

Rosson, M. B. (1985). The interaction of pronunciation rules and lexical representations in reading aloud. *Memory and Cognition*, *13*, 90–99.

Rosvold, H. E., Mirsky, A. F., Sarason, I., Bransome, E. D., & Beck, L. H. (1956). A continuous performance test of brain damage. *Journal of Consulting Psychology*, *20*(5), 343–350.

Rudy, J. W., & Sutherland, R. W. (1995). Configural association theory and the hippocampal formation: An appraisal and reconfiguration. *Hippocampus*, *5*, 375–389.

Rumelhart, D. E., Hinton, G. E., & Williams, R. J. (1986a). Learning internal representations by error propagation. In D. E. Rumelhart, J. L. McClelland, & PDP Research Group (Eds.), *Parallel distributed processing. Volume 1: Foundations* (Chap. 8, pp. 318–362). Cambridge, MA: MIT Press.

Rumelhart, D. E., Hinton, G. E., & Williams, R. J. (1986b). Learning representations by back-propagating errors. *Nature*, *323*, 533–536.

Rumelhart, D. E., & McClelland, J. L. (1986). On learning the past tenses of English verbs. In J. L. McClelland, D. E. Rumelhart, & PDP Research Group (Eds.), *Parallel distributed processing. Volume 2: Psychological and biological models* (pp. 216–271). Cambridge, MA: MIT Press.

Rumelhart, D. E., McClelland, J. L., & PDP Research Group (Eds.). (1986c). *Parallel distributed processing. Volume 1: Foundations*. Cambridge, MA: MIT Press.

Rumelhart, D. E., & Zipser, D. (1986). Feature discovery by competitive learning. In D. E. Rumelhart, J. L. McClelland, & PDP Research Group (Eds.), *Parallel distributed processing. Volume 1: Foundations* (Chap. 5, pp. 151–193). Cambridge, MA: MIT Press.

Saffran, E. M. (1997). Aphasia: Cognitive neuropsychological aspects. In T. E. Feinberg, & M. J. Farah (Eds.), *Behavioral neurology and neuropsychology* (pp. 151–166). New York: McGraw-Hill.

Saffran, E. M., & Schwartz, F. F. (1994). Of cabbages and things: Semantic memory from a neuropsychological perspective. In C. Umilta, & M. Moscovitch (Eds.), *Attention and performance XV* (pp. 507–536). Cambridge, MA: MIT Press.

Samsonovich, A., & McNaughton, B. L. (1997). Path integration and cognitive mapping in a continuous attractor neural network model. *Journal of Neuroscience*, *17*, 5900–5920.

Sanger, T. D. (1989). Optimal unsupervised learning in a single-layer linear feedforward neural network. *Neural Networks*, *2*, 459–473.

Saul, L. K., Jaakkola, T., & Jordan, M. I. (1996). Mean field theory for sigmoid belief networks. *Journal of Artificial Intelligence Research*, *4*, 61–76.

Sawaguchi, T., & Goldman-Rakic, P. S. (1991). D1 dopamine receptors in prefrontal cortex: Involvement in working memory. *Science*, *251*, 947–950.

Schacter, D. L. (1987). Implicit memory: History and current status. *Journal of Experimental Psychology: Learning, Memory, and Cognition*, *13*(3), 501–518.

Schacter, D. L. (1996). *Searching for memory: The brain, the mind, and the past.* New York: Basic Books.

Schacter, D. L., & Tulving, E. (1994). *Memory systems 1994.* Cambridge, MA: MIT Press.

Schmajuk, N. A., & DiCarlo, J. J. (1992). Stimulus configuration, classical conditioning, and hippocampal function. *Psychological Review, 99*(2), 268–305.

Schneider, W., & Shiffrin, R. M. (1977). Controlled and automatic human information processing: I. Detection, search, and attention. *Psychological Review, 84*, 1–66.

Schooler, C., Neumann, E., & Roberts, B. R. (1997). A time course analysis of Stroop interference and facilitation: Comparing normal individuals and individuals with schizophrenia. *Journal of Experimental Psychology: General, 126*, 169.

Schultz, W., Apicella, P., & Ljungberg, T. (1993). Responses of monkey dopamine neurons to reward and conditioned stimuli during successive steps of learning a delayed response task. *Journal of Neuroscience, 13*, 900–913.

Schultz, W., Apicella, P., Romo, R., & Scarnati, E. (1995). Context-dependent activity in primate striatum reflecting past and future behavioral events. In J. C. Houk, J. L. Davis, & D. G. Beiser (Eds.), *Models of information processing in the basal ganglia* (pp. 11–28). Cambridge, MA: MIT Press.

Schultz, W., Dayan, P., & Montague, P. R. (1997). A neural substrate of prediction and reward. *Science, 275*, 1593.

Schweighofer, N., Arbib, M., & Kawato, M. (1998a). Role of the cerebellum in reaching quickly and accurately: I. A functional anatomical model of dynamics control. *European Journal of Neuroscience, 10*, 86–94.

Schweighofer, N., Arbib, M., & Kawato, M. (1998b). Role of the cerebellum in reaching quickly and accurately: II. A detailed model of the intermediate cerebellum. *European Journal of Neuroscience, 10*, 95–105.

Seidenberg, M. (1993). Connectionist models and cognitive theory. *Psychological Science, 4*(4), 228–235.

Seidenberg, M. S. (1997). Language acquistion and use: Learning and applying probabilistic constraints. *Science, 275*, 1599.

Seidenberg, M. S., & McClelland, J. L. (1989). A distributed, developmental model of word recognition and naming. *Psychological Review, 96*, 523–568.

Sejnowski, T. J., & Churchland, P. S. (1989). Brain and cognition. In M. I. Posner (Ed.), *Foundations of cognitive science* (pp. 301–356). Cambridge, MA: MIT Press.

Seress (1988). Interspecies comparison of the hippocampal formation shows increased emphasis on the regio superior in the ammon's horn of the human brain. *J Hirnforsh, 29*, 335–340.

Servan-Schreiber, D., Cohen, J. D., & Steingard, S. (1997). Schizophrenic deficits in the processing of context: A test of a theoretical model. *Archives of General Psychiatry, 53*, 1105–1113.

Shadlen, M. N., & Newsome, W. T. (1994). Noise, neural codes, and cortical organization. *Current Opinion in Neurobiology, 4*, 569–579.

Shah, P., & Miyake, A. (1996). The separability of working memory resources for spatial thinking and language processing: An individual differences approach. *Journal of Experimental Psychology: General, 125*, 4–27.

Shallice, T. (1982). Specific impairments of planning. *Philosophical Transactions of the Royal Society (London) B, 298*, 199–209.

Shallice, T. (1988). *From neuropsychology to mental structure.* New York: Cambridge University Press.

Shallice, T., & Burgess, P. (1991). Higher-order cognitive impairments and frontal lobe lesions in man. In H. S. Levin, H. M. Eisenberg, & A. L. Benton (Eds.), *Frontal lobe function and dysfunction* (Chap. 6, pp. 125–138). New York: Oxford University Press.

Shastri, L., & Ajjanagadde, V. (1993). From simple associations to systematic reasoning: A connectionist representation of rules, variables, and dynamic bindings using temporal synchrony. *Behavioral and Brain Sciences, 16*, 417–494.

Shatz, C. J. (1996). Emergence of order in visual system development. *Proceedings of the National Academy of Sciences, 93*, 602.

Shepherd, G. M. (Ed.). (1990). *The synaptic organization of the brain.* Oxford: Oxford University Press.

Shepherd, G. M. (1992). *Foundations of the neuron doctrine.* New York: Oxford University Press.

Shepherd, G. M., & Brayton, R. K. (1987). Logic operations are properties of computer-simulated interactions between excitable dendritic spines. *Neuroscience, 21*, 151–166.

Sherman, S. M., & Koch, C. (1986). The control of retinogeniculate transmission in the mammalian lateral geniculate nucleus. *Experimental Brain Research, 63*, 1–20.

Shiffrin, R. M., & Schneider, W. (1977). Controlled and automatic human information processing: II. Perceptual learning, automatic attending, and a general theory. *Psychological Review, 84*, 127–190.

Singley, K., & Anderson, J. R. (1989). *The transfer of cognitive skill.* Cambridge, MA: Harvard University Press.

Sloman, S. A., & Rumelhart, D. E. (1992). Reducing interference in distributed memories through episodic gating. In A. Healy, S. Kosslyn, & R. Shiffrin (Eds.), *Essays in honor of W. K. Estes.* Hillsdale, NJ: Erlbaum.

Smolensky, P. (1986). Information processing in dynamical systems: Foundations of harmony theory. In D. E. Rumelhart, J. L. McClelland, & PDP Research Group (Eds.), *Parallel distributed processing. Volume 1: Foundations* (Chap. 5, pp. 282–317). Cambridge, MA: MIT Press.

Smolensky, P. (1990). Tensor product variable binding and the representation of symbolic structures in connectionist networks. *Artificial Intelligence, 46*, 159–216.

Snyder, L. H., Grieve, K. L., & Andersen, R. A. (1998). Separate body- and world-referenced representations of visual space in parietal cortex. *Nature, 394*, 887.

Spelke, E., Breinlinger, K., Macomber, J., & Jacobson, K. (1992). Origins of knowledge. *Psychological Review, 99*, 605–632.

Squire, L. R. (1987). *Memory and brain.* Oxford: Oxford University Press.

Squire, L. R. (1992). Memory and the hippocampus: A synthesis from findings with rats, monkeys, and humans. *Psychological Review, 99*, 195–231.

Squire, L. R., Shimamura, A. P., & Amaral, D. G. (1989). Memory and the hippocampus. In J. H. Byrne, & W. O. Berry (Eds.), *Neural models of plasticity: Experimental and theoretical approaches.* San Diego, CA: Academic Press.

St. John, M. F., & McClelland, J. L. (1990). Learning and applying contextual constraints in sentence comprehension. *Artificial Intelligence, 46*, 217–257.

Stroop, J. R. (1935). Studies of interference in serial verbal reactions. *Journal of Experimental Psychology, 18*, 643–662.

Stuart, G., & Sakmann, B. (1994). Active propagation of somatic action potentials into neocortical pyramidal cell dendrites. *Nature, 367*, 69–72.

Sur, M., Garraghty, P., & Roe, A. W. (1988). Experimentally induced visual projections into auditory thalamus and cortex. *Science, 242*, 1437–1441.

Surmeier, D. J., Baras, J., H. C. Hemmings, J., Narin, A. C., & Greengard, P. (1995). Modulation of calcium currents by a D1 dopaminergic protein kinase/phosphatase cascade in rat neostriatal neurons. *Neuron, 14*, 385–397.

Surmeier, D. J., & Kitai, S. T. (1999). D1 and D2 modulation of sodium and potassium currents in rat neostriatal neurons. *Progress in Brain Research, 99*, 309–324.

Sutherland, R. J., & Rudy, J. W. (1989). Configural association theory: The role of the hippocampal formation in learning, memory, and amnesia. *Psychobiology, 17*(2), 129–144.

Sutton, R. S. (1988). Learning to predict by the method of temporal diferences. *Machine Learning, 3*, 9–44.

Sutton, R. S. (1995). TD models: Modeling the world at a mixture of time scales. In A. Prieditis, & S. Russel (Eds.), *Proceedings of the Twelfth International Conference on Machine Learning* (pp. 531–539). San Francisco: Morgan Kaufmann.

Sutton, R. S., & Barto, A. G. (1981). Toward a modern theory of adaptive networks: Expectation and prediction. *Psychological Review, 88*(2), 135–170.

Sutton, R. S., & Barto, A. G. (1990). Time-derivative models of Pavlovian reinforcement. In J. W. Moore, & M. Gabriel (Eds.), *Learning and computational neuroscience* (pp. 497–537). Cambridge, MA: MIT Press.

Sutton, R. S., & Barto, A. G. (1998). *Reinforcement learning: An introduction.* Cambridge, MA: MIT Press.

Suzuki, W. A. (1996). The anatomy, physiology and functions of the perirhinal cortex. *Current Opinion in Neurobiology, 6*, 179.

Swindale, N. V. (1996). The development of topography in the visual cortex: A review of models. *Network: Computation in Neural Systems, 7*, 161–247.

Tamamaki, N. (1991). The organization of reciprocal connections between the subiculum, field CA1 and the entorhinal cortex in the rat. *Society for Neuroscience Abstracts, 17*, 134.

Tanaka, K. (1996). Inferotemporal cortex and object vision. *Annual Review of Neuroscience, 19*, 109–139.

Taraban, R., & McClelland, J. L. (1987). Conspiracy effects in word pronunciation. *Journal of Memory and Language, 26*, 608–631.

Tarr, M. J., & Bülthoff, H. H. (1995). Is human object recognition better described by geon structural descriptions or by multiple views? Comment on Biederman and Gerhardstein (1993). *Journal of Experimental Psychology: Human Perception and Performance, 21*, 1494.

Teitelbaum, P. (1967). *Physiological psychology; fundamental principles.* Englewood Cliffs, NJ: Prentice-Hall.

Tipper, S. P., & Behrmann, M. (1996). Object-centered not scene-based visual neglect. *Journal of Experimental Psychology: Human Perception and Performance, 22*, 1261.

Tootell, R. B. H., Dale, A. M., Sereno, M. I., & Malach, R. (1996). New images from human visual cortex. *Trends in Neurosciences, 19*, 481–489.

Touretzky, D. S. (1986). BoltzCONS: Reconciling connectionism with the recursive nature of stacks and trees. *Proceedings of the 8th Annual Conference of the Cognitive Science Society* (pp. 522–530). Hillsdale, NJ: Lawrence Erlbaum Associates.

Traub, R. D., & Miles, R. (1991). *Neuronal networks of the hippocampus.* Cambridge: Cambridge University Press.

Treisman, A. (1996). the binding problem. *Current Opinion in Neurobiology, 6*, 171.

Treisman, A. M., & Gelade, G. (1980). A feature-integration theory of attention. *Cognitive Psychology, 12*, 97–136.

Treves, A., & Rolls, E. T. (1994). A computational analysis of the role of the hippocampus in memory. *Hippocampus, 4*, 374–392.

Tulving, E. (1972). Episodic and semantic memory. In E. Tulving, & W. Donaldson (Eds.), *Organization of memory* (pp. 381–403). San Diego, CA: Academic Press.

Ullman, M. T., Corkin, S., & Pinker, S. (1997). A neural dissociation within language: Evidence that the mental dictionary is part of declarative memory, and that grammatical rules are processed by the procedural system. *Journal of Cognitive Neuroscience, 9*, 266–276.

Ullman, S. (1994). Sequence seeking and counterstreams: A model for bidirectional information flow in the cortex. In C. Koch, & J. L. Davis (Eds.), *Large-scale neuronal theories of the brain* (Chap. 12, pp. 257–270). Cambridge, MA: MIT Press.

Ungerleider, L. G., & Haxby, J. V. (1994). "What" and "where" in the human brain. *Current Opinion in Neurobiology, 4*, 157–165.

Ungerleider, L. G., & Mishkin, M. (1982). Two cortical visual systems. In D. J. Ingle, M. A. Goodale, & R. J. W. Mansfield (Eds.), *The analysis of visual behavior.* Cambridge, MA: MIT Press.

Van Essen, D. C., & Maunsell, J. H. R. (1983). Hierarchical organization and functional streams in the visual cortex. *Trends in Neurosciences, 6*, 370–375.

Van Orden, G. C., Pennington, B. F., & Stone, G. O. (1990). Word identification in reading and the promise of subsymbolic psycholinguistics. *Psychological Review, 97*(4), 488–522.

Vapnik, V. N., & Chervonenkis, A. (1971). On the uniform convergence of relative frequencies of events to their probabilities. *Theory of Probability and Its Applications, 16*, 264–280.

Vargha-Khadem, F., Gadian, D. G., Watkins, K. E., Connelly, A., Van Paesschen, W., & Mishkin, M. (1997). Differential effects of early hippocampal pathology on episodic and semantic memory. *Science, 277*, 376.

Vecera, S. P., & Farah, M. J. (1994). Does visual attention select objects or locations? *Journal of Experimental Psychology: General, 123*, 146–160.

Vecera, S. P., & O'Reilly, R. C. (1998). Figure-ground organization and object recognition processes: An interactive account. *Journal of Experimental Psychology: Human Perception and Performance, 24*, 441–462.

Vendrell, P., Junque, C., & Grafman, J. (1995). The role of prefrontal regions in the Stroop task. *Neuropsychologia, 33*, 341.

von der Malsburg, C. (1973). Self-organization of orientation-sensitive columns in the striate cortex. *Kybernetik, 14*, 85–100.

Wager, T. D., & O'Reilly, R. C. (submitted). Reconciling biology and function in the attentional role of the reticular nucleus of the thalamus.

Warrington, E. K., & McCarthy, R. (1983). Category-specific access dysphasia. *Brain, 106*, 859–878.

Warrington, E. K., & McCarthy, R. (1987). Categories of knowledge: Further fractionation and an attempted integration. *Brain, 110*, 1273–1296.

Warrington, E. K., & Shallice, T. (1984). Category specific semantic impairments. *Brain, 107*, 829–853.

Weigend, A. S., Rumelhart, D. E., & Huberman, B. A. (1991). Generalization by weight-elimination with application to forecasting. In R. P. Lippmann, J. E. Moody, & D. S. Touretzky (Eds.), *Advances in neural information processing systems, 3* (pp. 875–882). San Mateo, CA: Morgan Kaufmann.

Weliky, M., Kandler, K., & Katz, L. C. (1995). Patterns of excitation and inhibition evoked by horizontal connections in visual cortex share a common relationship to orientation columns. *Neuron, 15*, 541.

Werbos, P. (1974). *Beyond regression: New tools for prediction and analysis in the behavioral sciences.* PhD thesis, Harvard University.

White, E. L. (1989a). *Cortical circuits: Synaptic organization of the cerebral cortex, structure, function, and theory.* Boston: Birkhäuser.

White, H. (1989b). Learning in artificial neural networks: A statistical perspective. *Neural Computation, 1*, 425–464.

Wickelgren, W. A. (1969). Context-sensitive coding, associative memory, and serial order in (speech) behavior. *Psychological Review, 76*, 1–15.

Wickelgren, W. A. (1979). Chunking and consolidation: A theoretical synthesis of semantic networks, configuring in conditioning, S-R versus cognitive learning, normal forgetting, the amnesic syndrome, and the hippocampal arousal system. *Psychological Review*, *86*, 44–60.

Wickens, J. (1997). Basal ganglia: Structure and computations. *Network: Computation in Neural Systems*, *8*, 77–109.

Widrow, B., & Hoff, M. E. (1960). Adaptive switching circuits. *Institute of Radio Engineers, Western Electronic Show and Convention, Convention Record, Part 4* (pp. 96–104).

Williams, G. V., & Goldman-Rakic, P. S. (1995). Modulation of memory fields by dopamine d1 receptors in prefrontal cortex. *Nature*, *376*, 572–575.

Williams, M. S., & Goldman-Rakic, P. S. (1993). Characterization of the dopaminergic innervation of the primate frontal cortex using a dopamine-specific antibody. *Cerebral Cortex*, *3*, 199–222.

Williams, R. J., & Peng, J. (1990). An efficient gradient-based algorithm for on-line training of recurrent network trajectories. *Neural Computation*, *2*(4), 490–501.

Williams, R. J., & Zipser, D. (1989). A learning algorithm for continually running fully recurrent neural networks. *Neural Computation*, *1*(2), 270–280.

Wilson, C. J. (1990). Basal ganglia. In G. M. Shepherd (Ed.), *The synaptic organization of the brain* (Chap. 9, pp. 279–316). Oxford: Oxford University Press.

Wilson, F. A. W., Scalaidhe, S. P. O., & Goldman-Rakic, P. S. (1993). Dissociation of object and spatial processing domains in primate prefrontal cortex. *Science*, *260*, 1955–1957.

Wolpert, D. H. (1996a). The existence of a priori distinctions between learning algorithms. *Neural Computation*, *8*, 1391–1420.

Wolpert, D. H. (1996b). The lack of a priori distinctions between learning algorithms. *Neural Computation*, *8*, 1341–1390.

Yang, C. R., & Seamans, J. K. (1996). Dopamine D1 receptor actions in layer V-VI rat prefrontal cortex neurons in vitro: Modulation of dendritic-somatic signal integration. *Journal of Neuroscience*, *16*, 1922.

Yonelinas, A. P. (1994). Receiver-operating characteristics in recognition memory: Evidence for a dual-process model. *Journal of Experimental Psychology: Learning, Memory, and Cognition*, *20*, 1341–1354.

Young, A. W., & Burton, A. M. (1999). Simulating face recognition: Implications for modelling cognition. *Cognitive Neuropsychology*, *16*, 1–48.

Zemel, R. S. (1993). *A minimum description length framework for unsupervised learning*. PhD thesis, University of Toronto, Canada.

Zemel, R. S., Behrmann, M., Mozer, M. C., & Bavelier, D. (submitted). Experience-dependent perceptual grouping and object-based attention. *Journal of Experimental Psychology: Human Perception and Performance*.

Zemel, R. S., Mozer, M. C., & Hinton, G. E. (1989). TRAFFIC: A model of object recognition based on transformations of feature instances. In D. S. Touretsky, G. E. Hinton, & T. J. Sejnowski (Eds.), *Proceedings of the 1988 Connectionist Models Summer School* (pp. 452–461). San Mateo, CA: Morgan Kaufmann.

Zemel, R. S., Williams, C. K., & Mozer, M. C. (1995). Lending direction to neural networks. *Neural Networks*, *8*, 503.

Zilles, K. (1990). Anatomy of the neocortex: Cytoarchitecture and myleoarchitecture. In B. Kolb, & R. C. Trees (Eds.), *The cerebral cortex of the rat* (pp. 77–112). Cambridge, MA: MIT Press.

Zipser, D., & Andersen, R. A. (1988). A backpropagation programmed network that simulates response properties of a subset of posterior parietal neurons. *Nature*, *331*, 679–684.

Zipser, D., Kehoe, B., Littlewort, G., & Fuster, J. (1993). A spiking network model of short-term active memory. *Journal of Neuroscience*, *13*, 3406–3420.

Author Index

Abbott, L. F. 9, 26, 48
Abgueguen, I. 314
Abu-Mostafa, Y. 100
Ackley, D. H. 106, 166
Aertsen, A. 376
Aggleton, J. P. 319
Ahmed, A. 314
Ajjanagadde, V. 219
Alexander, G. E. 305, 385
Alexander, M. P. 327
Alfonso-Reese, L. A. 392, 407, 410
Allport, A. 211, 257, 268, 423
Allport, D. A. 208, 358, 365
Alonso, J. M. 231
Alvarez, P. 297
Amaral, D. G. 287, 288
Amari, S. 9
Amit, D. J. 9
Amitai, Y. 45
Andersen, R. A. 9, 10, 233, 234
Anderson, J. A. 9, 20
Anderson, J. R. 5, 166, 217, 224, 318, 379, 383, 410
Apicella, P. 170, 194, 195, 307
Arbib, M. 214
Arbisi, P. 306
Arieli, A. 376
Armony, J. L. 212, 416
Artola, A. 117, 169
Asanuma, C. 73
Ashby, F. G. 392, 407, 410
Atick, J. J. 9
Atkins, P. 330, 342
Audinat, E. 306
Awh, E. 383

Baddeley, A. D. 217, 299, 383, 406, 408
Baillargeon, R. 314
Baker, S. C. 406
Balkin, T. J. 381
Ballard, D. H. 20, 168
Balota, D. A. 383, 392
Banich, M. T. 114
Baras, J. 310
Barch, D. M. 312
Barlow, H. B. 11, 95
Barnes, C. A. 288
Barnes, J. M. 282
Barone, P. 189
Bartlett, F. C. 373
Barto, A. G. 193, 199, 202
Bashir, Z. 117
Basso, G. 224
Bates, E. A. xxv, 20, 120, 314
Bavelier, D. 243
Bear, M. F. 10, 114, 117, 170
Bechara, A. 194, 406
Beck, L. H. 303
Becker, S. 168, 278, 282, 298, 422
Beeman, D. 38, 70
Behrmann, M. 234, 243, 260, 268, 273, 278, 282, 298
Beiser, D. G. 213
Bell, A. J. 145
Berger, T. 306
Berndt, R. S. 327
Besner, D. 347, 349
Bialek, W. xxv, 66
Bianchi, L. 405
Biederman, I. 219, 221, 242, 243, 256
Bienenstock, E. L. 120, 144

Bishop, C. M. 20
Blasdel, G. G. 232
Bliss, T. V. P. 10, 116
Bolton, J. S. 73
Bortolotto, Z. A. 117
Boser, B. 242, 243, 244
Boss, B. D. 288
Bouchard, J. P. 416
Bower, J. M. 5, 9, 38, 70
Bransome, E. D. 303
Braun, A. R. 381
Braver, T. S. 216, 300, 301, 305, 306, 312, 320, 379, 383, 385, 392, 404, 406, 420
Brayton, R. K. 45, 66
Breinlinger, K. 120
Brocher, S. 117, 169
Brown, L. L. 213
Brown, M. W. 319
Brown, R. G. 213
Brown, T. H. 10
Bryson, A. E. 9, 159
Buchtel, H. A. 404
Bullock, D. 214
Bülthoff, H. H. 242
Burger, L. K. 377
Burgess, N. 297, 298, 320
Burgess, P. 405, 407
Burgund, E. D. 242
Burton, A. M. 417
Butler, R. W. 405

Camperi, M. 310
Caramazza, A. 327, 358
Carnevale, N. T. 38, 45, 70
Carpenter, G. 145

Carpenter, P. A. 307
Carter, C. S. 406, 420
Cauller, L. 45
Changeux, J. P. 300, 407
Chappell, M. 321
Chauvin, Y. 172
Cheng, P. 380
Chervonenkis, A. 178
Chiodo, L. 306
Chomsky, N. 11
Churchland, P. S. 3, 20, 28, 74
Cleeremans, A. 189, 190, 192
Cohen, A. 20
Cohen, J. D. xxi, 189, 210, 212, 216,
  260, 264, 266, 268, 300, 301, 303, 305,
  306, 307, 312, 320, 375, 379, 381, 383,
  385, 386, 387, 391, 392, 404, 406, 408,
  416, 420, 422, 423
Cohen, N. J. 219, 283, 285, 321
Colby, C. L. 168, 234
Coles, M. G. H. 406, 420
Collingridge, G. L. 10
Coltheart, M. 330, 342
Connelly, A. 215, 297
Conners, B. W. 114
Connors, B. 45
Contreras-Vidal, J. L. 214
Cooper, E. E. 242, 256
Cooper, L. N. 144
Corkin, S. xx
Coslett, H. B. 265
Cottrell, G. W. 178
Cowan, W. M. 288
Crepel, F. 306
Crick, F. 230, 269
Crick, F. H. C. 9, 73, 172
Curtis, B. 330, 342

Dale, A. M. 273
Damasio, A. R. 194, 327, 377, 406
Damasio, H. 194, 327, 377, 406
Daneman, M. 307
Das, A. 240
Daugherty, K. 351
Davies, C. H. 117
Dayan, P. 10, 95, 145, 168, 170, 193,
  198, 308
de Sa, V. R. 168
Dehaene, S. 300, 407

Dell, G. S. 377
DeLong, M. R. 385
Denker, J. S. 242, 243, 244
Depue, R. A. 306
Desai, N. S. 42, 154
Desimone, R. 82, 182, 189, 211, 233,
  257, 268, 273, 305, 306, 310, 319, 321,
  403, 423
DeVos, J. 314
Diamond, A. 314, 385, 404
Dias, R. 393, 394, 395, 397, 399, 400,
  402, 404
DiCarlo, J. J. 297
Dilmore, J. G. 310
Dolan, R. J. 406
Donchin, E. 406, 420
Douglas, R. J. 98
Douglas, R. M. 404
Doursat, R. 120
Doyon, J. 416
Duda, R. O. 143
Duhamel, J. R. 168, 234
Dumais, S. T. 325, 359, 422
Dunbar, K. 210, 381, 385, 386, 387,
  388, 391, 392, 404, 423
Duncan, J. 211, 257, 260, 268, 272,
  273, 423

Edelman, G. 17, 95
Eichenbaum, H. 321
Elman, J. L. xxv, 20, 120, 187, 314,
  351, 367
Engel, A. K. 221
Erickson, C. A. 189, 305, 306, 310,
  321, 403
Erlarson, R. 100
Ermentrout, G. B. 48, 310
Erwin, E. 234, 239, 240
Essick, G. K. 233
Everitt, B. J. 393

Farah, M. J. xxi, 20, 223, 233, 260, 264,
  265, 266, 268, 273, 327, 343, 358, 359,
  365, 404, 407, 417, 418, 422
Faust, M. E. 392
Felleman, D. J. 166
Fellous, J. M. 310
Field, D. J. 11, 95, 125, 126, 234, 235,
  241, 421

Fiez, J. A. 383
Fiser, J. 220
Floreano, D. 168
Fodor, J. 217
Forman, S. D. 312
Fox, P. T. 213, 416
Frackowiak, R. S. J. 383, 406
Francis, W. N. 353
French, R. M. 283
Friedman, A. 45
Friedman, R. B. 332
Friedrich, F. J. xxi, 20, 258, 259, 260,
  264, 265, 422
Frith, C. D. 383, 406
Fromkin, V. 377
Fukushima, K. 242, 243, 422
Fuster, J. 300
Fuster, J. M. 189, 305, 311, 385, 403,
  404, 407, 410

Gadian, D. G. 215, 297
Galland, C. C. 166, 167
Gao, J. H. 213, 416
Garraghty, P. 240
Gathercole, S. E. 407
Gaudreau, D. 416
Gazzaniga, M. S. 419
Gehring, W. J. 406, 420
Gelade, G. 221
Gelatt, C. D. 109
Geman, S. 120
Gerfen, C. R. 194
Gerhardstein, P. C. 242
Gershberg, F. B. 320
Ghahramani, Z. 95
Gilbert, C. D. 240
Gillund, G. 318
Glaser, M. O. 386, 390, 392
Glaser, W. R. 386, 390, 392
Gluck, M. A. 297
Glushko, R. J. 347, 349
Goddard, N. H. 290, 293
Goldberg, M. E. 168, 234
Goldman-Rakic, P. S. 189, 305, 306,
  311, 314, 385, 395, 403, 404, 408
Goodale, M. A. 232, 273
Goss, B. 406, 420
Graber, M. 314
Grabowski, T. J. 327, 377

Graf, P. 278
Grafman, J. 224, 387, 406, 408
Gray, C. M. 221
Graybiel, A. M. 194
Greengard, P. 310
Grieve, K. L. 234
Grossberg, S. 9, 11, 85, 94, 105, 106, 145, 214
Guitton, D. 404
Gutfreund, H. 9
Gutkin, B. G. 310
Gutnick, M. 45

H. C. Hemmings, J. 310
Hager, L. D. 404
Haller, M. 330, 342
Hare, M. 351
Hart, P. E. 143
Hasselmo, M. E. 297, 298, 313
Haxby, J. V. 273
Hayes, T. L. 306
Hebb, D. O. 9, 116, 289
Henderson, D. 242, 243, 244
Heron, C. 404
Herscovitch, P. 381
Hertz, J. xxv, 20, 114, 125, 146
Hetherington, P. A. 283
Hill, J. M. 405
Hillis, A. E. 358
Hillyard, S. A. 168
Hines, M. L. 38, 70
Hinton, G. E. xxii, 9, 10, 58, 64, 83, 95, 106, 145, 154, 159, 162, 165, 166, 167, 168, 176, 182, 183, 187, 223, 241, 297, 420
Hintzman, D. L. 318
Ho, Y. C. 9, 159
Hochreiter, S. 216, 306, 309
Hodges, J. R. 377, 393
Hodgkin, A. L. 46
Hoeffner, J. H. 280, 351, 352, 356, 357
Hoff, M. E. 151
Hofstadter, M. C. 314
Hollander, M. 351
Holyoak, K. J. 219, 380
Hopfield, J. J. 9, 106
Houk, J. C. 213
Howard, R. E. 242, 243, 244
Hua, S. E. 213

Hubbard, W. 242, 243, 244
Hubel, D. 231
Huberman, B. A. 178
Hummel, J. E. 219, 221
Humphreys, G. W. 272
Husain, M. 260
Huston, T. A. 385, 392
Huxley, A. F. 46

Ikeda, J. 288
Inhoff, A. W. 20
Ivry, R. B. 419

Jaakkola, T. 10, 145
Jackel, L. D. 242, 243, 244
Jacobs, R. A. 176
Jacobson, K. 120
Jacoby, L. L. 279, 319
Jaffe, D. B. 45
Jennings, J. M. 319
Jessell, T. M. 30, 114, 211
Joanisse, M. F. xxi
Johnson, M. H. xxv, 20, 120, 314
Johnson, M. J. 315, 317
Johnson-Laird, P. 380
Johnston, D. 38, 67, 70
Jonides, J. 306, 383, 406
Joordens, S. 278, 282, 298, 422
Jordan, M. I. 10, 145, 176, 187, 189
Joseph, J. P. 189
Junque, C. 387

Kairiss, E. W. 10
Kalat, J. W. 114
Kandel, E. R. 30, 114, 211
Kandler, K. 240
Kanne, S. M. 392
Karmiloff-Smith, A. xxv, 20, 120, 314
Katz, L. C. 240
Katz, S. 383
Kawato, M. 214
Kay, J. 168
Keenan, C. L. 10
Kehoe, B. 300
Keith, J. R. 118
Keller, J. B. 9, 144, 146, 236, 415
Kimberg, D. Y. 404, 407
Kinsbourne, M. 218, 419
Kintsch, W. 377
Kirkpatrick, S. 109

Kitai, S. T. 310
Koch, C. 230
Koechlin, E. 224
Koeppe, R. A. 383
Kohonen, T. 9, 11, 94, 105, 143, 146, 236
Konig, P. 221
Kortge, C. A. 283
Kosslyn, S. M. 20
Kreiter, A. K. 221
Krogh, A. xxv, 20, 114, 125, 146
Kubota, K. 305
Kučera, H. 353

LaBerge, D. 230, 269
Landauer, T. K. 325, 359, 422
LeCun, Y. 242, 243, 244
Lecuyer, R. 314
LeDoux, J. E. 212, 416
Legrenzi, M. S. 380
Legrenzi, P. 380
Leinbach, J. 351
Lemarie, C. 314
LeMasson, G. 9
Lenat, D. B. 209
Leon, A. 306
Leonard, B. W. 288
Levine, D. S. 407
Levitt, J. B. 305, 385
Levy, W. B. 297, 298
Lewis, D. A. 305, 306, 385
Lhermitte, F. 405
Lidsky, T. I. 213
Lin, L.-H. 288
Linsker, R. 9, 144, 146
Lisman, J. 117
Lisman, J. E. 117, 310
Littlewort, G. 300
Livingstone, M. 231
Ljungberg, T. 170, 194, 195, 307
Logothetis, N. K. 273
Lomo, T. 116
Lowe, D. G. 256
Luciana, M. 306
Lund, J. S. 305, 306, 385

MacDonald, M. C. 367
MacLeod, C. M. 385, 387, 388
Macomber, J. 120
MacWhinney, B. 351

Maginu, K. 9
Majani, E. 100
Malach, R. 273
Malenka, R. C. 31, 117, 170
Mandler, G. 278
Mangun, G. R. 419
Manning, F. J. 395
Marchman, V. A. 351
Marcus, G. F. 351, 420
Marr, D. 4, 20, 119, 241, 289, 291, 298
Marsden, C. D. 213
Marsolek, C. J. 242
Martin, K. A. C. 98
Mathis, D. A. 218, 419
Matthews, A. 314
Maunsell, J. H. R. 182
Maylor, E. 267
Mazzoni, P. 10
McCann, R. S. 347, 349
McCarthy, R. 358
McClelland, J. L. xxiii, 9, 10, 11, 14,
   17, 58, 64, 83, 90, 94, 106, 162, 167,
   178, 189, 190, 192, 210, 215, 219, 223,
   278, 280, 282, 286, 287, 290, 291, 292,
   293, 295, 315, 317, 318, 321, 324, 325,
   327, 328, 330, 331, 341, 342, 344, 347,
   351, 358, 359, 365, 366, 367, 368, 381,
   385, 386, 391, 392, 404, 417, 423
McCleod, P. 20
McCloskey, M. 219, 283, 285, 417
McCulloch, W. S. 8
McNaughton, B. L. 94, 215, 219, 286,
   287, 288, 289, 290, 297, 298, 417, 423
McRae, K. 283
Mel, B. A. 220
Meyer, D. E. 406, 420
Miikkulainen, R. 297, 298
Miles, R. 9
Miller, E. K. 189, 305, 306, 310, 319,
   321, 403
Miller, G. A. 222
Miller, K. D. 9, 144, 146, 236, 415
Milner, A. D. 232, 273
Milner, B. 405
Minsky, M. L. 9, 115, 158, 297
Mirsky, A. F. 303
Mishkin, M. 208, 215, 232, 233, 297,
   395
Miyake, A. 307, 383, 385

Mizumori, S. J. Y. 288
Moll, M. 297, 298
Montague, P. R. 170, 193, 308
Mood Edley, S. 194
Moran, J. 268
Mori, K. 288
Morris, R. G. M. 94, 289
Moscovitch, M. 278, 282, 298
Motter, B. C. 268
Movellan, J. R. 166, 280
Mozer, M. 383, 385
Mozer, M. C. 202, 218, 221, 241, 242,
   243, 260, 268, 272, 273, 419
Munakata, Y. 314, 315, 317, 381, 383,
   385, 404, 423
Munro, P. W. 144
Myers, C. E. 297

Nadel, L. 276, 289, 297
Narin, A. C. 310
Neal, R. N. 10, 145, 168
Nelson, S. B. 48
Neumann, E. 392
Newcombe, F. 405
Newell, A. 8, 11, 217, 379, 383, 410
Newsome, W. T. 47, 182
Nicoll, R. A. 31
Niki, H. 305
Noelle, D. 392
Noelle, D. C. 178
Noll, D. C. 306, 312, 383, 406
Norman, K. A. 287, 290, 295, 318, 319
Nowlan, S. J. 105, 143, 176
Nystrom, L. E. 306, 312, 383, 406

Obermayer, K. 234, 239, 240
Oeth, K. M. 306
Oja, E. 124, 125
Oka, S. 288
O'Keefe, J. 276, 297, 298
Olshausen, B. A. 11, 125, 126, 234,
   235, 241, 421
O'Reilly, R. C. xxi, 10, 11, 109, 158,
   162, 165, 166, 168, 172, 177, 178, 181,
   182, 183, 184, 202, 215, 216, 219, 233,
   269, 280, 286, 287, 290, 291, 292, 295,
   297, 301, 305, 306, 318, 320, 321, 351,
   356, 357, 379, 383, 385, 392, 404, 406,
   408, 417, 418, 423

Owen, A. M. 393, 406

Palmer, R. G. xxv, 20, 114, 125, 146
Papert, S. A. 9, 115, 158, 297
Paradiso, M. A. 114
Parisi, D. xxv, 20, 120, 314
Parker, D. B. 9, 159
Parsons, L. M. 213, 416
Patterson, K. 377
Patterson, K. E. 14, 324, 328, 330, 331,
   341, 342, 417
Paulesu, E. 383
Pearlmutter, B. A. 187
Pearlmutter, N. J. 367
Peng, J. 187
Penit-Soria, J. 306
Pennington, B. F. 330
Perlstein, W. M. 306, 406
Petersen, S. E. 383
Peterson, C. 166
Peterson, G. M. 288
Peterson, M. 243
Petrides, M. E. 385, 395, 406, 408
Phillips, W. 168
Piaget, J. 314
Picton, T. W. 168
Pinker, S. xx, 330, 331, 351, 420
Pitts, W. 8
Plaut, D. C. xxii, 14, 178, 324, 328,
   330, 331, 332, 333, 334, 338, 340, 341,
   342, 377, 417
Plunkett, K. xxv, 20, 120, 314, 351
Polkey, C. E. 393
Posner, M. I. xxi, 17, 20, 258, 259, 260,
   264, 265, 422
Prince, A. 351, 420
Prueitt, P. S. 407

Rafal, R. D. xxi, 258, 259, 260, 264,
   265, 422
Ragsdale, C. W. 194
Raichle, M. E. 383
Raife, E. A. 383
Rakic, P. 114
Rao, S. G. 305, 385
Rastle, K. 330
Reber, A. S. 189, 190
Recce, M. 297, 298
Redlich, A. N. 9
Reid, R. C. 231

Reike, F. xxv, 66
Rescorla, R. A. 151
Reznick, J. S. 314
Rissanen, J. 144
Robbins, T. W. 393, 394, 395, 397, 399, 400, 402, 404, 406
Roberts, A. C. 393, 394, 395, 397, 399, 400, 402, 404
Roberts, B. R. 392
Roberts, R. J. 404
Rodman, R. 377
Roe, A. W. 240
Rogers, R. D. 406
Rolls, E. T. 20, 297, 298
Romero, R. D. xxi, 260, 264, 266, 268, 422
Romo, R. 194
Rorsman, I. 405
Rosch, E. 16
Rosen, J. T. 351
Rosenblatt, F. 9
Rosenfeld, E. 20
Rosson, M. B. 341
Rosvold, H. E. 303
Rudy, J. W. 118, 158, 287, 292, 297, 321, 423
Ruffman, T. 314
Rumelhart, D. E. 9, 11, 17, 83, 90, 94, 105, 106, 128, 143, 159, 172, 178, 187, 223, 278, 282, 283, 297, 351
Rutherford, L. C. 42, 154

Saffran, E. 265
Saffran, E. M. 208, 327, 377
Sakmann, B. 45
Salama, G. 232
Samsonovich, A. 297, 298
Sanger, T. D. 125
Sarason, I. 303
Saul, L. K. 10, 145
Sawaguchi, T. 306
Scalaidhe, S. P. O. 395
Scarnati, E. 194
Schacter, D. 319
Schacter, D. L. 278, 318, 321
Schillen, T. B. 221
Schmajuk, N. A. 297
Schmidhuber, J. 216, 306, 309
Schneider, J. S. 213

Schneider, W. 217, 381, 407
Schooler, C. 392
Schulten, K. 234, 239, 240
Schultz, W. 170, 193, 194, 195, 307, 308
Schumacher, E. H. 383
Schwartz, F. F. 208, 377
Schwartz, J. H. 30, 114, 211
Schwarz, J. P. 383
Schweighofer, N. 214
Seamans, J. K. 310
Seidenberg, M. 11, 417
Seidenberg, M. S. xxi, 14, 324, 328, 330, 331, 341, 342, 351, 367, 417
Sejnowski, T. J. 20, 28, 58, 64, 74, 106, 145, 166, 170, 193, 308
Sen, K. 48
Sereno, M. I. 273
Seress 293
Servan-Schreiber, D. xxi, 189, 190, 192, 212, 260, 264, 266, 268, 300, 303, 306, 307, 312, 375, 385, 387, 391, 416, 422
Shadlen, M. N. 47
Shah, P. 307
Shallice, T. xxii, 20, 327, 330, 332, 333, 334, 338, 340, 341, 358, 375, 377, 405, 406, 407, 410
Shastri, L. 219
Shatz, C. J. 415
Sheinberg, D. L. 273
Shepherd, G. M. 9, 45, 66
Sherman, S. M. 230
Shiffrin, R. M. 217, 318, 381, 407
Shimamura, A. P. 287, 288, 320
Siegel, R. M. 233
Siegler, R. S. 315, 317
Simon, H. A. 8, 379, 410
Singer, W. 117, 169, 221
Singley, K. 224
Sitton, M. 268, 272, 273
Sloman, S. A. 283
Smith, E. E. 306, 383, 406
Smolensky, P. 107, 219
Snow, C. 351
Snyder, L. H. 234
Sompolinsky, H. 9
Spelke, E. 120
Squire, L. R. 276, 278, 287, 288, 297,

318, 321
St. John, M. F. 325, 366, 367, 368
Stanfield, B. B. 288
Stein, J. 260
Steingard, S. 303, 312
Sterkin, A. 376
Stone, G. O. 330
Strick, P. L. 385
Stroop, J. R. 385
Stryker, M. P. 9, 144, 146, 236, 415
Stuart, G. 45
Summers, B. A. 393
Sur, M. 240
Surmeier, D. J. 310
Sutherland, R. J. 158, 297
Sutherland, R. W. 297
Sutton, R. S. 193, 195, 199, 202, 308
Suzuki, W. A. 288
Svec, W. R. 377
Swindale, N. V. 234, 239, 240

Tamamaki, N. 288
Tanaka, K. 82, 83, 233, 241, 242, 246, 273
Taraban, R. 344, 347
Tarr, M. J. 242
Teitelbaum, P. 3
Tipper, S. P. 234, 273
Tootell, R. B. H. 273
Touretzky, D. S. 219
Tranel, D. 194, 406
Traub, R. D. 9
Treisman, A. 272
Treisman, A. M. 221
Treves, A. 297, 298
Tulving, E. 276, 289, 318
Tuma, R. 405
Turlejski, K. 288
Turrigiano, G. G. 42, 154
Tyler, L. K. 377

Ullman, M. 351
Ullman, M. T. xx
Ullman, S. 145
Underwood, B. J. 282
Ungerleider, L. G. 82, 182, 208, 232, 233, 273
Usher, M. 392

Van Essen, D. C. 166, 182

Van Orden, G. C. 330
Van Paesschen, W. 215, 297
van Steveninck, R. xxv, 66
Vapnik, V. N. 178
Varela, J. A. 48
Vargha-Khadem, F. 215, 297
Vecchi, M. P. 109
Vecera, S. P. xxi, 109, 233, 260, 268
Vendrell, P. 387
von der Malsburg, C. 105, 106, 236

Wager, T. D. 269
Wagner, A. R. 151
Waldron, E. M. 392, 407, 410
Walker, J. A. xxi, 258, 259, 260, 264, 265, 422
Wang, X. J. 310
Warland, D. xxv, 66
Warrington, E. K. 358

Watanabe, Y. 288
Watkins, K. E. 215, 297
Weigend, A. S. 178
Weliky, M. 240
Werbos, P. 9, 159
White, E. L. 72, 73, 95, 114, 166
White, H. 215, 417
Wickelgren, W. A. 220, 342
Wickens, J. 213
Widrow, B. 151
Wiesel, T. N. 231
Williams, C. K. 221
Williams, C. K. I. 260, 268
Williams, G. V. 305, 306, 385
Williams, M. S. 306
Williams, R. J. 9, 159, 187, 297
Willshaw, D. J. 9
Wilson, C. J. 194

Wilson, F. A. W. 395
Witherspoon, D. 279
Wolpert, D. H. 120, 178
Wu, S. M. 38, 67, 70
Wyble, B. 297, 298, 313

Xu, F. 351

Yang, C. R. 310
Yonelinas, A. P. 319
Yoshioka, T. 305, 385
Young, A. W. 417

Zemel, R. S. 10, 95, 144, 145, 168, 221, 241, 243, 260, 268
Zilles, K. 73, 95
Zipser, D. 9, 11, 94, 105, 128, 143, 187, 234, 300

Subject Index

A-not-B task, 314–318, 392, 404
    exploration, 315–317
Abstraction, 224, 385
Accessibility, 381
Accommodation, 66–69, 112
    channel, 36
act, 46, 50, 55, 459
act_avg, 285, 459
act_dif, 459
act_eq, 46, 50, 53, 459
act_fun, 51, 53, 460
act_gain, 46, 460
act_m, 156, 157, 459
act_p, 156, 157, 191, 459
Action potential, see Spike
Actions, 195–197, 307, 405
Activation, 24
    based processing, 380–384,
        392–395
        see also Active memory, Frontal
        cortex
    equilibrium, 56
    expected level (alpha), 43
    function, 24, 40–42, 45–48
        derivative, 160, 163, 164
        exploration, 49–54
    graded, 15
    in learning, 125
    in memory, see Active memory
    linear, 54, 152, 154
    phases, 156–157, 162–163,
        167–170, 177, 198–199, 310
    point neuron, 24, 38, 154
    rate coded, 46–48
    residual, 262, 263, 267, 298, 299

sigmoid, logistic, 40, 42, 47, 48,
        134, 154, 155
    spreading, 216, 278, 300, 312
    variable, see act
Activation based receptive field,
        247–250
Active memory, 206, 210, 212,
        214–217, 222, 223, 276, 277,
        299–314, 320, 403
    control, gating, 188–189, 277,
        306–313, 382, 385, 392, 395,
        406
    exploration, 301–305, 310–312
    noise, 302–303
    representations, 382–383, 395
    resetting, 311
    updating, 303–313
    see also Activation-based
        processing, Frontal cortex,
        Sequence learning
Actor, see Temporal differences learning
        (TD)
Adaptive critic (AC), see Temporal
        differences learning (TD)
Aggregation, of statistics, 432, 447
Agnosia, 233, 265
Alexia, see Dyslexia
Algorithm, 115
    backpropagation, see
        Backpropagation
    BCM, 144–145
    Boltzmann machine, 106, 166
    CHL, 165–166, 168
    clustering, 143
    competitive learning, 143

CPCA, see Conditional PCA
DBM, 165–166, 168
delta rule, see Delta rule
generative models, 145
GeneRec, see GeneRec
GRAIN, 10
Hebbian, see Hebbian learning
Hopfield network, 106
IAC, 106
ICA, 145
Infomax, 144
Kohonen, 143
kWTA, see k-Winners-take-all
level of analysis, 4
MDL, 144
mean field learning, 166
Oja, 124–125, 128
PCA, see Principal components
        analysis
recirculation, 162, 163
RL, see Reinforcement learning
SRN, see Sequence learning
TD, see Temporal differences
        learning
Winner-take-all (WTA), 105, 143,
        176
Alpha, α (expected activity level), 43,
        133–135
alpha_k, 43
Alternative uses task, 405
Ambiguous stimuli, 17, 92, 109, 111,
        158, 189, 192, 279, 297, 368,
        369, 373
Amnesia, 289–290
AMPA, 31

Amplification, 85, 89–92, 210
    exploration, 89–92
Amygdala, 212, 416
Annealing schedule, 109
Answer key, 20
Anti-saccade task, 404
Aphasia, 326–327
Apply button, 50, 430
Artificial intelligence, 4
Artificial neural networks (ANNs), 40
Associative
    learning, 11
    LTP/D, 115–118, 129–130,
        168–170, 175
Attention, 17, 211, 227–228, 257–272,
        407
    exploration, 261–272
    object-based, 227, 260, 267–268,
        272
    spatial, 221, 227, 234, 257–272
    thalamic, 212, 230, 269
Attractor, 86, 92–93, 108, 111, 210, 333
    basin, 86, 300, 303
    effects on generalization, 178, 180
    in active memory, 299
    in learning, 170
    in priming, 352
Automatic processing, 214, 217–218,
        381, 385–387, 408–409
Axon, 27, 29

Bálint's syndrome, 260
    exploration, 265–266, 271
Backpropagation, 9, 147, 158–162, 184,
        192
    biological implausibility, 9, 162,
        164
    derivation, 160–161
    learning rule, 159
    temporal, 196
    see also Task learning,
        Error-driven learning,
        Backpropagation, GeneRec
Basal ganglia, 72, 193–195, 213–214,
        307, 310, 382, 385
    Parkinson's disease, 213, 385, 393
Basin of attractor, 86, 300, 303
Basis functions, 16
Basket neuron, 72

Batch run, 140
Bayes formula, 61
Bayesian analysis, 10, 58–65
BCM algorithm, 144–145
Belief (probability), 59
β, see bias.wt
Bias
    in learning, 118–121, 134,
        175–178, 180–182, 184, 192
    input, 42, 44
    input in kWTA, 101
    weights, 42, 44, 80–81
        learning, 152–155, 159, 163
        variable, see bias.wt
Bias-variance dilemma, 120
bias.wt, 44, 157, 459
Bidirectional connectivity, 17, 72,
        85–93, 145, 177, 210, 288,
        329
    and parallel processing, 331
    attractors, 352
    effects on generalization, 178, 180
    in active memory, 215, 299,
        303–306, 308, 310, 314, 315,
        317
    in attention, 211, 268
    in error-driven learning, 163,
        166–167
    in pattern completion, 290
    see also Lateral connectivity
Binarization, 81
Binding
    hippocampal, 276, 289, 297,
        408–409
    problem, 220–222, 242–243, 255,
        269
Binding problem, 403
Biology
    basis of cognition, 3, 6, 9, 177, 379
    conditioning, 193–195
    cortex, 72–75
    detailed models, 5, 9–10
    frontal cortex, 305–306, 384–385
    hippocampus, 287–289
    implausibility of backpropagation,
        9, 162, 164
    language, 325–327
    learning, 115–118, 129–130,
        168–170, 175

    level of analysis, 6
    neurons, see Neuron
    visual system, 228–234
Blending in one-to-many mappings,
        190, 191, 279, 280, 298
Blobs, 231–232
Boltzmann machine, 106, 166
    deterministic (DBM), 165–166,
        168
Bootstrapping, 16, 18, 84, 89–93, 210
    exploration, 89–92
Bottom-up
    approach, 5–6
    processing, 17, 75–85, 162
Brain damage, 12
    agnosia, 233
    aphasia, 326–327
    basal ganglia, 385
    comparing patient and normal
        data, 264–265
    dyslexia, see Dyslexia
    frontal cortex, 189, 194, 305, 314,
        320, 375, 381, 391, 393–395,
        399, 401, 403–408
    generalized effects of, 264–265
    hippocampus, 278, 289–290, 297
    inferotemporal cortex, 233
    parietal, 233–234, 258, 260,
        264–266
    Parkinson's disease, 213, 385, 393
    schizophrenia, 306, 387, 391
    semantic deficits, 358–359
Broca's area, 326–327
Button (PDP++), 429
    Apply, 50, 430
    Cancel, 52, 430
    Clear, 51
    Init, 51
    NewInit, 58, 150
    Ok, 430
    ReInit, 58
    Revert, 50, 430
    Run, 50, 58
    Step, 56, 58
Button, synaptic, 29

Cable properties, 27
Calcium, 31, 32, 35, 36, 45
    in learning, 116

Cancel button, 52, 430

Canonical representations, 209, 223, 241–242, 317

Catastrophic interference, 219, 276, 283–285

Categories, 15, 76, 405

Categorization, dynamic, 380–381, 392–403, 407

Cell assembly, 8

Center surround receptive field, 229–230

Central processing unit (CPU), 24

Cerebellum, 213, 214, 416

Chain rule, 152, 158

Chandelier neuron, 72

Channels, 27
  accommodation, 36
  current equation, 37
  excitatory, 35, 37, 39
  inhibitory, 36, 37, 39
  leak, 36, 37, 39
  NMDA, 36
  voltage-gated, 28, 35, 36

Charge, 32

Chloride, 32, 35, 36, 45

Cingulate cortex, 212, 384, 406, 420

Clamping inputs, 56, 86

Cleanup, 333

Clear button, 51

Cluster plot, 77–79, 81–82, 84–85, 185, 192, 334, 362–363, 373–375

Clustering algorithms, 143

cnt_sum_se, 179

Coarse coding, 16, 82, 231

Cognitive
  architecture, 205, 214–219, 408–409
  level of analysis, 6
  neuroscience, 1
  psychology, 4, 8
  science, 4

Combinatorial representations, 139, 178, 342

Competition, 11, 17–18, 94–95, 139, 177, 352, 357, 404
  in attention, 17, 268
  in learning, 137, 143, 175–176, 180, 184, 192
  see also Inhibition, k-Winners-take-all (kWTA)

Competitive learning, 105, 143

Complete serial compound (CSC), 199, 200, 202, 309

Completion, pattern, 85, 87–89, 93, 210, 290, 292, 296, 297, 319, 333

Complexity, 4, 12, 13, 417–418, 422–423

Computational
  cognitive neuroscience, 1, 8–10
  level of analysis, 4
  modeling
    challenges, 13–14, 413–421
    contributions, 3–4, 12–13, 421–424

compute_i, 464

Computer metaphor, 4, 8, 15, 18, 24–25, 209, 217–218, 223, 324
  see also Production systems, Symbolic models

Concentration gradient, 34

Conditional PCA (CPCA), 116, 125–137, 143–145, 147–150, 155, 168, 171, 176–178, 181
  biology, 129–130, 175
  derivation, 128–129
  exploration, 130–132
  learning rule, 127, 128
  vs. PCA, 128, 131
  see also Model learning, Hebbian learning, Principal components analysis (PCA)

Conditional probability, 60, 129
  as correlation, 128, 133

Conditioning, 193–195
  exploration, 199–202
  second order, 195, 201
  see also Reinforcement learning, Temporal differences learning (TD)

Conductance, 33

Cones, 228

Conflict, 406

Conjunctive representations, 220–221, 223, 276, 291–292, 297, 342–343, 345, 347

Connection, 431, 438, 456

Connectionism, 9

Connectivity
  bidirectional, see Bidirectional

connectivity
  feedforward, 75–85
  lateral, see Lateral connectivity
  unidirectional, 75–85
  wrap-around, 236

Consciousness, 14–15, 18, 218–219, 381, 418, 419

Consolidation of memories, 289–290

Consonants, 328–329

ConSpec, 430, 431, 438, 440, 457

Constraint satisfaction, 16, 72, 106–112, 145, 151, 210, 268, 367, 375–376
  exploration, 110–112

Content-specific
  processing, 209–210
  representations, 25, 209–210, 219–224, 324, 325, 380

Context, 187, 284, 307
  for sequences, see Sequence learning
  internal, 210
  sensitivity, 24

Continua, 16
  in time, 186–187

Continuous performance tasks (CPT), 303, 304, 312

Contrast enhancement
  retinal, 228
  weights, 132–137, 139, 141, 150

Contrastive Hebbian learning (CHL), 165–166, 168
  see also GeneRec

Control
  of active memory, 188–189, 277, 306–313, 382, 385, 392, 395, 406
  of processing, 206, 214, 217–218, 381–382, 385–387, 403, 405–406, 408–409

Control panel, 49, 429, 430, 450–452
  process, 58, 432

Controlled processing, 206, 214, 217–218, 381–382, 385–387, 403, 405–406, 408–409
  see also Frontal cortex, Active memory control

Convolution, 47

Cooperation, 95

Correlations, 121–124, 138, 234–235, 238, 240
  matrix, 123
Cortex, 20, 71–75, 416
  areas, 72, 74
  cingulate, 212, 384, 406, 420
  frontal, *see* Frontal cortex
  functional layers, 72–75
  in memory, 276–287, 298–303
  inferotemporal, 232, 233, 241, 245, 305
  lobes, 211–212, 228
  neuron
    tuning curves, 82
    types, 72
  occipital, 212, 214, 228, 230, 326, 327
  parietal, *see* Parietal cortex
  posterior, 205, 206, 214–217, 222, 276, 277, 381, 383, 405
  prefrontal, *see* Frontal cortex
  six-layered structure, 72–75
  specializations, 211–212, 214–217
  temporal, 212, 214, 228, 326, 327
  unity of, 72, 276, 277
Cosine distance measure, 337
Credit assignment, 151
  temporal, 193
Cross entropy error (CE), 154–155, 160, 161, 196
CSS (script language), 429, 442–446, 448–452
Cued recall, 88, 290, 292, 319
Cumulative research, 14, 419
Current, 32, 34, 37
Cycles, 46, 50, 56

da, 56, 459, 465
Dead units, 140
Decision making, 379
  see also Higher-level cognition
Declarative representations, 218–219, 276, 381
Dedicated
  processing, 209–210
  representations, 25, 209–210, 219–224, 324, 325, 380
Deep dyslexia, 331–341
Deep networks, 181–186

exploration, 183–186
Degradation, graceful, 16
Delayed response task, 305
delta, δ, 159–165, 196–198, 309
Delta rule, 147, 150–158
  derivation, 152
  generalized, *see* Backpropagation
  learning rule, 151
  vs. temporal differences learning, 199
  see also Task learning, Error-driven learning, Backpropagation, GeneRec
Dendrites, 26, 31–32
  spine, 29
  tree, 42, 45
  voltage-gated channels, 45
Depolarization, 35
Depression, synaptic, 115–118, 129–130, 168–170, 175
Derivative, 38, 151–152, 160
  chain rule, 152, 158
  implicit, 163, 164
Descriptive theories, 11, 417
Detector, 23–27, 54–58, 69, 207
  as hypothesis testing, 58–65
  exploration, 54–58
  function vs. content, 24
  multiple roles, 84
  threshold, 26
Deterministic Boltzmann machine (DBM), 165–166, 168
  see also GeneRec
Deterministic processing, 47, 53, 166
Development, 18, 120, 314–315, 317, 382
Difference of Gaussians, 229
Diffusion, 27, 33–34
Digit recognition, 54–58, 76–85
Discounting of future rewards, 195
Discrete representations, 14, 383
Disengage deficit, 260, 264–266, 268, 317
Distance matrix, 77
Distinctions, emphasizing and deemphasizing, 73, 75–79, 81–82, 207, 227–228, 241–256
Distributed representations, 9, 11,

82–85, 90–92, 143, 177, 214, 216, 219–220, 223, 224, 227, 325, 366–367, 375
  combinatorial, 139, 178, 342
  exploration, 84–85, 90–92
  large scale, 208–209
  lexicon, 323–325, 329
  processing and memory, 206
  semantics, 358–360, 362, 364, 365
  see also Sparse distributed representations
div_gp_n, 43, 458
DNA, 18
Dopamine, 117, 193–195, 214, 306–310, 387, 396
Dot product distance measure, 337
Dreams, 381
Driving potential, 34
dt_net, 44, 461
dt_vm, 37, 45, 391, 461
dur, 46, 460
dwt, 123, 456
Dynamic categorization, 380–381, 392–403, 407
  exploration, 397–402
Dynamic principles, 206, 210–211
Dynamic range, 132
Dyslexia, 324, 326, 331–341
  deep, 331–341
  exploration, 335–341
  phonological, 331–333, 340
  surface, 331–333, 335–336, 338–339

e_rev, 45, 50, 52, 461
Edge detectors, 230–232, 234–235, 238–240, 245
Edit dialogs, 50, 429
Effective weight value, 134
Eigenvector, 124
Electricity, 32–33
Electrophysiology, 27, 32–40
  recording, 305, 384, 403
Emergent phenomena, 3–4, 14, 40, 211, 218–219, 257, 325, 382, 384, 419
  see also Reconstructionism
Encoding, memory, 290
End stopping, 245

Energy function, 106–107
Entropy, 108, 154
`Environment`, 55, 428, 431–432, 440, 441, 448–450
  `ScriptEnv`, 191
Environment, regularities, structure, 118, 324, 330–331, 341–342, 349–358, 420–421
Environmental dependency syndrome, 405
`EnviroView`, 55, 428, 431
Epilepsy, 89, 99
Episodic memory, 212, 276, 289, 297
Epoch, 131, 139, 428
`EpochProcess`, 428, 432, 441, 446, 448, 465
Epsilon (ϵ), see `lrate`
EPSP, 31
`eq_gain`, 46, 460
Equilibrium
  activations, 56
  membrane potential, 38–40, 65
  potential, 34
  weight, 124, 129
`err`, 176, 457
Error
  cross entropy (CE), 154–155, 160, 161, 196
  delta, δ, 159–165, 196–198, 309
  measure, 149, 154, 179, 191, 196
  minimizing, 151–152
  signals, 8, 147–148, 162–163, 165, 167–168, 406, 420
    see also Phases of error-driven learning
  summed squared (SSE), 149–151, 160, 196
Error-driven learning, 116, 147–172, 176–178, 297
  limitations, 157, 173–175, 182, 184
  vs. Hebbian, 173–175
    see also Task learning, Delta rule, Backpropagation, GeneRec
Euclidean distance, 77
`Event`, 55, 428, 431
Event related potentials (ERP), 168
`EventSpec`, 428, 431
Evolution, 17, 94–95, 119, 120, 166, 326

Exceptions, 324, 330–331, 341–342, 349–358
  regularities in, 331, 341
Excitation, 31
  and inhibition, separation, 32, 41
  inputs, 31, 65
  net input, 41–45
  synaptic input channel, 35, 37, 39
Excitatory neuron, 32, 41, 72
Executive control, 206, 214, 217–218, 381–382, 385–387, 403, 405–406, 408–409
Exiting from simulation, 54
Expectation
  in infant testing, 314–316
  in learning, 156, 167–168
    see also Phases of error-driven learning
Explanatory theories, 11, 417
Explicit representations, 189, 218–219
Explorations, 1, 20
  installing, 427
    see also Projects
`ext`, 86, 459
External input, 86
Extinction
  in attention, 266
  in conditioning, 193, 201
Extracellular space, 35

Familiarity, 282, 319
Family trees task, 182–186
Fatigue, neural, 66–69, 112
Feature-based representations, see Distributed representations
Feedback inhibition, 93–100
Feedforward
  connectivity, 75–85
  inhibition, 93–100
Feedforward connectivity, 72
Fick's first law, 34
Finite state automaton (FSA), 189–193
Flexibility, 380, 403–404
  vs. specialization, 209, 219
Fluency, 403, 405
`fm_hid`, 188
`fm_prv`, 188
fMRI, 1, 208, 306, 312, 325, 384, 419
Fovea, 228, 231

Fractal, 7, 8, 208, 416
Free energy, 108
Free recall, 319
Frequency-based probabilities, 60
Frontal cortex, 14, 193–195, 205, 206, 212, 214–218, 222, 223, 277, 300, 305–314, 319, 320, 325, 381–392, 408–409
  biology, 305–306, 384–385
  context representations, 189, 307
  damage, 189, 194, 305, 314, 320, 375, 381, 391, 393–395, 399, 401, 403–408
  exploration, 310–312, 315–317, 388–391, 397–402
  in language, 326, 327
  in memory, see Active memory
  in sequences, 189
  representations, 382–383, 395
    see also Sequence learning

`g_bar`, 45, 50–53, 461
GABA, 31, 72
Gain
  activation, 46, 48, 92, 387
  weight, 134–135
Ganglion retinal neurons, 229
Gating, 188–189, 277, 306–313, 382, 385, 392, 395, 406
Gaze, 314–316
Generalization, 83, 178–181, 224, 243, 255–256, 324, 340, 342, 347–349, 375, 420–421
  and simplicity, 120
  exploration, 179–181
  of invariance mapping, 254
  statistic, 180
Generalized delta rule, see Backpropagation
Generative models, 145
Generativity, 224
GeneRec, 10, 148, 162–171, 176–178
  biology, 166–170, 175
  derivation, 163–165
  exploration, 170–171
  learning rule, 163
  phases, 156–157, 162–163, 167–170, 177, 198–199, 310
  relation CHL, DBM, 165–166

see also Task learning,
    Error-driven learning,
    Backpropagation,
    Recirculation
Genetic constraints, 18, 119, 177, 314,
    326
Geons, 256
Global maxima/minima, 108
Glutamate, 31, 35, 72
    metabotropic receptors, 117
Goals, 380–383, 403, 405–407
Goodness, 108
Graceful degradation, 16, 66
Gradedness, 15–16, 66, 317
    in learning, 18
Gradient descent, 151–152
    see also Error-driven learning,
        Task learning, Delta rule,
        Backpropagation, GeneRec
GRAIN model, 10
Grammar, 186, 366
    finite state, Reber, 189–193
    see also Syntax
Grandmother cell, 82
GraphLog, 50, 56, 429, 433, 442
    clearing, 51
    number viewing, 50
GridLog, 80, 82, 86, 91, 316, 429,
    433, 446

Hard clamping, 88
Harmony, 107–112
hebb, 176, 179, 183, 286, 457
Hebbian learning, 8, 9, 11, 115–150,
    157, 171, 176–178, 181, 184,
    192, 290, 316, 352
    exploration, 130–132
    limitations, 149–150, 173–175,
        184
    normalization, 124–125, 128
    vs. error-driven, 173–175
    see also Model learning, Principal
        components analysis (PCA),
        Conditional PCA
Hemispatial neglect, 233–234, 260,
    264–266
    exploration, 264–266
Heterarchical representations, 125–127
Hidden

cortical area, 74
layer, 72–75
    in learning, 158
    see also Transformations
layers, multiple, 181–186
Hierarchical representations, 125–127,
    206–210, 212, 227, 242–256,
    343
    exploration, 246–255
    of goals, 382
Higher-level association areas, 208
Higher-level cognition, 313, 379–410,
    421
Higher-order representations, 302–303
Hippocampus, 14, 205, 206, 212,
    214–217, 219, 223, 276–277,
    287–298, 318–320, 325
    binding, 276, 289, 297, 408–409
    biology, 287–289
    damage, 278, 289–290, 297
    exploration, 293–296
    role in spatial memory, 276, 297
Homunculus, 12, 217, 240, 307, 317,
    382
Hopfield networks, 106
Hypercolumn, 232, 236
Hypothesis testing, 58
    in learning, 18
    null hypothesis, 46
Hysteresis, 66–69, 198

I_net, 37, 50, 459
Iconifying windows, 50
ID/ED task, 393–403
    exploration, 397–402
    see also Dynamic categorization,
        Wisconsin card sorting task
        (WCST)
Ill-posed problems, 118
Imagery, 85
Imaging, 1, 208, 306, 312, 325, 384, 419
Implementational level of analysis, 4
Implicit
    expectations, 167–168
    learning, 189–190
    representations, 218–219
Independent components analysis
    (ICA), 145
Indeterminacy, 13, 418

Inference, 216, 300–301
Inferotemporal cortex, 232, 233, 241,
    245, 305
    damage, 233
Inflectional morphology, 324, 350
    see also Past tense
Information maximization, 144
Inhibition, 17, 31, 72, 93–106, 317,
    403–404
    and excitation, separation, 32, 41,
        71, 72
    benefits of, 94–95
    enabling modulatory effects, 271
    exploration, 95–100
    feedback, 93–100
    feedforward, 93–100
    function, 94, 100
    in attention, 17, 268
    in constraint satisfaction, 109
    in perseveration, 314
    inputs, 31, 65
    of inhibition, 96
    of return, 266–267
    shunting, 36
    synaptic input channel, 36, 37, 39
    thermostat model, 93, 94
    see also Competition,
        k-Winners-take-all (kWTA)
Inhibitory neuron, 32, 41, 72, 93
Init button, 51
Inner product distance measure, 337
Input-output mapping, 147–148, 158
Inputs, 23, 26, 66
    clamping, 56
    cortical area, 74
    excitatory, 31
    inhibitory, 31
    layer, 72–75
    scaling, 44
    weighting, 63
Insight problems, 158
Installing the software, 427
Integrate-and-fire model, 23, 26
Integration
    in learning, 119, 206, 214–217,
        283, 382
    neural, 26
    of inputs, 63

Interactive activation and competition (IAC), 106
Interactive approach, 5–6
Interactivity, *see* Bidirectional connectivity
Interblobs, 231
Interference, 206, 246, 254, 255, 282–284, 344, 385, 390
    catastrophic, 219, 276, 283–285
    exploration, 284–286, 293–296
    in active memory, 216, 277, 299–301, 305
    in hippocampus, 277, 284, 287, 292, 296
Interleaved learning, 119, 206, 214–217, 283, 382
Interneurons, 32, 41, 72, 93
Interpretation, 207
Introspection, 14
Intuition, 16
Invariance, 207
    location, 228, 233, 343, 345–347
    mapping, generalization, 254
    rotational, 233
    size, 228, 233
    spatial, 228, 233, 241–256
        exploration, 246–255
Inversion, of sensory input, 118
Ionotropic receptors, 30
Ions, 27, 32
    calcium, 32, 35, 36, 45
    chloride, 32, 35, 36, 45
    potassium, 32, 35, 36, 45
    sodium, 32, 35, 45
IPSP, 31
Isolated representations, 216, 300, 303, 304, 385, 397

Joint probability, 60

k, 285, 387, 464
k-Winners-take-all (kWTA), 94, 100–106, 177, 236, 387
    average-based, 102, 139
    exploration, 103–105
    in learning, 137, 143–145, 166, 175–176, 180, 184
    nested, 244, 246
    see also Competition, Inhibition

Knowledge, *see* Representations
    real world, 209
Kohonen networks, 105, 143, 236

Language, 212, 218–219, 323–377
    aphasia, 326–327
    Broca's area, 326–327
    direct pathway, 330–333, 335–341
    distributed representations, *see* Distributed representations: lexicon, semantics
    dyslexia, *see* Dyslexia
    exceptions, 324, 330–331, 341–342, 349–358
    in higher-level cognition, 383
    indirect pathway, 330–333, 335–341
    inflectional morphology, 324, 350
    lexicon, 323
    orthographic representations, 324, 329–350
    overregularization, 324, 350–358
    past tense, 324, 350–358
    phonological representations, 324, 327–358
    reading, *see* Reading
    regularities, 118, 324, 330–331, 341–342, 349–358, 420–421
    semantic representations, 324–327, 329–341, 349–358, 365, 367–368
    syntax, 325–327, 365–376
    Wernicke's area, 326–327
    word frequency, 330–331
Latent semantic analysis, 358–360
    exploration, 361–365
Lateral connectivity, 85, 87–89, 288
    in active memory, 299, 304–306, 308, 310, 314, 315, 317
    in pattern completion, 290
    see also Bidirectional connectivity
Layer
    hidden, 72–75
    input, 72–75
    output, 72–75
Layer, 431, 437–439, 463
    number of units, 437
LayerSpec, 430, 431, 439, 464
Leabra, 11, 19, 42

    summary, 177–178
leabra++, 427–433, 455–465
    installing, 427
Leak current, 52, 57–58, 65, 81, 82, 88–93, 96, 98, 100, 101, 104, 105
    channel, 36, 37, 39
Learning, 18–19, 382
    activation dynamics, 125
    associative, Hebbian, *see* Hebbian learning
    bias weights, 152–155, 159, 163
    biology, 115–118, 129–130, 168–170, 175
    conditioning, *see* Conditioning
    curve, 149
    delayed, *see* Reinforcement learning
    error-driven, *see* Error-driven learning
    expectation, 156, 167–168
        see also Phases of error-driven learning
    hidden layers, 158
    implicit, 189–190
    integrative, interleaved, 119, 206, 214–217, 283, 382
    model, *see* Model learning
    overview, 115–116
    phases, 156–157, 162–163, 167–170, 177, 198–199, 310
    positive feedback, 137
    rate, 123, 128, 131, 141, 214–215, 276–277, 286, 287
        parameter, ϵ, *see* lrate
    reinforcement, *see* Reinforcement learning
    self-organizing, 115, 127, 137–142
    separating, 206, 214–217
    sequences, *see* Sequence learning
    statistics, 119
    task, *see* Task learning
    temporal, *see* Temporal differences learning
    trial-and-error, 18
Least mean squares (LMS), *see* Delta rule
Lesions, *see* Brain damage
Levels of analysis, 4–6

Lexicon, 323, 330
LGN, 212, 228, 230
Likelihood, 61
Limbic system, 194, 212
Line detector, 121–122, 130–132,
        135–142, 179–181
Linear
        activation function, 54, 152, 154
        weight value, 134
List learning, 282
        AB–AC, 282–287
                exploration, 284–286, 293–296
        length, strength effects, 319
lmix, 176, 457
Local maxima/minima, 108
Localist representations, 9, 82–84, 86,
        87, 95, 104, 105, 143, 183,
        334, 369, 373, 417, 419
        exploration, 84–85
Logic, 15, 65, 380
Logistic, 40, 42, 47, 48, 134, 154, 155
Logs (PDP++), 429, 433
Long-term depression (LTD), 115–118,
        129–130, 168–170, 175
Long-term potentiation (LTP), 115–118,
        129–130, 168–170, 175
Loop counter, 432
lrate, 123, 128, 131, 141, 160, 179,
        214, 286, 457
Luce choice ratio, 58

Magnocellular, 230
Mapping
        input-output, 147–148, 158
        one-to-many, 190, 191, 279, 280,
        298
Markov sequence, 187
Marr's levels of analysis, 4
Mean field learning, 166
Membrane
        cable properties, 27
        neural, 27
        potential, 26, 38, 41
        potential, computing, 37
Memory, 275–321
        active, see Active memory
        amnesia, 289–290
        consolidation, 289–290
        cortical, 276–287, 298–303

declarative, 276
distributed, 206
dual-process models, 319
embedded, 206
encoding, retrieval, 290
episodic, 212, 276, 289, 297
frontal, see Frontal cortex
hippocampus, see Hippocampus
multiple systems, 275, 318
priming, see Priming
procedural, 276, 277
recognition, 318–319
semantic, 276, 277, 280, 289
spatial, 276, 297
Mental (internal) models, 118–119, 140,
        145, 234
Menus (PDP++), 429
Metabotropic receptors, 30, 117
mGlu, 31
Microtubules, 30
Midpoint method, 165
Minimizing error, 151–152
        see also Error-driven learning,
                Task learning, Delta rule,
                Backpropagation, GeneRec
Minimizing windows, 50
Minimum description length (MDL),
        144
Minus phase, 156–157, 162–163,
        167–170, 177, 198–199, 310
Mixtures of experts, 176
Model learning, 115, 118–146,
        176–178, 277
        exploration, 130–132
        other approaches, 142–145
        vs. task learning, 173–175
        see also Hebbian learning,
                Principal components
                analysis (PCA), Conditional
                PCA
Modulatory inputs, 271
Monitoring, 403, 406
MonitorStat, 432
Motor control, 213–214, 384, 385, 404
Mouse buttons
        left, 50, 429, 431, 433
        middle, 57, 431, 433, 438
        right, 433
Multiple constraint satisfaction, 16, 72,

        106–112, 145, 151, 210, 268,
        367, 375–376
Mutual support, 85, 88, 210
Mutually exclusive hypotheses, 59
Myelin, 29

Nativism, 18, 120
Negative feedback loop, 93
Neglect, 233–234, 260, 264–266
Neighborhood, 341
Neocortex, see Cortex
net, 44, 50, 57, 459
Net current, 37
Net input, 40, 41, 154
        computing, 42–45
        time averaging, 43
Net potential, 34
NetView, 49, 428, 431, 437, 438
        moving within, 440
Network, 71
        semantic, 109
Network, 428, 431, 437, 438
Neurobiology, see Biology
Neuroimaging, 1, 208, 306, 312, 325,
        384, 419
Neuromodulators, 117, 193, 298, 306,
        312, 416
        dopamine, 117, 193–195, 214,
                306–310, 387, 396
Neuron, 23–70
        axon, 27
        basket, 72
        cell body, 27
        chandelier, 72
        channels, 27
        cortical, 72
        dedicated processing, 25
        detector model, see Detector
        excitatory, 32, 41, 72
        exploration, 49–58
        inhibitory, 32, 41, 72
        inputs, 16, 26, 66
        integration, 26
        membrane, 27
        nucleus, 27
        output, 26, 42
        point, 24, 38, 154
        pyramidal, 24, 72

receptors, 26, 28–32, 46, 116–117, 228
self-regulation, 66–69
specialization of, 25
spiny stellate, 72
weights, 26
Neuron doctrine, 8
Neurotransmitters (NT), 28, 30–31
dopamine, 117, 193–195, 214, 306–310, 387, 396
GABA, 31, 36
glutamate, 31, 35
NewInit button, 58, 150
NMDA, 31
channel, 36
mediated LTP/D, 115–118, 129–130, 168–170, 175
Nodes of Ranvier, 29
Noise
and active memory, 302–303, 383
implications for processing, 66
in constraint satisfaction, 108–109, 112, 237
in learning curves, 170
spike timing, 47
noise_var, 53, 303, 462
Noisy X-over-X-plus-1 (Noisy XX1) function, 47–48, 50, 53, 54
Non-accidental properties, 256
Nonlinear
activation, 40, 48, 92
bidirectionality effects, 92, 182
discriminations, 158, 297
Normalization
activation parameters, 45
Hebbian learning, 124, 128
net input, 43
Noun phrase, 366
Null hypothesis, 46, 64

Object recognition, 212, 227–228, 232–233, 241–257, 324, 343, 349
exploration, 246–255
Object-based attention, 227, 260, 267–268, 272
Objective function
model learning, 127
reinforcement learning, 195

task learning, 151
Objective probabilities, 59, 62
Objects (PDP++), 427
Occipital cortex, 212, 214, 228, 230, 326, 327
see also V1, V2, V4
Ocular dominance columns, 231–232
Ohm's law, 33, 37
Oja's Hebbian learning rule, 124–125, 128
Ok button, 430
One-to-many mapping, 190, 191, 279, 280, 298
One-to-one connectivity, 90
Optimality approaches, 5
Orthographic representations, 324, 329–350
Outcome, as target state, 156, 167–168
see also Phases of error-driven learning
Output
cortical area, 74
layer, 72–75
neural, 23, 26, 42
rate code, 42
target, 148, 156
Overregularization, 324, 350–358
exploration, 353–357

Paired associates learning, 282
Paired-pulse facilitation, 31
Parallel distributed processing (PDP), 9, 15, 24
Parallel search, 109
Parameter
act_fun, 51, 53, 460
act_gain, 46, 460
alpha_k, 43
compute_i, 464
div_gp_n, 43, 458
dt_net, 44, 461
dt_vm, 37, 45, 391, 461
dur, 46, 460
e_rev, 45, 50, 52, 461
eq_gain, 46, 460
err, 176, 457
fm_hid, 188
fm_prv, 188
g_bar, 45, 50–53, 461

hebb, 176, 179, 183, 286, 457
k, 285, 387, 464
lmix, 176, 457
lrate, 123, 128, 131, 141, 160, 179, 214, 286, 457
noise_var, 53, 303, 462
normalized, 45
savg_cor, 134, 136, 137, 141, 458
thr, 45, 46, 460
v_bar, 45
v_m_r, 46, 460
v_rest, 45, 461
vs. variable, 428
wt_gain, 134, 136, 137, 141, 150
wt_off, 135–137, 141, 150
wt_scale, 44, 286, 303, 304, 308, 457
wt_sig, 134, 135, 457
Parameter fitting, 13, 418
Parietal cortex, 212, 214, 228, 233–234, 258, 260, 264–266, 326, 327
damage, 233–234, 258, 260, 264–266
exploration, 261–268
Parkinson's disease, 213, 385, 393
Parsimony, 12
in learning, 118–122, 144
Parvocellular, 230
Past tense, 324, 350–358
exploration, 353–357
Pathways
specialized, 206–208, 211–212, 227–228, 323–324
Patients, see Brain damage
Pattern
associator, 148–150
completion, 85, 87–89, 93, 210, 290, 292, 296, 297, 319, 333
exploration, 88–89, 294–296
overlap, 83, 149, 216, 285, 286, 294, 301
separation, 276, 284, 286, 290–292, 296, 297
exploration, 294
Pattern, 55, 428, 431
PDP++, 427–433
installing, 427

PDP++ Root, 49, 54, 58, 436, 443, 445
PDPLog, 429, 433
pdw, 456
Perception, 212, 220–224, 227–273
Perceptron, 8
Perseveration, 314–317, 393–395, 401, 403–404, 407
Phases of error-driven learning, 156–157, 162–163, 167–170, 177, 198–199, 310
Phonological
    dyslexia, 331–333, 340
    loop, 383
    representations, 324, 327–358
Photoreceptors, 228–229
Phrase structure, 366
Physical reductionism, 2–3
Pixel, 7, 55, 77, 119, 121, 126, 138, 228, 234, 235, 237, 245, 254, 414
Plus phase, 156–157, 162–163, 167–170, 177, 198–199, 310
Point neuron, 24, 38, 154
Positive feedback, 89–92
    in learning, 137
Posner spatial cuing task, 17, 258
Posterior (Bayesian), 61
Posterior cortex, 205, 206, 214–217, 222, 276, 277, 381, 383, 405
Postsynaptic, 28
Potassium, 32, 35, 36, 45
Potential, 32
    equilibrium, reversal, driving, 34
    membrane, 26, 41
    membrane equilibrium, 38–40, 65
    negative resting, 35
    net, 34
Potentiation, synaptic, 115–118, 129–130, 168–170, 175
Predictions, importance of, 12, 423
Prefrontal cortex, see Frontal cortex
Presynaptic, 28
Priming, 276, 278–279, 298
    long-term, weight-based, 276–282
        exploration, 279–282
    short-term, activation-based, 276, 278, 298–299
        exploration, 298–299

Principal components analysis (PCA), 116, 122–125
    demonstration, 124
    sequential (SPCA), 125–127
    see also Model learning, Hebbian learning, Conditional PCA
Principles, 6, 10, 13, 19
    dynamic, 210–211
    level of analysis, 6
    structural, 206–210
Prior (Bayesian), 61, 144
Probabilities, 59, 129
    conditional, 60, 128, 129, 133
    frequency-based, 60
    joint, 60
    posterior, 61
    prior, 61
Problem solving, 379
    see also Higher-level cognition
Procedural
    memory, 276, 277
    representations, 218
Process, 428, 432, 441, 442, 446, 465
    control panel, 58, 432, 442
Processing
    activation-based, 380–384, 392–395
    content-specific, dedicated, 209–210
    controlled vs. automatic, 214, 217–218, 381, 385–387, 408–409
    see also Controlled processing
    deterministic, 47, 53, 166
    distributed, 206
    embedded, 206
    speed, 386
    stochastic, 47, 53, 166
    weight-based, 380–381, 392–395
Production systems, 8, 25, 209, 217, 382–383, 407
    see also Computer metaphor, Symbolic models
Project
    ab.proj.gz, 315–317
    ab_ac_interference.proj.gz, 284–286
    act_maint.proj.gz, 301–305

act_priming.proj.gz, 298–299
amp_top_down.proj.gz, 89–90
amp_top_down_dist.proj.gz, 90–92
attn_simple.proj.gz, 261–268
bidir_xform.proj.gz, 86–87
cats_and_dogs.proj.gz, 110–111
creating, 435–452
detector.proj.gz, 54–58
dyslex.proj.gz, 335–341
ed_id.proj.gz, 397–402
family_trees.proj.gz, 183–186
fsa.proj.gz, 190–193
generec.proj.gz, 170–171
hebb_correl.proj.gz, 121–122, 130–132, 135–137
hip.proj.gz, 293–296
inhib.proj.gz, 95–100, 103–104
inhib_digits.proj.gz, 104–105
loc_dist.proj.gz, 84–85
model_and_task.proj.gz, 179–181
necker_cube.proj.gz, 111–112
objrec.proj.gz, 246–255
objrec_multiobj.proj.gz, 269–272
pat_assoc.proj.gz, 148–150, 156–158
pat_complete.proj.gz, 88–89
pfc_maint_updt.proj.gz, 310–312
pt.proj.gz, 353–357
rl_cond.proj.gz, 199–202
self_org.proj.gz, 138–142
self_reg.proj.gz, 68–69
sem.proj.gz, 361–365
sg.proj.gz, 370–375
ss.proj.gz, 344–349
stroop.proj.gz, 388–391

transform.proj.gz, 79–82
unit.proj.gz, 49–54
v1rf.proj.gz, 237–240
wt_priming.proj.gz,
        279–282
Projection, 42
    of world onto senses, 118
Projection, 431, 438, 439
ProjectionSpec, 430, 431, 438,
        439
Prototypes, 15, 16
Punishments, *see* Conditioning,
        Reinforcement learning
Pyramidal neuron, 24, 72

Quitting from simulation, 54

Rate code, 42, 46–48, 53
Rational analysis, 5
Re-representation, *see* Transformations
Re-write rules, 366
Reaction time, 258, 261, 278, 282, 388,
        389
Reading, 324, 326, 329–350
    direct route, 349
    division of labor, 331–332, 339,
        341
    dyslexia, *see* Dyslexia
    exploration, 335–341, 344–349
    indirect route, 349
    latencies, 349
    nonwords, 324, 331–332,
        340–342, 347–349
Recall
    cued, 290, 292, 319
    free, 319
Receiving weights, 55
Receptive field, 229–230, 237–239, 245,
        247, 253, 361, 438
    activation based, 247–250
    and attention, 268
    probe, 251–252
    spatially localized, 245, 256
    V1, 126–127
Receptors, 26, 28–32, 46, 116–117, 228
Recirculation, 10, 162–164
    see also GeneRec
Recognition memory, 318–319
Reconstructionism, 3–4, 14, 419

Recurrence, *see* Bidirectional
        connectivity
Recursion, 223–224
    equations, 39, 196
Reductionism, 2–3, 14, 418–419
Refractory period, 29
Regularities, 118, 324, 330–331,
        341–342, 349–358, 420–421
Regularization, 118–121, 134, 175–178,
        180–182, 184, 192
Reinforcement learning, 186, 187,
        193–202, 307, 312, 313
    exploration, 199–202
    see also Temporal differences
        learning (TD), Conditioning
ReInit button, 58
Release failures, 31
REM sleep, 381
Renormalization, 132–137, 141
Representations, 25, 69, 76
    accessibility, 381
    active memory, 382–383, 395
    canonical, 209, 223, 241–242, 317
    categorical, 15, 76, 405
    coarse-coded, 16, 82, 231
    combinatorial, 139, 178, 342
    comparing, 222
    conjunctive, 220–221, 223, 276,
        291–292, 297, 342–343, 345,
        347
    content-specific, dedicated, 25,
        209–210, 219–224, 324, 325,
        380
    context, *see* Context
    declarative, 218–219, 276, 381
    discrete, 14, 383
    distributed, *see* Distributed
        representations
    explicit, 189, 218–219
    feature-based, *see* Distributed
        representations
    frontal, 382–383, 395
    goals, 380–383, 403, 405–407
    heterarchical, 125–127
    hierarchical, 125–127, 206–210,
        212, 227, 242–256, 343
    hierarchical relationships, 222–223
    higher-order, 302–303
    implicit, 218–219

    isolated, 216, 300, 303, 304, 385,
        397
    localist, 9, 82–84, 86, 87, 95, 104,
        105, 143, 183, 334, 369, 373,
        417, 419
    object, 212, 227–228, 232–233,
        241–257, 324, 343, 349
    orthographic, 324, 329–350
    phonological, 324, 327–358
    procedural, 218
    redundant, 222
    semantic, 324–327, 329–341,
        349–358, 365, 367–368
    topographic, *see* Topographic
        representations
    visual, 212, 227–272
Rescorla-Wagner rule, 151, 199
Resistance, 33
Resonance, 16, 85, 88
Resting potential, 35
Retina, 228–229
    contrast enhancement, 228
Retinotopic organization, 230, 231
Retrieval, memory, 290, 292, 319
Reuptake, 30
Reversal potential, 34
Revert button, 50, 430
Rewards, *see* Conditioning,
        Reinforcement learning
    absorbing, 198, 311
Rods, 228
Rules, 118, 324, 330–331, 341–342,
        349–358, 420–421
Run button, 50, 58

Saturation
    activation, 40, 48, 92
    weight changes, 130, 134,
        155–156, 165
savg_cor, 134, 136, 137, 141, 458
Scaling, 6–8, 42, 236, 416–417
    input, 44
Schizophrenia, 306, 387, 391
ScriptEnv, 191, 448
Scripts (PDP++), 429, 433, 436–437,
        442–446, 448–452
    language, 429, 442–446, 448–452
Selection, 17, 94–95
    see also Competition, Inhibition

Selection (PDP++), 438
Selectivity, 81, 132, 134, 137, 139, 207
Self-organizing learning, 115, 127,
        137–142
    exploration, 138–142
Self-regulation, neural, 66–69
Semantic
    deficits, 358–359
    memory, 276, 277, 280, 289
    network, 109
    representations, 324–327,
        329–341, 349–358, 365,
        367–368
        exploration, 361–365
        from word co-occurrence,
        358–365
Sending weights, 86
Separation, pattern, 276, 284, 286,
        290–292, 296, 297
Sequence learning, 186–193, 307
    biological basis, 189
    context updating, 188–189
    exploration, 189–193, 370–375
    network configuration, 452–453
    see also Active memory
Sequences
    Markov, 187
Sequential principal components
        analysis (SPCA), 125–127
Serial processing, 14
Set point behavior, 93, 99–100
SettleProcess, 441, 465
Settling, 56, 86, 162
Shift-click, 57, 431, 433, 438
Shunting inhibition, 36
Sigmoid, 40, 42, 47, 48, 134, 154, 155
    derivative, 155, 160
Similarity structure, 75–79, 81–82
Simple cells, 230
Simple recurrent network (SRN), see
        Sequence learning
Simplification, 4, 13, 414–417
Simulated annealing, 109
Simulations, 20
    installing, 427
    quitting, 54
    see also Projects
Sleep, 230, 381
SOAR, 11

Sodium, 32, 35, 45
Sodium-potassium pump, 35, 36
Soft clamping, 88, 110
Soft weight bounding, 130, 134,
        155–156, 165
Software, installing, 427
Sparse distributed representations, 95,
        143, 216, 234, 276, 284, 286,
        290–292
Spatial
    attention, 221, 227, 234, 257–272
    cuing task, 17, 258
    frequency, 231
    invariance, 228, 233, 241–256
    memory, 276, 297
    processing, 212, 227, 232–234
Spec, 428
Specialization
    areas, 72, 74–75, 177, 211–212,
        214–217, 227–228, 286, 304
    neurons, 25
    pathways, 206–208, 211–212,
        227–228, 323–324
    vs. flexibility, 209, 219
Speed of processing, 386
Spike, 28, 29, 38, 42, 53
    computing, 45–46
    timing, randomness, 47, 53
Spines, dendritic, 29, 45
Spiny stellate neuron, 72
Spreading activation, 216, 278, 300, 312
Squared error, 149–151, 160, 196
Statistical models, 10
Statistics
    closest event, 280, 281, 447
    cnt_sum_se, 179
    learning, 119
    max da, 465
    PDP++, 429, 432, 442, 447–448,
        450
    sum_se, 149
    Unique pattern (unq_pats), 140,
        180
    Wrong on, 270
Stem completion, 278–282, 298
Step button, 56, 58
Stepping grain, 156
Stochastic processing, 47, 53, 166
    see also Noise

Strategic processing, 206, 214, 217–218,
        381–382, 385–387, 403,
        405–406, 408–409
    see also Higher-level cognition
Stress, 108
Stroop task, 382, 383, 385–392, 395,
        404
    exploration, 388–391
Structural principles, 206–210
Structure, 118, 324, 330–331, 341–342,
        349–358, 420–421
    levels, 6
Subcortical areas, 72–75, 193–195,
        212–214, 230, 306–307, 385
    see also Basal ganglia, Thalamus
Subjective probabilities, 59, 62
Subroutines, 223–224
Substantia Nigra (SN), 193–195
sum_se, 149
Summed squared error (SSE), 149–151,
        160, 196
    error count, 179
Supervisory attentional system (SAS),
        407
Surface dyslexia, 331–333, 335–336,
        338–339
Symbolic models, 8, 209, 219, 223,
        241–242, 324, 330, 366,
        379–380, 382–383
    see also Computer metaphor,
        Production systems
Symmetric weights, 86, 107, 165–167
Synapse, 26, 29–31
    efficacy, 26, 27, 31
    excitatory input, 35
    inhibitory input, 36
    modification, 115–118, 129–130,
        168–170, 175
Syntax, 325–327, 365–376
    exploration, 370–375

targ, 157, 459
Target output, 148, 156
Task learning, 116, 147–172, 176–178,
        277
    vs. model learning, 173–175
    see also Error-driven learning,
        Delta rule, Backpropagation,
        GeneRec

Task variation, 317
Teaching signals, 156, 167–168
Template matching, 82
Temporal, *see* Time
Temporal cortex, 212, 214, 228, 326, 327
Temporal differences learning (TD), 193–202
    derivation, 196
    exploration, 199–202
    in active memory control, 308–313, 395–397, 406
    phase-based, 198–199
    vs. delta rule, 199
    see also Reinforcement learning, Conditioning
Text comprehension, 408
`TextLog`, 429, 433
Thalamus, 72, 212, 228, 230, 269, 307
Theories, descriptive vs. explanatory, 11, 417
Θ, *see* `thr`
`thr`, 45, 46, 460
Threshold
    detector, 26
    error, 149
    high, 291
    parameter, *see* `thr`
    soft, 48
    spike, 28, 38, 42, 46, 53
Tick (time step), 192, 200
Time
    averaging, 43
    constant
        `dt_vm`, 37
        `dt_net`, 44
    continuous, 186–187
    learning over delays, *see* Reinforcement learning
    summation, 43
Tip-of-the-tongue, 16
Top-down
    approach, 4–6
    processing, 17, 85–93, 162, 385, 392
Topographic representations, 143, 240
    V1, 231–232, 236–237
        exploration, 237–240
Tower of Hanoi/London task, 405, 406

Tradeoffs, 206, 209, 213–217, 219, 286, 292, 300, 304, 343
Training set, 151
`TrainProcess`, 428, 432, 448
Trajectories
    continuous, 186–187
Transformations, 72, 73, 185, 207–209, 227–228, 241–256
    bidirectional, 85–87
    exploration, 79–87, 246–255
    learning, 158
    sequences, 253
    unidirectional, 75–85
Trial, 428
Trial-and-error learning, 18, 309, 313, 382, 395–397
`TrialProcess`, 428, 432, 441, 446–448, 465
Tripartite functional organization, 205, 214–217
Tuning curves of cortical neurons, 82
Turing test, 14

U-shaped curve, 350–358
    exploration, 353–357
Unidirectional connectivity, 75–85
Unified theories of cognition, 11, 12
Unit, 23–70
    as population of neurons, 7, 42, 46, 48
    dead, loser, 140
    exploration, 49–58
    weights, 26
`Unit`, 428, 431, 459, 460
    number in a layer, 437
`UnitSpec`, 52, 428, 430, 431, 438, 460, 462

V1, 126–127, 212, 230–232, 234–241
    exploration, 237–240
    pinwheel, 232, 239
    singularity, 232, 239
    topography, 231–232, 236–237
V2, 212, 233
V4, 212, 233
`v_bar`, 45
`v_m`, 37, 50, 459
`v_m_r`, 46, 460
`v_rest`, 45, 461

Value function, 195–196
Variable
    `act`, 46, 50, 55, 459
    `act_avg`, 285, 459
    `act_dif`, 459
    `act_eq`, 46, 50, 53, 459
    `act_m`, 156, 157, 459
    `act_p`, 156, 157, 191, 459
    β, *see* `bias.wt`
    `bias.wt`, 44, 157, 459
    `da`, 56, 459, 465
    `dwt`, 123, 456
    `ext`, 86, 459
    `I_net`, 37, 50, 459
    `net`, 44, 50, 57, 459
    `pdw`, 456
    `targ`, 157, 459
    `v_m`, 37, 50, 459
    vs. parameter, 428
    `wt`, 43, 55, 135, 456
Variable binding, 209
Variance
    as information, 144
    vs. bias, 120
Ventral tegmental area (VTA), 193–195, 214, 306–307
Verb phrase, 366
Vesicles, 30
View window, 428
Visual
    cortex, *see* V1, V2, V4, Occipital cortex
    pathways, 15, 228–234
    representations, 212, 227–272
    search, 271
Voltage-gated channels, 28, 35, 36, 39, 45, 117
    in dendrites, 45
Vowels, 328

Weighted average, 39
Weights, 26, 27, 31, 63
    based memory, 210, 276–298, 314
    based processing, 380–381, 392–395
    contrast enhancement, 132–137, 139, 141, 150
    decay, 165, 175
    equilibrium, 124, 129

gain, 134–135

in memory, 210, 276–298, 314

learning, *see* Learning

linking/sharing, 244

receiving, 55

renormalization, 132–137, 141

sending, 86

soft bounding, 130, 134, 155–156, 165

symmetric, 86, 107, 165–167

updating, 123

variable, *see* wt

Wernicke's area, 326–327

What vs. where, 15, 227, 232–234, 315, 403

Wickelfeatures, 342, 343

Windows

Control panel, 49, 429, 430, 450–452

edit dialogs, 50, 429

EnviroView, 428, 431

GraphLog, 429, 433

GridLog, 429, 433

iconifying, minimizing, 50

NetView, 49, 428, 431

PDP++ Root, 49, 54, 58, 436, 443, 445

TextLog, 429, 433

Winner-take-all (WTA), 105, 143, 176

see also k-Winners-take-all (kWTA)

Wisconsin card sorting task (WCST), 392–393, 404, 407

see also Dynamic categorization, ID/ED task

Word superiority effect, 17, 89, 90, 106

Working memory, *see* Active memory

Wrap-around connectivity, 236

wt, 43, 55, 135, 456

wt_gain, 134, 136, 137, 141, 150

wt_off, 135–137, 141, 150

wt_scale, 44, 286, 303, 304, 308, 457

wt_sig, 134, 135, 457

X-over-X-plus-1 (XX1) function, 46

XOR task, 158

DATE DUE

OhioLINK		
MAY 1 6 2006		
MAY 1 5 2006		
OhioLINK		
APR 1 9 REC'D		
LINK		
FEB 2 4 REC'D		
MAR 2 4 2011		
GAYLORD		PRINTED IN U.S.A.

SCI QP 360.5 .074 2000

O'Reilly, Randall C.

Computational explorations
  in cognitive neuroscience